THORACIC IMAGING
Pulmonary and Cardiovascular Radiology

SECOND EDITION

THORACIC IMAGING
Pulmonary and Cardiovascular Radiology

SECOND EDITION

W. RICHARD WEBB, MD

Professor Emeritus of Radiology and Biomedical Imaging
Department of Radiology and Biomedical Imaging
University of California, San Francisco
San Francisco, California

CHARLES B. HIGGINS, MD

Distinguished Professor of Radiology
Department of Radiology
University of California, San Francisco
San Francisco, California

. Wolters Kluwer | Lippincott Williams & Wilkins
Health

Philadelphia · Baltimore · New York · London
Buenos Aires · Hong Kong · Sydney · Tokyo

Acquisitions Editor: Charles W. Mitchell
Product Manager: Ryan Shaw
Vendor Manager: Alicia Jackson
Senior Manufacturing Manager: Benjamin Rivera
Senior Marketing Manager: Angela Panetta
Design Coordinator: Doug Smock
Production Service: SPi Technologies

Library of Congress Cataloging-in-Publication Data

Webb, W. Richard (Wayne Richard), 1945-
    Thoracic imaging : pulmonary and cardiovascular radiology / W. Richard Webb and Charles B. Higgins. —2nd ed.
        p. ; cm.
    Includes bibliographical references and index.
    ISBN 978-1-45111-089-0 (hardback : alk. paper)
    1. Chest—Radiography. 2. Cardiopulmonary system—Diseases—Diagnosis. 3. Cardiopulmonary system—Radiography. I. Higgins, Charles B. II. Title.
    [DNLM: 1. Cardiovascular Diseases—diagnosis. 2. Lung Diseases—diagnosis. 3. Diagnostic Imaging—methods. 4. Radiography, Thoracic—methods. WF 975]

    RC941.W295   2011
    617.5′407572—dc22

                                                                                    2010026154

Care has been taken to confirm the accuracy of the information presented and to describe generally accepted practices. However, the authors, editors, and publisher are not responsible for errors or omissions or for any consequences from application of the information in this book and make no warranty, expressed or implied, with respect to the currency, completeness, or accuracy of the contents of the publication. Application of the information in a particular situation remains the professional responsibility of the practitioner.

The authors, editors, and publisher have exerted every effort to ensure that drug selection and dosage set forth in this text are in accordance with current recommendations and practice at the time of publication. However, in view of ongoing research, changes in government regulations, and the constant flow of information relating to drug therapy and drug reactions, the reader is urged to check the package insert for each drug for any change in indications and dosage and for added warnings and precautions. This is particularly important when the recommended agent is a new or infrequently employed drug.

Some drugs and medical devices presented in the publication have Food and Drug Administration (FDA) clearance for limited use in restricted research settings. It is the responsibility of the health care provider to ascertain the FDA status of each drug or device planned for use in their clinical practice.

To purchase additional copies of this book, call our customer service department at (800) 638-3030 or fax orders to (301) 223-2320. International customers should call (301) 223-2300.

Visit Lippincott Williams & Wilkins on the Internet: at LWW.com. Lippincott Williams & Wilkins customer service representatives are available from 8:30 am to 6 pm, EST.

                                                    10 9 8 7 6 5 4 3 2 1

To Jack and Cole, my Grandsons, who learn and teach every day
—W. Richard Webb

To the many fellows who have contributed to our progress
in developing new cardiovascular imaging techniques
—Charles B. Higgins

CONTRIBUTORS

Michael B. Gotway, MD
Scottsdale Medical Imaging
An Affiliate of Southwest Diagnostic Imaging, Ltd
Clinical Associate Professor
Diagnostic Radiology/Biomedical Imaging and Pulmonary/
    Critical Care Medicine
Department of Radiology
University of California
San Francisco, California
Adjunct Professor
Department of Biomedical Informatics
Arizona State University
Tempe, Arizona

Charles B. Higgins, MD
Distinguished Professor of Radiology
Department of Radiology
University of California, San Francisco
San Francisco, California

Karen G. Ordovas, MD
Assistant Professor
Radiology and Biomedical Imaging
University of California San Francisco
San Francisco, California

Gautham P. Reddy, MD, MPH
Professor and Vice Chair for Education
Department of Radiology
University of Washington Medical Center
Seattle, Washington

W. Richard Webb, MD
Professor Emeritus of Radiology and Biomedical Imaging
Department of Radiology and Biomedical Imaging
University of California, San Francisco
San Francisco, California

PREFACE

Our goal in writing *Thoracic Imaging: Pulmonary and Cardiovascular Radiology* was to provide, in a single volume, a comprehensive but easy-to-digest discussion of the title topic and to review the use and interpretation of chest radiographs and advanced imaging techniques (e.g., spiral computed tomography [CT], high-resolution CT, magnetic resonance imaging [MRI], and magnetic resonance angiography).

We have tried to be thorough without being exhaustive. Rather than referencing specific studies, we have summarized what we consider to be the most important and pertinent information and have provided numerous tables to make key facts easily available to the reader. More than 2,100 illustrations demonstrate important radiographic findings and the typical appearances of the various disease entities one might encounter in current clinical practice. The second edition provides current updates on a number of topics and also provides improved and additional illustrations.

Imaging of the lungs and mediastinum requires an understanding of both plain radiography and CT. Although in many situations CT has assumed a preeminent role, knowledge of chest radiographs and their utility is essential to the radiographic assessment of patients with suspected pulmonary disease. We have attempted to review and illustrate both the plain radiographic and the CT findings of most abnormalities and disorders. Other imaging modalities, such as MRI and radionuclide imaging, are also discussed in situations in which they play a significant role.

Chapters in the pulmonary radiology section of this book are organized according to important radiographic findings, anatomic regions, clinical problems, or disease states, as is appropriate to an approach to diagnosis and differential diagnosis. Radiographic and CT techniques are not described in detail (e.g., there is no chapter specifically on techniques), but these are reviewed in context in various chapters. In most cases, normal radiographic and CT findings are reviewed where appropriate to the understanding of specific abnormal findings or diseases.

Cardiovascular imaging has transitioned nearly completely in the past two decades from dependence on x-ray angiography for definitive diagnosis to noninvasive tomographic imaging techniques. Therefore, *Thoracic Imaging* emphasizes the use of tomographic imaging for the evaluation of cardiovascular morphology and function. The currently employed tomographic techniques are echocardiography, MRI, and CT. Although echocardiography is the most frequently used imaging modality for the evaluation of cardiac disease, it is not included in this volume. Many books encompassing all aspects of echocardiography already exist, so inclusion of it would be not only repetitious but also incomplete because of the intended size of this book. Another practical consideration is that echocardiography is rarely practiced by radiologists.

Frequently, the initial radiographic study used in patients with cardiovascular disease is the thoracic radiograph. Two chapters describe a systematic approach to the evaluation of the thoracic radiograph in acquired and congenital heart disease. The major tomographic imaging technique employed by radiologists in the evaluation of cardiac disease is MRI. The use and interpretation of MRI are described in several chapters covering the various categories of cardiovascular diseases. MRI and CT have become increasingly important in the evaluation of ischemic heart disease in the past few years. Individual chapters describe the current capabilities of MRI and CT in ischemic heart disease.

W. Richard Webb, M.D.
Charles B. Higgins, M.D.

CONTENTS

Congenital Bronchopulmonary Lesions

W. RICHARD WEBB

A variety of congenital abnormalities may involve the bronchi, lung and it vascular supply. They often have characteristic plain film and computed tomography (CT) findings. Congenital abnormalities of the aorta and great vessels are reviewed in Chapter 35.

BRONCHIAL ANOMALIES

Anomalies of bronchial anatomy include abnormal origin, absent branches, supernumerary branches, and congenital diverticula (Table 1-1). Minor variation in subsegmental bronchial anatomy is common but clinically insignificant; a detailed knowledge of subsegmental bronchial anatomy is not necessary for clinical practice. Variation in segmental bronchial anatomy is less frequent and not often of significance.

Tracheal Bronchus

A tracheal bronchus is present in about 0.1% of the population. It usually arises from the right tracheal wall, at or within 2 cm of the tracheal bifurcation. It supplies a variable portion of the medial or apical right upper lobe, most often the apical segment (Fig. 1-1); in occasional cases, the entire right upper lobe bronchus arises from the trachea (Fig. 1-2). When a right-sided tracheal bronchus is present, the azygos arch is seen above the tracheal bronchus. Tracheal bronchus is sometimes referred to as a "pig bronchus" or "bronchus suis" as it is common in pigs and other cloven-hoofed animals.

In most cases, this anomaly is insignificant. However, recurrent infection or bronchiectasis may result, since the tracheal bronchus is often slightly narrowed at its origin. A left tracheal bronchus, supplying the apical posterior segment of the left upper lobe, is rarely present; it is much less common than a right-sided tracheal bronchus. The term "tracheal bronchus" is sometimes used to refer to a displaced bronchus, supplying a part of the upper lobe, even if it does not arise from the trachea.

Accessory Cardiac Bronchus

Accessory cardiac bronchus is a supernumerary bronchus with an incidence of about 0.1%. It arises from the medial wall of the bronchus intermedius or right lower lobe bronchus and extends inferiorly and medially toward the mediastinum or heart. In some cases, the cardiac bronchus is a short, blind-ending bronchial stump without associated alveolar tissue, and it may terminate in the mediastinum. In others, a longer branching bronchus is present, associated with rudimentary lung tissue (Fig. 1-3). In most cases, this anomaly is an incidental finding; occasionally, chronic infection or hemoptysis is associated.

Bronchial Isomerism

Bronchial isomerism refers to bilateral symmetry of the bronchi and associated pulmonary lobes. It may be isolated or associated with a variety of anomalies, particularly congenital heart disease. Bronchial anatomy may be bilaterally right sided (associated with asplenia) or left sided (associated with polysplenia).

TABLE 1.1 Bronchial Anomalies

Variations in subsegmental branching
  Common but insignificant
Tracheal bronchus
  Incidence 0.1%
  Arises from right tracheal wall; rare on left
  Usually supplies apical segment of right upper lobe
  Rarely supplies entire right upper lobe
  Increased incidence of infection or bronchiectasis
Accessory cardiac bronchus
  Incidence 0.1%
  Arises from medial wall of bronchus intermedius
  Usually blind ending or supplies rudimentary lung
  May terminate in the mediastinum
  Increased incidence of infection or hemoptysis
Bronchial isomerism
  Symmetrical bronchial anatomy
  Bilateral right- or left-sided bronchial anatomy
  Associated with congenital heart disease, other anomalies

FIG. 1.1. Tracheal bronchus. A: Coronal CT reconstruction shows a tracheal bronchus (*Tr Br*) arising from the right tracheal wall just above the carina. The azygos arch (*Azygos*) is visible above the bronchus. **B:** CT (1.25-mm slice thickness) shows the origin of the tracheal bronchus. As in this case, slight narrowing at the origin of the bronchus is common. The bronchus supplies the apical segment of the right upper lobe. **C:** The tracheal carina is seen slightly below (**B**). **D:** Below (**C**), the main right upper lobe bronchus (*RUL*) gives rise to the anterior (*Ant Seg*) and posterior (*Post Seg*) segmental bronchi.

BRONCHIAL ATRESIA

Bronchial atresia is a developmental defect characterized by local narrowing or obliteration of a lobar, segmental, or subsegmental bronchus (Table 1-2). It is most common in the left upper lobe, followed by the right upper and right middle lobes; it is less common in the lower lobes. This entity is usually detected incidentally in adults and is undoubtedly related to congenital lobar emphysema (CLE). Patients usually have no symptoms, but lung distal to the obstruction may occasionally become infected. In patients with chronic infection, resection may be necessary.

The lobe or segment distal to the bronchial obstruction usually remains aerated because of collateral ventilation

A   B

FIG. 1.2. Tracheal bronchus in a patient with pneumonia. **A:** Coronal reconstruction shows the entire right upper lobe bronchus (*RUL*) arising from the right tracheal wall above the carina. The apical segmental bronchus extends superiorly. **B:** Transaxial CT shows the right upper lobe bronchus (*arrow*) giving rise to anterior and posterior segments. Patchy areas of increased lung opacity reflect the presence of pneumonia.

A   B

FIG. 1.3. Accessory cardiac bronchus. **A:** Coronal CT reconstruction shows an accessory cardiac bronchus (*CB*) arising from the medial aspect of the bronchus intermedius (*BI*), to supply a small region of lung. **B:** Transaxial image shows the cardiac bronchus (*CB*) arising from the medial wall of the bronchus intermedius (*BI*). (*Figure continues.*)

C

D

FIG. 1.3. (*Continued.*) **C:** Slightly below (**B**), the cardiac bronchus (*arrow*) is seen medial to the bronchus intermedius. **D:** Below (**C**), the bronchus supplies a small segment of lung separated from the lower lobe by an accessory fissure (*arrows*).

(Figs. 1-4 and 1-5). In 90% of cases, air trapping in the distal lung results in decreased perfusion; radiographs and CT show the affected lung to be hyperlucent and hypovascular. Affected lung is often increased in volume, resulting in mediastinal shift or shift of a fissure. In 80% of cases, mucus accumulates within dilated bronchi distal to the obstruction, resulting in a tubular, branching, or ovoid density (mucous plug or *mucocele*). Mucus within dilated bronchi usually appears low in attenuation. Expiratory radiographs or CT scans show air trapping (see Fig. 1-5B).

The combination of these typical radiographic or CT findings in a young patient is strongly suggestive of the diagnosis. Bronchoscopy may be warranted to rule out another cause of bronchial obstruction, such as tumor.

TABLE 1.2 Bronchial Atresia
Narrowing or obliteration of a lobar, segmental, or subsegmental bronchus
Left upper lobe > right upper lobe > right middle lobe > lower lobes
Detected incidentally in adults
Infection may occur
Mucous plug distal to obstructed bronchial segment
Distal lung
Lucent
Increased in volume
Decreased vessel size
Air trapping on expiration
Rule out obstructing tumor

CONGENITAL LOBAR EMPHYSEMA

CLE, also known as congenital lobar hyperinflation, is characterized by marked overinflation of a lobe (Table 1-3). Most cases present within the first month of life; symptoms of respiratory distress are typical. Presentation after the first month may occur.

Most cases of CLE are associated with partial or complete bronchial obstruction occurring as a result of (a) deficient cartilage; (b) external compression, usually by an anomalous vessel or bronchogenic cyst; or (c) luminal abnormalities such as mucosal folds. Some cases are unassociated with bronchial obstruction.

CLE is most common in the left upper lobe, followed by the right middle lobe and right upper lobe. Only a few percent

FIG. 1.4. Bronchial atresia. **A:** Chest radiograph in a young patient with bronchial atresia involving the left upper lobe. The left upper lobe is increased in volume, with mediastinal shift toward the right side. The lobe is lucent, and its vascularity is decreased. **B:** Transaxial CT shows the left upper lobe to be increased in volume, with mediastinal shift to the right, hyperlucent, and hypovascular. Branches of the left upper lobe bronchus are dilated, and one branch contains a mucous plug (*arrows*). **C:** Coronal reconstruction shows the hyperlucent and hypovascular left upper lobe with focal atresia of its apical-posterior segmental branch (*arrow*). Distal bronchi are dilated.

occur in the lower lobes. Radiographs typically show marked overinflation and air trapping in the affected lobe. However, in neonates, the affected lobe may sometimes appear opaque because of retained fetal lung fluid. Mediastinal shift away from the abnormal lobe often occurs, and normal lobes are reduced in volume. Resection is often necessary.

It is reasonable to assume that cases of CLE that go unrecognized at birth may be diagnosed years later as bronchial atresia.

A   B

FIG. 1.5. Bronchial atresia. **A:** CT shows a branching mucous plug (*white arrow*) in the location of the posterior segmental bronchus of the right upper lobe. Lung distal to the bronchus (*black arrows*) is hyperlucent and hypovascular. Mediastinal shift to the left side is present. **B:** Expiratory CT shows air trapping in the lung distal to the obstructed bronchus. Normal lung increases significantly in attenuation relative to (**A**).

PULMONARY BRONCHOGENIC CYST

Bronchogenic cysts are foregut duplication cysts and result from abnormal development of the lung bud. They are lined by pseudostratified ciliated columnar epithelium, typical of bronchi. The cyst wall may also contain smooth muscle, mucous glands, or cartilage. Bronchogenic cysts are filled with fluid, which can be serous, hemorrhagic, or highly viscous and gelatinous because of its high protein content.

Bronchogenic cysts may be mediastinal or pulmonary. Mediastinal bronchogenic cysts are much more common than pulmonary cysts. They are discussed along with mediastinal masses in Chapter 8.

Pulmonary bronchogenic cysts are most common in the medial lung and the lower lobes (Table 1-4). They are sharply circumscribed and round or oval. The cyst wall may calcify. Rarely, the cyst may contain milk of calcium and appear dense. Cysts may slowly increase in size; a rapid increase in size is unusual unless infection occurs.

About half of fluid-filled bronchogenic cysts appear to be low in attenuation on CT (0 to 20 HU) (Fig. 1-6). However, as with mediastinal bronchogenic cysts, the CT attenuation of a pulmonary bronchogenic cyst is variable. High CT numbers (40 to 80 HU), suggesting a solid mass, can be seen. Such cysts contain bloody or thick, proteinaceous fluid. Typically, the cyst wall appears very thin on CT or is invisible. A bronchogenic cyst may sometimes appear to be related to a small bronchus.

Infection eventually occurs in 75% of cases. In the presence of acute infection, a rapid increase in size of the cyst may be seen. Also, the outer cyst wall may become less well defined because of surrounding lung inflammation. During or after infection, a cyst may contain air (Fig. 1-7; see also Fig. 9-29 in Chapter 9) or a combination of air and fluid (with an air-fluid level). When the cyst contains air, its wall appears very thin.

TABLE 1.3 Congenital Lobar Emphysema

Partial or complete bronchial obstruction caused by:
  Deficient cartilage
  External compression
  Luminal abnormalities
Some cases unassociated with bronchial obstruction
Left upper lobe > right middle lobe > right upper
  lobe > lower lobes
Respiratory distress in neonates
Presentation after first month uncommon
Marked overinflation of lobe
Air trapping
Sometimes the abnormal lobe retains fetal lung
  fluid
Resection often necessary

TABLE 1.4 Pulmonary Bronchogenic Cyst

Foregut duplication cyst
Lined by bronchial epithelium
Fluid contents can be serous, hemorrhagic, or viscous
Less common than mediastinal bronchogenic cyst
Most common in medial lung and lower lobes
Sharply circumscribed and round or oval
Thin wall; occasionally calcifies
Contents 0–20 HU in half; often 40–80 HU; milk of calcium
  rare
Infection occurs in 75%
  Rapid increase in size
  Blurring of outer edge
  Air-fluid level
  Air in cyst may remain after infection

FIG. 1.6. Pulmonary bronchogenic cyst. A sharply marginated round nodular opacity (*arrow*) is visible in the right lower lobe. This measured 0 HU in attenuation. This appearance is typical of a fluid-filled bronchogenic cyst.

CONGENITAL CYSTIC ADENOMATOID MALFORMATION (CONGENITAL PULMONARY AIRWAY MALFORMATION)

Congenital cystic adenomatoid malformation (CCAM), also termed congenital pulmonary airway malformation (CPAM) consists of a multicystic, intralobar mass of disorganized lung tissue, derived primarily from bronchioles. About 70% present during the first week of life, but 10% are diagnosed after the first year, and rare cases in adults have been reported.

CCAM/CPAM can involve an entire lobe. Lower lobes are most often involved, but any lobe can be affected. The CCAM/CPAM communicates with the bronchial tree and is supplied by the pulmonary artery; systemic arterial supply is rarely present.

FIG. 1.7. Pulmonary bronchogenic cyst. A thin-walled, sharply marginated, air-filled bronchogenic cyst is visible in the left lung. The presence of air within the cyst indicates prior infection.

TABLE 1.5	Congenital Cystic Adenomatoid Malformation (CCAM)

Also known as Congenital Pulmonary Airway Malformation (CPAM)
Multicystic, intralobar mass of disorganized lung tissue
70% present in first week; 10% after first year
Respiratory distress in neonates; recurrent infection in adults
Most common in lower lobe

Three primary types
Type 1 (65%)
   One or more cysts, >2 cm in diameter
   May appear initially as solid mass
   Large air-filled multicystic lesion
   Sometimes with air fluid levels
   May occupy the entire hemithorax
Type 2 (20%–25%)
   Multiple cysts <2 cm in diameter
   May appear initially as solid mass
   Air-filled multicystic mass or focal consolidation
   Associated renal and cardiac abnormalities
   Often a poor prognosis
Type 3 (10%)
   Microscopic (<3–5 mm) cysts
   Appears as solid mass
Two additional types proposed, based on histology, each a few percent of cases
Type 0
   Small cysts
   Similar to Type 3 in appearance
Type 4
   Large cysts
   Similar to Types 1 and 2 in appearance

CCAMs are typically classified into three primary types (Types 1 to 3), which have different histology, gross pathologic findings, radiographic appearance, and prognosis (Table 1-5).

Type 1 CCAMs (65% of cases) contain one or more cysts more than 2 cm in diameter (Fig. 1-8). They usually appear radiographically as a large, air-filled multicystic lesion, sometimes with air-fluid levels, which may occupy the entire hemithorax.

Type 2 CCAMs (20% to 25% of cases) contain multiple cysts less than 2 cm in diameter. They present radiographically as an air-filled multicystic mass or a solid mass or area of consolidation (see Fig. 1-9). This type may be associated with a poor prognosis because of associated renal and cardiac abnormalities.

Type 3 CCAMs (10% of cases) contain microscopic (less than 3 to 5 mm) cysts and present radiographically as a solid mass.

Two additional types of CCAM have been proposed, Types 0 and 4, based on histopathologic findings and the type of airway epithelium involved in the malformation. The term CPAM (congenital pulmonary airway malformation) has been suggested to encompass this expanded classification. Types 0 and 4 CCAM/CPAM each account for a few percent of cases. Type 0 CCAM/CPAM is associated with small cysts,

FIG. 1.8. Type 1 congenital cystic adenomatoid malformation. A multicystic lesion is visible in the right lower lobe. This is a typical appearance of Type 1 CCAM in an adult.

as in Type 3. Type 4 CCAM/CPAM is associated with large cysts, as is Type 1; its radiographic and CT appearance is the same as for Type 1 or 2.

Sonography can be used for prenatal diagnosis. Findings include polyhydramnios, fetal hydrops, and a solid or cystic mass in the fetal thorax. Fetal surgery may be attempted.

In infancy, CCAM/CPAM presents as a space-occupying lesion. Symptoms of respiratory distress are common. In neonates, CCAM/CPAM usually presents as a solid mass regardless of its type. Types 1 and 2 may become air filled over a period of days to weeks. They are often associated with progressive air trapping and mediastinal shift to the opposite side.

The treatment of choice is excision of the affected lobe. The prognosis of neonates with CCAM/CPAM is adversely affected by large size, underdevelopment of uninvolved lung (i.e., the presence of associated lung hypoplasia), and the presence of associated fetal hydrops or other congenital anomalies.

In adults, CCAM/CPAM usually presents as an air-filled or air- and fluid-filled cystic or multicystic mass. Most adults present with recurrent pneumonia, although recurrent pneumothorax has also been associated. Occasionally, bronchiolo-alveolar carcinoma may arise in relation to a CCAM/CPAM.

PULMONARY ARTERIOVENOUS MALFORMATION

Congenital arteriovenous malformation (AVM), also known as arteriovenous fistula, likely results from deficient

FIG. 1.9. Type II congenital cystic adenomatoid malformation. A solid mass (*black arrow*) is visible in the right lower lobe of a neonate. An opacified vessel is visible within the mass (*white arrow*). Type II CCAM may present as an air-filled or fluid-filled mass.

formation or abnormal dilation of pulmonary capillaries due to a developmental defect in the capillary wall. From 35% to 67% of cases are associated with Osler-Weber-Rendu syndrome (*hereditary hemorrhagic telangiectasia*), in which AVMs are found in the skin, mucous membranes, and viscera (Table 1-6). Also, AVMs may rarely occur in patients with hepatopulmonary syndrome or as a result of trauma.

Pulmonary arteriovenous fistulas slowly enlarge over time and are usually first diagnosed in adulthood. More than two thirds of AVMs are found in the lower lobes, and they are typically subpleural in location. Fistulas are multiple in 35% of patients and bilateral in 10%.

Simple and Complex Arteriovenous Malformations

A *simple AVM* is a single, dilated vascular sac connecting one artery and one vein (Figs. 1-10 and 1-11). It is

TABLE 1.6	**Pulmonary Arteriovenous Malformation (AVM)**

35%–67% associated with Osler-Weber-Rendu syndrome
Multiple in 35%
Bilateral in 10%
Single AVM less often symptomatic than multiple AVM (35% vs. 60%)
Symptoms: cyanosis, dyspnea, and hemoptysis
Complications: rupture and paradoxical embolization
Simple AVM: one feeding artery and one draining vein
Complex AVM: multiple feeding vessels
Most common in lower lobes, subpleural
Diagnosis by morphology at CT
Treatment by embolization

A

B

C

FIG. 1.10. Simple arteriovenous malformation. **A:** Chest radiograph shows a nodule in the subpleural right lower lobe (*large white arrow*) with a large feeding vessel (*small arrows*). **B:** CT slice shows a fistula in the subpleural lung with a feeding vessel. **C:** On an arteriogram, a single feeding artery (*large arrow*) supplies a simple malformation drained by a single vein (*small arrows*). As is typical, the fistula is subpleural in location.

A

B

C

FIG. 1.11. Simple arteriovenous malformation (AVM). **A:** A well-defined, smooth, round, 3-cm nodule is visible on chest radiograph in the left lower lobe. **B:** Contrast-enhanced CT shows a densely opacified fistula in the subpleural lung. Its feeding artery is also visible on this slice. **C:** Pulmonary arteriogram shows an AVM and a single feeding artery.

most frequent and accounts for the bulk of cases of AVM. *Complex AVMs*, which have more than one feeding artery, are rare.

Radiographically, a simple fistula appears as a peripheral, well-defined round, oval, lobulated, or serpentine opacity. Large vessels (feeders) extending centrally toward the hilum are usually visible (see Figs. 1-10, 1-11, and 1-12). Enlargement of fistulas over a period of months or years is common and a rapid increase in size can occur.

On CT, a simple AVM is visible as a smooth, sharply defined, round, or elliptical nodule, almost always in a subpleural location (see Figs. 1-12 and 1-13). Arteriovenous fistulas characterized by a tangle of tortuous, dilated vessels are seen as lobulated, serpiginous masses and can often be suspected as being vascular simply by their morphology. In both instances, the feeding pulmonary artery branch and draining pulmonary vein are dilated, and with fistulas of significant

size (larger than 1 to 2 cm), the feeders are easily recognizable. In general, the feeders are about half the diameter of the fistula.

Spiral CT is highly accurate in demonstrating AVMs and their architecture (see Figs. 1-10, 1-11, and 1-12). In most cases, morphologic findings are sufficient for diagnosis of AVM (see Figs. 1-12B and E), but contrast infusion may be used for confirmation (see Fig. 1-12C). Following the bolus injection of contrast, pulmonary AVMs show rapid contrast opacification and washout, occurring in phase with opacification and washout of the main pulmonary artery and right ventricle.

In general, AVMs appearing less than 2 cm in diameter on chest radiographs are asymptomatic. Single fistulas are less commonly symptomatic (35%) or associated with positive physical findings (70%) than are multiple fistulas (60% and 85%, respectively). An AVM results in a right to left

(text continues on page 14)

A

B

C

E

D

FIG. 1.12. Multiple arteriovenous malformations (AVMs) in a 30-year-old woman with Osler-Weber-Rendu syndrome. **A:** Chest radiograph shows a nodule in the right upper lobe (*arrow*). **B:** Spiral CT with 1.25-mm slices shows a well-defined subpleural nodule with a feeding vessel (*arrow*), representing a vein. This appearance is typical of an AVM. **C:** With contrast injection, dense opacification of the fistula and feeding vein is seen. **D:** Coronal reconstruction shows the subpleural fistula, feeding artery, and draining vein. **E:** Multiple other fistulas were visible. A small fistula (*arrow*) in the lower lobe may be diagnosed based on its morphology. (*Figure continues.*)

FIG. 1.12. (*Continued.*) **F:** Arteriogram performed at the time of embolization shows the fistula in (**C**) to opacify (**G**). The fistula shown in (**F**) has been occluded by wire coils. **H:** T2-weighted MRI of the brain shows findings of infarction (*arrow*). This is a common complication of AVMs.

FIG. 1.13. Multiple arteriovenous malformations (AVMs) in a 19-year-old woman with Osler-Weber-Rendu syndrome. **A:** Multidetector spiral HRCT obtained with 1.25-mm slices shows three small subpleural nodules (*arrows*). **B:** A maximum intensity projection (MIP) image at the same level shows the small AVMs (*arrows*) with feeding vessels. **C–E:** Transaxial (**C**), coronal (**D**), and sagittal (**E**) MIP images show other subpleural fistulas (*arrows*).

FIG. 1.14. Osler-Weber-Rendu syndrome with multiple arteriovenous malformations (AVMs) is shown on CT and pulmonary hemorrhage. Patchy areas of ground-glass opacity (*arrows*) in the left lung represent blood due to rupture of an AVM.

shunt, and cyanosis is common, depending on the size of the shunt. The most frequent symptoms occurring in patients with AVMs are dyspnea, palpitation, hemoptysis, and chest pain. Stroke (see Fig. 1-12H) may be associated with polycythemia, and paradoxical embolization through the AVM from systemic veins is a serious and potentially fatal complication. Rupture can result in pulmonary hemorrhage (Fig. 1-14) or hemothorax (Fig. 1-15). Without treatment, approximately 25% of patients with AVMs experience worsening of symptoms, and 50% of them will eventually die as a result of complications.

The use of pulmonary arteriography is generally limited to patients having embolization of the fistula (see Fig. 1-12F and G). Transcatheter occlusion of fistulas using wire coils is the treatment of choice for simple AVMs, and is generally reserved for fistulas having an arterial feeder greater than 3 mm in diameter. Recanalization of an AVF may occasionally occur after coil embolization. Complex AVMs (Fig. 1-16) are more often symptomatic that simple fistulas, because of a larger shunt. They are more difficult to treat because many feeders may be present, but wire coil embolization may be successful.

A

FIG. 1.15. Arteriovenous malformation (AVM) and hemothorax in a young woman with acute chest pain and shortness of breath. **A:** CT shows a right pleural effusion with a region of high attenuation indicating clot. A rounded lesion opacified by contrast is visible in the lung periphery (*arrow*). This appearance suggests AVM. **B:** Arteriogram shows a simple AVM in the lung periphery. Wire-coil embolization was performed, with resolution of the symptoms.

B

A

B

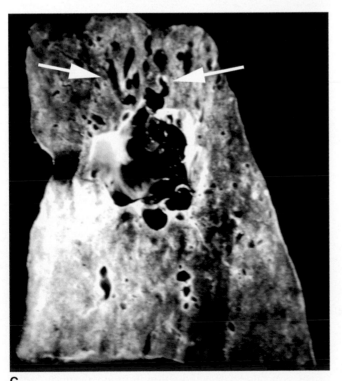

C

FIG. 1.16. Complex arteriovenous malformation in a patient with cyanosis. **A:** An ill-defined opacity is visible in the retrocardiac left lower lobe. **B:** Arteriogram shows a malformation with multiple feeding arteries (*arrows*). **C:** Left lower lobectomy specimen shows the fistula and its complex arterial supply (*arrows*).

A

B

C

FIG. 1.17. Pulmonary aplasia in a child. **A:** CT through the upper chest shows opacification of the right hemithorax and shift of the trachea to the right side. **B:** Just distal to the tracheal carina, the left main bronchus (*large arrow*) and a small right-sided bronchus (*small arrow*) are visible. There is marked shift of the mediastinum to the right, with left lung herniating across the midline. **C:** At a lower level, the bronchi to the left lung (*large arrow*) and the small right-sided bronchus (*small arrow*) are both visible. The heart is displaced into the posterior right hemithorax.

Pulmonary Telangiectasia

Pulmonary telangiectasia is an uncommon form of AVM characterized by innumerable very small fistulas scattered throughout both lungs. Symptoms are common and progressive, and cyanosis is present in all patients. Unlike simple AVMs, pulmonary telangiectasia is typically discovered by 10 years of age. Radiographs can be normal. If abnormal, radiographic findings are often limited to an abnormal pattern of pulmonary vessels, including (a) a coarse spidery appearance of pulmonary vessels, (b) vascular tortuosity, and (c) areas of hypervascularity. On angiograms, beaded or tortuous vessels, small aneurysmal sacs, or multiple ill-defined areas of vascular blush are visible. Treatment of this condition is difficult and prognosis is poor. Surgery is not possible because of the multiplicity of lesions.

PULMONARY AGENESIS, APLASIA, AND HYPOPLASIA

Agenesis and Aplasia

Pulmonary agenesis and aplasia are nearly the same, and a distinction is not usually necessary. *Pulmonary agenesis* represents complete absence of a lung, its bronchi, and

its vascular supply. *Pulmonary aplasia* is characterized by complete absence of a lung and its vascular supply, but a rudimentary bronchus is present (Fig. 1-17), ending in a blind pouch (Table 1-7). Either side may be affected. Associated congenital anomalies are often present. Pulmonary agenesis and aplasia are usually associated with a poor prognosis, with few patients surviving to adulthood.

Radiographically, pulmonary agenesis and aplasia result in opacification of a hemithorax and marked mediastinal shift (see Fig. 1-17). The heart is displaced into the posterior hemithorax on the side of agenesis or aplasia, along with other mediastinal structures. On lateral radiographs, the anterior chest appears abnormally lucent because of herniation of the remaining lung into the opposite hemithorax. CT demonstrates absence of the lung and pulmonary artery with marked mediastinal shift. In patients with agenesis, bronchi are also absent.

Hypoplasia

Pulmonary hypoplasia represents abnormal lung development associated with a reduction in lung volume and often a decrease in the number of alveoli and bronchial divisions (see Table 1-7). There may also be anomalous lobes or segments, or they may be reduced in number. Hypoplasia is associated with other anomalies in *hypogenetic lung*

TABLE 1.7 Pulmonary Agenesis, Aplasia, and Hypoplasia

Agenesis and Aplasia
   Occur on either side
   Mediastinal herniation into affected hemithorax
   Congenital anomalies associated
   Poor prognosis
Agenesis: absence of a lung and its bronchi and vascular supply
Aplasia: absence of a lung and its vascular supply; a rudimentary bronchus is present
Hypoplasia
   Abnormal lung development
   Decreased alveoli and bronchial divisions
   Deficient lobes or segments may be present
   Causes:
      Hypogenetic lung (Scimitar) syndrome
      Proximal interruption of pulmonary artery
      Lung compression during development

TABLE 1.8 Hypogenetic Lung (Scimitar) Syndrome

Four features typical (although each not always present):
   Hypoplasia of the lung with abnormal segmental or lobar anatomy
   Hypoplasia of the ipsilateral pulmonary artery
   Anomalous pulmonary venous return (scimitar vein)
   Anomalous systemic arterial supply to lower lobe
Almost always on the right side
Mediastinal shift toward the hypoplastic lung
Reduced size of ispilateral pulmonary artery
Anomalous (scimitar) vein usually paralleling right heart border
Congenital heart disease in 25% (e.g., atrial septal defect and patent ductus arteriousus)
Symptoms: recurrent infection and dyspnea

(scimitar) syndrome. It may also result from abnormal lung development due to deficient vascular supply (e.g., *proximal interruption of the pulmonary artery*) or lung compression during gestation [e.g., congenital diaphragmatic hernia (Fig. 1-18), space-occupying lesions, cystic adenomatoid malformation, sequestration, thoracic deformity, or oligohydramnios]. In patients with lung hypoplasia, the prognosis depends on the degree of abnormality and associated anomalies.

The pulmonary artery supplying the lung is reduced in size or absent (see Fig. 1-18E). On radiographs or CT, the size of pulmonary vessels may appear reduced on the affected side. Mediastinal shift toward the hypoplastic lung occurs with hypogenetic lung syndrome and proximal interruption of the pulmonary artery. Mediastinal shift may or may not be present when hypoplasia results from an ipsilateral space-occupying lesion.

HYPOGENETIC LUNG (SCIMITAR) SYNDROME

A rare anomaly, almost always occurring on the right side, hypogenetic lung syndrome is characterized by (a) hypoplasia of the lung with abnormal segmental or lobar anatomy, (b) hypoplasia of the ipsilateral pulmonary artery, (c) anomalous pulmonary venous return to the inferior vena cava (or right atrium, hepatic veins, etc.), and (d) anomalous systemic arterial supply to a portion of the hypoplastic lung, usually the lower lobe (Table 1-8). Although these four features often coexist, hypogenetic lung syndrome shows considerable variation in the degree to which each feature is expressed. Patients may exhibit some features of this syndrome but not others.

This syndrome is usually diagnosed in patients less than 30 years of age, and more than half have symptoms. Recurrent respiratory infections and dyspnea on exertion are most common. Congenital heart lesions, most commonly septal defects and patent ductus arteriosus, are associated in 25%. Surgical treatment involves implantation of the anomalous vein into the left atrium.

Radiographically, the appearance of scimitar syndrome is often characteristic (Fig. 1-19). The hypoplastic lung is recognizable because of dextroposition of the heart, mediastinal shift to the right side, and right diaphragmatic elevation. CT may show abnormal bronchial anatomy on the side of the hypoplastic lung.

Hypoplasia of the pulmonary artery may be recognizable by the decreased size of vessels within the hypoplastic lung. Because most of the pulmonary blood flow must traverse the normal artery on the side opposite the hypoplastic lung, the opposite pulmonary artery appears enlarged, further increasing the contrast between the right and left vasculature.

When the anomalous vein is visible radiographically, it appears as a broad arcuate band at the right lung base, paralleling the right heart border and extending to the diaphragmatic surface (see Figs. 1-19 and 1-20). This venous shadow often resembles a scimitar, hence the nickname of this syndrome. In nearly two thirds of patients, the scimitar vein drains the entire right lung. On CT, the scimitar vein is located in close relation to the major fissure. Left-sided scimitar syndrome, with the anomalous vein entering the coronary sinus, is rarely seen.

Systemic arteries, usually multiple and arising below the diaphragm, typically supply the lower lobe. These may be visible using CT (see Fig. 1-19D and E).

In some patients, findings of the scimitar syndrome may be associated with "horseshoe lung." Horseshoe lung is a rare congenital malformation in which an isthmus of pulmonary parenchyma extends from the right lung base across the midline behind the pericardium and fuses with the base of the left lung. Horseshoe lung may occur in the absence of scimitar syndrome.

(text continues on page 20)

FIG. 1.18. Pulmonary hypoplasia in a baby with congenital diaphragmatic hernia. **A:** Chest radiograph shows opacification of the right hemithorax with mediastinal shift to the right. **B:** CT shows mediastinal shift, opacification of the right hemithorax, and both main bronchi. The right lung is airless. **C:** Coronal MRI shows herniation of the liver into the right hemithorax. No aerated right lung is visible, but rudimentary lung is visible at the apex of right hemithorax (*arrow*). **D:** 3D MR angiogram shows a normal left pulmonary artery (*arrows*). The right pulmonary artery is not clearly seen. **E:** Transaxial MR shows a small right pulmonary artery (*arrow*).

FIG. 1.19. Scimitar syndrome. **A:** Plain radiograph shows displacement of the heart toward the right side and elevation of the right hemidiaphragm, because of right lung hypoplasia, and the anomalous pulmonary vein paralleling the right heart border (*arrows*). **B:** CT at the level of the right upper lobe bronchus shows the anomalous pulmonary vein (*arrow*). Shift of the anterior mediastinum toward the right is visible (*small arrows*). The right pulmonary artery is smaller than the left. **C:** At the lower level, the scimitar vein (*arrow*) is visible in relation to the major fissure, which appears thickened. Mediastinal shift is also visible. **D:** Near the right diaphragm, the scimitar vein (*large arrow*) is within the major fissure. A septum in the posteromedial right lung (*small arrows*) is at the site of systemic arterial supply to the lower lobe. **E:** Soft tissue window scan at the level of the right hemidiaphragm shows the scimitar vein (*large arrow*) entering the inferior vena cava (*IVC*). A systemic artery (*small arrow*) supplies the lower lobe. **F:** Coronal reconstruction shows the scimitar vein (*arrow*) to best advantage.

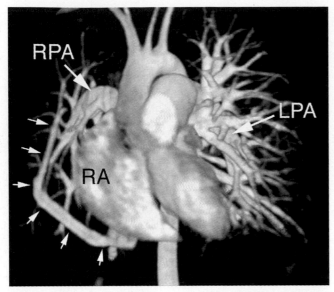

FIG. 1.20. 3D MR angiogram in scimitar syndrome. The right pulmonary artery (*RPA*) is smaller than the left (*LPA*). The scimitar vein (*small arrows*) parallels the border of the right atrium (*RA*) and drains into the inferior vena cava.

TABLE 1.9	Proximal Interruption of the Pulmonary Artery

Congenital absence of a main pulmonary artery
Almost always on the side opposite the aortic arch (i.e., usually the right)
Hypoplastic ipsilateral lung
Reduced size of ipsilateral pulmonary vessels
Lung vascular supply derived from bronchial arteries
Mediastinal shift toward the hypoplastic lung
Congenital heart disease common (tetralogy of Fallot and septal defects)

PROXIMAL INTERRUPTION OF THE PULMONARY ARTERY

This anomaly can closely resemble hypogenetic lung syndrome. In proximal interruption of the pulmonary artery, the proximal portion of a main pulmonary artery, usually the right, fails to develop (Table 1-9). The ipsilateral lung is hypoplastic because of deficient growth but has a normal number of lobes and segments, and bronchial anatomy

A

B

C

FIG. 1.21. Proximal interruption of the right pulmonary artery. **A:** Chest radiograph shows mediastinal shift to the right with small right pulmonary vessels and a large left pulmonary artery (*arrow*). **B:** Contrast-enhanced CT shows the ascending aorta (*Ao*) and a large left pulmonary artery (*LPA*), but the right pulmonary artery is absent. Large bronchial arteries (*arrows*) supply the right lung. **C:** Lung window scan shows hypoplasia of the right lung and small right lung vessels.

is normal. Vessels within the lung appear small (Fig. 1-21), whereas those on the opposite side are much larger. The lung vascular supply is derived from hypertrophied bronchial arteries (see Fig. 1-21B). This entity is often associated with congenital heart disease, most typically tetralogy of Fallot and septal defects. This anomaly usually occurs on the side opposite the aortic arch (Fig. 1-22). When the interrupted pulmonary artery and aorta are ipsilateral, the incidence of congenital heart disease is higher than when they are not.

UNILATERAL PULMONARY VEIN ATRESIA

In unilateral pulmonary vein atresia, another rare entity, long segments of the pulmonary veins of one lung are congenitally atretic (Table 1-10). The involved lung can be normal in size or hypoplastic, and it often shows increased interstitial densities and interlobular septal thickening because of venous stasis, edema, and fibrosis (Fig 1-23). The ipsilateral pulmonary artery may appear small (Fig 1-23B). Radionuclide imaging shows decreased perfusion. Angiography shows decreased size of the ipsilateral pulmonary artery, peripheral pruning, contrast stasis, and nonvisualization of the pulmonary veins. Symptoms include hemoptysis and infection.

PULMONARY VEIN VARIX

Dilation of a pulmonary vein branch (pulmonary vein varix) can be congenital or acquired (Table 1-11). One or more veins appear dilated or tortuous near the point they enter the left atrium. With congenital varices, symptoms are usually absent, although rupture rarely occurs.

TABLE 1.10 Pulmonary Vein Atresia

Pulmonary veins of one lung atretic
Lung hypoplastic or normal in volume
Reduced size of ispilateral pulmonary artery
Increased interstitial opacities in affected lung

Acquired varices are associated with chronically elevated left atrial pressure, as in mitral stenosis. These most commonly involve the right inferior pulmonary vein. On plain radiographs, these are visible through the right part of the heart shadow and often appear rounded and sharply defined. They may mimic the appearance of a lung nodule, leading to further evaluation. CT is diagnostic.

ANOMALOUS PULMONARY VEIN DRAINAGE

Anomalous pulmonary vein drainage involves drainage of a pulmonary vein branch into the right atrium, coronary sinus, or systemic vein, producing a left-to-right shunt (Table 1-12).

Partial anomalous pulmonary venous drainage is present in about 0.5% of the population and is usually asymptomatic. The anomalous vein may drain into various vascular structures. On the right, the most common are the superior vena cava (Fig. 1-24), azygos vein, inferior vena cava, and right atrium. On the left, drainage may be through the left brachiocephalic vein, persistent left superior vena cava (vertical vein; Fig. 1-25), or coronary sinus. Drainage may also be below the diaphragm.

A

B

FIG. 1.22. Proximal interruption of the left pulmonary artery in a patient with right aortic arch. **A:** Chest radiograph shows mediastinal shift to the left. **B:** Contrast-enhanced CT shows the ascending aorta (*Ao*), a right-sided descending aorta (*DA*), and a large right pulmonary artery (*RPA*), but the left pulmonary artery is absent. Large bronchial arteries (*arrows*) supply the hypoplastic left lung.

A   B

FIG. 1.23. Unilateral pulmonary vein atresia. **A:** Scout view from a CT shows the right lung to be small, with mediastinal shift to the right and elevation of the right hemidiaphragm, and increased interstitial markings on the right. **B:** Contrast-enhanced CT shows the right inferior pulmonary vein to be absent (*black arrow*). The right superior pulmonary vein was also absent. The right lung is hypoplastic with mediastinal shift to the right, and the right pulmonary artery is much smaller than the left (*large arrow*). A small right pleural effusion is present. **C:** High-resolution CT shows interlobular septal thickening in the hypoplastic right lung.

C

Total anomalous pulmonary venous drainage must be associated with a septal defect and is best considered to be a type of congenital heart disease.

BRONCHOPULMONARY SEQUESTRATION

Bronchopulmonary sequestration is a congenital malformation resulting from abnormal budding of the foregut and its associated structures during the period that lung, bronchi, and pulmonary vessels are developing. Pathologically, sequestration represents an area of disorganized pulmonary parenchyma without normal pulmonary arterial or bronchial communications (i.e., it is sequestered from bronchi and pulmonary arteries). Sequestration usually receives its blood supply from branches of the thoracic or abdominal aorta, and aortography is usually necessary before surgical excision in order to visualize these arterial branches. Fatal hemorrhage can occur if these systemic arteries are accidentally cut during surgery. There are two forms of sequestration—intralobar and extralobar. Although they share some features, they

(*text continues on page 25*)

TABLE 1.11 Pulmonary Vein Varix
Congenital
Usually asymptomatic
Acquired
Associated with elevated left atrial pressure (e.g., mitral stenosis)
Usually on the right
Mimics a lung nodule

TABLE 1.12 Anomalous Pulmonary Venous Drainage
Pulmonary vein drainage into the right atrium, coronary sinus, or systemic vein
Left to right shunt
Partial: 0.5%, usually asymptomatic
Total: septal defect present

A   B

FIG. 1.24. Partial anomalous pulmonary vein drainage in a patient with a tracheal bronchus. **A:** The tracheal bronchus is visible arising from the right tracheal wall (*arrow*). **B:** At a lower level, a right superior pulmonary vein (*v*) branch enters the superior vena cava (*S*).

FIG. 1.25. Partial anomalous pulmonary vein drainage. **A:** A left pulmonary vein (*arrow*) enters a left superior vena cava (vertical vein). **B:** At a higher level, the left superior vena cava (*arrow*) is visible lateral to the aortic arch. **C:** The left superior vena cava (*arrow*) drains into the left brachiocephalic vein (*bv*).

FIG. 1.26. Intralobar sequestration in a young woman with recurrent left lower lobe pneumonia. **A, B:** Patchy consolidation is visible in the left lower lobe (*arrows*). **C:** Angiogram shows several branches (*small arrows*) of the descending aorta resulting in opacification of the sequestration (*Seq*). Drainage is into the azygos vein (*large arrow*).

TABLE 1.13 Intralobar Sequestration
More common than extralobar sequestration
Within visceral pleura of lobe
65% at left base
No pulmonary artery or bronchial supply
Arterial supply from thoracic aorta in 75%
Drainage via pulmonary veins in most
Presentation in older children or adults
Recurrent infection
Imaging appearances:
Homogeneous and well-defined mass lesion
Cystic or multicystic air- and fluid-filled lesion
Hyperlucent and hypovascular region of lung
Combination of these

differ significantly in several important clinical and radiographic characteristics.

Intralobar Sequestration

Intralobar sequestration is the more common of these two malformations. In this anomaly, sequestered lung lies within the visceral pleura of one of the lobes. It occurs most often on the left side, and approximately two thirds are found adjacent to the diaphragm in relation to the posterior basal segment of the left lower lobe (Table 1-13). In almost 75% of cases, the arterial supply of an intralobar sequestration is from the descending thoracic aorta; others receive supply from branches of the abdominal aorta or from intercostal arteries. These systemic arteries often enter the lung via the inferior pulmonary ligament. Usually venous drainage is by pulmonary veins, but drainage into the azygos or hemiazygos system is not uncommon.

Intralobar sequestration usually presents in adults or older children. Acute or recurrent infection is most common as a presenting complaint (Fig. 1-26). Hemoptysis may occur. The systemic arterial to pulmonary venous shunt produced by interlobar sequestration is usually small and clinically insignificant. However, cases resulting in congestive heart failure have been reported. Bilateral sequestrations may occur. Connection to the esophagus is rarely seen. Association with other anomalies is uncommon.

Uncomplicated intralobar sequestration can have a variety of appearances. It may appear as (a) a homogeneous and well-defined mass lesion (Fig. 1-27), (b) a cystic or multicystic air and fluid-filled lesion, (c) a hyperlucent and hypovascular region of lung (Fig. 1-28), or (d) a combination of these. Hyperlucency is common in uncomplicated sequestration due to air trapping; this may be difficult to

(text continues on page 28)

A   B

FIG. 1.27. Intralobar sequestration presenting as a mass. **A and B:** Contrast-enhanced CTs show a mass lesion posterior to the descending aorta. Large vessels are visible within the mass. An artery (*art*) can be seen arising from the aorta, supplying the sequestration. Venous drainage (*v*) is into the azygos vein (*az*).

FIG. 1.28. Intralobar sequestration presenting as a hyperlucent lesion. **A:** Digital radiograph shows normal-appearing lungs. **B:** CT shows a lucent lesion (*white arrows*) at the right lung base. Pulmonary artery branches are draped over the surface of the lucency. A large, abnormal vessel (*black arrow*) is visible with the region of lucency, but fewer vessels are seen in the lesion than the surrounding lower lobe. **C:** At a lower level, the lucent lesion (*white arrows*) and abnormal vessel (*black arrow*) are visible. **D:** Contrast-enhanced scan at a lower level shows the abnormal vessel (*arrow*) arising from the descending aorta. **E:** Maximum intensity coronal reconstruction shows the abnormal aortic branch (*arrows*) supplying the right lung base. **F:** Minimum intensity coronal reconstruction shows the hyperlucency intralobar sequestration (*arrows*) and its supplying vessel.

FIG. 1.29. Bilateral intralobar sequestrations supplied by a single anomalous branch of the descending aorta (subtracted arteriogram).

A

B

C

D

FIG. 1.30. Extralobar sequestration in a neonate. **A:** Chest radiograph shows a soft tissue mass at the left base (*arrows*). **B, C:** Contrast-enhanced CTs show a soft tissue mass with arterial supply (*arrows*) from the aorta. **D:** Aortogram performed via umbilical artery catheter shows anomalous arteries supplying the left base.

TABLE 1.14 Extralobar Sequestration

Within its own pleural envelope
90% at left base
No pulmonary artery or bronchial supply
Arterial supply from abdominal aorta in most
Drainage via systemic (e.g., azygos or hemiazygos)
    veins in most
Presentation in infancy in most
Presents as mass lesion; infection is rare
Imaging appearances:
    Homogeneous and well-defined mass lesion
    May contain fluid-filled cystic areas
    Rarely contains air

TABLE 1.15 Comparison of Intralobar and Extralobar Sequestration

	Intralobar Sequestration	Extralobar Sequestration
Patient age	Adult or older child	Infant or child
Symptoms	Infection common	Infection rare
Morphology	Within a lobe	Within its own pleural envelope
Location	65% at left base	90% at left base
Arterial supply	Thoracic or abdominal aorta	Usually abdominal aorta
Venous drainage	Usually pulmonary veins	Usually systemic veins
Appearance	Commonly contains air	Rarely contains air

recognize on chest radiographs but is commonly seen at CT (see Fig. 1-28). The presence of mucous or fluid-filled cysts with air-fluid levels can be seen with or without infection. In such cases, a sequestration can closely mimic lung abscess. Rarely, bilateral sequestrations may be seen. These often are supplied by a single artery (Fig. 1-29).

On CT, bronchi and normal pulmonary arteries can be shown draped over the lesion (see Fig. 1-28) but do not enter a sequestration. With contrast-enhanced spiral CT, the supplying systemic arteries are often visible (see Figs. 1-27 and 1-28). If not, aortography can be used to confirm the diagnosis. The draining veins can also be identified following contrast infusion.

Extralobar Sequestration

Extralobar sequestration represents an anomaly in which the sequestered tissue is enclosed within its only pleural envelope; it is less common than intralobar sequestration. Approximately 90% of cases are present at the left lung base, contiguous with the left hemidiaphragm (Table 1-14). Arterial supply is usually from the abdominal aorta and drainage is almost always by means of systemic veins (inferior vena cava, azygos, hemiazygos, or portal veins), producing a left-to-right shunt. Rarely, they may be located within the diaphragm or immediately below the diaphragm in the upper abdomen.

Extralobar sequestration is often diagnosed in infancy (unlike intralobar sequestration) (Table 1-15). It is detected incidentally or presents as a mass lesion (Fig. 1-30). Unlike intralobar sequestration, infection is rare. Associated congenital anomalies, particularly diaphragmatic abnormalities and ipsilateral lung hypoplasia, are common. Because of its complete pleural envelope, extralobar sequestration rarely becomes infected.

Radiographically and on CT, extralobar sequestration appears as a sharply-marginated mass lesion, which does not contain air (unlike intralobar sequestration) (see Figs. 1-30

and 1-31). It is usually homogeneous in appearance but may contain cystic areas. Its supplying artery may be seen on CT. If not, aortography may be needed for diagnosis.

ANOMALOUS SYSTEMIC ARTERIES WITHOUT SEQUESTRATION (SYSTEMIC ARTERIAL MALFORMATION)

Systemic arteries may supply normal basal segments of lung (Table 1-16). Although these lesions can be thought of as representing systemic AVMs, they are unassociated with the large, dilated vascular sac typically seen with pulmonary AVMs. Rather, the arteriovenous communications in patients with systemic arterial malformations usually represent normal capillaries.

This lesion is probably best thought of as anomalous systemic arterial supply to an area of lung due to persistence of an embryonic aortic branch. The pulmonary parenchyma in the region supplied by the anomalous artery is normal, as are bronchial communications (Fig. 1-32). The pulmonary artery supply to these areas can be normal or absent.

A relationship may exist between systemic arterial malformations and pulmonary sequestration, and both these lesions represent different points on the spectrum of anomalies affecting the pulmonary artery, systemic arteries, and bronchial development. Some cases have been reported in which intralobar sequestration on one side

TABLE 1.16 Systemic Artery Malformation

Arterial supply to lung from thoracic or abdominal aorta
Lung normal
Bronchi normal
Pulmonary artery normal or absent in affected region
Pulmonary vein drainage normal
Symptoms: Congestive heart failure or hemoptysis

A

B

C

FIG. 1.31. Extralobar sequestration in an adult. PA (**A**) and lateral (**B**) chest radiographs show a mass (*arrows*) at the left base. **C:** Contrast-enhanced CT shows opacified vessels (*black arrow*) within the mass (*white arrows*).

coexists with systemic arterial malformation on the other. In such cases, both lesions are typically supplied by the same aortic branch.

Because systemic arterial malformation results in a left-to-left arterial shunt, left ventricular enlargement and congestive heart failure can occur. Hemoptysis may also occur. However, most patients have no symptoms. If the anomalous vessel supplies an area of lung also supplied by the pulmonary artery, treatment involves ligation or embolization of the anomalous vessel.

A

B

C

FIG. 1.32. Anomalous systemic arteries without sequestration in a patient with hemoptysis. **A:** Radiograph of the right lower lobe appears normal. **B:** Pulmonary arteriogram shows an area of lung (∗) without pulmonary artery supply. **C:** An abnormal arterial branch (*arrows*) from the descending aorta supplies this region of lung.

SELECTED READING

Desir A, Ghaye B. Congenital abnormalities of intrathoracic airways. Radiol Clin North Am 2009; 47:203–225.

Dines DE, Arms RA, Bernatz PE, Gomes MR. Pulmonary arteriovenous fistulas. Mayo Clin Proc 1974; 49:460–465.

Do KH, Goo JM, Im JG, et al. Systemic arterial supply to the lungs in adults: spiral CT findings. Radiographics 2001; 21:387–402.

Fitch SJ, Tonkin ILD, Tonkin AK. Imaging of foregut cysts. Radiographics 1986; 6:189–201.

Ghaye B, Szapiro D, Fanchamps JM, Dondelinger RF. Congenital bronchial abnormalities revisited. Radiographics 2001; 21:105–119.

Griffin N, Devarai A, Goldstraw P, et al. CT and histopathological correlation of congenital cystic pulmonary lesions: a common pathogenesis? Clin Radiol 2008; 63:995–1005.

Ikezoe J, Murayama S, Godwin JD, et al. Bronchopulmonary sequestration: CT assessment. Radiology 1990; 176:375–379.

Lee EY, Boiselle PM, Cleveland RH. Multidetector CT evaluation of congenital lung abnormalities. Radiology 2008; 247:632–648.

Mata JM, Caceres J, Lucaya J, Garcia-Conesa JA. CT of congenital malformations of the lung. Radiographics 1990; 10:651–674.

McAdams HP, Kirejczyk WM, Rosado-de-Christenson ML, Matsumoto S. Bronchogenic cyst: imaging features with clinical and histopathologic correlation. Radiology 2000; 217:441–446.

Patz EF Jr, Müller NL, Swensen SJ, Dodd LG. Congenital cystic adenomatoid malformation in adults: CT findings. J Comput Assist Tomogr 1995; 19:361–364.

Rappaport DC, Herman SJ, Weisbrod GL. Congenital bronchopulmonary diseases in adults: CT findings. AJR Am J Roentgenol 1994; 162:1295–1299.

Remy J, Remy-Jardin M, Wattinne L, Deffontaines C. Pulmonary arteriovenous malformations: evaluation with CT of the chest before and after treatment. Radiology 1992; 182:809–816.

Roehm JOF, Jue KL, Amplatz K. Radiographic features of the scimitar syndrome. Radiology 1966; 86:856–859.

Rosado-de-Christenson ML, Stocker JT. Congenital cystic adenomatoid malformation. Radiographics 1991; 11:865–886.

Sener RN, Tugran C, Savas R, Alper H. CT findings in scimitar syndrome. AJR Am J Roentgenol 1993; 160:1361.

Shenoy SS, Culver GJ, Pirson HS. Agenesis of lung in an adult. AJR Am J Roentgenol 1979; 133:755–757.

Shimohira M, Hara M, Masanori K, et al. Congenital Pulmonary Airway Malformation: CT-pathologic correlation. J Thorac Imaging 2007; 22:149–153

Yamanaka A, Hirai T, Fujimoto T, et al. Anomalous systemic arterial supply to normal basal segments of the left lower lobe. Ann Thorac Surg 1999; 68:332–338.

Consolidation and Atelectasis

W. RICHARD WEBB

ecognizing consolidation and atelectasis is fundamental to an understanding of pulmonary radiology.

AIR-SPACE CONSOLIDATION

Air-space consolidation represents replacement of alveolar air by fluid, blood, pus, cells, or other substances. *Alveolar consolidation* and *parenchymal consolidation* are synonyms for air-space consolidation.

Radiographic Findings

Radiographic and computed tomography (CT) abnormalities indicating the presence of air-space consolidation include the following:

- Homogeneous opacity obscuring vessels
- Air bronchograms
- Ill-defined or fluffy opacities
- "Air alveolograms"
- Patchy opacities
- "Acinar" or air-space nodules
- Preserved lung volume
- Extension to the pleural surface
- "CT angiogram" sign

Homogeneous Opacity Obscuring Vessels

With complete replacement of alveolar air, homogeneous opacification of the lung results. Vessels within the consolidated lung are invisible (Fig. 2-1A).

Air Bronchograms

In patients with consolidation, air-filled bronchi are often visible on plain radiographs or CT, appearing lucent compared with opacified lung parenchyma (see Fig. 2-1). This finding is termed an *air bronchogram*.

With some causes of consolidation, air bronchograms may not be visible. This usually occurs because of central bronchial obstruction (e.g., by cancer or mucus) or filling of bronchi in association with the underlying pathologic process. For example, pulmonary infarction often results in

consolidation without air bronchograms because of blood filling the bronchi. In patients with bronchopneumonia, bronchi may be filled with mucus or pus.

If air bronchograms are visible within an area of consolidation, bronchial obstruction is unlikely (but not ruled out) as its cause. Although air bronchograms are considered a classic sign of air-space consolidation, they may also be seen in the presence of confluent interstitial disease.

Ill-defined or Fluffy Opacities

Consolidation often results in opacities with ill-defined margins (Figs. 2-2 and 2-3), in contrast to the relatively sharp margins of a lung mass. This results from patchy local spread of disease with variable involvement of alveoli at the edges of the pathologic process.

Air Alveolograms

If lung consolidation is not confluent, small focal lucencies representing uninvolved lung may be visible (see Fig. 2-2). These have been termed "air alveolograms," but this is a misnomer as alveoli are too small to see radiographically. Nonetheless, these lucencies reflect incomplete lung consolidation.

Patchy Opacities

Variable consolidation in different lung regions results in patchy areas of increased opacity (see Fig. 2-3). Pulmonary vessels may be obscured or poorly defined.

Patchy consolidation visible on chest radiographs sometimes appears to be lobular or multilobular on CT (i.e., involving individual pulmonary lobules; Fig. 2-4). Some lobules appear abnormally dense while adjacent lobules appear normally aerated.

"Acinar" or Air-space Nodules

An acinus is the largest unit of lung structure in which all airways participate in gas exchange. Anatomically, it is located distal to a terminal bronchiole and is supplied by a first-order respiratory bronchiole. Acini average 7 to 8 mm in diameter.

The terms *acinar nodule* and *air-space nodule* are used to describe poorly margined rounded opacities, usually

(*text continues on page 35*)

FIG. 2.1. Consolidation: homogeneous opacity obscuring vessels, air bronchograms, and the CT angiogram sign. **A:** Right lung consolidation due to pulmonary edema. Air bronchograms are visible bilaterally within the consolidated lung and pulmonary vessels are obscured. **B:** Enhanced CT in a patient with right middle and lower lobe pneumonia shows homogeneous consolidation, preserved lung volume, air bronchograms (*black arrows*), and opacified vessels (*white arrows*), appearing denser than surrounding consolidated lung (i.e., the "CT angiogram" sign).

FIG. 2.2. Consolidation: ill-defined, fluffy opacities with "air alveolograms." **A:** Detailed view of incomplete right lower lobe consolidation shows fluffy, ill-defined opacity containing small rounded lucencies. These lucencies have been termed air alveolograms, although they do not correspond to alveoli. **B:** Ill-defined fluffy consolidation (*white arrows*) is visible on CT in a patient with right lower lobe pneumonia. Small focal lucencies (*black arrows*) within the area of consolidation are "air alveolograms."

A   B

FIG. 2.3. Consolidation: patchy opacities. **A:** Chest radiograph in a patient with pulmonary edema due to renal failure shows patchy perihilar consolidation. **B:** Patchy areas of fluffy consolidation are seen on CT. The fluffy margins are due to variable involvement of alveoli at the edges of the pathologic process.

A   B

FIG. 2.4. Consolidation: patchy opacities with lobular consolidation. **A, B:** Contrast-enhanced HRCT in a patient with bronchopneumonia and lobular consolidation. Individual lobules are consolidated while others appear normal. Centrilobular arteries (*white arrow*) and bronchi (*black arrows*) are visible within consolidated lobules. **C:** Coronal reconstruction also shows the lobular distribution of the patchy lung opacities.

C

A   **B**

FIG. 2.5. Consolidation: acinar or air-space nodules. **A:** Chest radiograph shows a patchy left upper lobe pneumonia. Ill-defined nodular opacities less than 1 cm in diameter (*arrows*) are visible on the edge of the area of denser consolidation. These represent air-space or acinar nodules. **B:** CT (5-mm slice thickness) in a patient with bilateral consolidation. Air bronchograms are visible in the left lower lobe. Patchy consolidation and ground-glass opacities are present. Air-space nodules are visible in the right middle lobe (*arrows*) and the right lower lobe. These nodules are ill-defined, 5 to 10 mm in diameter, and centrilobular in distribution.

5 to 10 mm in diameter, that occur due to focal consolidation (Fig. 2-5). Although these nodules approximate the size of acini, they tend to be centrilobular and peribronchiolar rather than acinar. They may be seen as the only finding of consolidation or may be seen in association with larger areas of consolidation, usually at the edges of the more abnormal lung.

These nodular opacities are more easily seen on high-resolution CT (HRCT) than on chest radiographs. On HRCT, their centrilobular location is usually visible. This appearance is described further in Chapter 10.

Preserved Lung Volume

In the presence of consolidation, because alveolar air is replaced by something else (e.g., fluid), the volume of affected lung tends to be preserved (see Fig. 2-1B). Although some volume loss may be seen in patients with consolidation, it is usually of a minor degree. Alternatively, in some patients with consolidation, the lobe is expanded.

Extension to Pleural Surfaces

Pathologic processes resulting in consolidation often spread from alveolus to alveolus until reaching a fissure or pleural surface (see Fig. 2-5B). The pleural surface prevents further spread. When extension to a pleural surface occurs, the process may appear lobar, as in lobar pneumonia.

CT Angiogram Sign

A unique finding seen on CT in patients with consolidation is the "CT angiogram" sign. This sign is present if normal-appearing

opacified vessels are visible within the consolidated lung following the infusion of intravenous contrast (see Figs. 2-1B and 2-6). Although opacified vessels are sometimes seen within a lung mass, they usually appear compressed or distorted.

FIG. 2.6. Consolidation: the CT angiogram sign. Contrast-enhanced CT in a patient with pneumonia shows focal consolidation. Opacified arteries (*arrows*) appear denser than consolidated lung (i.e., the CT angiogram sign). The consolidation borders on the major fissure posteriorly and appears segmental.

Differential Diagnosis

In general, the differential diagnosis of air-space consolidation is based on a consideration of the substance that is replacing alveolar air:

1. Water (e.g., the various types of pulmonary edema)
2. Blood (e.g., pulmonary hemorrhage)
3. Pus (e.g., pneumonia)
4. Cells (e.g., bronchioloalveolar carcinoma, lymphoma, eosinophilic pneumonia, organizing pneumonia [bronchiolitis obliterans organizing pneumonia or BOOP], hypersensitivity pneumonitis)

5. Other substances (e.g., lipoprotein in alveolar proteinosis, lipid in lipoid pneumonia).

Patients with consolidation may be divided into two primary groups for the purpose of diagnosis: those with diffuse or bilateral consolidation and those with focal consolidation.

Diffuse Consolidation

Diffuse consolidation has a number of possible causes (Table 2-1), and the clinical history is often more important than the radiographic findings in making the diagnosis.

TABLE 2.1   Differential Diagnosis of Diffuse Consolidation

Water (edema) (see Chapter 11)	Chemotherapy
Hydrostatic (cardiogenic) pulmonary edema	Leukemia
Heart failure	Low platelets
Left atrial or pulmonary venous obstruction	Collagen-vascular disease and immune complex
Volume overload	vasculitis
Low intravascular oncotic pressure	Systemic lupus erythematosus most common
Hypoalbuminemia	Behçet's syndrome
Liver disease	Henoch-Schönlein purpura
Renal failure	Antiphospholipid syndrome
Increased permeability (noncardiogenic) pulmonary edema	Goodpasture's syndrome
With diffuse alveolar damage (acute respiratory distress	Idiopathic pulmonary hemosiderosis
syndrome [ARDS])	Trauma
Acute interstitial pneumonia	Vasculitis
Aspiration of gastric acid	Wegener's granulomatosis
Drugs	Churg-Strauss granulomatosis
Fat embolism	Microscopic polyangiitis
Infection and sepsis	**Pus (pneumonia)**
Near-drowning	Bacterial pneumonia
Pneumonia	Pneumonia in an immunosuppressed patient
Radiation	Tuberculosis
Shock	Nontuberculous mycobacteria
Toxic fumes or gases	Fungal pneumonia (histoplasmosis, aspergillosis most
Trauma	common)
Without diffuse alveolar damage	Atypical organisms
Any cause of ARDS, in a mild form	Virus
Drug reactions	*Pneumocystis*
Hantavirus pulmonary syndrome	**Cells**
Transfusion reaction	Neoplasm
Mixed types of edema	Bronchioloalveolar carcinoma
Air embolism	Lymphoma and other lymphoproliferative diseases
High-altitude pulmonary edema	Eosinophilic pneumonia or other eosinophilic diseases
Neurogenic pulmonary edema	Organizing pneumonia (BOOP)
Posttransplantation edema	Hypersensitivity pneumonitis
Postpneumonectomy	Idiopathic interstitial pneumonias
Reexpansion edema	Nonspecific interstitial pneumonia
Reperfusion edema	Desquamative interstitial pneumonia
Tocolytic therapy	Sarcoidosis
Hydrostatic and permeability edema	**Other substances**
Blood (hemorrhage) (see Chapter 19)	Alveolar proteinosis (lipoprotein)
Aspiration of blood	Lipoid pneumonia (lipid)
Bleeding diathesis	
Anticoagulation	

Nonetheless, several patterns of diffuse consolidation may suggest possible causes.

Pattern and Differential Diagnosis

Perihilar "bat-wing" consolidation shows central consolidation with sparing of the lung periphery (Figs. 2-7 and 2-8). It is most typical of pulmonary edema (hydrostatic or permeability). This pattern also may be seen with pulmonary hemorrhage, pneumonias (including bacteria and atypical pneumonias such as *Pneumocystis jiroveci (P. carinii)* pneumonia [PCP] and viral pneumonia), and inhalational lung injury. In patients with pulmonary edema, a perihilar distribution is most often present when rapid accumulation of fluid has occurred. Relative sparing of the lung periphery has been attributed to better lymphatic clearance of edema fluid in this region, although the exact mechanism is unclear and undoubtedly varies with the disease.

Peripheral subpleural consolidation is the opposite of a bat-wing pattern (i.e., a reverse bat-wing pattern). Consolidation is seen adjacent to the chest wall, with sparing of the perihilar regions. It is most often seen in a patients with a chronic lung disease (also the reverse of what is true of a bat-wing pattern). It is classically associated with eosinophilic lung diseases, particularly eosinophilic pneumonia (Fig. 2-9A), but may also occur with organizing pneumonia (BOOP) (see Fig. 2-9B), sarcoidosis, radiation pneumonitis, lung contusion, or bronchioloalveolar carcinoma. Peripheral consolidation need not always appear peripheral on the frontal (posteroanterior [PA] or anteroposterior [AP])

FIG. 2.7. Perihilar "bat-wing" consolidation in pulmonary edema. Chest radiograph in a patient with pulmonary edema due to renal failure (note the dialysis catheter in the right atrium) shows a distinct perihilar bat-wing pattern of consolidation. The lung periphery is spared. Note the lucency at the level of the minor fissure (*arrow*) because of sparing of peripheral lung adjacent to the fissure.

A

B

FIG. 2.8. Perihilar "bat-wing" consolidation in pulmonary edema. **A:** Chest radiograph shows a distinct perihilar predominance of consolidation. The heart is enlarged. **B:** CT shows sparing of the lung periphery.

radiograph; it may be peripheral in the anterior or posterior lung and overlie the parahilar regions.

Diffuse patchy consolidation (Fig. 2-10) may be seen with any pneumonia (bacterial, mycobacterial, fungal, viral, PCP); pulmonary edema (see Fig. 2-3A) (hydrostatic and permeability); acute respiratory distress syndrome (ARDS); pulmonary hemorrhage syndromes; aspiration; inhalational diseases; eosinophilic diseases; and diffuse bronchioloalveolar carcinoma. The patchy opacities may correspond to consolidation of lobules, subsegments, or segments.

Diffuse air-space nodules as a prominent feature of consolidation are typical of endobronchial spread of disease (Fig. 2-11). This appearance is seen in patients with endobronchial spread of infection such as tuberculosis (TB) or *Mycobacterium avium* complex (MAC), bacterial bronchopneumonia,

A

FIG. 2.10. Diffuse patchy consolidation in a patient with viral pneumonia.

and neoplasm, while pulmonary edema and hemorrhage are much less likely than in patients with diffuse abnormalities.

Pattern and Differential Diagnosis

Focal consolidation may represent pneumonia; postobstructive pneumonia; aspiration; bronchioloalveolar carcinoma; lymphoma or other lymphoproliferative disease; infarction; hemorrhage due to trauma, pulmonary embolism, or diseases such as Wegener's granulomatosis; pulmonary infarction; radiation pneumonitis; organizing pneumonia (BOOP);

B

FIG. 2.9. Peripheral subpleural (reverse bat-wing) consolidation. **A:** Chest radiograph in a patient with chronic eosinophilic pneumonia shows areas of consolidation in the subpleural lung. The perihilar regions are spared. **B:** CT in a patient with BOOP shows patchy areas of consolidation in the subpleural lung.

viral pneumonia (cytomegalovirus [CMV], measles), endobronchial spread of bronchioloalveolar carcinoma, pulmonary hemorrhage, or sometimes aspiration.

Diffuse homogeneous consolidation is most typical in patients with pulmonary edema, ARDS, pulmonary hemorrhage, pneumonias (including viral and PCP), alveolar proteinosis, and extensive atelectasis.

Focal Consolidation

The most likely causes of focal consolidation include pneumonia, atelectasis with or without bronchial obstruction,

FIG. 2.11. Diffuse air-space nodules in bronchopneumonia. Multiple small nodular opacities are typical of spread of infection through the airways. This represented a bacterial bronchopneumonia, but other organisms such as TB, MAC, fungus, or viruses may be involved.

TABLE 2.2 **Differential Diagnosis of Focal Consolidation**

Water (edema) (uncommon)
Papillary muscle rupture with mitral prolapse (right upper lobe)
Edema in a patient with
  Pulmonary artery obstruction (e.g., pulmonary embolism)
  Hypoplastic pulmonary artery
  Swyer-James syndrome
Decubitus position
Reexpansion edema
Pulmonary vein occlusion
Systemic to pulmonary artery shunt (congenital or acquired)
Bland aspiration
Atelectasis with drowned lung

Blood (hemorrhage)
Contusion
Infarction
Aspiration of blood
Vasculitis

Pus (pneumonia)
Bacterial
Tuberculosis or nontuberculous mycobacterial
Fungal
Virus (uncommon)
Pneumocystis (uncommon)
Aspiration pneumonia
Atelectasis with postobstructive pneumonia

Cells
Neoplasm
  Bronchioloalveolar carcinoma
  Lymphoma and other lymphoproliferative diseases
Eosinophilic pneumonia or other eosinophilic diseases
Organizing pneumonia (BOOP)
Sarcoidosis

Other substances
Lipoid pneumonia (lipid)

A

B

FIG. 2.12. Lobar consolidation with expansion. **A:** A patient with right upper lobe consolidation due to *Klebsiella* pneumonia shows downward bowing of the minor fissure (*arrows*) because of lobar expansion. **B:** Bronchioloalveolar carcinoma involving the left upper lobe with posterior bulging (*arrows*) of the left major fissure.

eosinophilic pneumonia; atelectasis; or rarely focal edema. The appearance of focal consolidation may also result from confluent interstitial disease, as in patients with sarcoidosis. The appearance or pattern of focal or multifocal consolidation may be helpful in differential diagnosis.

Lobar consolidation is most typical of pneumonia (including *S. pneumoniae*, *Klebsiella* (Fig. 2-12A), *Legionella*, and TB) and abnormalities associated with bronchial obstruction.

Lobar consolidation with pneumonia often occurs because of interalveolar spread of disease via the *pores of Kohn* (small holes in the alveolar walls). This type of spread continues until a fissure or pleural surface is reached. Organisms associated with spread of pneumonia via the pores of Kohn are characterized by thin secretions (thus passing easily through the pores). The presence of an incomplete fissure may lead to a lobar pneumonia becoming bilobar (or trilobar) (see Fig. 2-1B).

Lobar consolidation resulting from interalveolar spread of disease can also be seen with lymphoma and bronchioloalveolar carcinoma (see Fig. 2-12B). The term *lepidic growth* is used to describe the local interalveolar spread of tumors such as bronchioloalveolar carcinoma, using alveolar walls as a scaffold.

Bronchial obstruction with postobstructive pneumonia or atelectasis also commonly results in lobar consolidation. The differential diagnosis is that of bronchial obstruction and includes neoplasm, lymph node enlargement, inflammatory lesions, stricture, and foreign body.

Lobar consolidation is uncommonly the result of vascular abnormalities. Right upper lobe consolidation representing pulmonary edema may occur in patients with acute myocardial infarction resulting in papillary muscle rupture and mitral valve prolapse; it occurs because a jet of regurgitant blood is directed into the right superior pulmonary vein. Focal pulmonary hemorrhage may lead to a lobar consolidation. Lobar consolidation is uncommon with pulmonary embolism.

Lobar expansion in association with lobar consolidation suggests infection, particularly by *Klebsiella* (see Fig. 2-12A) or *Pneumococcus*, TB, bronchial obstruction with postobstructive pneumonia, or consolidation associated with neoplasm (see Fig. 2-12B).

Round or spherical consolidation is most typical of bronchioloalveolar carcinoma, lymphoma or lymphoproliferative disease, or pneumonia (i.e., *round pneumonia*). A round or spherical pneumonia is typical of organisms that spread via the pores of Kohn and progress to being lobar, such as *S. pneumoniae, Klebsiella, Legionella*, or TB (Fig. 2-13). Such diseases begin in at a single site and result in an enlarging ill-defined

FIG. 2.13. Spherical consolidation due to pneumonia. **A:** On the initial radiograph, a patient with *Legionella* pneumonia shows a poorly defined area of consolidation (*arrows*) in the right upper lobe. This may be termed "round pneumonia." **B:** Over the next several days, the spherical consolidation increases in size because of local interalveolar spread. This appearance may be seen in the early stages of lobar pneumonias. **C:** Further progression results in consolidation of the right upper lobe, marginated by the minor fissure (*arrows*). **D:** A lateral view at the same time as **C** shows upper lobe consolidation marginated by the major and minor fissures (*arrows*). Partial right middle lobe consolidation is also present.

sphere of consolidation as more and more alveoli become involved. As the growing sphere reaches a pleural surface or fissure and cannot spread further, it becomes lobar.

Segmental (or subsegmental) consolidation may be diagnosed if a wedge-shaped opacity of more than a few centimeters in size is visible with the apex of the wedge pointing toward the hilum (see Figs. 2-6 and 2-14). This finding suggests an abnormality related to a segmental (or subsegmental) bronchus or artery, such as bronchial obstruction due to mucus or tumor, bronchopneumonia, focal aspiration, or pulmonary embolism with infarction.

Focal patchy consolidation is typical of pneumonias, endobronchial spread of TB, or endobronchial spread of tumor such as bronchioloalveolar carcinoma (see Fig. 2-2). CT may show a pattern of lobular consolidation. Centrilobular nodules are seen in some cases (see Fig. 2-4).

Patchy consolidation is typical of bronchopneumonia. Pneumonias associated with this pattern (e.g., *Staphylococcus, Haemophilus, Pseudomonas*) are characterized by thick and tenacious secretions and spread via airways rather than the pores of Kohn. Infected secretions are typically present within the bronchi. Bronchopneumonia is also known as *lobular pneumonia* because of its tendency to involve individual lobules. *Mycoplasma pneumonia* often results in this pattern.

Time Course in Diagnosis

Rapidly appearing consolidation (a few hours) suggests atelectasis with drowned lung, aspiration, pulmonary edema, pulmonary hemorrhage, infarction, or rapidly progressing pneumonia, particularly in an immunocompromised host.

FIG. 2.14. Segmental consolidation. A patient with pneumonia shows consolidation of the lateral segment of the right middle lobe. The segmental bronchus is seen within the consolidated lung as an air bronchogram. The medial segment, adjacent to the right heart border, is normally aerated. The consolidated segment borders posteriorly on the major fissure.

Of these, only pulmonary edema and drowned lung may clear quickly. Occasionally, a lymphoproliferative neoplasm progresses within hours.

Longstanding (chronic) consolidation (4 to 6 weeks) with little change suggests eosinophilic pneumonia, BOOP, bronchioloalveolar carcinoma, lymphoma, lipoid pneumonia, or some indolent pneumonias such as fungal infections. Recurrent processes (e.g., recurrent pulmonary edema, pulmonary hemorrhage, or aspiration) may appear to be chronic if radiographs are obtained only during the acute episodes.

SILHOUETTE SIGN

The borders of soft tissue structures such as the mediastinum, hila, and hemidiaphragms are visible on chest radiographs because they are outlined by adjacent air-containing lung. When consolidated lung (or a soft tissue mass) contacts one of these structures, its border becomes invisible or is poorly marginated. This is termed the "silhouette" sign. The silhouette sign is used to diagnose the presence of a lung abnormality (i.e., consolidation, atelectasis, mass) and localize it to a specific lobe or lung region (Figs. 2-15 to 2-20).

On the frontal (PA or AP) radiograph, obscuration (in radiologic parlance, "silhouetting") of specific contours may be related to abnormalities in specific lobes. Specific contours and their corresponding lobes are illustrated in Figure 2-15 and listed below:

Right superior mediastinum (i.e., superior vena cava [SVC]) = right upper lobe (see Fig. 2-16)
Right heart border = right middle lobe (common; see Fig. 2-17) or medial right lower lobe (less common). This appearance may be mimicked by pectus excavatum.
Right hemidiaphragm = right lower lobe (see Fig. 2-18)
Left superior mediastinum (e.g., aortic arch) = left upper lobe (see Fig. 2-19B)
Left heart border = lingular segments of left upper lobe (see Fig. 2-19)
Left hemidiaphragm or descending aorta = left lower lobe (see Fig. 2-20)
Caveat: The diaphragmatic contour seen on the frontal (PA or AP) radiograph represents the dome, or the highest point, of the diaphragm. The diaphragmatic dome is relatively anterior, and lower lobe consolidation may be posterior to it (see Fig. 2-21); in this case, the hemidiaphragm may remain visible.

The silhouette sign is also used on the lateral projection:

Posterior margin of the heart or posterior left hemidiaphragm = left lower lobe (see Fig. 2-20); hiatal hernia may mimic this.
Anterior right hemidiaphragm = right middle lobe
Posterior right hemidiaphragm = right lower lobe (see Figs. 2-18 and 2-21)

(text continues on page 44)

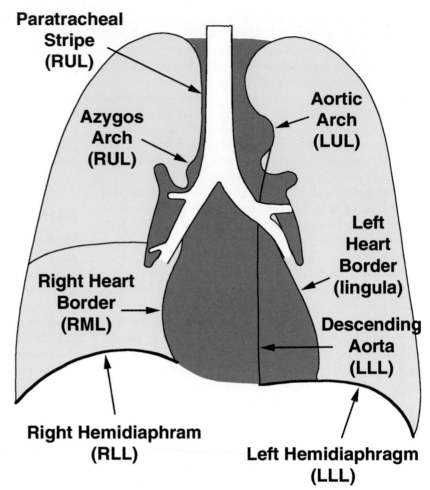

Paratracheal Stripe (RUL)

Aortic Arch (LUL)

Azygos Arch (RUL)

Left Heart Border (lingula)

Right Heart Border (RML)

Descending Aorta (LLL)

Right Hemidiaphram (RLL)

Left Hemidiaphragm (LLL)

FIG. 2.15. Anatomic relationships used with the silhouette sign. Obscuration of the borders shown in this diagram are associated with consolidation of the listed lobes. *RUL*, right upper lobe; *RML*, right middle lobe; *RLL*, right lower lobe; *LUL*, left upper lobe; *LLL*, left lower lobe.

A

B

FIG. 2.16. The silhouette sign in right upper lobe pneumonia. **A:** Consolidation of the right upper lobe obscures (i.e., silhouettes) the border of the right superior mediastinum and superior vena cava. The upper part of the right hilum is also invisible. **B:** On the lateral view, the consolidated upper lobe is outlined superiorly by the upper aspect of the major fissure (*black arrows*). Inferiorly, it is outlined by the minor fissure (*white arrows*). (*Figure continues.*)

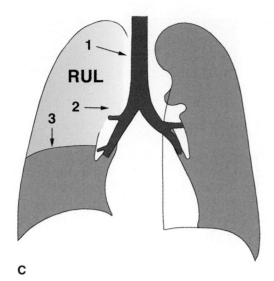

FIG. 2.16. (*Continued.*) **C:** Typical findings of right upper lobe consolidation: (*1*) obscuration of the right superior mediastinum, (*2*) obscuration of the superior right hilum, and (*3*) opacity marginated inferiorly by the minor fissure.

FIG. 2.17. The silhouette sign in right middle lobe pneumonia. **A:** Consolidation of the right middle lobe obscures ("silhouettes") the right heart border (i.e., it is not clearly seen). In contrast, the left heart border is sharply marginated. The right hemidiaphragm appears sharply marginated. The pneumonia is marginated by the minor fissure (*arrow*). **B:** On the lateral view, middle lobe consolidation is visible, marginated above by the minor fissure (*large arrows*); inferiorly, it is marginated by the major fissure (*small arrows*). **C:** Typical findings of right middle lobe consolidation: (*1*) the right heart border is obscured, (*2*) the opacity is marginated superiorly by the minor fissure, and (*3*) the right diaphragm remains visible.

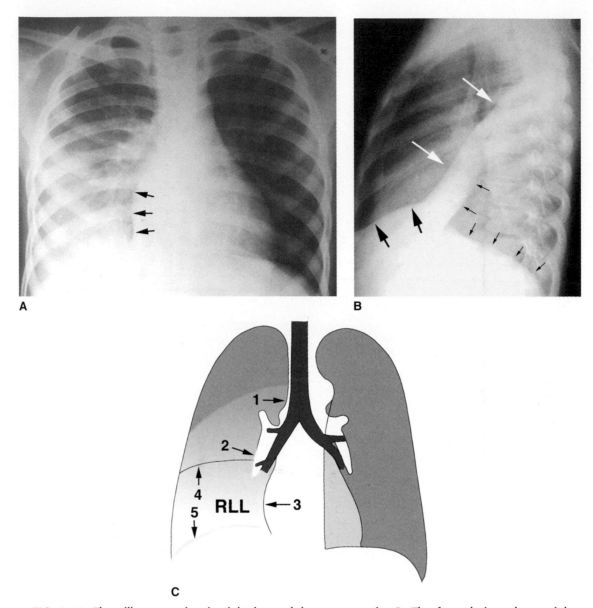

FIG. 2.18. The silhouette sign in right lower lobe pneumonia. **A:** The frontal view shows right lower lobe consolidation with obscuration of the diaphragm. The right heart border (*arrows*) remains visible as an edge. **B:** On the lateral view, complete right lower lobe consolidation is visible, outlined anteriorly by the major fissure (*white arrows*). The right hemidiaphragm (*large black arrows*) is sharply marginated anterior to the consolidated lobe but is invisible posteriorly. The posterior left heart border and left hemidiaphragm are sharply marginated (*small black arrows*). **C:** Typical findings of right lower lobe consolidation: (*1*) the superior mediastinum is well seen; (*2*) the inferior right hilum is obscured; (*3*) the right heart border remains visible; (*4*) the right hemidiaphragm is obscured; and (*5*) the right minor fissure remains visible as a line.

If the border of a specific structure remains visible, absence of the silhouette sign may be used to indicate that an abnormality is *not* in that location. For example, if a lung abnormality is visible at the medial right base but the right heart border remains visible, the lesion is not likely to be in the middle lobe.

There are two caveats regarding the silhouette sign:

1. The silhouette sign does not always work. Correlate it with other findings.
2. The presence of volume loss (i.e., atelectasis) may alter these specific relationships.

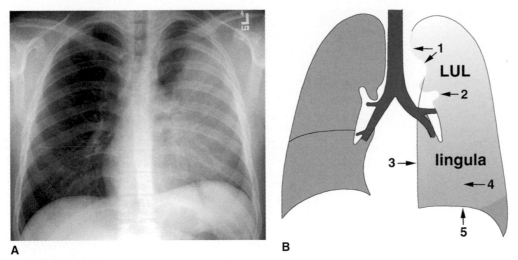

A

B

FIG. 2.19. The silhouette sign in left upper lobe pneumonia. **A:** The left heart border is obscured because of lingular consolidation. The left superior mediastinum remains sharply marginated because the medial portions of the anterior and apical segments of the left upper lobe remain aerated. **B:** Typical findings of left upper lobe (*LUL*; and lingular) consolidation: (*1*) the left superior mediastinum and aortic arch are obscured; (*2*) the superior left hilum is obscured; (*3*) the descending aorta remains visible; (*4*) the left heart border is obscured; and (*5*) the left hemidiaphragm remains visible.

A

B

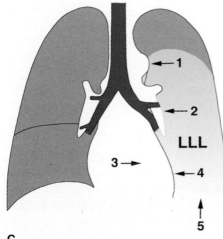

C

FIG. 2.20. The silhouette sign in left lower lobe pneumonia. **A:** The left hemidiaphragm is partially obscured by left lower lobe consolidation (*arrows*). **B:** On the lateral view, a portion of the left hemidiaphragm (*arrow*) also is obscured. **C:** Typical findings of left lower lobe (*LLL*) consolidation: (*1*) the left superior mediastinum and aortic arch remain visible; (*2*) the inferior left hilum is obscured; (*3*) the descending aorta is obscured; (*4*) the left heart border remains visible; and (*5*) the left hemidiaphragm is obscured.

A   B

FIG. 2.21. The silhouette sign (lateral radiograph) in right lower lobe pneumonia. **A:** There is focal right lower lobe consolidation, which appears to be segmental. The right hemidiaphragm is sharply defined because the consolidated lung is located posterior to the dome of the diaphragm. **B:** The lateral view shows consolidation (*white arrows*) that obscures the posterior aspect of the right hemidiaphragm (*black arrows*). The dome of the right diaphragm (seen on the frontal projection) is sharply marginated.

ATELECTASIS

The term *atelectasis* means "incomplete stretching" in Greek. It is used to indicate loss of volume of lung tissue associated with a decrease in the amount of air it contains. It is synonymous with collapse.

Types of Atelectasis

Four different types or mechanisms of atelectasis are recognized (Table 2-3).

FIG. 2.22. Drowned lung in acute bronchial obstruction by mucus. The right lung is nearly airless, but volume loss is minimal. Slight shift of the trachea and mediastinum to the right is visible. Air bronchograms are invisible because of central bronchial obstruction.

TABLE 2.3 Types of Atelectasis

Resorption (obstructive) atelectasis
Caused by airway obstruction and resorption of alveolar gas
Occurs within 24 hours
More rapid when breathing oxygen
May result in drowned lung with little volume loss
Collateral ventilation may prevent collapse
With large airway obstruction, air bronchograms are often absent

Relaxation (passive) atelectasis
Atelectasis due to pleural effusion, pneumothorax, or mass
Lung density need not be increased

Adhesive atelectasis
Atelectasis caused by loss of lung surfactant
Typical of respiratory distress syndrome of the newborn, acute respiratory distress syndrome, radiation pneumonitis

Cicatricial atelectasis
Atelectasis caused by lung fibrosis

Resorption (Obstructive) Atelectasis

Resorption atelectasis occurs when alveolar gas is absorbed by circulating blood and not replaced by inspired air. It occurs in the presence of airway obstruction. The obstructed airway may be the trachea, main bronchi, lobar bronchi, or multiple small bronchi or bronchioles. Small bronchial or bronchiolar obstruction by mucus resulting in resorption atelectasis is common after surgery and general anesthesia.

Bronchial obstruction usually results in lung becoming airless within 24 hours. Since oxygen is absorbed from the alveoli more rapidly than other inspired gases, resorption atelectasis occurs much more quickly when the patient is breathing pure oxygen; it may occur within minutes. Rapid resorption atelectasis may also occur in the presence of an endobronchial lesion acting as a one-way valve.

In the presence of bronchial obstruction, resorption of gas may be accompanied by rapid transudation of fluid from the circulating blood into the interstitium and alveoli (because of reduced interstitial and alveolar pressure). When this happens, lung becomes airless (consolidated) with only a minor reduction in lung volume (see Fig. 2-22). This occurrence is termed *drowned lung*. If the bronchial obstruction is relieved, the lung rapidly returns to normal density in most cases. This occurrence is common in ICU patients with mucous plugging or retention of secretions.

Obstruction of a main bronchus will cause atelectasis of a lung. Air bronchograms are often absent in an obstructed and collapsed lung (see Fig. 2-22). In a patient with a collapsed lung resulting from obstruction of small peripheral bronchi by secretions, air bronchograms are usually visible.

Obstruction of a lobar or smaller bronchus may or may not result in atelectasis, depending on the absence or presence of *collateral ventilation* or collateral air drift. Collateral ventilation is aeration of a lung lobe or segment from adjacent alveoli (usually via the pores of Kohn) rather than from its supplying bronchus. Collateral ventilation between adjacent lobes may occur in the presence of incomplete fissures. Collateral ventilation between smaller lung units (e.g., segments) occurs more readily. The presence of lung disease, such as pneumonia, may prevent collateral ventilation.

Relaxation (Passive) and Compression Atelectasis

The lung is elastic and stretches to fill the thoracic cavity because of negative intrapleural pressure. The presence of pneumothorax, pleural effusion, or a mass lesion allows the lung to decrease in volume or *relax* to its natural size, which is smaller than the thoracic cavity. This is termed *relaxation atelectasis* or *passive atelectasis* (Fig. 2-23). The term *compressive atelectasis* can also be used to describe this occurrence, although it implies a reduction in lung volume beyond its normal relaxed state.

A   B

FIG. 2.23. Relaxation (compression) atelectasis. **A:** Contrast-enhanced CT in a patient with a right pleural effusion shows right lower lobe *(RLL)* atelectasis. The right lower lobe is airless. Fluid in the major fissure allows the aerated right middle lobe *(RML)* to float anteriorly. Little if any mediastinal shift is present because the increased volume of the effusion is compensated for by the decreased volume of the lower lobe. **B:** Right pneumothorax with relaxation atelectasis of the right lung. Despite its reduction in volume *(arrows)*, the right lung is not abnormally dense. Vessels in the right lung appear reduced in size compared to those on the left. This reflects reduced lung perfusion. The right lower lobe maintains its contact with the mediastinum because of the inferior pulmonary ligament. Air is seen within the minor fissure, separating the lobes.

FIG. 2.24. Cicatricial atelectasis in a patient with chronic right middle lobe collapse (right middle lobe syndrome) leading to fibrosis. **A:** Frontal chest radiograph shows poor definition of the right heart border, typical of right middle lobe consolidation. There is little increase in opacity at the right base. **B:** Lateral view shows volume loss in the right middle lobe with downward bowing of the minor fissure (*white arrows*) and anterior displacement of the major fissure (*black arrows*). Crowded air bronchograms are visible within the collapsed lobe. **C, D:** CT scans at two levels show a typical appearance for right middle lobe collapse, having a triangular configuration (*white arrows*). The right middle lobe bronchus (*black arrows*) is patent, and air bronchograms are visible within the collapsed lobe. Collapse in the absence of bronchial obstruction is typical of right middle lobe syndrome. The dilated air bronchograms may indicate reversible bronchiectasis.

When lung collapses in the presence of pneumothorax, a significant increase in lung density need not be visible (see Fig. 2-23B). Approximately half of the density of lung is blood, and a reduction in lung volume typically results in a reduction in lung perfusion and a decrease in lung density. Until the lung becomes very small, its density does not significantly increase unless consolidation also occurs.

Adhesive Atelectasis

Surfactant reduces the surface tension of alveolar fluid and tends to prevent lung collapse as the alveoli decrease in volume with expiration. Deficiency of surfactant allows alveoli to collapse, so-called *adhesive atelectasis*. This is most typical of respiratory distress syndrome of the newborn but is also seen in patients with ARDS, acute radiation pneumonitis, or hypoxemia, and in the postoperative period.

Cicatricial Atelectasis

This term refers to loss of lung volume occurring in the presence of lung fibrosis. It may be focal, lobar (Fig. 2-24), or diffuse, depending on the disease responsible. Findings of fibrosis are typically present.

RADIOGRAPHIC FINDINGS OF ATELECTASIS

Radiographic findings of atelectasis are usually considered as direct or indirect (Table 2-4). For practical purposes, the diagnosis is based on a combination of these findings.

Direct Signs of Atelectasis

Direct signs of atelectasis indicate loss of volume in an abnormal lobe.

Displacement of Interlobar Fissures

Displacement of interlobar fissures is the best sign of atelectasis (see Figs. 2-24 to 2-26) but is not always visible. The appearance of fissure displacement reflects the specific

TABLE 2.4 Radiographic Signs of Atelectasis

Direct signs: due to lobar volume loss
Displacement of fissures
Crowding of vessels
Indirect signs: secondary to volume loss
Diaphragmatic elevation
Mediastinal shift
Compensatory overinflation of normal lung
Hilar displacement
Reorientation of the hilum or bronchi
Approximation of the ribs
Increased lung opacity
Absence of air bronchograms
Shifting granuloma sign

lobe involved. Specific patterns of lobar atelectasis are described below.

Crowding of Vessels or Bronchi

Crowding of vessels or bronchi in a given lobe reflects volume loss and is useful in diagnosis if a shift of fissures is not visible. Crowded air bronchograms may be seen in the presence of collapsed and consolidated lung (see Fig. 2-24B to D). Crowded vessels may be visible on radiographs if volume loss is present without consolidation. Vascular crowding in collapsed and consolidated lung is commonly seen on CT following contrast infusion.

Indirect Signs of Atelectasis

Indirect signs of atelectasis are those not directly due to lobar volume loss but occurring secondary to it.

Diaphragmatic Elevation

Diaphragmatic elevation occurs because of ipsilateral volume loss (see Figs. 2-25 to 2-27). It is more common with lower lobe atelectasis than upper lobe atelectasis, although it may be difficult to see if the lower lobe is consolidated.

FIG. 2.25. Signs of atelectasis in right upper lobe collapse. The right hemidiaphragm is elevated. The minor fissure is displaced and bowed upward (*large white arrow*). The right hilum is elevated compared to the left, and the descending pulmonary artery is rotated outward (*small white arrows*), being more easily seen than normal. The thin triangular opacity at the dome of the right hemidiaphragm (*black arrow*) is a so-called juxtaphrenic peak, which may be seen in upper lobe atelectasis.

A

B

FIG. 2.26. Signs of atelectasis in left upper lobe collapse. **A:** The left hilum is elevated. The left main and left upper lobe bronchi (*arrows*) are elevated and appear more horizontal than normal. The left hemidiaphragm is higher than the right and a slight increase in opacity is seen in the left upper lung. **B:** Lateral radiograph in the same patient as (**A**) shows marked anterior displacement of the major fissure (*arrows*). As the left upper lobe loses more volume, it appears thinner on the lateral view and less dense on the frontal radiograph.

A

B

FIG. 2.27. Left lung atelectasis due to TB with bronchostenosis. **A:** The position of the superior aspect of the stomach bubble (*large black arrow*) indicates elevation of the left hemidiaphragm. Marked leftward shift of the trachea (*Tr*), azygoesophageal recess (*Az*), and right heart border (*H*) is present. Air bronchograms (*white arrow*) are visible in the left upper lobe. **B:** CT shows narrowing of the left main bronchus (*black arrow*). The anterior mediastinum (*Ant*) and azygoesophageal recess (*Az*) are shifted to the left. Air bronchograms are not visible at this level.

Diagnosis is based on knowledge of normal diaphragmatic position or comparison to prior radiographs.

The right hemidiaphragm is up to 2 cm higher than the left in 90% of normal persons. In about 10% of normal persons, the right hemidiaphragm is more than 3 cm higher than the left, the hemidiaphragms are at the same level, or the left hemidiaphragm is higher than the right.

Mediastinal Shift

Mediastinal shift often occurs with lobar atelectasis (see Figs. 2-27 and 2-28A). Shift of the upper mediastinum usually occurs with upper lobe collapse (see Fig. 2-27A) and is most easily recognized by shift of the trachea. Shift of the lower mediastinum predominates with lower lobe atelectasis (see Fig. 2-28A). This may be manifested by shift of the heart, anterior junction line, posterior junction line, or azygoesophageal interface. Shift of normal lung across the midline in a patient with atelectasis is sometimes referred to as lung herniation.

Compensatory Overinflation

Compensatory overinflation of normal lung on the same side as atelectasis appears as increased volume and decreased density of lung, associated with splaying of vessels. Decreased lung density is easiest to see on CT.

Hilar Displacement

Hilar displacement may occur in the presence of upper or lower lobe atelectasis (see Figs. 2-25 and 2-26). The hilum is elevated in the presence of upper lobe collapse and depressed if lower lobe collapse is present. The left hilum is higher than the right in most normals. If the hila appear to be at the same level, right upper lobe collapse or left lower lobe collapse may be present.

Reorientation of the Hilum or Bronchi

Reorientation of the hilum or bronchi occurs in association with hilar displacement. With upper lobe collapse, the hilum rotates outward and the descending pulmonary artery and bronchi are less vertical than normal and more easily seen (see Fig. 2-25). The left main bronchus may appear elevated and more horizontal than normal in the presence of left upper lobe collapse (see Fig. 2-26A). With lower lobe collapse, the hila are depressed and the bronchi appear more vertical than normal.

Approximation of the Ribs

The ipsilateral ribs may appear closer together in the presence of ipsilateral volume loss (see Fig. 2-28A). Although this finding may be seen in patients with collapse, other findings of atelectasis will always be seen; never base a diagnosis

on this sign alone. Rotation of the patient may mimic this appearance.

Increased Lung Opacity

An increase in lung opacity or attenuation may be seen, but this is nonspecific. It may reflect replacement of alveolar air by fluid (i.e., drowned lung) or, when extreme, compressed, and airless lung tissue (see Figs. 2-24 to 2-28).

Absence of Air Bronchograms

In a patient with lung consolidation, the absence of air bronchograms suggests central bronchial obstruction (see Figs. 2-22 and 2-28). However, air bronchograms are sometimes seen in the presence of a (partially) obstructing central bronchial lesion (see Fig. 2-27A) or resorption atelectasis resulting from small peripheral mucous plugs (see Fig. 2-1A).

In patients with atelectasis and air bronchograms, the air-filled bronchi may appear dilated on plain radiographs or CT because of the collapse, simulating bronchiectasis. This is termed *reversible bronchiectasis* (an oxymoron) as it disappears following reexpansion of the lobe. Bronchiectasis is defined as irreversible bronchial dilatation.

Mucous Bronchograms

In the presence of bronchial obstruction, CT may show low-attenuation mucus within obstructed bronchi (see Fig. 2-28D). Mucus-filled bronchi may appear dilated. This may be due to large mucous plugs or reversible bronchiectasis.

Shifting Granuloma Sign

Shift in the location of a parenchymal lesion visible on prior films may be seen in the presence of atelectasis.

Indirect Signs Seen With Specific Types of Atelectasis

Other indirect signs of atelectasis associated with specific types of atelectasis are described below, and include the following:
Golden's S sign: right upper lobe atelectasis
Juxtaphrenic peak: upper lobe atelectasis
Luftsichel sign: upper lobe atelectasis (usually the left upper lobe)
Flat waist sign: left lower lobe atelectasis
Comet-tail sign: rounded atelectasis

ATELECTASIS OF AN ENTIRE LUNG

Lung atelectasis usually results from obstruction of a main bronchus by an endobronchial lesion (or intubation of the

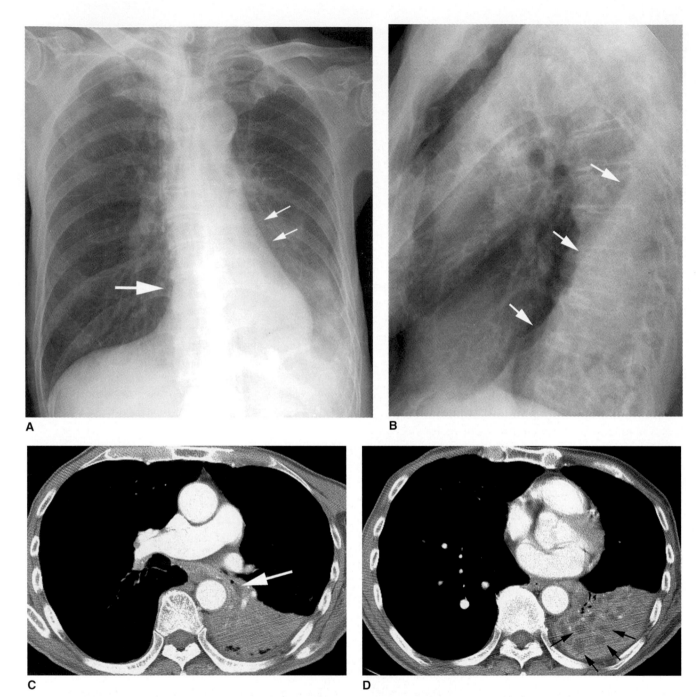

FIG. 2.28. Left lower lobe atelectasis due to mucous plugging. **A:** Chest radiograph shows consolidation at the left base with obscuration of the left hemidiaphragm. The heart is displaced to the left (*large arrow*). The left interlobar pulmonary artery is poorly defined, as is typical in left lower lobe atelectasis. There is flattening of the left heart border (*white arrows*) due to leftward rotation of the heart and great vessels, termed the "flat waist" sign. The left ribs appear closer together than the right. **B:** Lateral view shows left lower lobe atelectasis with posterior displacement of the major fissure (*arrows*). **C:** Obstruction of the left lower lobe bronchus (*arrow*) is due to mucus. Mucus in the obstructed bronchus appears lower in attenuation than surrounding consolidated lung. Consolidation borders on the major fissure, which is displaced posteriorly. The mediastinum is shifted to the left. **D:** At a lower level, mucous bronchograms (*arrows*) are visible. The mucus-filled bronchi are dilated, but this represents "reversible bronchiectasis."

opposite main bronchus), obstruction of small peripheral bronchi by secretions, or large ipsilateral pneumothorax or pleural effusion.

Bronchial Obstruction With Lung Collapse

With bronchial obstruction, the ipsilateral diaphragm is elevated, shift of both the upper and lower mediastinum to the side of atelectasis is present, the ipsilateral ribs appear too close together, and the lung is increased in density in comparison to the opposite side (see Fig. 2-27). The cause of bronchial obstruction may be evident. Absence of air bronchograms suggests a central obstruction; visible air bronchograms suggest peripheral small airway obstruction.

In the presence of bronchial obstruction with acute collapse, alveoli may rapidly fill with fluid, resulting in drowned lung. In this case, little mediastinal shift may be seen (see Fig. 2-22). If complete opacification of a hemithorax occurs acutely with significant mediastinal shift to the opposite side, pleural effusion is the likely diagnosis; if complete opacification of a hemithorax occurs acutely without significant mediastinal shift to the opposite side, drowned lung is the likely diagnosis.

Pneumothorax With Lung Collapse

Pneumothorax causes the lung to collapse centrally toward the hilum and mediastinum. The shape of the collapsed lung usually is maintained (see Fig. 2-23B). Because of the inferior pulmonary ligament, the lower lobe usually maintains its contact with the paracardiac mediastinum and diaphragm.

Until collapse is complete and the lung becomes airless, it may appear normal in density or relatively lucent despite its small size (see Fig. 2-23B). This occurs because of reduced lung perfusion associated with volume loss. Some shift of the mediastinum to the opposite side is typical in patients with a sizable pneumothorax regardless of the presence of tension.

Pleural Effusion With Lung Collapse

Massive pleural effusion results in relaxation or compressive atelectasis of the lung, a variable degree of mediastinal shift to the opposite side (depending on the size of the effusion and the degree of collapse), and variable opacification of the hemithorax (depending on the extent of residual aerated lung).

Large pleural effusion may result in loss of lung volume without complete lung opacification. Because a free effusion in an upright patient predominantly occupies the inferior hemithorax, the lower lobe is usually more compressed, contains less air, and appears denser than the upper lobe.

Collapsed lung is tethered at the hilum, and the lower lobe maintains its relationship with the mediastinum because of the inferior pulmonary ligament (see Fig. 2-23A). However, fluid often separates the peripheral part of the lobe from the chest wall and enters the major fissure or major and minor fissures, allowing adjacent lobes to float apart. These findings are difficult to recognize on chest radiographs unless the lung remains partially aerated. On CT obtained with contrast infusion, collapsed lobes opacify and appear denser than fluid in the pleural space. On unenhanced CT, the collapsed lung usually appears slightly denser than fluid.

LOBAR ATELECTASIS

Specific appearances are associated with collapse of an individual lobe or lobes in combination. These appearances may be modified by the degree of volume loss, the degree of lung consolidation occurring in association with volume loss, and the presence of pleural effusion or pneumothorax.

Lobar collapse usually results from bronchial obstruction (resorption atelectasis). Lobar cicatricial atelectasis is less common but may be associated with chronic infection. Several general rules apply to lobar atelectasis:

1. Atelectasis usually results in bowing of a fissure toward the collapsing lobe.
2. An atelectatic lobe generally assumes the shape of a triangle or pyramid, with the apex of the triangle or pyramid at the hilum.
3. Unless atelectasis is severe or pleural effusion or pneumothorax is present, a collapsed upper or lower lobe maintains its contact with the costal (peripheral) pleural surface. The middle lobe, on the other hand, commonly loses its costal pleural contact with atelectasis.
4. Because atelectasis is associated with decreased lung perfusion and blood volume, collapse does not result in increased lung density unless the lobe is moderately reduced in volume or air-space consolidation is associated with the volume loss.
5. With total lobar collapse, and in the absence of consolidation or drowned lung, collapsed lobes are very thin and may be difficult to recognize en face as an area of increased density.
6. Collapsed and airless lung often appears densely opacified on CT following contrast infusion.
7. Hilar masses causing collapse usually appear less dense than collapsed lung on contrast-enhanced CT.

The Normal Interlobar Fissures

Recognition of lobar collapse is fundamentally based on knowledge of the normal positions of the interlobar fissures. They are described in greater detail in Chapter 26.

Major (Oblique) Fissure

On the right, the major fissure separates the upper and middle lobes from the lower lobe. On the left, it separates the upper lobe from the lower lobe. The major fissures originate posteriorly above the level of the aortic arch, near the level of the fifth thoracic vertebra, and angle anteriorly and inferiorly, nearly parallel to the sixth rib (Fig. 2-29). Posteriorly, the superior aspect of the left major fissure is cephalad to the right in 75%. They terminate along the anterior diaphragmatic pleural surface of each lung, several centimeters posterior to the anterior chest wall. The right and left fissures may be identified by noting their relationships to the right or left hemidiaphragms or posterior ribs. The major fissures are not clearly seen on frontal (PA or AP) radiographs unless there is lower lobe volume loss.

On CT, the orientation of the major fissures varies at different levels. In the upper thorax, the major fissures angle posterolaterally from the mediastinum. Within the lower thorax, the major fissures angle anterolaterally from the mediastinum (Fig. 2-30A). The fissure may be seen as a linear opacity on thin slices. Alternatively, its position may be localized by recognizing a 1- to 2-cm avascular band within the lung (i.e., lung adjacent to the fissure containing only small vessels) having a typical orientation.

Minor (Horizontal) Fissure

The minor or horizontal fissure separates the superior aspect of the right middle lobe from the right upper lobe. On frontal (PA or AP) radiographs, the minor fissure or a portion is visible in 50% to 80% of the cases, appearing as a roughly horizontal line, generally at or near the level of the anterior fourth rib (see Fig. 2-29). Its contour is variable, but its lateral

part is often visible inferior to its medial part. Medially, the fissure usually appears to arise at the level of the right hilum and interlobar pulmonary artery.

On the lateral radiograph, the anterior part of the fissure often appears inferior to its posterior part. The posterior part of the fissure may be seen to end at the major fissure or may project posterior to it.

On CT, the minor fissure tends to parallel the scan plane and is usually difficult to see. Characteristically, the position of the minor fissure can be inferred because of a broad avascular region in the anterior portion of the right lung, anterior to the major fissure, at the level of the bronchus intermedius. The minor fissure may be seen as a discrete line, similar to the appearance of the major fissure, when thin slices are obtained.

When visible, the minor fissure is variable in appearance, depending on its orientation. Because the minor fissure often angles caudally, the lower lobe, middle lobe, and upper lobe may all be seen on a single CT scan (see Fig. 2-30B). If this is the case, the major and minor fissures can have a similar appearance, with the major fissure being posterior and the minor fissure anterior; in this situation, the lower lobe is most posterior, the upper lobe is most anterior, and the middle lobe is in the middle.

If the minor fissure is concave caudally, it can sometimes be seen in two locations or can appear ring-shaped, with the middle lobe between the fissure lines or in the center of the ring and the upper lobe anterior to the most anterior part of the fissure.

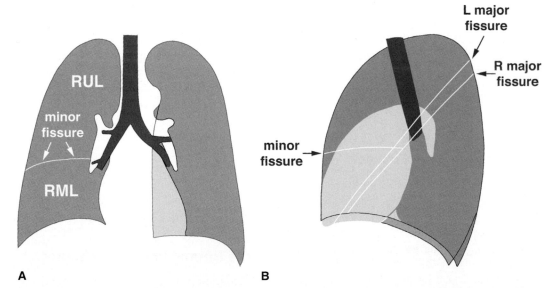

FIG. 2.29. Normal appearances of the fissures on chest radiographs. **A:** Frontal projection. The major fissures are not normally visible. The minor fissure is visible in 50% to 80% of cases, appearing as a roughly horizontal line, generally at or near the level of the anterior fourth rib. Medially, it arises at the level of the interlobar pulmonary artery, and its lateral part is often inferior to its medial part. **B:** Lateral projection. The major fissures originate posteriorly above the level of the aortic arch, near the level of the fifth thoracic vertebra. Posteriorly, the superior aspect of the left major fissure is cephalad to the right in 75%. They terminate along the anterior diaphragmatic pleural surface of each lung, several centimeters posterior to the anterior chest wall.

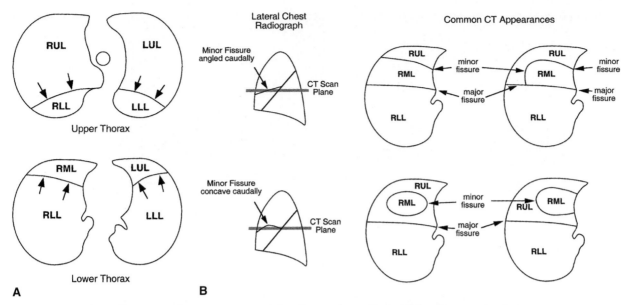

FIG. 2.30. Normal appearances of the fissures on CT. **A:** Major fissures. In the upper thorax, the major fissures angle posterolaterally from the mediastinum. In the lower thorax, the major fissures angle anterolaterally. **B:** Minor fissure. The appearance of the minor fissure on CT is related to its orientation as seen on the lateral chest radiograph.

Right Upper Lobe Atelectasis

Frontal (PA or AP) Radiograph

On the frontal radiograph, the minor fissure bows upward (Table 2-5; see Figs. 2-25 and 2-31A) in the presence of right upper lobe atelectasis. The medial aspect of the lobe maintains its relationship to the hilum, and its lateral aspect (marginated by the minor fissure) rotates upward toward the upper mediastinum in a clockwise fashion.

A collapsed and consolidated right upper lobe obscures the superior mediastinal contours. With complete collapse, the upper lobe is pancaked against the upper mediastinum. It may have a concave margin laterally, representing the displaced minor fissure, or may have a convex lateral edge, mimicking the appearance of mediastinal widening.

In patients with right upper lobe collapse associated with bronchogenic carcinoma (the right upper lobe is the most common site for lung cancer) or other mass lesion producing bronchial obstruction, a characteristic appearance may be seen, termed *Golden's S sign*. This sign refers to a combination of upward bowing of the lateral aspect of the minor fissure due to volume loss, with downward bulging of the medial fissure due to the presence of a hilar mass (see Fig. 2-31A). This combination results in a shallow reverse-S appearance. Although described as a sign of right upper lobe collapse, a similar appearance may be seen in any lobe if the bordering fissure is visible in profile.

Shift of the trachea toward the right may be seen as a result of right upper lobe volume loss. The hilum is typically elevated, the bronchus intermedius rotates outward, appearing less vertical than normal (see Fig. 2-25).

With upper lobe atelectasis, a finding termed the *juxtaphrenic peak* may be seen on the frontal (PA or AP) radiograph (see Fig. 2-25). This appears as a small sharp triangular opacity near the dome of the ipsilateral hemidiaphragm. It is related to stretching of an inferior accessory fissure or folds or septa on the undersurface of the lung adjacent to the phrenic nerves or inferior pulmonary ligament.

Lateral Radiograph

On the lateral radiograph, the minor fissure bows upward and rotates superiorly, being anchored at the hilum (see Fig. 2-31B). The superior portion of the major fissure bows anteriorly in a similar fashion, and the lobe assumes the

TABLE 2.5 Radiographic Findings of Right Upper Lobe Atelectasis

Frontal radiograph
Ill-defined increase in opacity in the upper thorax
Apparent right mediastinal widening
Silhouetting of the right upper mediastinum
Tracheal shift to the right
Upward bowing and displacement of the minor fissure
Golden's S sign
Elevation of the hilum
Outward rotation of the hilum or bronchus
Right-sided juxtaphrenic peak

Lateral radiograph
Upward displacement and bowing of the minor fissure
Anterior displacement and bowing of the upper major fissure

A   B

C   D

FIG. 2.31. Right upper lobe collapse with Golden's S sign. **A:** PA chest radiograph in a patient with a right hilar carcinoma shows elevation of the lateral aspect of the minor fissure (*white arrow*) due to atelectasis and downward convexity of the medial fissure (*black arrows*) due to the hilar mass. Right upper mediastinal contours are obscured because of adjacent consolidation. The right hemidiaphragm is also elevated. **B:** The lateral view shows upward bowing of the minor fissure (*white arrows*), with the anterior aspect of the fissure being most displaced. There is anterior displacement of the upper portion of the major fissure (*black arrows*). The right upper lobe assumes the shape of a wedge as it loses volume. The collapsed upper lobe maintains its contact with the hilum and anterior chest wall. **C:** CT shows anterior rotation and bowing of the minor fissure (*small white arrows*) outlining the collapsed right upper lobe. The hilar mass results in bulging of the posterior aspect of the major fissure (*large white arrow*), resulting in the CT equivalent of the S sign. The right upper lobe bronchus is obstructed (*black arrow*). **D:** CT with a lung window setting at a higher level shows the collapsed and consolidated upper lobe (*RUL*) outlined laterally by the minor fissure (*black arrows*) and posteriorly by the anteriorly displaced major fissure (*small white arrows*). A tongue of lung extending medial to the collapsed lobe represents a portion of superior segment of lower lobe. This may result in a luftsichel sign visible on a plain radiograph. *ML*, middle lobe; *RLL*, right lower lobe. **E:** Diagram of right and left upper lobe collapse on CT. In some cases, lung extending medial to the collapsed lobe may result in a luftsichel sign, as seen on a chest radiograph.

E

shape of a progressively thinner wedge as it loses volume. The collapsed upper lobe maintains its contact with the anterior chest wall. With marked upper lobe volume loss, a very thin dense wedge may be seen, associated with anterior displacement of the entire major fissure.

Computed Tomography

On CT, the minor fissure rotates anteriorly and medially as the upper lobe progressively flattens against the mediastinum, marginating its lateral aspect (see Fig. 2-31C). The collapsed lobe appears thinner near the hilum than in the apex unless a hilar mass is present. The lobe is usually triangular in cross section. The major fissure outlines the posterior margin of the collapsed lobe and may be bowed anteriorly (see Fig. 2-31D and E). In the presence of a hilar mass, an appearance similar to Golden's S sign is visible with posterior bulging of the fissure.

Left Upper Lobe Atelectasis

Frontal (PA or AP) Radiograph

On the frontal radiograph, an ill-defined increase in lung density is typically visible, being most obvious in the upper portion of the hemithorax (Table 2-6). Increased lung opacity is usually associated with obscuration of the left superior mediastinum and left cardiac margin (because of the silhouette sign; Figs. 2-32A and 2-33A). However, with marked collapse, the left upper lobe may become very thin and difficult to recognize as being abnormally dense, and the silhouette sign may not be clearly seen (see Fig. 2-26A and B). If the lingular segments of the left upper lobe remain aerated, the left heart border may remain well defined. On the other hand, if lingular collapse is unassociated with collapse of the apical posterior and anterior segments of the upper lobe, only the left heart border is obscured.

In the presence of upper lobe atelectasis and anterior shift of the major fissure, the superior segment of the lower lobe expands to occupy the apex of the hemithorax. On the frontal radiograph, the superior segment may insinuate itself between the upper lobe and the mediastinum, resulting in

an interface where lucent lung contacts collapsed lung. This interface is often crescentic in appearance and has been termed the "luftsichel" *sign* (luftsichel means "air crescent" in German; see Fig. 2-33A). The luftsichel sign is less common with right upper lobe collapse.

If the expanded superior segment does not reach the apex of the hemithorax (usually because upper lobe volume loss is not marked), the airless upper lobe may result in the appearance of a crescentic soft tissue–density shadow over the lung apex (termed an *apical cap*), mimicking apical pleural thickening or effusion, Pancoast tumor, or an extrapleural fluid collection (Fig. 2-34). This appearance has been termed *peripheral* upper lobe atelectasis. It may also be seen on the right.

As on the right, left upper lobe collapse may be associated with a left-sided juxtaphrenic peak (see Fig. 2-33A). Elevation of the left hilum may be seen; the left main bronchus may appear elevated and more horizontal than normal; and leftward shift of the upper mediastinum and trachea is typically present.

Lateral Radiograph

On the lateral radiograph, left upper lobe atelectasis results in progressive anterior displacement of the major fissure along a line paralleling the anterior chest wall (see Figs. 2-26B, 2-32B, and 2-33B). Lung anterior to the displaced fissure appears abnormally dense. With complete collapse, a very thin dense band may be seen along the anterior chest wall. The left hilum and bronchi may be displaced anteriorly.

Computed Tomography

On CT, the major fissure rotates anteromedially with upper lobe collapse (see Fig. 2-32C). If lingular segments remain aerated, the appearance closely mimics that of right upper lobe collapse. The luftsichel sign is associated with a V-shaped appearance at the posterior margin of the collapsed lobe, with the superior segment of the lower lobe extending medial to the collapsed lobe (see Fig. 2-31E).

Right Middle Lobe Atelectasis

Frontal (PA or AP) Radiograph

On the frontal radiograph, the minor fissure is usually invisible in the presence of middle lobe atelectasis; it rotates downward (as shown on the lateral view) and is no longer tangent to the X-ray beam (Table 2-7). Depending on the amount of consolidation and the degree of volume loss, increased lung opacity may be seen, obscuring the right heart border (see Figs. 2-24A and 2-35A). With marked volume loss, increased density may not be visible (see Fig. 2-24A), or the right heart border may appear normal. A lordotic radiograph may be helpful in showing the displaced minor fissure and area of increased density, but this is uncommonly used in clinical practice for making this diagnosis.

With middle lobe collapse, volume loss may not be sufficient to cause hilar displacement or mediastinal shift.

TABLE 2.6 **Radiographic Findings of Left Upper Lobe Atelectasis**

Frontal radiograph
Ill-defined increase in opacity in the upper thorax (decreasing with increased collapse)
Silhouetting of the left upper mediastinum
Tracheal shift to the left
Luftsichel sign
Apical cap
Elevation of the hilum
Outward rotation of the hilum or bronchus
Juxtaphrenic peak

Lateral radiograph
Anterior bowing and displacement of the major fissure

FIG. 2.32. Left upper lobe atelectasis associated with bronchostenosis. **A:** The frontal radiograph shows tracheal shift to the left (*large black arrow*), elevation of the left hilum (*white arrow*), an ill-defined increase in lung density, and obscuration of the left superior mediastinum and cardiac border. The edge of the aortic arch, a relatively posterior structure, remains well defined. The left main bronchus (*small black arrows*), faintly outlined by a stent in its lumen, is elevated and appears more horizontal than is normal. The inferior left heart border remains sharply defined because of marked volume loss. **B:** On the lateral view, the left upper lobe is dense and there is anterior displacement of the major fissure (*black arrows*) paralleling the anterior chest wall. The stent within the left main bronchus (*white arrow*) is visible. **C:** CT shows anterior bowing and anteromedial displacement of the major fissure (*white arrows*). The left main bronchus (*black arrow*) is narrowed. A relative decrease in the density of the left lower lobe is due to compensatory hyperexpansion.

Chronic right middle lobe atelectasis may not resolve even if its original cause is alleviated. The presence of chronic inflammation or infection, bronchiectasis, and fibrosis may prevent reexpansion (i.e., cicatricial atelectasis). The occurrence of chronic nonobstructive middle lobe collapse is often termed *right middle lobe syndrome* (see Fig. 2-24). It was originally described as occurring in association with tuberculous hilar lymph node enlargement resulting in transient bronchial obstruction. Typically the right middle lobe bronchus appears patent, and dilated air bronchograms are visible in the collapsed lobe.

Lateral Radiograph

On the lateral radiograph, middle lobe collapse results in upward bowing and displacement of the inferior major fissure and downward displacement of the minor fissure, resulting in a thin wedge-shaped opacity with its apex at the hilum (see Fig. 2-35B).

The appearance of right middle lobe collapse on the lateral view may mimic fluid within the major fissure. However, with fissural fluid the lower edge of the opacity is often convex downward instead of concave downward, as is typical of middle lobe collapse. If a minor fissure is seen as separate from a similar wedge-shaped opacity, occurring in a normal position, fissural fluid may be diagnosed.

Computed Tomography

On CT, as the middle lobe loses volume, the minor fissure, which normally is difficult to see because it lies in the plane of scan, rotates downward and medially and becomes visible on CT. The collapsed lobe assumes a triangular shape, with one

A   **B**

FIG. 2.33. Left upper lobe collapse due to bronchogenic carcinoma. **A:** Frontal chest radiograph shows increased density in the left upper lobe region, but a crescentic lucency (*small white arrows*) in the medial aspect of the left lung apex represents insinuation of the aerated superior segment of the lower lobe, the so-called luftsichel sign. Other findings of left upper lobe collapse include tracheal shift (*large white arrow*), elevation of the left main bronchus (*small black arrows*), and a juxtaphrenic peak (*large black arrow*). A left hilar mass represents the carcinoma. **B:** Anterior displacement and bowing of the major fissure (*arrows*) are visible on the lateral view.

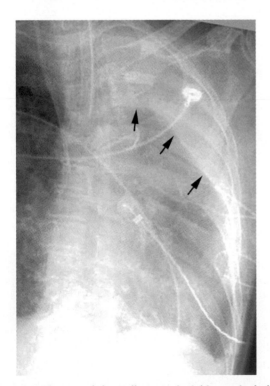

FIG. 2.34. Left upper lobe collapse mimicking apical pleural thickening. A crescentic soft tissue opacity at the left apex represents collapsed upper lobe outlined inferiorly by the aerated superior segment of the lower lobe (*arrows*). This appearance is sometimes termed peripheral atelectasis.

side of the triangle abutting the mediastinum and anchored at the hilum (Fig. 2-36). The apex of the triangle is directed laterally. The upper lobe is anterolateral to the collapsed lobe, and the lower lobe borders it posterolaterally (i.e., the middle lobe is in the middle). These aerated lobes usually contact each other lateral to the collapsed middle lobe and separate it from the lateral chest wall.

Lower Lobe Atelectasis

Findings of lower lobe collapse are identical on the right and left.

Frontal (PA or AP) Radiograph

With moderate atelectasis, the major fissure may not be visible on the frontal radiograph (see Fig. 2-28A). With further volume loss, the major fissure rotates toward the mediastinum,

TABLE 2.7 **Radiographic Findings of Middle Lobe Atelectasis**

Frontal radiograph
Minor fissure is invisible
Increased lung opacity (decreasing with increased collapse)
Silhouetting of the right heart border

Lateral radiograph
Downward bowing and displacement of the minor fissure
Anterior bowing and displacement of the inferior major fissure
Wedge of consolidated lung anchored at the hilum

A   B

FIG. 2.35. Right middle lobe collapse. **A:** On the frontal radiograph, ill-defined middle lobe consolidation obscures the right heart border. **B:** The lateral view shows downward displacement of the minor fissure (*white arrows*) and anterior displacement of the major fissure (*black arrows*). The collapsed middle lobe appears to be a thin wedge-shaped opacity with its apex at the hilum.

A   B

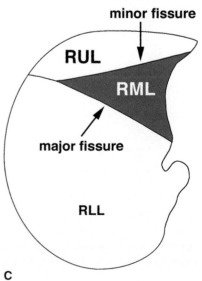

FIG. 2.36. CT of right middle lobe collapse. **A:** CT through the inferior right hilum shows anterior displacement of the major fissure (*large arrow*) and downward displacement of the minor fissure (*small arrows*). The minor fissure is less well defined because of its greater obliquity relative to the scan plane. The collapsed and consolidated middle lobe (*RML*) has a typical triangular configuration. *RUL*, right upper lobe; *RLL*, right lower lobe. **B:** At a lower level the collapsed lobe appears bandlike, outlined by the upper and lower lobes. **C:** Diagram of right middle lobe collapse on CT.

C

resulting in the typical triangular or wedge-shaped opacity of lower lobe collapse (Table 2-8; Fig. 2-37A). Often the upper portion of the major fissure is best seen. The apex of the triangle is at the hilum, and its base is at the diaphragm. Because of the inferior pulmonary ligament, the medial surface of the lower lobe maintains its contact with the mediastinum. With total atelectasis, a thin wedge of consolidated lung may be seen adjacent to the thoracic spine (Fig. 2-38A).

Lower lobe collapse usually results in downward displacement of the hilum (see Figs. 2-37A and 2-38A). The interlobar pulmonary artery is commonly invisible or poorly defined because of adjacent lower lobe consolidation. Obscuration of the diaphragm may be present on frontal or lateral radiographs.

Mediastinal shift is commonly present. Leftward shift and rotation of the heart with left lower lobe atelectasis may result

TABLE 2.8 **Radiographic Findings of Lower Lobe Atelectasis**

Frontal radiograph
Major fissure becomes visible (upper portion best seen)
Triangular opacity
Downward bowing of the minor fissure (right lower lobe atelectasis)
Downward displacement of the hilum
Invisibility of the interlobar pulmonary artery
Obscuration of the diaphragm
Shift of the heart
Flat-waist sign (left lower lobe atelectasis)

Lateral radiograph
Obscuration of the posterior diaphragm
Posterior bowing of the major fissure (lateral radiograph)

A

B

C

FIG. 2.37. Right lower lobe atelectasis secondary to bronchogenic carcinoma. **A:** Frontal radiograph shows the typical triangular appearance of right lower lobe atelectasis marginated by the major fissure (*black arrows*). The upper portion of the major fissure is most sharply defined. The right hilum (*white arrow*) is displaced downward, and the interlobar pulmonary artery is poorly seen. **B:** There is narrowing of the bronchus intermedius. Opacified arteries are visible within the collapsed right lower lobe. Posterior rotation of the major fissure (*arrow*) causes it to be well seen on the frontal radiograph. **C:** At a lower level, the major fissure (*arrow*) is displaced posteriorly.

FIG. 2.38. Marked left lower lobe atelectasis secondary to bronchogenic carcinoma. **A:** On the frontal radiograph, a thin wedge of consolidated lung (*arrows*) is seen adjacent to the spine. This represents the collapsed lower lobe. The heart is displaced to the left. **B:** Lateral view shows a vague opacity (*arrows*) in the region of the lower lobe. **C, D:** CT shows obstruction of the lower lobe bronchus (*black arrow*) and marked posteromedial rotation of the major fissure (*white arrows*). **E:** Diagram of CT appearances of lower lobe atelectasis. With progressive atelectasis (*left to right*), the major fissure rotates posteriorly.

in a straightening of the left mediastinal border, including the left heart margin, aorta, and pulmonary artery. This has been termed the "flat waist" *sign* (see Fig. 2-28A).

Right lower lobe atelectasis may result in downward displacement of the minor fissure seen on the frontal radiograph.

Lateral Radiograph

In its early stages, lower lobe collapse results in posterior and downward displacement of the major fissure seen on the lateral view (see Fig. 2-28B). However, with more severe atelectasis, the lateral aspect of the major fissure rotates posterior and medially, and the fissure may become invisible on the lateral view (see Fig. 2-38B). Increased density overlying the lower spine may be the only visible abnormality (normally the thoracic spine appears less dense in the inferior chest than at higher levels; this may not be true in the presence of lower lobe atelectasis or consolidation). On the lateral view, the hilum and bronchi may be displaced posteriorly.

Computed Tomography

On CT, the major fissure rotates posteromedially from the hilum with collapse, it may be displaced posteriorly, or both (see Figs. 2-28, 2-37, and 2-38). The collapsed lobe contacts the posterior mediastinum and posteromedial chest wall and maintains contact with the medial diaphragm.

Combined Collapse of Right Middle and Lower Lobes

This occurs in patients with obstruction of the bronchus intermedius. On the frontal and lateral radiographs, both the displaced major and minor fissures may be variably visible, outlining the consolidated lung. On the frontal view, both the right heart border and diaphragm often appear obscured (Fig. 2-39). This appearance may closely mimic that of right lower lobe collapse associated with an elevated hemidiaphragm or subpulmonic pleural effusion. Absence of a visible minor fissure at a higher level and obscuration of the right heart border favors combined collapse.

Combined Collapse of Right Middle and Upper Lobes

This combination cannot be explained by a single bronchial lesion, an occurrence termed the "double lesion" *sign*. This most commonly occurs when lung cancer involves the hilum, with invasion of both the upper and middle lobe bronchi while the lower lobe bronchus remains patent; it may also be seen with multiple isolated bronchial lesions, as in a patient with mucous plugging.

On the frontal radiograph, right upper lobe opacification obscures the right superior mediastinum while right middle lobe opacification obscures the right heart border

A   B

FIG. 2.39. Combined right middle and right lower lobe atelectasis. **A:** The superior aspect of the major fissure (*large arrows*) is visible, marginating the collapsed lower lobe. The major fissure merges inferiorly with the minor fissure (*small arrows*), which is displaced inferiorly. The right middle and lower lobes remain partially aerated. **B:** One day later, both the middle and lower lobes are consolidated (drowned lung). The major (*large arrows*) and minor (*small arrows*) fissures sharply marginate consolidated (drowned) lung. Both the right heart border and diaphragm are obscured.

FIG. 2.40. Combined right middle and right upper lobe atelectasis in a patient with right hilar bronchogenic carcinoma. **A:** Right-sided volume loss is present with mediastinal shift to the right. The upper mediastinal contour and right heart border are partially obscured and poorly defined. The right hemidiaphragm is elevated and a juxtaphrenic peak is visible (*arrow*). **B:** The lateral view shows anterior displacement of the major fissure (*arrows*) because of collapse of both right upper (*RUL*) and middle (*RML*) lobes. Both lobes are homogeneously consolidated. This appearance mimics that of left upper lobe collapse.

(Fig. 2-40A). Since both lobes anterior to the major fissure are collapsed, the appearance of combined middle and upper lobe collapse on the lateral radiograph is identical to that of left upper lobe atelectasis (see Fig. 2-40B).

SEGMENTAL ATELECTASIS

Segmental (or subsegmental) atelectasis may occur secondary to obstruction of segmental (or subsegmental) bronchi by tumor, mucus, or inflammatory disease. Typically wedge-shaped opacities are seen radiating outward from the hilum or involving the peripheral lung, with the base of the wedge touching the pleural surface. Indirect findings of volume loss are typically absent because of the small amount of lung tissue involved.

PLATELIKE OR DISCOID ATELECTASIS

Linear areas of atelectasis, a few millimeters to 1 cm thick and at least several centimeters in length, commonly occur in patients with decreased depth of breathing or diminished diaphragmatic excursions. They tend to occur at the lung bases, several centimeters above and parallel to the diaphragm (Fig. 2-41). They cross segmental boundaries. They may also occur in the medial infrahilar regions, typically angled upward from the mediastinum at about a 45-degree angle. They are thought to occur because of

decreased ventilation of lung associated with retained secretions. Bronchial obstruction is not a cause. They are of little clinical significance but serve as a marker of poor ventilatory function.

ROUNDED ATELECTASIS

The term "rounded atelectasis" refers to the presence of focal rounded lung collapse. In some patients, it is associated with invagination of the visceral pleura with folding or rolling of the collapsed lung. It usually occurs in the presence of pleural thickening or effusion, and likely results from local restriction of lung expansion. It is most commonly associated with asbestos exposure, empyema, tuberculous effusions, renal failure, and pleural neoplasm but may occur with pleural effusion of any cause. On plain radiographs, rounded atelectasis may mimic neoplasm, but its CT appearance is often characteristic.

To suggest the diagnosis of rounded atelectasis on the basis of chest radiographs or CT, the opacity should be (a) round or elliptical; (b) associated with an ipsilateral pleural abnormality, either effusion or pleural thickening; (c) peripheral in location, having significant contact with the abnormal pleural surface; (d) associated with curving of pulmonary vessels or bronchi into the edge of the lesion (the so-called "comet-tail" sign); and (e) associated with volume loss in the affected lobe (Figs. 2-42 and 2-43; Table 2-9). If each of these

FIG. 2.41. Disk atelectasis. Frontal (**A**) and lateral (**B**) radiographs show disk atelectasis (*arrows*) at the lung bases, roughly paralleling the hemidiaphragms. **C:** HRCT at the right base shows linear areas of atelectasis (*small arrows*). When these are oriented parallel to the plane of scan, large areas of opacity may be seen (*large arrow*).

criteria for rounded atelectasis is met, a confident diagnosis can usually be made.

Rounded atelectasis is most common in the posterior lower lobes; this location is typical of patients with free pleural effusion (see Figs. 2-42 and 2-43). In patients with bilateral effusions, it may be bilateral or symmetrical. Rounded atelectasis in patients with pleural fibrosis may be anterior in location (Figs. 2-44 to 2-46).

On chest radiographs, posteriorly located rounded atelectasis usually appears ill-defined on the frontal projection and well-defined and elliptical on the lateral view, having extensive pleural contact. It is most often seen several centimeters above a blunted posterior costophrenic angle

(see Fig. 2-43). Vessels may be seen curving into its inferior edge, representing the comet-tail sign.

Rounded atelectasis may have acute or obtuse angles where it contacts the pleura. Since rounded atelectasis represents collapsed lung parenchyma, it can show significant enhancement on CT following the intravenous injection of contrast agents. Air bronchograms may be visible within the collapsed lung.

Atypical examples of rounded atelectasis are often encountered in patients who have pleural thickening and fibrosis rather than pleural effusion (see Fig. 2-45). Such cases may show rounded atelectasis that is irregular in shape, unassociated with the comet-tail sign, separated from the pleural surface, or anterior in location.

FIG. 2.42. Typical rounded atelectasis associated with pleural effusion. CT scans at two adjacent levels (**A, B**) show characteristic findings of rounded atelectasis. An elliptical opacity is visible (*ra*), which is peripheral in location and has significant contact with the pleural surface in contiguity with a right pleural effusion. Vessels (*small black arrows*) curve into the edge of the lesion (i.e., the so-called comet-tail sign). Posterior displacement of the major fissure (*large white arrows*) indicates volume loss in the right lower lobe. For comparison, note the location of the normal left major fissure (*small white arrows*). Because these findings are typical, follow-up should be sufficient.

FIG. 2.43. Typical rounded atelectasis associated with pleural effusion. **A:** Frontal chest radiograph shows blunting of the right costophrenic angle due to pleural effusion. An ill-defined opacity (*ra*) at the right base represents rounded atelectasis. Note the presence of mediastinal shift to the right. **B:** On the lateral view, a well-defined elliptical opacity (*ra*) is seen posteriorly, having extensive pleural contact. This location, several centimeters above the blunted posterior costophrenic angle (*black arrow*), is characteristic of rounded atelectasis in patients with effusion. Curving of vessels (*white arrows*) into the inferior aspect of the opacity reflects the comet-tail sign. The appearance in this case is sufficiently characteristic to allow follow-up.

TABLE 2.9	CT and Radiographic Findings of Rounded Atelectasis

Round or elliptical opacity
Associated with an ipsilateral pleural abnormality
Peripheral in location
Extensive contact with the abnormal pleural surface
Comet-tail sign
Volume loss
Posterior, paravertebral lower lobe in patients with effusion
Atypical appearances when associated with pleural fibrosis
Dense opacification on CT after contrast infusion

Rounded atelectasis is seen in as many as 10% of patients with asbestos exposure, usually due to visceral or parietal pleural thickening or plaques, diffuse pleural thickening, or sometimes exudative effusion, and it often appears atypical.

FIG. 2.44. Anterior rounded atelectasis associated with pleural fibrosis in a patient with prior TB. **A:** CT shows left pleural thickening anteriorly (*black arrows*). The area of rounded atelectasis (*ra*) is irregular in shape but contacts the pleural surface and is associated with the comet-tail sign (*white arrows*). **B:** At a lower level, anterior displacement of the major fissure (*white arrow*) indicates volume loss in the upper lobe.

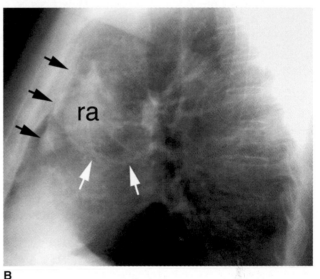

FIG. 2.45. Anterior rounded atelectasis in a patient with asbestos-related pleural thickening. **A:** Frontal chest radiograph shows a mass overlying the right hilum. This appearance suggests bronchogenic carcinoma. **B:** Lateral chest radiograph shows anterior pleural thickening and calcification (*black arrows*). A comet-tail sign (*white arrows*) is seen adjacent to the area of rounded atelectasis (*ra*). The area of rounded atelectasis does not appear to contact the anterior chest wall.

Atypical cases of rounded atelectasis may represent a diagnostic problem because lung cancer has an increased incidence in asbestos-exposed individuals. Needle biopsy may be necessary to exclude carcinoma.

SELECTED READING

Batra P, Brown K, Hayashi K, Mori M. Rounded atelectasis. J Thorac Imaging 1996; 11:187–197.
Blankenbaker DG. The luftsichel sign. Radiology 1998; 208:319–320.

A   B

FIG. 2.46. Atypical rounded atelectasis in a patient with asbestos-related pleural thickening. **A:** CT using a soft tissue window shows anterior pleural thickening with calcification (*arrows*). Irregular lung masses are also visible. **B:** CT with a lung window setting shows bilateral masses. Although there is some evidence of the comet-tail sign on each side, the right-sided mass does not contact the pleural surface, and the left-sided mass is very irregular in contour. Biopsy of each mass was negative, and follow-up CT showed no change.

Davis SD, Yankelevitz DF, Wand A, Chiarella DA. Juxtaphrenic peak in upper and middle lobe volume loss: assessment with CT. Radiology 1996; 198:143–149.

Felson B. The roentgen diagnosis of disseminated pulmonary alveolar diseases. Semin Roentgenol 1967; 2:3–21.

Genereux GP. Pattern recognition in diffuse lung disease: a review of theory and practice. Med Radiogr Photogr 1985; 61:2–31.

Kattan KR, Wlot JF. Cardiac rotation in left lower lobe collapse: "the flat waist sign." Radiology 1976; 118:275–279.

Naidich DP, Ettinger N, Leitman BS, McCauley DI. CT of lobar collapse. Semin Roentgenol 1984; 19:222–235.

Reed JC, Madewell JE. The air bronchogram in interstitial disease of the lungs: a radiological-pathological correlation. Radiology 1975; 116:1–9.

Rohlfing BM. The shifting granuloma: an internal marker of atelectasis. Radiology 1977; 123:283–285.

Shah RM, Friedman AC. CT angiogram sign: incidence and significance in lobar consolidations evaluated by contrast-enhanced CT. AJR Am J Roentgenol 1998; 170:719–721.

Westcott JL, Cole S. Plate atelectasis. Radiology 1985; 155:1–9.

Woodring JH. The computed tomography mucous bronchogram sign. J Comput Tomogr 1988; 12:165–168.

Woodring JH, Reed JC. Types and mechanisms of pulmonary atelectasis. J Thorac Imaging 1996; 11:92–108.

Woodring JH, Reed JC. Radiographic manifestations of lobar atelectasis. J Thorac Imaging 1996; 11:109–144.

Lung Cancer and Bronchopulmonary Neoplasms

W. RICHARD WEBB

LUNG CARCINOMA

Lung carcinoma is the most common fatal malignancy in both men and women. In the United States, it accounts for 14% to 15% of all new cancers and 26% to 30% of all cancer deaths. Lung cancer is more common in men than women, but at present its incidence is decreasing in men and increasing in women.

RISK FACTORS FOR LUNG CANCER

Tobacco smoking accounts for 80% to 90% of lung cancers. In smokers, the risk of lung cancer correlates with younger age at the onset of smoking, the duration and cumulative amount of exposure, and the depth of inhalation. Heavy smoking is associated with a 20- to 30-fold increase in lung cancer risk compared to nonsmokers. A decrease in risk following smoking cessation has been demonstrated. Well-differentiated squamous cell carcinoma, small cell carcinoma, large cell carcinoma, and to a lesser extent adenocarcinoma all demonstrate an increased incidence with increasing cigarette consumption. About 25% of lung cancers in nonsmokers have been attributed to second-hand smoke.

Increasing age is associated with an increased risk of lung cancer. Lung cancers are rare in patients under age 30.

Occupational exposures to various substances have been linked to lung cancer; as many as 10% of lung cancer cases may be due to occupational exposure. Agents associated with occupational lung cancer include arsenic, nickel, chromium, asbestos, beryllium, cadmium, chromium, mustard gas, pesticides, and radon or uranium.

Asbestos exposure is the best-recognized occupational risk for lung cancer and is the most frequent exposure in the general population (Fig. 3-1). A dose–response relationship between the severity and duration of asbestos exposure and the likelihood of developing lung cancer is well established, although the risk of exposure depends not only on the amount of asbestos to which one is exposed but also the fiber type (increased risk with amphibole fibers), the industrial use of asbestos, the conditions of exposure, and the presence of asbestosis. The risk of lung cancer in a

heavily exposed asbestos worker is about five times that of a nonexposed subject. Also, smoking is a synergistic risk in asbestos-exposed subjects: the risk of lung cancer in an asbestos worker who is a heavy smoker is about 20 times that of a nonsmoking asbestos worker and 100 times that of a nonexposed nonsmoker (Table 3-1).

Diffuse pulmonary fibrosis has been associated with a 10-fold increase in the risk of lung cancer. In addition, patients with focal lung scarring, particularly as a result of tuberculosis, can develop a carcinoma in association with areas of fibrosis or scarring. Although this is infrequent, cases of carcinoma arising in areas of focal scarring, so-called scar carcinoma, are encountered in clinical practice.

Chronic obstructive lung disease (chronic bronchitis and emphysema) is a risk factor for developing lung cancer, independent of cigarette smoking. In both chronic obstructive pulmonary disease (COPD) and diffuse pulmonary fibrosis, proposed mechanisms of increased cancer risk include decreased clearance of inhaled carcinogens and epithelial metaplasia.

Genetic predisposition plays a role in the development of lung cancer. In general, relatives of subjects with lung cancer have a higher risk of developing lung cancer (about twofold) than the general population. An increased risk of lung cancer has been associated with specific oncogenes, chromosome defects, specific HLA antigens, enzyme defects, and defects in proteins normally produced by tumor suppressor genes.

CELL TYPES OF LUNG CANCER

Lung carcinomas have been classified by the World Health Organization (WHO) based on their light-microscopic appearances (Table 3-2). The large majority of lung cancers are classified by WHO criteria as one of four major histologic types: squamous cell carcinoma, adenocarcinoma, small cell carcinoma, and large cell carcinoma. Numerous subtypes of these four major tumors have also been defined, but most of these are unimportant from a radiologic or clinical standpoint.

These cell types are not absolutely distinct. As many as 50% of lung tumors have mixed appearances, and the most

A
B

FIG. 3.1. Lung cancer associated with asbestos exposure. **A:** Chest radiograph shows a large left lung mass (*M*) representing lung cancer. Bilateral pleural thickening with calcification is also visible (*arrows*). **B:** CT shows a left lung mass (*M*) and bilateral localized calcified pleural plaques (*arrows*) typical of asbestos exposure.

differentiated feature of the carcinoma is used to define its cell type. Many tumors classified as one histologic type (e.g., large cell carcinoma) using light microscopy and the WHO system would be reclassified if electron microscopy were used. Cytologic examination uncommonly allows a specific cell type to be determined; cytologic diagnosis of lung cancer is usually limited to the designation *nonsmall cell lung carcinoma (NSCLC)* or *small cell carcinoma.*

Preinvasive Lesions

These lesions are dysplastic or localized and include atypical adenomatous hyperplasia (AAH), squamous dysplasia and carcinoma in situ, and diffuse idiopathic pulmonary neuroendocrine cell hyperplasia (described below along with carcinoid tumors).

AAH represents a bronchioloalveolar proliferation that resembles but does not meet the criteria for bronchioloalveolar carcinoma (BAC). Its incidence ranges from 5% to 20%. Most lesions are 5 mm or less in diameter, and lesions are often multiple. AAH is most often found incidentally in pathologic specimens but may mimic lung carcinoma radiographically (particularly on CT), leading to resection. On

CT, AAH typically appears as a small nodule of ground-glass opacity.

Squamous Cell Carcinoma

Until recently, squamous cell carcinoma was the most common cell type of lung carcinoma; it currently accounts for about 30% of cases. It is strongly associated with cigarette smoking (Table 3-3).

Squamous cell carcinoma frequently (65%) arises in main, lobar, or segmental bronchi. In this location, tumor growth

TABLE 3.2 Classification of Lung Carcinoma and Important Subtypes From the 1999/2004 WHO Classifications

Preinvasive lesions
  Atypical adenomatous hyperplasia
Squamous cell carcinoma
Adenocarcinoma
Bronchioloalveolar carcinoma
  Nonmucinous
  Mucinous
Adenocarcinoma, mixed subtype
Small cell carcinoma
Large cell carcinoma
  Large cell neuroendocrine carcinoma
Adenosquamous carcinoma
Carcinoma with pleomorphic, sarcomatoid, or sarcomatous
  elements
Carcinoid tumor
  Typical carcinoid tumor
  Atypical carcinoid tumor
Carcinomas of salivary gland type
  Adenoid cystic carcinoma
  Mucoepidermoid carcinoma

(Modified from **Travis WD**. Pathology of lung cancer. Clin Chest Med 2002; 23:65–81.)

TABLE 3.1 Increased Risk of Lung Cancer Associated With Smoking and Asbestos Exposure

Risk Factor	Comparison Group	Relative Risk
Heavy asbestos exposure	No asbestos exposure	5:1
Heavy smoking	Nonsmoker	20:1
Heavy smoking and heavy asbestos exposure	No smoking history and no asbestos exposure	100:1

TABLE 3.3	Squamous Cell Carcinoma

30% of lung cancer cases
Strongly associated with cigarette smoking
65% arise in main, lobar, or segmental bronchi
    Endobronchial mass
    Bronchial obstruction
    Infiltration of bronchial wall
    Local invasion
    Hilar mass
    Atelectasis and consolidation common
30% present as solitary nodule or mass
    Cavitation relatively common
Metastasizes late
Relatively good prognosis

results in obstruction of the bronchial lumen, infiltration of the bronchial wall, and invasion of the adjacent lung or vessels. This tumor tends to cause symptoms early in its course because of its proximal and endobronchial location and may be detected using sputum cytology before being radiographically visible. Early metastasis is uncommon, and it has a relatively good 5-year survival rate.

A polypoid endobronchial mass or bronchial obstruction is frequently seen (Fig. 3-2A). Hilar mass is also common due to the central location of the tumor, with local invasion

and involvement of hilar lymph nodes (see Fig. 3-2B). Atelectasis (Fig. 3-3), consolidation, mucoid impaction, and bronchiectasis are common radiographic findings, reflecting the presence of bronchial obstruction (see Table 3-3). Only about 30% of squamous cell carcinomas present in the lung periphery as a lung nodule. Central necrosis and cavitation (Fig. 3-4) are more common than with other cell types.

Adenocarcinoma

Adenocarcinoma is the most common cell type of lung cancer and accounts for 30% to 35% of lung cancer cases (Table 3-4). As with squamous cell cancer, it is related to cigarette smoking, although its association with smoking is relatively weak. Adenocarcinoma is thought to arise from bronchiolar or alveolar epithelium and is characterized by glandular differentiation. Invasion of lung parenchyma is usually present. Early metastasis is more common than with squamous cell carcinoma, particularly to the central nervous system and adrenal glands. Seventy-five percent originate in the lung periphery, presenting as a solitary pulmonary nodule (Fig. 3-5). In a few cases, adenocarcinoma originates within large airways. It is most common in the upper lobes. It is often associated with fibrosis; it may arise in relation to preexisting lung fibrosis (i.e., a scar carcinoma) or may result in a desmoplastic reaction in surrounding lung.

A

B

FIG. 3.2. Squamous cell carcinoma with an endobronchial and hilar mass. **A:** CT shows a polypoid mass (*arrow*) within the right lower lobe bronchus, typical of squamous cell carcinoma. **B:** At a slightly lower level, the bronchial lumen appears obstructed and local invasion has resulted in a hilar mass (*M*).

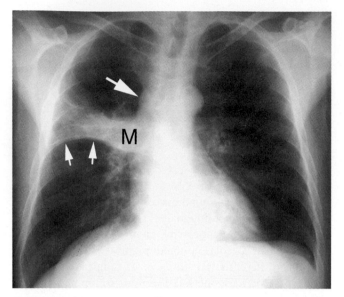

FIG. 3.3 Squamous cell carcinoma with bronchial obstruction and atelectasis. Chest radiograph shows a right hilar mass (*M*) with upward bowing of the minor fissure (*small arrows*). This combination results in Golden's S sign. Mediastinal lymph node enlargement is also present (*large arrow*).

Adenocarcinomas often appear ill defined on chest radiographs because of their irregular margin (see Fig. 3-5A). On high-resolution CT, adenocarcinoma presenting as a solitary nodule may appear round or lobulated. They frequently have an irregular and spiculated margin because of associated lung fibrosis (see Fig. 3-5B). When occurring in a subpleural location, this may result in thin linear extensions to the pleural surface (i.e., a *pleural tail*; see Fig. 3-5C). Air

TABLE 3.4 Adenocarcinoma
30%–35% of lung cancer cases (most common cell type)
Weak association with smoking
Early metastases common
75% present as peripheral lung nodule
Common in the upper lobes
Associated with lung fibrosis
Often appear spiculated

bronchograms may be visible within the nodule using CT; although central necrosis is common, cavitation visible on radiographs or CT is uncommon. When adenocarcinoma arises from the wall of a central bronchus, it is radiographically indistinguishable from squamous cell carcinoma.

Bronchioloalveolar Carcinoma

BAC is a well-differentiated subtype of adenocarcinoma that also tends to occur in the lung periphery (Table 3-5). In the current WHO classification, BAC is defined as unassociated with invasion of pleura, vessels, or lung stroma. Using this restrictive definition, BAC is relatively uncommon, accounting for fewer than 5% of lung malignancies. It has a very good prognosis when localized, with a 5-year survival rate approaching 100%.

BAC spreads as a thin layer of cells, using the alveolar or bronchiolar walls as a framework or scaffold. This pattern of growth is termed *lepidic*. Other types of adenocarcinoma usually invade and destroy lung parenchyma as they grow, a pattern termed *hilic*.

Nonmucinous and *mucinous* subtypes of BAC occur in about equal numbers. These cell types correlate with radiographic appearance.

A

B

FIG. 3.4. Squamous cell carcinoma with a cavitary lung mass. **A:** On a chest radiograph, a large, thick-walled cavitary mass is visible in the right upper lobe. **B:** CT shows the cavity to have a thick and nodular wall. This is typical of cavitary carcinoma. This would be considered a T2 carcinoma.

A

B

C

FIG. 3.5. Typical appearances of adenocarcinoma. **A:** Chest radiograph in a patient with adenocarcinoma shows an ill-defined nodule in the left lung apex (*arrow*). Adenocarcinomas often appear ill defined on radiographs because of their irregular and spiculated edge. **B:** High-resolution CT in a patient with adenocarcinoma in the left upper lobe shows a solitary lung nodule with an irregular and spiculated edge. Spiculation usually results from lung fibrosis associated with the tumor. This tumor would be classified as a T1 carcinoma in the lung cancer staging system. **C:** High-resolution CT in a patient with adenocarcinoma presenting as a solitary nodule in the posterior right upper lobe. The nodule appears lobulated and spiculated. Extensions to the pleural surface (*arrows*) are termed pleural tails. They result from fibrosis with a puckering of the visceral pleural surface.

BAC most commonly presents as solitary nodule (60%) and radiographically may be indistinguishable from adenocarcinoma. BAC presenting as a solitary nodule is usually the nonmucinous subtype of BAC. Because of its lepidic growth pattern, radiographs and CT usually show a very ill-defined nodule (Fig. 3-6). On HRCT, localized BAC appears as a ground-glass opacity nodule, sometimes associated with regions of soft tissue attenuation (Fig. 3-7), and often contains air bronchograms or bubbly lucencies. The bubbly lucencies represent cystic air-filled areas within the tumor termed *pseudocavitation* (see Fig. 3-6B).

TABLE 3.5	Bronchioloalveolar Carcinoma

Subtype of adenocarcinoma
Noninvasive tumor characterized by lepidic growth
60% present as a solitary nodule
    Usually nonmucinous cell type
    Ill-defined nodule of ground-glass opacity
    Air bronchograms and cystic areas (pseudocavitation)
    Excellent prognosis
40% appear as diffuse or patchy consolidation and/or nodules
    Mucinous cell type
    Lung consolidation due to mucus filling alveoli
    CT angiogram sign
    Poor prognosis

In 40% of cases, BAC presents with diffuse or multifocal lung involvement having the appearance of lung consolidation or multiple ill-defined nodules (Figs. 3-8 and 3-9; see Fig. 3-22). This appearance is typical of the mucinous subtype of BAC. It is unclear whether this pattern results from multicentric origin of the tumor or endobronchial spread. Although lepidic growth is present in such patients, with tumor cells lining alveolar walls, mucin produced by the tumor fills the alveoli, resulting in the radiographic appearance of consolidation. The CT angiogram sign, in which opacified vessels are visible within consolidated lung, is often seen if CT is obtained with contrast infusion (see Chapter 2). Patients with diffuse BAC can present with profuse watery sputum production, termed *bronchorrhea*, as a result of extensive mucin production. Diffuse BAC has a poor prognosis.

Adenocarcinoma, mixed subtype

Adenocarcinomas having some characteristics of BAC are common and classified as adenocarcinoma, mixed subtype. They are sometimes referred to as minimally-invasive adenocarcinoma with BAC. These tumors have a prognosis intermediate between invasive adenocarcinoma and BAC. They may resemble either tumor radiographically, appearing as a solid nodule, a nodule of ground-glass opacity, a nodule of mixed attenuation, or as a diffuse or multifocal abnormality.

Small Cell Carcinoma

Small cell carcinoma is the third most common histologic variety of primary lung cancer (15% to 20% of cases) and is made up of small cells, similar in size to lymphocytes, that have scanty cytoplasm (Table 3-6). It is thought to originate from neuroendocrine cells, and electron microscopy shows neurosecretory granules in many cases of small cell carcinoma. Along with carcinoid tumor and atypical carcinoid tumor, small cell carcinoma is considered to be a type of *neuroendocrine carcinoma* and is described further below. It is a common cause of paraneoplastic syndromes. It is strongly associated with smoking.

A

B

FIG. 3.6. Focal bronchioloalveolar carcinoma (BAC). **A:** Chest radiograph shows a very ill-defined nodule (*arrow*) in the left lung. **B:** CT with 5-mm slice thickness shows an ill-defined, irregular, spiculated nodule, containing both air bronchograms and bubbly lucencies. This appearance is typical of focal BAC.

A   B

FIG. 3.7. Focal bronchioloalveolar carcinoma. **A:** CT with 5-mm slice thickness shows an ill-defined nodule. **B:** High-resolution CT shows the nodule to be largely of ground-glass opacity. This appearance is typical of carcinoma having lepidic growth.

A   B

FIG. 3.8. Diffuse bronchioloalveolar carcinoma. **A:** Chest radiograph shows consolidation at the right lung base (*arrow*). **B:** CT with 5-mm slice thickness shows multiple areas of consolidation, with air bronchograms, and numerous ill-defined nodules. These nodules are typically centrilobular; they represent air-space or acinar nodules and are common with diffuse bronchioloaveolar carcinoma.

FIG. 3.9. Diffuse bronchioloalveolar carcinoma involving both upper lobes, with air-space consolidation and air bronchograms.

TABLE 3.6 Small Cell Carcinoma
15%–20% of lung cancers
Strongly associated with smoking
Neuroendocrine carcinoma
Paraneoplastic syndromes commonly associated
Most occur in main or lobar bronchi
Extensive peribronchial invasion
Large hilar or parahilar mass
Bronchial narrowing
Lymph node enlargement
Metastases at diagnosis in >90%
Prognosis very poor

Small cell carcinoma tends to occur in the main or lobar bronchi and is associated with extensive peribronchial invasion and a large hilar or parahilar mass (Fig. 3-10). Endobronchial tumor masses are less common than with squamous cell carcinoma, but the large tumor mass frequently compresses bronchi (Fig. 3-11). Atelectasis may be associated. This tumor is commonly associated with marked mediastinal lymph node enlargement (Fig. 3-12). It is a common cause of superior vena cava (SVC) syndrome. Presentation as a lung nodule is very uncommon, accounting for less than 5% of cases.

Although the tumor is relatively radiosensitive, its prognosis is very poor because of the frequent presence of distant metastases at the time of diagnosis. Small cell lung cancer is not generally considered amenable to surgical treatment. Over 90% of cases are Stage IV at diagnosis. Reported cases of small cell carcinoma that present as lung nodules or masses, and that have been cured at surgery, may in fact represent misclassified cases of atypical carcinoid.

Large Cell Carcinoma

The term large cell carcinoma is used to describe tumors that do not show squamous or adenomatous differentiation or have typical features of small cell carcinoma. Distinction from poorly differentiated squamous cell or adenocarcinoma can be difficult, and in fact many cases classified as large cell carcinoma on the basis of light microscopy are reclassified as other cell types if electron microscopy is used.

Large cell carcinoma accounts for 10% of lung cancers (Table 3-7). It tends to present as a large peripheral mass; more than 60% are larger than 4 cm at presentation (Fig. 3-13). It is similar to adenocarcinoma in its radiologic characteristics (except for its large size), histologic ultrastructure, and survival statistics. As with adenocarcinoma, it tends to metastasize early and has a poor prognosis. It is strongly associated with smoking.

Large cell neuroendocrine carcinoma is an important subtype of large cell carcinoma, differing histologically from other neuroendocrine tumors such as small cell carcinoma and atypical carcinoid tumor. As with small cell carcinoma, it has a very poor prognosis.

Adenosquamous Carcinoma

Adenosquamous carcinoma has mixed histologic characteristics of both adenocarcinoma and squamous cell carcinoma. If light microscopy is used for classification, adenosquamous carcinoma accounts for a few percent of lung cancers at most. If electron microscopy is used, as many as one third of all lung cancers have mixed characteristics. These tumors usually present as masses in the lung periphery and are indistinguishable from adenocarcinoma or large cell carcinoma. Metastases are common. Adenosquamous carcinomas are aggressive and have a poor prognosis.

A

B

FIG. 3.10. Small cell carcinoma. **A:** Chest radiograph show a large right hilar mass (*arrows*). **B:** CT shows the large mass (*M*). Interstitial thickening characterized by interlobular septal thickening in the middle lobe indicates local lymphangitic spread of tumor.

FIG. 3.11. Small cell carcinoma. Contrast-enhanced CT shows a large hilar mass (*M*). Tumor surrounds and narrows the bronchus intermedius (*large arrow*) and extends into the subcarinal space. Pericardial thickening (*small arrows*) is likely due to local invasion. A left pleural effusion is also present.

FIG. 3.12. Small cell carcinoma. CT following contrast infusion shows extensive mediastinal lymph node enlargement typical of small cell carcinoma. The superior vena cava (*arrow*) is displaced anteriorly and markedly narrowed by lymph node mass (*M*) in the pretracheal space. A large anterior mediastinal lymph node mass (*A*) is also visible. A right pleural effusion is also present.

Carcinoma With Pleomorphic, Sarcomatoid, or Sarcomatous Features

This disparate group of tumors includes those characterized pathologically by a combination of epithelial and mesenchymal tissues (e.g., giant cell carcinoma, carcinosarcoma, pulmonary blastoma). These tumors are rare and may present as polypoid endobronchial masses or large lung masses. Their prognosis is poor.

Carcinoid Tumor

Carcinoid tumor originates from neuroendocrine cells in the bronchial wall. It is classified as typical or atypical carcinoid tumor. *Typical carcinoid tumor* is a low-grade malignancy and accounts for a few percent of all primary lung malignancies. This tumor most often occurs in the central bronchi, resulting in an endobronchial mass, and is locally invasive. Metastases are relatively uncommon. *Atypical carcinoid tumor* is a more aggressive variant and has a poorer prognosis. Typical carcinoid tumor, atypical carcinoid tumor, large cell neuroendocrine carcinoma, and small cell carcinoma are considered to be different types of neuroendocrine carcinoma.

TABLE 3.7 Large Cell Carcinoma

10% of lung cancers
Strongly associated with smoking
Overlap with other cell types
Usually present as a large peripheral mass (>4 cm)
Metastasizes early
Prognosis poor

Carcinoid tumors are discussed in detail below because of their distinct clinical and radiographic appearances.

Carcinomas of Salivary Gland Type

Salivary gland type carcinomas, also referred to as bronchial gland carcinomas, include adenoid cystic carcinoma (cylindroma) and mucoepidermoid carcinoma. These are similar to salivary gland tumors in their histologic characteristics and arise from glands in the tracheal or bronchial wall. These tumors account for much less than 1% of tracheobronchial malignancies. As with carcinoid tumors, they are locally invasive and uncommonly metastasize, and are discussed in detail below.

RADIOGRAPHIC APPEARANCES OF LUNG CANCER

In most patients with lung cancer, the findings on chest radiographs are sufficiently characteristic to suggest the diagnosis and lead to appropriate clinical and imaging evaluation. Although lung cancer can manifest in a variety of ways, a short list of radiographic abnormalities is commonly seen. These abnormalities reflect the location and manner in which lung cancer arises and the sites to which it most commonly spreads. Such abnormalities include the presence of a lung nodule, evidence of bronchial obstruction with collapse or consolidation of a lobe or lung, a hilar or mediastinal mass, and benign or malignant pleural effusion.

Although the frequency of these findings varies according to the cell type of the tumor (Table 3-8), each of the

A   **B**

FIG. 3.13. Large cell carcinoma. A: Chest radiograph shows a large left lung mass. **B:** On contrast-enhanced CT, a large mass occupies the left lung. A left pleural effusion is also present.

four major cell types of lung carcinoma (squamous cell carcinoma, adenocarcinoma, small cell carcinoma, large cell carcinoma) can show similar findings. Radiographic findings associated with carcinoid tumor and the bronchial gland carcinomas are discussed later in this chapter because of their somewhat different biological behavior and X-ray appearances.

Solitary Pulmonary Nodule or Mass

Approximately one third of lung cancers present radiographically as a solitary pulmonary nodule or lung mass.

A solitary pulmonary nodule (see Figs. 3-5 to 3-7) is usually defined as being visible as a focal opacity on chest radiographs or CT and is

1. Relatively well-defined
2. At least partially surrounded by lung
3. Roughly spherical
4. 3 cm or less in diameter

Similar lesions larger than 3 cm in diameter are usually referred to using the term *mass* (see Figs. 3-1, 3-4, and 3-13).

This measurement is also used to distinguish a T1 carcinoma (3 cm or less in diameter) from a T2 carcinoma (larger than 3 cm).

Among lung cancers presenting as a solitary nodule or mass, the most common cell types are adenocarcinoma (40% of cases), squamous cell carcinoma (20%), large cell carcinoma (15%), and BAC (10%). Since BAC is considered to be a subtype of adenocarcinoma, the adenocarcinomas account for half of the cases (see Figs. 3-5 to 3-7). Large cell carcinoma typically results in a mass (see Fig. 3-13) that at diagnosis is larger than that seen with other cell types, averaging nearly twice the diameter of adenocarcinoma or BAC. Small cell carcinoma uncommonly results in a solitary nodule.

Lung cancers presenting as a solitary pulmonary nodule may have specific radiographic appearances that suggest the diagnosis (Table 3-9); if a combination of radiologic, clinical, and laboratory information is used, malignant pulmonary nodules can be diagnosed in over 90% of patients. The radiographic assessment of a solitary pulmonary nodule is a common and important problem; this topic is discussed in greater detail in Chapter 9. The differential diagnosis of a solitary nodule is reviewed in Table 9-1 in Chapter 9.

TABLE 3.8 Plain Radiologic Findings in Lung Cancer by Cell Type[a]

Finding	Squamous (%)	Adencarcinoma (%)	Small Cell (%)	Large Cell (%)
Peripheral nodule or mass	30	**75**	5	**65**
Atelectasis	**40**	10	20	15
Consolidation	20	15	20	25
Hilar enlargement	**40**	20	**80**	30
Mediastinal mass	<5	<5	**15**	**10**
Pleural effusions	5	5	5	5
No abnormalities	5	<5	0	0
Multiple abnormalities	35	30	65	45

[a]Boldface findings are those most helpful in differentiating cell types. Percentages are approximate.

TABLE 3.9 Typical Radiographic Characteristics of Lung Cancer Presenting as a Solitary Pulmonary Nodule

Diameter >2 cm
Most common in the upper lobes
Ill-defined, irregular, or spiculated margin
Lobulated or irregular in shape
Containing air bronchograms or bubbly lucencies (pseudocavitation)
Cavitation with a thick (>15 mm) and nodular wall
Cavitation without an air-fluid level
Satellite nodules absent
Calcification absent or not typical of a benign pattern
Enhancement of ≥15 HU following contrast infusion
Doubling time of 30–200 days (although BAC may be very slow growing, i.e., doubling time >1,000 days)

Superior Sulcus (Pancoast) Tumor

Tumors arising at or near the lung apex are termed *superior sulcus carcinoma*, *thoracic inlet carcinoma*, or simply *apical carcinoma*. The term *Pancoast tumor* is best reserved for patients with some (although not necessarily all) manifestations of the Pancoast syndrome. Approximately 5% of lung cancers occur in the superior sulcus; any cell type may be responsible.

Superior sulcus tumors are commonly associated with symptoms because of their propensity to invade structures in the thoracic inlet, including the brachial plexus, cervicothoracic sympathetic ganglia, subclavian artery and vein (Fig. 3-14), and vertebral column. *Pancoast syndrome* results from involvement of the brachial plexus and sympathetic ganglia and consists of the combination of

1. Pain in the shoulder
2. Radicular pain along the distribution of the eighth cervical and first and second thoracic nerves, sometimes associated with wasting of the small muscles of the hand
3. Horner's syndrome, consisting of ptosis, miosis, and hemifacial anhidrosis

Classic Pancoast syndrome is uncommon. Most superior sulcus tumors present with shoulder or scapular pain that radiates down the arm and may be associated with ulnar neuropathy. Horner's syndrome is present in only about

FIG. 3.14. Superior sulcus tumor. **A:** Chest radiograph shows a mass (*arrows*) at the right lung apex. **B:** CT following contrast injection via the right arm shows the tumor (*T*) occupying the lung apex. Obstruction of the right subclavian vein (*arrow*) is associated with numerous venous collaterals in the chest wall. **C:** Coronal CT reformation shows the apical mass (*arrows*) extending along the chest wall.

A

FIG. 3.15. Superior sulcus tumor appearing as an apical cap with bone destruction and invasion of the brachial plexus. **A:** A right apical Pancoast tumor (*white arrow*) mimics pleural thickening. The underlying rib is partially destroyed (*black arrow*). **B:** CT shows a mass occupying the right apex, with focal rib destruction (*arrow*). **C:** T1-weighted MRI shows a mass in the right apex, with invasion of the brachial plexus (*white arrow*). The normal left brachial plexus is identified for comparison (*black arrow*).

25% of patients; atrophy or weakness of the hand muscles is uncommon. Rib or vertebral body invasion is common in patients with superior sulcus tumors.

Radiographic findings include an apical mass (60%; see Fig. 3-14), unilateral or asymmetrical apical pleural thickening ("apical cap," 40%; Fig. 3-15A), and bone destruction (25%). Asymmetry in the thickness of an apical cap exceeding 5 mm is considered suggestive. The presence of an apical cap may reflect diseases other than carcinoma (Table 3-10).

TABLE 3.10 Differential Diagnosis: Apical Cap/Apical Mass

Normal apical cap: Unilateral or bilateral apical caps, usually <5 mm in thickness, are each seen in 10% of normals on chest radiographs. These represent apical lung scars unassociated with tuberculosis, although their etiology is unclear.

Extrapleural fat: Extrapleural fat deposition can result in smooth, symmetrical apical caps. This can be seen in normals, obese patients, and patients with Cushing's syndrome or those receiving steroids.

Inflammatory disease (tuberculosis): Apical caps associated with inflammatory disease (particularly TB) are rarely the only abnormality visible. Associated upper lobe fibrosis, volume loss, lung destruction, or other evidence of inflammatory disease is usually present. The cap is often quite irregular in appearance because of adjacent lung abnormalities and in one study ranged from 5 to 27 mm in thickness (mean 16.5 mm). In patients with TB, thickened extrapleural fat accounts for most of the apical cap, variably associated with thickening of the pleura and atelectatic lung.

Superior sulcus carcinoma

Neural tumor or other posterior mediastinal mass: These are typically localized masses.

Mesothelioma: Diffuse pleural thickening is often seen.

Mediastinal hemorrhage: Mediastinal blood can dissect laterally in the extrapleural space over the lung apex, resulting in a smooth apical cap. This can be seen with traumatic aortic rupture and is more common on the left.

Radiation fibrosis: Radiation therapy can result in apical lung fibrosis mimicking an apical cap. This is most common following head and neck or supraclavicular node radiation.

Peripheral upper lobe collapse: Peripheral upper lobe collapse is said to be present when the peripheral part of a collapsed upper lobe is pancaked against the apical pleural surface (see Fig. 2-34). It has been reported in a variety of conditions, including inflammatory diseases and bronchial obstruction.

Superior sulcus carcinomas, even if invasive, can be treated using a combination of radiation and en bloc resection of the tumor and adjacent chest wall; 5-year survival rates as high as 30% to 35% have been reported using this approach. Contraindications to this combined therapy generally include (1) tumor involvement of the great vessels above the lung apex, principally the subclavian artery or vein; (2) extensive brachial plexus invasion; (3) extensive vertebral body or spinal canal invasion; (4) clinical evidence of recurrent laryngeal nerve or phrenic nerve involvement; (5) involvement of the mediastinum, including the trachea or esophagus; and (6) distant metastases. Some patients may have restaging of an extensive tumor following chemotherapy to determine whether resection is possible.

MRI in the sagittal or coronal planes is advantageous in imaging apical tumors. It is more accurate than CT in diagnosing apical chest wall invasion and its extent. MRI is often obtained preoperatively in patients with superior sulcus carcinoma to define the relationship of the tumor to great vessels and the brachial plexus (Figs. 3-15 and 3-16). The radiographic assessment of chest wall invasion and superior sulcus tumor is discussed in detail in the section on lung cancer staging below.

A

B

C

FIG. 3.16. MRI of superior sulcus tumor. **A:** Coronal T1-weighted image shows an apical mass (*M*) with extension into the chest wall. **B:** Sagittal T1-weighted MRI shows the mass (*M*) occupying the lung apex. The left subclavian artery (*arrow*) appears normal. **C:** More laterally, the mass (*M*) invades the chest wall (*small arrow*) with narrowing of the left subclavian artery (*large arrow*).

TABLE 3.11 Differential Diagnosis of Bronchial Narrowing or Obstruction

Congenital (bronchial atresia, bronchogenic cyst, cartilage deficiency)
Primary malignant tumor
   Lung carcinoma
   Carcinoid and atypical carcinoid
   Salivary gland type carcinoma
   Sarcoma
Metastatic tumor
Lymphoma
Benign bronchial tumor (e.g., hamartoma)
Papilloma or papillomatosis
Granulomas
   Infectious (e.g., tuberculosis, fungal infection)
   Noninfectious (e.g., sarcoidosis, Wegener's granulomatosis)
Inflammatory stricture (many causes)
Malacia
   Postinflammatory
Polychondritis
Foreign body
Mucous plug
Infiltrative diseases (e.g., amyloidosis)
Compression by enlarged lymph nodes (many causes)
Broncholithiasis
Traumatic hematoma or bronchial fracture
Postoperative (e.g., lung transplantation)

Airway Abnormalities

Airway abnormalities are common in lung cancer. The segmental bronchi are most often involved by the primary tumor, followed in frequency by the lobar bronchi and the main bronchi. The trachea is rarely involved as the site of origin.

Radiographs or CT can show evidence of bronchial narrowing or obstruction, or abnormalities secondary to bronchial obstruction, such as mucous plugging, air trapping, atelectasis, or obstructive pneumonia. Although lung cancer is a common cause of bronchial obstruction, the differential diagnosis is long and should be kept in mind (Table 3-11).

Bronchial Abnormalities

Bronchial abnormalities sometimes can be recognized on chest radiographs in patients with lung cancer, but CT is much more sensitive. Abnormalities include

1. Narrowing or tapering of the bronchial lumen, a finding that reflects the tendency of lung carcinomas to infiltrate along the bronchial wall (Fig. 3-17A); a tapered narrowing, or "rat-tail," appearance of the bronchial lumen is highly suggestive of carcinoma.
2. Sharp cutoff of the bronchial lumen (see Fig. 3-17B)
3. An endobronchial mass, sessile, irregular, or polypoid in appearance (see Figs. 3-2A and 3-17C)
4. Bronchial wall thickening, most easily seen involving the posterior wall of the right upper lobe bronchus or bronchus intermedius (see Figs. 3-17D and 3-24B)

5. Smooth luminal narrowing caused by bronchial wall infiltration or bronchial compression by an extrinsic mass (see Figs. 3-17E and 3-24B).

CT is commonly used to identify bronchial abnormalities in patients with lung cancer, in conjunction with bronchoscopy. CT can serve to identify the bronchi involved by the mass, thus guiding bronchoscopy, and can better assess the presence and degree of tumor extension outside the bronchus.

Generally speaking, the CT findings of an endobronchial lesion, an abrupt bronchial occlusion, or bronchial wall irregularities correlate closely with what is seen at bronchoscopy, but the appearances of smooth luminal narrowing or tapered bronchial occlusion can be seen with either endobronchial disease or extrinsic mass.

Mucous Plugging

Rarely, an obstructing or partially obstructing tumor causes retention of mucus distal to the obstruction, while the lobe remains aerated because of collateral ventilation. This can result in a mucous plug or plugs visible on radiographs or CT (Fig. 3-18). It can be recognized on plain film or CT by its typical branching, "finger-in-a-glove," or clustered-grape appearance. On CT, mucous plugs appear low in attenuation.

More common causes of mucous plugging include asthma, allergic bronchopulmonary aspergillosis, and cystic fibrosis. In patients with these diseases, however, mucous plugs are usually multiple and bilateral. In a patient with focal mucous plugging, bronchoscopy is advisable to rule out an obstructing lesion. In addition to lung cancer, focal mucous plugging can result from benign tumors, strictures, or congenital bronchial atresia.

Air Trapping

An obstructing or partially obstructing carcinoma rarely causes air trapping within the lung distal to the tumor. If a lobar bronchus is involved, the volume of the lobe may be increased. If the lesion involves a main bronchus, the distal lung is of normal or slightly decreased volume on inspiration, but on expiration air trapping will be recognized. In some patients, bronchial obstruction and air trapping can be detected because of hypovascularity of the involved lobe or lung; poorly ventilated lung tends to be poorly perfused.

Tracheal Carcinoma

Less than 1% of lung carcinomas arise in the trachea. Squamous cell carcinoma and carcinomas of mucous gland origin (adenoid cystic carcinoma) occur in nearly equal numbers. Squamous cell carcinomas arise most commonly in the distal trachea (Fig. 3-19), near the carina, and may cause obstruction of a main bronchus; adenoid cystic carcinoma is most common in the proximal trachea and often arises from the posterior or lateral tracheal wall.

FIG. 3.17. Bronchial abnormalities in lung cancer. A: The left upper lobe bronchus is obstructed and shows a tapered narrowing or rat-tail appearance (*arrow*). Left upper lobe atelectasis is also present. **B:** Left upper lobe carcinoma (*arrow*) associated with sharp cutoff of the bronchial lumen. **C:** A polypoid carcinoma (*arrow*) is visible in the right lower lobe bronchus, outlined by a crescent of air. **D:** Thickening of the posterior wall of the right upper lobe bronchus (*arrows*) associated with right hilar carcinoma. This usually indicates bronchial infiltration. **E:** Narrowing of the left upper lobe and anterior segment bronchi (*arrows*) by a left hilar carcinoma. This may be caused by tumor infiltrating the bronchial wall or compression by an extrinsic mass.

A   B

FIG. 3.18. Mucous plugs in a patient with carcinoma and bronchial obstruction. **A:** Mucous plugs (*arrows*) fill lower lobe bronchi. Note that the mucus-filled bronchi lie adjacent to opacified pulmonary arteries. The distal lung remains aerated. **B:** At a higher level, a hilar mass (*M*) is associated with obstruction of the right lower lobe bronchus.

Radiographic studies may be important in suggesting the diagnosis, because symptoms are often late and nonspecific. Radiographic findings are similar to those seen with tumors affecting the bronchi. However, findings of obstructive pneumonitia or air trapping are not seen unless there is secondary involvement of a main bronchus. Focal tracheal narrowing associated with thickening of the right paratracheal stripe, a focal endotracheal lesion, or mediastinal mass are most commonly seen on radiographs (Fig. 3-20A). Invasion of the mediastinum may occur. If the mass extends posteriorly, esophageal obstruction can result (see Fig. 3-20B). If a tracheal lesion is suspected on plain radiographs, evaluation using CT and bronchoscopy is appropriate. Surgery can be curative if the diagnosis is made prior to mediastinal invasion. Tracheal tumors are also discussed in Chapter 22.

Atelectasis, Consolidation, and Diffuse Parenchymal Involvement

Obstructive Atelectasis and Consolidation

Almost half of all lung cancers demonstrate atelectasis and/or consolidation as a result of obstruction of the lobar, main, or segmental bronchi. Atelectasis is common; a segment, lobe, or entire lung may be involved (see Fig. 3-3). Infection with pneumonia or lung abscess can also result.

The degree of volume loss associated with obstructive atelectasis is variable. The affected lung may be completely airless and reduced to its minimum volume. Alternatively,

FIG. 3.19. Polypoid squamous cell carcinoma of the trachea. A rounded mass (*arrow*) is visible at the level of the carina.

A

FIG. 3.21. Obstructive pneumonia with mucous bronchograms. In a patient with a right hilar carcinoma, right lower lobe consolidation is associated with minimal volume loss. This is typical of obstructive pneumonia. Mucous bronchograms (*arrows*) are visible.

B

FIG. 3.20. Squamous cell carcinoma of the trachea with mediastinal invasion and esophageal involvement. **A:** Plain radiograph shows tracheal displacement to the right by a large mediastinal mass (*arrow*). Focal tracheal narrowing by an endobronchial mass is present. **B:** Esophagogram shows esophageal compression and narrowing (*arrows*) because of invasion by the tumor.

the obstructed lobe or lung may become filled with desquamated material, mucus, and fluid and lose little of its volume. In both instances the absence of air bronchograms is suggestive of obstruction (see Chapter 2).

Obstructive pneumonia is a common manifestation of bronchial obstruction in lung cancer and is visible in about 35% of patients with squamous cell carcinoma. This term refers to the presence of obstructive atelectasis, bronchial dilatation and mucous plugging, fibrosis, and parenchymal consolidation by lipid-filled macrophages and inflammatory cells. This entity is sometimes referred to as *endogenous lipoid pneumonia* or "golden pneumonia" because of its yellow color at gross pathology. Infection need not be present. On chest radiographs, lung consolidation and volume loss are typically present. On CT, bronchial obstruction by tumor, lung consolidation, and dilated fluid- or mucus-filled bronchi within the consolidated lung ("mucous bronchograms") are commonly seen, particularly when contrast infusion is used (Fig. 3-21). Air bronchograms are usually absent. However, air bronchograms are sometimes seen in the presence of a partially obstructing central bronchial lesion associated with collapse and consolidation. Areas of necrosis within the tumor mass or lung are sometimes visible using CT.

Typically, a lung carcinoma involves a single bronchus, resulting in collapse of the segment, lobe, or lung distal to the lesion. It has been suggested that the collapse of two segments or lobes that cannot be explained by the presence of a single endobronchial lesion (e.g., the right upper and middle lobes, with the lower lobe being normal) indicates that a benign process is much more likely than lung cancer. This association of two or more endobronchial lesion with benign disease has been termed the "double-lesion sign" (see Fig. 2-40 in Chapter 2). Rarely, a hilar lung carcinoma produces a double-lesion sign by arising in one bronchus and invading or compressing another. In any patient with persisting bronchial obstruction, regardless of what segments or lobes are involved, CT and bronchoscopy are advisable.

Consolidation in Bronchioloalveolar Carcinoma

Forty percent of BAC show radiographic findings of diffuse lung involvement by tumor; these are typically the mucinous subtype of BAC. Although most patients show a combination of findings, the predominant radiographic pattern of diffuse BAC is

1. Patchy, lobar, or diffuse consolidation, with air bronchograms (60%; see Figs. 3-8, 3-9, and 3-22A)

2. Multiple ill-defined nodules (30%; see Figs. 3-8B, 3-22B and C)

3. Patchy, lobar, or diffuse ground-glass opacity (10%)

Consolidation in patients with BAC is usually indistinguishable from pneumonia on plain films. However, in some patients, consolidation is associated with adjacent linear opacities or a spiculated margin, reflecting the same type of fibrotic response seen in patients with BAC who present with a solitary nodule.

On CT, the consolidation seen in patients with BAC is typically low in attenuation; this largely reflects the presence of watery fluid and mucus produced by the tumor. If a contrast agent is infused, enhancing pulmonary vessels can be seen within areas of consolidation; this has been termed the "CT angiogram sign" and reflects the low density of the consolidated lung (see Fig. 2-6 in Chapter 2). The CT angiogram sign is typical of BAC and should alert you to the possibility of this diagnosis, but it can also be seen with any other cause of consolidation, particularly when rapid contrast infusion

A

B

FIG. 3.22. Diffuse bronchioloalveolar carcinoma (BAC). **A:** BAC with bilateral lung consolidation. **B:** BAC with bilateral small ill-defined nodules. **C:** High-resolution CT in the same patient as in (**B**). shows diffuse small nodules.

C

FIG. 3.23. Lymphangitic spread of lung carcinoma. High-resolution CT shows typical findings of unilateral interlobular septal thickening (*black arrows*) and thickening of the peribronchovascular interstitium (*white arrows*). A right pleural effusion is also present.

is used. In BAC, lung consolidation is not associated with bronchial obstruction; however, air bronchograms may be absent because of fluid within the bronchi.

Ill-defined nodules associated with BAC reflect focal areas of consolidation and have characteristics typical of air-space nodules (see Figs. 3-8B and 3-22B). They usually measure from 5 mm to 1 cm in diameter but can be larger. On CT, they are usually centrilobular in location.

Lymphangitic Spread of Tumor

Lung carcinoma commonly spreads via the lymphatic system. Diffuse involvement of the pulmonary lymphatics results in the appearance of lymphangitic spread of carcinoma, often in association with hilar node enlargement and pleura effusion. The classic plain film appearance is a unilateral or asymmetrical increase in pulmonary interstitial markings, which may be associated with Kerley's B lines; however, atypical appearances are common. High-resolution CT typically shows interlobular septal thickening (Fig. 3-23), thickening of the peribronchovascular interstitium, and thickening of fissures.

Lymph Node Enlargement

Hilar and mediastinal node enlargement is detected radiographically in up to 35% of lung cancers at diagnosis, although 50% have evidence of node metastasis at surgery. The diagnosis of hilar and mediastinal mass and lymph node enlargement is discussed in detail in other chapters.

Hilar Mass or Lymph Node Enlargement

Hilar enlargement visible on radiographs can reflect the primary tumor arising in a central location (usually this results in a poorly marginated hilar mass that may be large; Fig. 3-24) or metastases to hilar lymph nodes from a peripheral lung primary (usually a well-defined hilar mass; Fig. 3-25). Hilar mass is common in squamous cell carcinoma. Enlargement of hilar lymph nodes in association with a central mass

A

B

FIG. 3.24. Right hilar carcinoma in a patient with asbestos exposure. **A:** Chest radiograph shows an ill-defined right hilar mass (*arrows*). This is typical of carcinoma originating in the hilum. Pleural thickening and calcification typical of asbestos exposure are visible. **B:** A large, poorly marginated right hilar mass surrounds and narrows the right upper lobe bronchus. This appearance is most typical of small cell carcinoma.

FIG. 3.25. Left hilar lymph node enlargement (*arrow*) due to metastasis from a peripheral cancer. The hilar mass is sharply marginated.

is characteristic of small cell carcinoma (see Table 3-8). Hilar enlargement is the first detectable radiographic finding in 10% to 15% of cases of lung cancer. Airway abnormalities (narrowing or obstruction) are common, but not invariably, seen in patients with a hilar mass or lymph node enlargement.

Mediastinal Mass or Lymph Node Enlargement

Mediastinal lymph node metastases are common in patients with lung carcinoma, occurring in up to 40% of patients at diagnosis, depending on the size, location, and cell type of the primary tumor. In patients with a small lung nodule as the only presenting finding, mediastinal metastases are found in approximately 20%. CT is most accurate in making this diagnosis.

Mediastinal lymph node enlargement is an uncommon plain film abnormality at initial presentation (see Table 3-8).

When visible radiographically, lymph node enlargement is usually limited to the middle mediastinum and is associated with a visible lung or hilar mass. The most common sites of mediastinal node enlargement seen on plain radiographs are the right paratracheal mediastinum for right-sided tumors and the aorticopulmonary window for left-sided tumors. The subcarinal lymph nodes are also commonly involved but are difficult to recognize on plain radiographs unless they are quite large. It is unusual for mediastinal lymph nodes to be involved radiographically without involvement of the hilum.

In some patients with lung carcinoma, a mediastinal mass may be the first and only presenting abnormality, occurring in the absence of a visible lung mass. Isolated mediastinal masses are usually associated with small cell carcinoma or poorly differentiated carcinoma.

Pleural Abnormalities

Pleural Effusions or Masses

Small pleural effusions are common in patients with lung cancer; pleural effusion occurs in 5% to 15% of patients. They can result from pleural metastases, lymphatic obstruction in the hilum or mediastinum, or inflammatory lung disease associated with bronchial obstruction. The term *malignant effusion* should be reserved for effusions containing malignant cells. The presence of a pleural effusion, particularly when bloody, indicates a poor prognosis in lung cancer, but only a malignant effusion rules out surgical treatment.

Decubitus radiographs, ultrasound, and CT are sensitive methods of detecting pleural effusion. On CT, the presence of pleural thickening or nodularity in association with effusion should be considered highly suspicious for malignancy. However, malignant effusions commonly occur without visible pleural thickening. Extensive involvement of the pleural space mimicking malignant mesothelioma is sometimes seen, particularly in patients with adenocarcinoma.

A   **B**

FIG. 3.26. Cavitary squamous cell carcinoma with pneumothorax shown on chest radiograph (**A**) and CT (**B**).

FIG. 3.27. Pneumothorax ex vacuo in small cell carcinoma obstructing the right upper lobe bronchus. **A:** Chest radiograph shows a right hilar mass and right upper lobe collapse associated with an apical pneumothorax (*arrows*). **B:** CT shows right upper lobe (*RUL*) collapse capped by a pneumothorax (*arrows*). The right upper lobe bronchus is obstructed and invisible. This appearance is typical of pneumothorax ex vacuo.

Pneumothorax

Spontaneous pneumothorax is rare with bronchogenic carcinoma and usually results from direct invasion of the visceral pleura or cavitation (Fig. 3-26). Occasionally airway obstruction due to a proximal endobronchial lesion causes rupture of a subpleural bulla, producing a pneumothorax.

Pneumothorax ex vacuo is an unusual occurrence in lung cancer. It occurs in the presence of acute lobar collapse due to bronchial obstruction. A sudden decrease in intrapleural pressure around the collapsed lobe results in gas being drawn from blood and tissues into the pleural space. Radiographs or CT scans show a crescentic gas collection localized to the pleural space surrounding the collapsed lobe (Fig. 3-27). It is most common with right upper lobe tumors and resolves with alleviation of the obstruction.

Missed Lung Cancer

Lung cancers presenting as a solitary nodule may be difficult to see on chest radiographs. The *conspicuity* of a lesion is determined by (1) the sharpness of its edge, (2) the visual complexity of the region in which it is seen, (3) its size, and (4) its density. Cancers are usually missed on chest radiographs because of their poor conspicuity, being ill-defined, located in areas that are complex and difficult to evaluate (e.g., in the lung apex, in the perihilar lung regions, in the posterior costophrenic angle, and projected below the dome of the diaphragm), or small.

Lung cancers smaller than 5 mm are very difficult to see on chest radiographs, but many missed cancers are not small. Missed cancers average about 1.5 cm in diameter but may be more than 3 cm. On chest radiographs, most (80%) missed cancers are in an upper lobe, with the right upper lobe being the most common site (50% of missed cancers). Lung cancers are more commonly missed in women than in men. Lateral radiographs may show the lesion better than frontal films.

Cancers may be missed when films are interpreted prospectively, but visible in retrospect. This does not imply malpractice. The detection rate on plain films for nodules 1 cm in diameter ranges from 40% to 90%. In patients with inconspicuous lesions, as many as 25% of visible lung cancers are missed by experienced observers, even if they know a cancer is present.

Cancers may also be missed using CT, even when the purpose of the scan is lung cancer screening and the reader's suspicion is high. Missed cancers may be small and endobronchial or may present as solitary nodules. Missed solitary nodules are usually small (often less than 3 mm), indistinguishable from adjacent vessels or other lung disease (e.g., old tuberculosis), poorly defined and of ground-glass opacity, or may mimic air-space consolidation or pleural thickening. Cancers missed on CT are often present in a lower lobe. The presence of other significant abnormalities on the CT scan may distract the observer. Missing something because the reader sees something else that is more obvious is termed *satisfaction of search*.

CLINICAL MANIFESTATIONS OF LUNG CANCER

Lung cancer is more common in men and most frequently presents in patients in their 50s and 60s. It is uncommon in patients less than 30 years of age. The clinical manifestations of lung carcinoma result from the following:

1. Local tumor growth
2. Intrathoracic metastases
3. Extrathoracic metastases
4. A paraneoplastic syndrome

Local Tumor Growth and Intrathoracic Metastases

Symptoms associated with lung cancer are largely nonspecific and are present in a minority of patients when the tumor is first detected radiographically (Table 3-12). Most patients with cancer are smokers and have a history of chronic cough; any change in their pattern of cough or sputum production should be considered significant.

Symptoms are most common in patients with central carcinomas involving large bronchi or mediastinal structures, and in patients with tumors metastatic to hilar or mediastinal lymph nodes. Symptoms of central carcinoma can include the following:

1. Bronchial obstruction with cough, hemoptysis, wheezing, dyspnea, or fever due to postobstructive pneumonia
2. Hoarseness from involvement of the recurrent laryngeal nerve
3. SVC syndrome resulting from mediastinal invasion or metastases
4. Dysphagia from esophageal invasion or compression
5. Chylothorax from involvement of the thoracic duct
6. Diaphragmatic paralysis from involvement of the phrenic nerve

Peripheral lung cancers can be associated with pleural or chest wall invasion, resulting in chest pain, dyspnea, or cough. At autopsy, about 10% of patients with lung cancer have chest wall involvement by direct extension. Peripheral carcinomas in the superior sulcus can produce Pancoast syndrome.

Superior Vena Cava Syndrome

Obstruction or narrowing of mediastinal vessels as a result of mediastinal invasion or lymph node metastases is a relatively common manifestation of lung cancer. Because of its location and relatively thin wall, the SVC is particularly susceptible to involvement by tumor. SVC obstruction is associated with the *SVC syndrome*. About 65% to 85% of cases of SVC syndrome are caused by lung carcinoma. Symptoms and signs of SVC syndrome include the following:

1. Facial fullness, flushing, and cyanosis
2. Headache
3. Edema of the upper extremities
4. Prominent veins on the face and upper chest

Other common causes of SVC syndrome include granulomatous diseases such as histoplasmosis or tuberculosis involving the mediastinum (granulomatous mediastinitis), and venous thrombosis.

Extrathoracic Metastases

Small cell carcinoma grows rapidly and tends to metastasize early. Adenocarcinoma may grow slowly but metastasizes early. Squamous cell carcinoma may grow rapidly but tends to metastasize late.

Hematogenous spread to many sites has been reported with lung cancer, but the central nervous system, bones, liver, and adrenal glands are most commonly involved. Such metastases preclude successful surgical resection. The use of imaging studies to detect distant metastases in lung cancer patients is discussed below.

Paraneoplastic Syndromes

Paraneoplastic syndromes are disorders associated with malignant neoplasms but not directly related to the physical effects of the primary tumor. Such syndromes are present in 10% of patients with lung carcinoma (20% of those with small cell carcinoma) and result from the production of hormones or peptides by the tumor, antigen–antibody interactions resulting from tumor products, or neurovascular mechanisms. They may precede pulmonary findings by months or even years. A large variety of manifestations have been reported.

Hypertrophic Pulmonary Osteoarthropathy

Digital clubbing and hypertrophic pulmonary osteoarthropathy (HPO) are the most common cutaneous disorders. Eighty percent of cases of HPO in adults are due to lung

TABLE 3.12 Symptoms in Patients with Lung Cancer

Symptom	Patients With Symptom (%)
Cough	75
Dyspnea	60
Chest pain	45
Hemoptysis	35
Hypertrophic pulmonary osteoarthropathy	10
Hoarseness	10
Wheezing	2

cancer. Squamous cell carcinoma is most commonly associated with HPO; HPO is uncommon with small cell carcinoma. Relief of symptoms typically follows resection of the primary neoplasm. Pulmonary osteoarthropathy may precede discovery of the lung neoplasm by up to 2 years.

Vascular Disorders

Thrombophlebitis has an increased incidence in lung cancer patients and is most common with adenocarcinoma.

Endocrine Disorders

Cushing's syndrome, resulting from tumor secretion of ectopic adrenocorticotrophic hormone (ACTH), consists of weakness, hyperglycemia, polyuria, and hypokalemic alkalosis; in patients with lung cancer it is typically of rapid onset and progression. It can be associated with any cell type of tumor. Cushing's syndrome is most common in patients with carcinoid tumor, and approximately 30% of patients with an ectopic cause of this syndrome have a bronchial carcinoid tumor. Small cell carcinoma is associated with Cushing's syndrome in less than 5% of cases, at least partially because of the short life expectancy of patients with this tumor.

Hypercalcemia associated with lung cancer is most common with squamous cell carcinoma. Occasionally it is associated with bone metastases, but it is more often due to production of a peptide similar to parathyroid hormone. Other mediators such as prostaglandin have also been implicated in hypercalcemia.

Inappropriate antidiuretic hormone secretion, resulting in hyponatremia, is usually associated with small cell carcinoma. Although 50% of patients with small cell carcinoma have elevated levels of antidiuretic hormone, only 10% to 15% have hyponatremia, and less than 5% of patients have symptoms attributable to this syndrome.

Neuromuscular Syndromes

Neuromuscular syndromes associated with lung cancer may result from immunologic mechanisms. Small cell carcinoma is most commonly responsible. Symptoms may precede the diagnosis of the tumor or may be the first sign of recurrence.

Eaton-Lambert syndrome is characterized by proximal muscle weakness similar to myasthenia gravis, with the exception that muscle strength increases (rather than decreases) with use. Hyporeflexia and autonomic dysfunction are also parts of this syndrome. Small cell carcinoma is the most common malignant tumor associated with Eaton-Lambert syndrome; it can also be seen with extrathoracic tumors, and approximately 50% of cases are not associated with a detectable tumor. This syndrome apparently results from the production of anti–calcium channel antibodies, which impairs the release of acetylcholine.

Peripheral neuropathy is associated with small cell carcinoma and less often with squamous cell carcinoma and adenocarcinoma. Antineuronal nuclear antibodies are likely involved. Chronic intestinal pseudoobstruction, limbic encephalitis, necrotizing myelopathy, and visual paraneoplastic syndrome also occur with small cell carcinoma and are associated with antineuronal nuclear antibodies. Symptoms from the neuropathy may precede the discovery of the carcinoma by years; however, in most cases, advanced disease is present.

Other neuromuscular manifestations include subacute cerebellar degeneration (ataxia, vertigo, uncoordination) and dementia.

STAGING OF LUNG CANCER

In patients with lung cancer, both the cell type of the tumor and the tumor extent affect prognosis and survival following treatment. However, the anatomic extent of the tumor at diagnosis is usually most important in determining what therapeutic approach will be chosen. Imaging studies play a fundamental role in determining the extent of tumor, or in other words, its anatomic stage.

Lung cancer is staged using a TNM classification, which is based on a combination of findings: the location and morphologic characteristics of the primary tumor (T), the presence or absence of hilar, mediastinal, or other lymphadenopathy (N), and the presence or absence of distant metastases (M). In 2009, revisions to the TNM staging system, which had been in use since 1997 (TNM5) were recommended, based on evaluation of a large number of lung cancer patients from around the world. The revised staging system (TNM7) is shown in detail in Tables 3-13 and 3-14 and in Figure 3-28A. Using this classification, excellent correlations can be made between tumor stage and survival after treatment (see Fig. 3-28B).

Use of the TNM system is most appropriate for patients with nonsmall cell lung cancer (NSCLC). Small cell carcinoma has a very poor prognosis regardless of tumor stage and is often associated with metastases at the time of diagnosis. However, staging of early small cell carcinoma using the TNM classification is recommended.

The manner in which NSCLC is treated is fundamentally based on the tumor stage, although treatment may vary in individual cases, depending on a variety of factors such as the histology and genetics of the tumor, and is subject to continued reassessment in clinical trials. Stage I and II tumors are usually treated by resection, sometimes with adjuvant chemotherapy; Stage IIIA tumors are often treated by radiation or chemotherapy followed by resection (if anatomically possible); Stage IIIB by radiation, chemotherapy, or both; and Stage IV by chemotherapy (Table 3-15).

In radiologic lung cancer staging, it is most important to determine which patients have localized disease and are likely to benefit from surgical resection, and alternatively, which patients have extensive disease not amenable to surgical

TABLE 3.13 TNM Staging of Lung Cancer (TNM 7, 2009)

T	Primary tumor
T0	No evidence of a primary tumor
T1	A tumor that is
	a. 3 cm or less in greatest diameter
	T1a ≤ 2 cm
	T1b > 2 cm but ≤ 3 cm
	b. Surrounded by lung or visceral pleura
	c. Without invasion proximal to a lobar bronchus (i.e., not involving main bronchus)
T2	A tumor with any of the following features:
	a. Larger than 3 cm and less than or equal to 7 cm in greatest diameter
	T2a > 3 cm but ≤ 5 cm
	T2b > 5 cm but ≤ 7 cm
	b. Invades the visceral pleura
	c. Involves a main bronchus ≥ 2 cm distal to the carina
	d. Associated with atelectasis or obstructive pneumonia, extending to the hilum, but involving less than the entire lung
T3	A tumor with any of the following features:
	a. Larger than 7 cm (i.e., $T3_{>7}$)
	b. Associated with additional tumor nodule(s) in the same lobe (i.e., $T3_{Satell}$)
	c. Invades chest wall, diaphragm, phrenic nerve, mediastinal pleura, or parietal pericardium (i.e., $T3_{Inv}$)
	d. Involves the main bronchus <2 cm distal to the carina, without involvement of the carina (i.e., $T3_{Centr}$)
	e. Associated with atelectasis or obstructive pneumonia of an entire lung (i.e., $T3_{Centr}$)
T4	A tumor of any size with any of the following features:
	a. Invasion of the heart, great vessels, trachea, carina, recurrent laryngeal nerve, esophagus, or vertebral body (i.e., $T4_{Inv}$)
	b. Additional tumor nodule(s) in another ipsilateral lobe (i.e., $T4_{Ipsi Nod}$)
N	**Regional lymph nodes**
N0	No regional lymph node metastases
N1	Metastases to ipsilateral peribronchial, perihilar, or intrapulmonary nodes, including direct extension
N2	Metastases to ipsilateral mediastinal nodes or subcarinal nodes
N3	Metastases to contralateral hilar or mediastinal lymph nodes, or scalene or supraclavicular lymph nodes
M	**Distant metastases**
M0	Metastases absent
M1	Metastases present
M1a	Intrathoracic metastases, with either
	a. tumor nodules in the contralateral lung (i.e., $M1a_{Contr Nod}$)
	b. tumor with pleural nodules or malignant pleural effusion (i.e., $M1a_{Pl Dissem}$) (pleural effusion not obviously associated with metastases has no effect on stage)
M1b	Distant metastases

(Modified from **Rami-Porta R, Crowley JJ, Goldstraw P**. The revised TNM staging system for lung cancer. Ann Thorac Cardiovasc Surg 2009; 15:4–9 and **Detterbeck FC, Boffa DJ, Tanoue LT**. The new lung cancer staging system. Chest 2009; 136:260–271.)

TABLE 3.14 Lung Cancer Staging Groups (TNM7, 2009)

Stage Groups	T	N	M
Ia	T1a,b	N0	M0
Ib	T2a	N0	M0
IIa	T1a,b	N1	M0
	T2a	N1	M0
	T2b	N0	M0
IIb	T2b	N1	M0
	T3	N0	M0
IIIa	T1-3	N2	M0
	T3	N1	M0
	T4	N0,1	M0
IIIb	any T	N3	M0
	T4	N2	M0
IV	any T	any N	M1a,b

(Modified from **Rami-Porta R, Crowley JJ, Goldstraw P**. The revised TNM staging system for lung cancer. Ann Thorac Cardiovasc Surg 2009; 15:4–9 and **Detterbeck FC, Boffa DJ, Tanoue LT**. The new lung cancer staging system. Chest 2009; 136:260–271.)

treatment. Generally speaking, tumors are considered to be unresectable if they are classified as T4, N3, or M1. An exception are invasive T4 carcinomas without or with hilar lymph node metastases; such tumors are often restaged after chemotherapy or radiation, and treated surgically if significant reduction in tumor volume and extent makes resection possible.

Different surgeons have different anatomic criteria for considering a tumor to be unresectable, and a careful and detailed discussion of the radiographic findings with the surgeon is necessary. Generally, you should be reluctant to make a dogmatic statement about resectability solely on the basis of the radiographic findings (which in themselves may be nonspecific). The results of imaging studies must be considered in the framework of what diagnostic or therapeutic options are available.

Primary Tumor (T Descriptor)

The primary tumor is classified using one of four T designations. Each designation delineates criteria for tumors originating in, or involving, the lung or bronchial tree.

T1 Carcinoma

A T1 carcinoma usually presents as a small peripheral nodule (defined as 3 cm or less) surrounded by lung or the visceral pleura (see Fig. 3-5B). In the 2009 staging system, T1 tumors presenting as a lung nodule are subclassified into those ≤2 cm (T1a) and those >2 cm but ≤3 cm (T1b), although these classifications do not affect the tumor stage. A tumor limited to a lobar bronchus is also considered to be T1 (see Fig. 3-17C). T1 tumors are easily resectable.

FIG. 3.28. Revised lung cancer staging classifications (TNM7). **A:** Lung cancer stage related to combinations of T, N, and M. To determine the stage, find the correct T class and go across the square until reaching the appropriate N class. M1 indicates Stage IV regardless of T or N. **B:** Five-year survival rates according to combinations of T, N, and M determined clinically (rather than pathologically). Survival decreases from the top left to bottom right of the diagram.

T2 Carcinoma

A lung mass larger than 3 cm, but 7 cm or less in diameter (see Fig. 3-4) is classified as T2, as is a tumor invading the visceral pleura. In the 2009 system, T2 carcinomas presenting as a mass are subdivided into those greater than 3 cm but ≤5 cm (T2a) and those greater than 5 cm but ≤7 cm (T2b). Tumor involving a main bronchus 2 cm or more from the carina or associated with atelectasis or obstructive pneumonia extending to the hilum is also classified as T2. Presentation as a lung mass and bronchial lesion are both common. T2 tumors are resectable.

T3 Carcinoma

In the 2009 staging system, a tumor greater than 7cm in diameter is classified as T3 (T3$_{>7}$), as is a tumor associated with small tumor nodule(s) (i.e., satellite nodules) in the

TABLE 3.15 Lung Cancer Treatment Related to Stage

Stage	Common Treatment
I	Resection
II	Resection
IIIA	Radiation or chemotherapy followed by resection
IIIB	Radiation and/or chemotherapy
IV	Chemotherapy

same lobe (T3$_{Satell}$) (Fig. 3-29). Tumors of any size that invade the chest wall (Fig. 3-30), diaphragm, mediastinal pleura, or parietal pericardium, without invasion of mediastinal structures are also considered T3 (T3$_{inv}$). A tumor involving a main bronchus less than 2 cm from the carina or associated with atelectasis or obstructive pneumonia of an entire lung is T3 (T3$_{Centr}$). These tumors are resectable with difficulty in many cases.

T4 Carcinoma

T4 carcinomas may present as a lung nodule, mass, or bronchial lesion resulting in one of the following:

1. Invasion of the chest wall with involvement of great vessels or vertebral body (T4$_{inv}$)
2. Invasion of the mediastinum with involvement of mediastinal fat, the heart, great vessels, trachea, or esophagus (T4$_{inv}$)
3. Invasion the tracheal carina in a patient with an airway tumor (T4$_{inv}$)
4. Additional nodule(s) in a different ipsilateral lobe (T4$_{Ipsi\ Nod}$)

FIG. 3.29. Right lower lobe carcinoma with a satellite nodule. This is classified as T3.

FIG. 3.30. Chest wall invasion classified as T3 in the lung cancer staging system. **A, B:** A small peripheral carcinoma is associated with pleural thickening (*white arrows*). The tumor has an obtuse angle at the point it contacts the pleura. These findings suggest chest wall invasion, but their specificity is limited. Also, tumor can be seen invading and thickening extrapleural soft tissues (*black arrow* in **B**).

Resectability of the Primary Tumor: Radiographic Assessment

When determining the primary tumor extent and T classification, several key observations need to be made, including the size of the tumor, its location within a bronchus, and its association with atelectasis or consolidation. However, of most importance in determining respectability is assessment of the specific features that indicate a T4 lesion.

Chest Wall Invasion

Direct invasion of the pleura and chest wall by a peripheral lung carcinoma may or may not indicate that the tumor is unresectable. Only extensive chest wall invasion rules out surgery.

Unless obvious rib destruction is present, the diagnosis of chest wall invasion on plain radiographs is difficult. However, several plan film findings suggest invasion. Pleural thickening adjacent to a lung mass suggests invasion but is nonspecific. Tumors with extensive contact with the pleural surface are more likely invasive than those with minimal contact. A tumor that appears to flatten out against the pleura (i.e., it appears sessile, lenticular, or crescentic in profile) may be invasive.

The accuracy of CT in diagnosing chest wall invasion is 70% to 80%, although sensitivity and specificity values vary from 40% to 90% in different studies. CT findings of value in the diagnosis of chest wall invasion (Figs. 3-31 and 3-32) include the presence of the following:

1. Obtuse angles or pleural thickening at the point of contact between tumor and pleura
2. More than 3 cm of contact between tumor and the pleural surface (5 cm of contact is more specific but less sensitive)
3. A ratio of the tumor diameter to the length of pleural contact by the tumor exceeding 0.5 (the higher this ratio, the more specific this finding)
4. Invisibility of extrapleural (chest wall) fat planes at the point tumor contacts chest wall

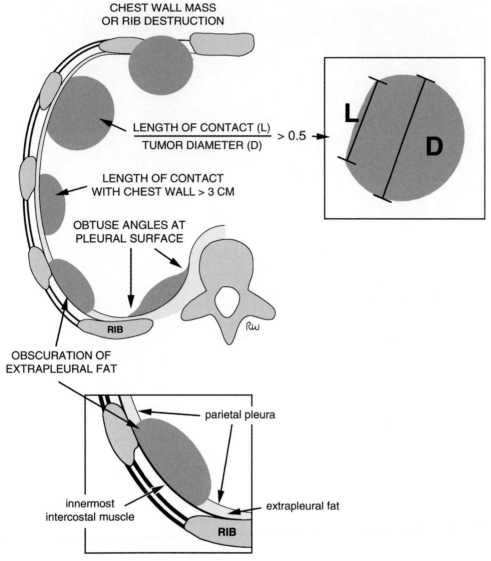

CHEST WALL MASS
OR RIB DESTRUCTION

$$\frac{\text{LENGTH OF CONTACT (L)}}{\text{TUMOR DIAMETER (D)}} > 0.5$$

LENGTH OF CONTACT
WITH CHEST WALL > 3 CM

OBTUSE ANGLES AT
PLEURAL SURFACE

RIB

OBSCURATION OF
EXTRAPLEURAL FAT

parietal pleura

innermost
intercostal muscle

extrapleural fat

RIB

EXTRAPLEURAL FAT INVASION - Detail View

FIG. 3.31. CT findings of chest wall invasion.

5. A mass involving the chest wall
6. Rib destruction

The only definite findings of chest wall invasion include rib destruction or chest wall infiltration or mass. Otherwise, invisibility of the extrapleural fat plane (sensitivity 85%, specificity 85%) and a ratio of tumor diameter to pleura contact exceeding 0.9 (sensitivity 85%, specificity 80%) are most accurate in predicting invasion (Table 3-16; see Fig. 3-32).

The demonstration of motion of the tumor relative to the chest wall during respiration indicates that no invasion is present; alternatively, the absence of motion during respiration suggests that invasion is present. This may be assessed using fluoroscopy, sonography, or dynamic spiral CT.

The extent of chest wall invasion adjacent to a lung tumor may be better shown using MRI than CT because of the better contrast between tumor and chest wall fat and muscle that can be obtained using MRI.

In patients with superior sulcus tumors, vertebral body invasion (Fig. 3-33A) and invasion of the great vessels above the lung apex (see Fig. 3-16) generally prevent surgical resection, although patients with such abnormalities may be restaged after radiation or chemotherapy. MRI in the sagittal or coronal planes can be advantageous in imaging apical tumors and is more accurate than CT in diagnosing chest wall invasion and its extent in this region. In patients with a superior sulcus tumor who are being considered for resection, MRI is recommended to determine the extent of chest wall invasion and possible involvement of the subclavian artery (Fig. 3-16) or brachial plexus (see Figs. 3-15 and 3-33B).

FIG. 3.32. CT findings of chest wall invasion in three patients. **A:** CT at three adjacent levels shows a lenticular mass having more than 3 cm of contact with the chest wall, obtuse angles at the point it contacts the chest wall (*white arrows*), and rib destruction (*black arrow*). **B:** There is extensive pleural contact, with the length of contact (*L*) being 5 cm. The tumor diameter (*D*) equals the length of pleural contact (i.e., their ratio is 1). Normal fat is seen in intercostal spaces (*small white arrows*), while these fat planes are invisible where the tumor contacts the chest wall (*small black arrows*). **C:** Chest wall invasion by lung cancer with rib destruction and a large chest wall mass.

TABLE 3.16 Accuracy of CT Findings for Diagnosing Chest Wall Invasion

CT Finding	Sensitivity (%)	Specificity (%)
Obtuse angles at pleural surface	60	75
Length of contact with chest wall		
>3 cm	95	40
>4 cm	90	55
>5 cm	75	70
Ratio of:		
Length of contact/tumor diameter		
>0.5	100	35
>0.7	90	60
>0.9	85	80
Obliteration of chest wall fat plane	85	85
Chest wall mass	33	100
Rib destruction	16	100

(Modified from **Ratto GB, Piacenza G, Frola C, et al**. Chest wall involvement by lung cancer: computed tomographic detection and results of operation. Ann Thorac Surg 1991; 51:182–188.)

Mediastinal Invasion

Contiguous invasion of the mediastinum by tumor, with involvement of the heart, great vessels, trachea, or esophagus, generally precludes resection, as does significant invasion of mediastinal fat. Invasion of the mediastinal pleura or parietal pericardium, or limited fat invasion, does not prevent resection.

On plain radiographs, findings that suggest mediastinal invasion include the presence of a mediastinal mass, extensive contact of tumor with the mediastinum (Fig. 3-34A), or diaphragmatic paralysis, which in turn implies involvement of the phrenic nerve.

CT is more accurate than plain radiographs in assessing mediastinal invasion. However, some caution in interpreting CT is necessary. Contiguity of tumor mass with the mediastinal pleura or thickening of the mediastinal pleura does not necessarily indicate mediastinal invasion. Also, not all findings indicative of mediastinal invasion indicate unresectability.

CT findings (Fig. 3-35A) usually regarded as indicating "definite" or "gross" mediastinal invasion and

A   **B**

FIG. 3.33. CT and MRI diagnosis of chest wall invasion. **A:** Vertebral invasion by lung carcinoma is shown using CT. Tumor (*T*) invades the vertebral body (*small arrow*) and spinal canal (*large arrow*). **B:** T1-weighted MRI shows brachial plexus invasion by a superior sulcus tumor (*white arrows*). Tumor (*black arrow*) surrounds the brachial plexus.

unresectability (although they are not 100% accurate) include the following:

1. Extensive replacement of mediastinal fat by soft-tissue mass (see Figs. 3-34B and 3-36)
2. Mass surrounding mediastinal vessels, trachea, or esophagus
3. Mass resulting in obvious invasion of one of these structures (see Fig. 3-36)

In lung cancer patients who do not have gross mediastinal invasion, additional CT findings may be of value in predicting that invasion of the mediastinum and mediastinal structures is present. These CT findings (see Figs. 3-35B and 3-37) include the following:

1. Tumor contact of more than 3 cm with the mediastinum
2. Tumor contact with more than one fourth (90 degrees) of the circumference of the aorta or other mediastinal structures
3. Obliteration of the fat planes that are normally seen adjacent to the aorta or other mediastinal structures
4. Compression of mediastinal structures by a mass
5. Mediastinal pleural or pericardial thickening

A   **B**

FIG. 3.34. Mediastinal invasion by lung cancer. **A:** Chest radiograph shows extensive contact of tumor with mediastinum. **B:** CT shows extensive contact of tumor with mediastinum and a mediastinal mass (*arrow*) contiguous with the lung tumor, with soft tissue replacing mediastinal fat.

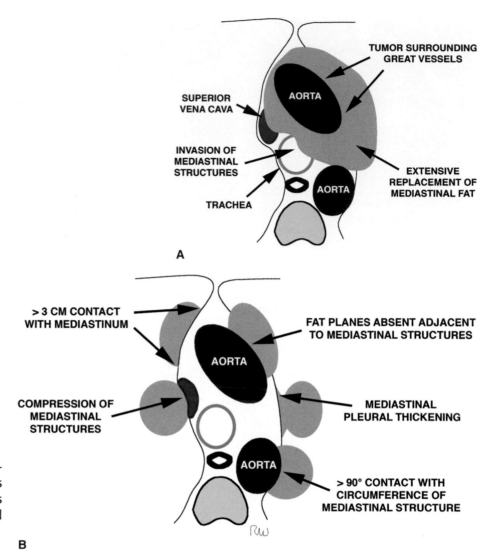

A

B

FIG. 3.35. CT findings of mediastinal invasion. **A:** Definite findings of mediastinal invasion. **B:** Less specific findings of mediastinal invasion.

FIG. 3.36. Mediastinal and superior vena cava (SVC) invasion by lung cancer. Tumor (*T*) has invaded mediastinal fat anterior to the carina. Invasion of the SVC with a tumor thrombus (∗) in its lumen is also visible.

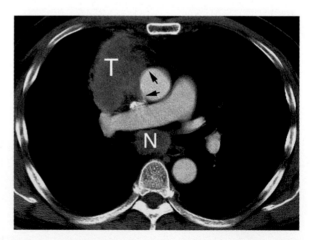

FIG. 3.37. Mediastinal invasion by lung cancer. A right upper lobe tumor (*T*) shows more than 3 cm of contact with the mediastinum, replaces mediastinal fat, obliterates the fat plane adjacent to the aorta, and contacts more than one fourth of its circumference (*arrows*). An enlarged subcarinal lymph node (*N*) is also seen.

TABLE 3.17 Accuracy of CT Findings for Diagnosing Mediastinal Invasion

CT Finding	Sensitivity (%)	Specificity (%)
Contact with mediastinum >3 cm	80	55
Contact with aorta >1/4 circumference	85	75
Absent mediastinal fat plane	90	10
Compression of mediastinal structure	35	75
Mediastinal pleural or pericardial thickening	40	80

(Modified from **Glazer HS, Kaiser LR, Anderson DJ, et al.** Indeterminate mediastinal invasion in bronchogenic carcinoma: CT evaluation. Radiology 1989; 173:37–42.)

The first three findings are highly sensitive but have poor specificity (Table 3-17). Because of the high sensitivity of these three findings, if they are all absent, the tumor will likely be resectable, even if mediastinal invasion is present. MRI does not have a great advantage in the diagnosis of mediastinal invasion unless the patient cannot have contrast-enhanced CT.

Tracheal and Central Bronchial Lesions

Although tumor masses that cause total lung collapse or consolidation or involve the proximal bronchus may be difficult to treat surgically, they are not generally considered unresectable unless they involve the tracheal carina or trachea (Figs. 3-19 and 3-38). In this situation, it is difficult to perform a pneumonectomy, resect the tumor, and surgically close the remaining airway. However, some surgeons may excise tumors that involve the carina or even the distal trachea, reanastomosing the tracheal stump to the remaining bronchus or bronchi.

In some patients, CT can demonstrate the relationship of a proximal tumor mass to the main bronchus, carina, or trachea (Fig. 3-19). CT findings that suggest carinal involvement include bronchial wall thickening that extends to the carina, or carinal thickening, blunting, or nodularity. However, bronchoscopy is more accurate in making this diagnosis. On bronchoscopy, minimal mucosal involvement by tumor can be diagnosed, while on CT or plain radiographs, only discrete masses are visible. Bronchoscopic confirmation of an apparent carinal or tracheal tumor is usually necessary unless the findings are gross.

Nodules in the Ipsilateral Lung

The presence of tumor nodules in a different ipsilateral lobe than the primary tumor indicates T4 but does not prevent resection. Since benign nodules are common, it should not be assumed that any nodule seen on CT represents a tumor. Also, a second primary lung cancer in a different lobe (a synchronous primary tumor) does not indicate T4.

Lymph Node Metastases (N Descriptor)

Descriptors of lymph node metastasis remain unchanged in the new staging system. N0 indicates the absence of lymph node metastases.

Hilar Lymph Node Metastases

The presence of a hilar mass on radiographs or CT may reflect a primary bronchial tumor with local extension (T1–T4 depending on its location) or hilar lymph node metastases (N1; see Fig. 3-25). Hilar involvement by a carcinoma does not generally affect resectability. However, the presence of hilar tumor often means that a pneumonectomy rather than lobectomy needs to be performed. In patients with poor respiratory function who cannot tolerate a pneumonectomy, the presence of hilar metastases may make them inoperable despite the fact that the tumor itself is technically resectable.

CT is superior to plain radiographs in evaluating the pulmonary hila. CT findings of bronchial obstruction or narrowing correlate closely with bronchoscopic findings (see Fig. 3-17). CT is quite accurate in showing hilar lymph enlargement; generally a least (short axis) lymph node diameter of 1 cm is used to distinguish normal from abnormal lymph nodes. However, the sensitivity and specificity of CT for the diagnosis of hilar lymph node metastases are limited, respectively, by the presence of microscopic metastases in normal sized nodes and enlarged lymph nodes that are benign hyperplastic. Very large (more than 2 cm) hilar lymph nodes in a lung cancer patient usually are associated with metastases.

FIG. 3.38. Tracheal invasion by a right hilar carcinoma. Right lung atelectasis is due to a carcinoma arising in the right main bronchus. Tumor invades the trachea (*arrow*), precluding resection.

A   B

FIG. 3.39. Mediastinal lymph node metastases from small cell carcinoma. **A, B:** A large right hilar mass (*M*) is associated with lymph node enlargement in the subcarinal space (*S*), pretracheal space (*P*), anterior mediastinum (*A*), and the contralateral mediastinum (*large arrows*). Right pleural thickening and effusion (*small arrows*) are due to pleural metastases. The large bulky mediastinal nodes and contralateral nodes (N3) preclude resection.

Assessment of Mediastinal Lymph Nodes

Because large or bulky mediastinal masses in patients with lung cancer are considered unresectable by most surgeons, a patient who has a mediastinal mass visible on plain radiographs (indicating its large size) is not likely a surgical candidate. In such patients, CT followed by mediastinoscopy or biopsy should be performed to confirm the presence of mediastinal disease.

CT is helpful in detecting lymph node enlargement in patients with lung carcinoma who have normal plain radiographs. By convention, a short axis (least diameter) lymph node diameter of 1 cm is commonly used on CT to distinguish normal from abnormal nodes. The short axis of a mediastinal lymph node rather than its long axis correlates most closely with the actual lymph node diameter and volume measured pathologically. However, normal lymph node size varies with the lymph node group being assessed (see Chapter 8). An upper limit of 1.5 cm is usually used for the nodes in the subcarinal space (see Fig. 3-37). Lymph nodes containing metastases are quite variable in size, although those larger than 2 cm are nearly always involved by tumor (Fig. 3-39).

The accuracy of CT in predicting the presence or absence of mediastinal node metastases on the basis of node diameter is limited by two factors. On the one hand, the sensitivity of CT in diagnosing lymph node metastases is reduced by the common occurrence of microscopic lymph node metastases not resulting in increased lymph node size; on the other hand, specificity is reduced by the presence of enlarged benign hyperplastic lymph nodes, particularly in patients with squamous cell carcinoma.

A number of studies evaluating the accuracy of CT in diagnosing mediastinal node metastases from lung carcinoma have been performed. An assessment of the accuracy of CT in diagnosing mediastinal metastases must be based on a correlation of CT findings with surgical exploration (total nodal sampling) and histologic analysis. When total nodal sampling is performed, the average accuracy of CT ranges from about 67% to 79%, with a sensitivity of 60% to 79%. Improvements in CT technology and attempts to refine the criteria for determining nodes to be normal or abnormal have had little effect on accuracy.

Furthermore, in patients who have enlarged mediastinal nodes on CT, nodal metastases found at surgery are not always in the nodes that appear large on CT. Thus, the sensitivity of CT in diagnosing mediastinal node metastases on a patient-by-patient basis is higher than its sensitivity in detecting metastases in a specific node or node group (about 40%). In general, MR is similar to CT in its ability to detect and define mediastinal lymph nodes, and its accuracy in diagnosing mediastinal metastases is similar to that of CT.

Stage and Resectability

Ipsilateral mediastinal or subcarinal node metastases are classified N2 and are considered potentially resectable, usually following preoperative chemotherapy, but this remains the subject of investigation. Contralateral hilar or mediastinal node metastases or supraclavicular or scalene lymph node metastases are considered N3 and unresectable (see Fig. 3-39). Treatment usually includes chemotherapy.

The American Joint Committee on Cancer (AJCC) and the Union Internationale Contre le Cancer (UICC) have proposed a numeric system for localizing intrathoracic lymph nodes for the purpose of lung cancer staging (described in detail in Chapter 8); this represents a modification of the system devised by the American Thoracic Society. According to the AJCC/UICC system of lymph node localization ("lymph node stations") in patients with lung cancer, the tracheal midline is used to distinguish ipsilateral nodes from contralateral nodes, although this is somewhat arbitrary and does not necessarily correlate with pathways of lymphatic spread or ease of resection of the abnormal lymph nodes. In the 2009 modification of the TNM staging system (TNM7), a simplification of this numerical system into nodal zones has been recommended. These include only four N2 zones (upper, aortopulmonary, subcarinal, and lower) and two N1 zones (hilar and peripheral).

The survival of patients with nodal metastases can be stratified into three groups by the number and location of nodal zones involved. Involvement of a single N1 zone has a 5-year survival of 48%; multiple N1 zones and a single N2 zone have a 5-year survival rates of 35% and 34%, respectively; multiple N2 zones have a 5-year survival of 20%.

CT and Mediastinoscopy

CT is helpful in determining which patients should have mediastinoscopy prior to surgery. In general, patients who have enlarged mediastinal lymph nodes seen on CT have mediastinoscopy prior to surgery; patients with normal-sized mediastinal lymph nodes on CT often have surgery without mediastinoscopy. This approach, however, varies among surgeons, and some perform mediastinoscopy routinely.

CT is also used as a guide for invasive procedures performed before an attempt at curative resection. Although mediastinoscopy is generally regarded as the gold standard of preoperative mediastinal evaluation, routine mediastinoscopy through a suprasternal incision does not evaluate all mediastinal compartments or lymph node groups. A significant percentage (up to 30%) of patients with lung carcinoma who have a negative mediastinoscopy prove to have mediastinal nodal metastases at surgery.

Routine mediastinoscopy can evaluate pretracheal lymph nodes, nodes in the anterior subcarinal space, and lymph nodes extending anterior to the right main bronchus (Fig. 3-40A). Lymph nodes in the anterior mediastinum (prevascular space), aortopulmonary window, and posterior portions of the mediastinum (e.g., posterior subcarinal space, azygoesophageal recess) are generally inaccessible using this technique (see Fig. 3-40B), although some of these can be evaluated using a left parasternal mediastinoscopy (Chamberlain procedure). CT can serve to guide the mediastinoscopist to the most suspicious lymph nodes. It may also suggest that needle aspiration biopsy, transbronchoscopic needle aspiration biopsy, or parasternal mediastinotomy would be appropriate.

Positron Emission Tomography

The use of positron emission tomography (PET) following injection of 2-[fluorine-18]-fluoro-2-deoxy-D-glucose (FDG) is becoming routine for lung cancer staging where available. PET is significantly more sensitive and specific (80%

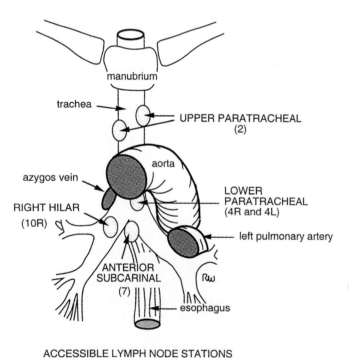

FIG. 3.40. Mediastinal nodes accessible (**A**) and inaccessible (**B**) at routine mediastinoscopy performed through a suprasternal incision, as viewed from the front. Numbers indicate the corresponding AJCC/UICC lymph node stations (see Chapter 8).

FIG. 3.41. Mediastinal lymph node metastasis diagnosed using FDG-PET. A metabolically active left upper lobe carcinoma (*small arrow*) is associated with a lymph node metastasis (*large arrow*) in the aortopulmonary window. High activity is also seen in the myocardium and brain.

to 95%) in diagnosing mediastinal lymph node metastases in lung cancer than is CT (60% to 70% sensitivity and specificity; Fig. 3-41). Lymph node metastases may be diagnosed using PET when lymph nodes appear normal on CT.

PET may also be used to diagnose a lung nodule as malignant, with similar sensitivity and specificity (see Chapter 9). Scans are evaluated quantitatively using the *standardized uptake value* (SUV), which compares the activity of a lesion to that of other tissues. A SUV of more than 2.5 is usually used to diagnose lung cancer or metastases; benign lesions have a lower SUV. Because of the high sensitivity of PET, mediastinoscopy can be reserved for patients with a positive scan. However, the anatomic resolution of PET is quite limited, and it should be combined with CT when staging the mediastinum.

Metastases (M Descriptor)

M0 indicated the absence of metastases. In the 2009 system, metastases (M1) are subclassified as either intrathoracic or extrathoracic (distant), although these classifications do not affect the tumor stage (Stage IV). Intrathoracic metastases, subclassified as M1a, include (a) tumor nodule(s) in the contralateral lung (M1a$_{Contr\ Nod}$), (b) pleural tumor nodules or malignant pleural effusion (M1a$_{Pl\ Dissem}$). Distant metastases are subclassified as M1b. Distant metastases are present at diagnosis in 10% to 35% of patients with NSCLC; they are most common with adenocarcinoma or large cell carcinoma.

Tumor Nodules in the Contralateral Lung

As with nodules in the same lobe as the primary tumor, or the same lung, contralateral pulmonary nodules seen on CT may be benign, and cannot be assumed to represent metastases. Also keep in mind that a contralateral lung tumor may represent a synchronous primary lung cancer.

Malignant Pleural Effusion and Pleural Nodules

In a patient with lung carcinoma, pleural effusion can occur for a variety of reasons, including pleural invasion, obstructive pneumonia, and lymphatic or pulmonary venous obstruction by the tumor. Although the presence of effusion indicates a poor prognosis, only patients who have tumor cells in the pleural fluid (i.e., a *malignant effusion*) or on pleural biopsy are considered to have unresectable disease. Patients with other causes of effusion are considered to have resectable lesions despite their poor prognosis; nonmalignant effusion has no effect on stage classification. Usually plain radiographs are sufficient for the diagnosis of pleural effusion, leading to thoracentesis or pleural biopsy. On CT, the presence of pleural thickening or pleural nodules in association with pleural effusion should be considered highly suspicious for malignancy (see Chapter 26). However, malignant effusions can occur without pleural thickening (Fig. 3-42), and pleural thickening can be seen in many cases of benign exudative pleural effusion.

In patients with a lung cancer involving the pleural surface, small pleural nodules may indicate the presence of pleural dissemination. They may be seen in the peripheral pleural space or within a fissure, and with or without a pleural effusion.

Distant metastases

Approximately 60% to 65% of patients with small cell carcinoma have detectable distant metastases at diagnosis, and many of the rest have microscopic metastases. Distant metastases rule out surgery; patients are treated with chemotherapy and have a poor prognosis.

Common sites of extrathoracic spread in patients with NSCLC include the adrenal glands, liver, bone, and brain.

History, physical examination (including a detailed neurologic evaluation), and blood tests (including liver function tests and serum calcium and alkaline phosphatase determinations) are used to suggest possible metastatic sites but are limited in accuracy. Imaging studies including radionuclide bone scanning with technetium 99m-methylene diphosphonate, contrast-enhanced brain and abdominal CT, brain and abdominal MRI, abdominal ultrasound, and FDG-PET are used to confirm organ-specific involvement as suggested by the clinical findings, although recommendations vary. Whole-body PET scanning is particularly useful in assessing distant metastases, except for those involving the brain (because of the high background activity of brain).

Adrenal metastases are present in up to 20% of patients with NSCLC at diagnosis and are often the only site of

FIG. 3.42. Malignant effusion in lung cancer. A: Chest radiograph shows a large left pleural effusion with mediastinal shift to the right. **B:** CT shows a tapered obstruction (rat-tail appearance) of the left lower lobe bronchus associated with left lower lobe collapse. There is no evidence of pleural thickening.

extrathoracic spread. Because of this, a chest CT in patients with lung cancer should be extended to encompass the upper abdomen. However, adrenal adenomas are common (3% to 5%) in the general population, and as many as 65% of small (less than 3 cm) adrenal masses in patients with lung cancer represent an adrenal adenoma rather than a metastasis. Although CT without contrast infusion and enhanced CT with delayed images can be helpful in distinguishing benign and malignant adrenal lesions, they may be nonspecific. Other methods of evaluating an adrenal mass include FDG-PET (which is highly accurate), chemical-shift MRI, and biopsy.

Liver metastases are present in 5% to 15% of cases. Their appearance on routine staging CT is often nonspecific and difficult to distinguish from cysts, hemangiomas, or other lesions without further imaging. However, isolated liver metastases are uncommon. CT, MRI, or FDG-PET may be used for diagnosing liver metastases.

Skeletal metastases are present at diagnosis in 5% to 20% of patients with lung carcinoma; they are present at autopsy in up to 30%. Squamous cell carcinoma and large cell carcinoma tend to cause osteolytic lesions, while small cell carcinoma and adenocarcinoma produce osteolytic or osteoblastic metastases. The bones most commonly involved are the vertebrae, pelvic bones, and proximal long bones. Metastases to the distal extremities are unusual, but lung carcinoma is the most common cause of distal metastases. Radionuclide imaging should be reserved for patients with symptoms or biochemical abnormalities and has a high false-positive rate (40%). FDG-PET scanning also allows detection of metastases and has a lower false-positive rate.

Central nervous system metastases are common and are often symptomatic (although the symptoms may be vague). However, asymptomatic brain metastases occur in up to 15% of patients with NSCLC and have a higher incidence with adenocarcinoma and large cell carcinoma than with other cell types. Consequently, routine brain CT or MRI is recommended in asymptomatic patients with these tumors. With other cell types, imaging is usually limited to patients with symptoms. PET is less valuable.

CARCINOID TUMOR

About 25% of all primary lung tumors can be considered to be neuroectodermal carcinomas in that they arise from neuroectodermal cells, contain secretory granules, and can produce active peptides; this group includes typical carcinoid tumor, atypical carcinoid tumor, small cell carcinoma, and large cell neuroendocrine carcinoma. These tumors reflect a spectrum of abnormalities ranging from typical carcinoid tumor (which has a good prognosis) to small cell carcinoma (which has a poor prognosis; Table 3-18).

Typical Carcinoid Tumor

Carcinoid tumors account for 1% to 2% of tracheobronchial neoplasms. They are considered the best-differentiated type of neuroectodermal carcinoma.

Typical carcinoid tumors are slowly growing and locally invasive. They metastasize to regional lymph nodes in 5% to 15% of cases, and a lesser number of patients have distant metastases.

Typical carcinoid tumors occur most commonly in patients 40 to 60 years of age (mean age, 45 to 55). However, they are not uncommon in patients younger than 20 years, and this tumor tends to occur in a younger population than other lung carcinomas. It is slightly more common in women. There is no association with smoking.

Approximately 80% of typical carcinoid tumors occur centrally, in the main, lobar, or segmental bronchi; 1% are intratracheal. Involvement of lobar bronchi (75% of those with airway lesions) is most common (Fig. 3-43). Because of associated bronchial obstruction, symptoms are common, occurring in approximately 75% of cases; they include cough, fever, and wheezing. These tumors are highly vascular, and hemoptysis is

TABLE 3.18 Features Distinguishing the Neuroendocrine Carcinomas

	Typical Carcinoid	Atypical Carcinoid	Small Cell Carcinoma
Mean age (year)	45–50	60	>60
Male:female ratio	0.8:1	2:1	4:1
Smoking history	Uncommon	Common	Very common
Symptoms	75%	50%	90%
Regional metastases	5%–15%	40%–60%	>90%
Distant metastases	Rare	20%	>90%
5-year survival	90%–95%	50%–70%	>5%
Endobronchial mass	80%	10%	20%
Lung nodule or mass	20%	90%	20%
Large hilar mass	50%	10%	80%

a common presenting complaint. Peripheral carcinoid tumors may be asymptomatic. Patients who have central carcinoid tumors associated with bronchial obstruction tend to present at a younger age than patients with peripheral lesions.

Nearly half of typical carcinoid tumors are associated with radiographic findings of bronchial obstruction, primarily atelectasis or consolidation, typically limited to a lobe or segment (see Fig. 3-43A). Atelectasis and consolidation are often intermittent, and recurrent episodes of infection can result in bronchiectasis or lung abscess. Bronchiectasis is present pathologically in more than one third of patients but is less often visible on radiographs. Air trapping related to bronchial obstruction is sometimes seen.

Central tumors, with or without findings of obstruction, may be visible as discrete mass lesions in or near the hila. These masses, which are usually less than 4 cm in diameter, can be difficult to recognize without CT. In many cases, these tumors have a large endobronchial component and appear on CT as intraluminal masses (see Fig. 3-43B and C) with a convex margin pointing toward the hilum. Also, lesions that are largely endobronchial can expand the bronchus as they grow, typically resulting in a flaring of the bronchial lumen at the point of obstruction. Because they are highly vascular, dense enhancement may be seen on CT (see Fig. 3-43D).

A peripheral nodule or mass, not associated with findings of obstruction, is present in approximately 20% of patients (Fig. 3-44). These nodules are often well defined, round or oval, and slightly lobulated.

Calcification and ossification may be seen on plain films in a patient with carcinoid tumor. On CT, calcification of central carcinoid tumors is seen in nearly 40%. Calcifications may be large.

Radionuclide imaging with somatostatin analogs (e.g., octreotide) may be used to localize an occult carcinoid tumor in a patient with Cushing's syndrome or carcinoid syndrome or to diagnose metastases (Fig. 3-45).

Local extension of typical carcinoid tumors beyond the bronchial wall is common, and endoscopic removal of visible tumor is not usually curative. Surgical resection is the treatment of choice. Peripheral carcinoid tumors can be excised using wedge resection or segmentectomy. For central

endobronchial lesions, a sleeve resection may be performed to avoid pneumonectomy or lobectomy. In this procedure, a segment of bronchus containing the tumor is resected and the two bronchial stumps are sutured together.

For patients treated surgically, the prognosis is good. The 10-year survival rate of patients treated by surgery is as high as 90%. Following resection, distant metastasis is more common than local recurrence at the primary site. Bone metastases, either lytic or blastic, can occur.

Clinical Syndromes Associated With Carcinoid Tumor

Carcinoid tumors are capable of producing a number of active neuroendocrine peptides, and several clinical syndromes have been associated with this tumor. Typically, metastases are present before these syndromes become manifest; it is unusual for a small localized tumor to produce a sufficient amount of active peptides to result in clinical manifestations.

Carcinoid syndrome occurs in 2% to 5% of patients with pulmonary carcinoid tumor. It is most common in the presence of liver metastases. The carcinoid syndrome consists of flushing, fever, nausea, diarrhea, hypotension, and wheezing; it results from secretion of 5-hydroxytryptamine and other active agents such as bradykinin and prostaglandins. Cardiac valvular lesions and heart murmurs associated with this syndrome may be limited to the left side of the heart because of high concentrations of active substances in the pulmonary venous blood; cardiac valvular abnormalities associated with gastrointestinal carcinoid tumors usually involve the right side of the heart. Some other symptoms are said to help distinguish bronchial carcinoid syndrome from that resulting from intestinal tumors; these include severe flushing, facial edema, lacrimation, salivation, rhinorrhea, and diaphoresis.

Cushing's syndrome can result from production of ACTH or ACTH-releasing hormone by the tumor. It is uncommon, being seen in about 2% of cases (Fig. 3-46). Approximately 1% of cases of Cushing's syndrome are produced by bronchial carcinoid. Other syndromes associated with bronchial carcinoid tumor include Zollinger-Ellison syndrome, hyperinsulinemia, and acromegaly.

A

B

C

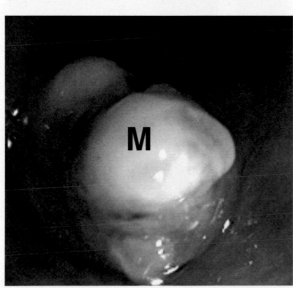

E

FIG. 3.43. Typical carcinoid tumor presenting as an endobronchial mass in a 30-year-old patient with recurrent left lower lobe pneumonia. **A:** Chest radiograph shows left lower lobe atelectasis (*arrows*). **B:** CT at a later date shows a lobulated endobronchial mass (∗) associated with obstruction of the left lower lobe bronchus. **C:** Contrast-enhanced CT at the same level shows enhancement of the tumor (*large arrow*) and its relationship to the left upper lobe bronchus (*LUL*) and the interlobar left pulmonary artery (*LPa*). **D:** Coronal reformation shows the mass (∗) obstructing the proximal left lower lobe bronchus (*LLL*). The left upper lobe bronchus (*LUL*) is normal. **E:** Bronchoscopic photograph shows the endobronchial mass (*M*) protruding from the left lower lobe bronchus. This mass appeared highly vascular and bled easily.

FIG. 3.44. Typical carcinoid tumor presenting as a lung mass. A well-defined and sharply margin-ated rounded mass is visible in the left lower lobe on the chest radiograph (**A**) and CT (**B**).

Atypical Carcinoid Tumor

Approximately 10% to 25% of carcinoid tumors can be classified as *atypical carcinoid tumor* because of histologic features suggesting a more aggressive behavior, includ-ing an increased frequency of mitoses and the presence of necrosis. These tumors are considered to be intermediate between typical carcinoid tumor and small cell carcinoma in differentiation, the incidence of metastases, and mortality. Lymph node metastases are present in approximately 50% of

patients. Patients with atypical carcinoid tend to be slightly older than those with typical carcinoid, and men outnumber women. There is an association with smoking.

Atypical carcinoid tumors tend to present as a lung nodule or mass, round or ovoid, lobulated, and somewhat larger than those seen with typical carcinoid tumor (10 cm or smaller). An endobronchial mass resulting in obstruc-tion and atelectasis is less common than that with typical carcinoid tumor, occurring in about 10%.

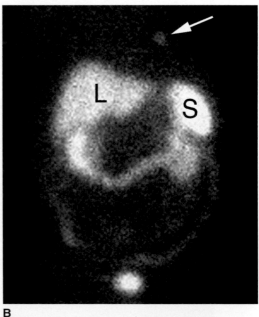

FIG. 3.45. Lymph node metastasis in a patient following resection of a carcinoid tumor. **A:** Chest CT shows an enlarged left mediastinal lymph node (*arrow*). **B:** Octreotide radionuclide scan shows increased activity in the lymph node (*arrow*). The liver (*L*) and spleen (*S*) are indicated for orientation.

A   B

FIG. 3.46. Metastatic carcinoid tumor with Cushing's syndrome. **A:** CT shows mediastinal widening and fat deposition (lipomatosis; *arrows*) secondary to Cushing's syndrome. A sclerotic vertebral metastasis (∗) is visible. **B:** At a lower level, enlarged mediastinal lymph nodes (*arrows*) reflect metastatic tumor.

These tumors have a worse prognosis than typical pulmonary carcinoids, and a more aggressive surgical approach is usually employed (lobectomy, sometimes with radiation or chemotherapy). Surgical cures have been reported, and 5-year survival rates range from 50% to 70%. As with typical carcinoid tumor, they can be associated with various clinical syndromes.

Neuroendocrine (Carcinoid) Tumorlets

Very small nodular collections or tumorlets of neuroendocrine cells may be seen in the walls of small airways in patients with chronic lung diseases such as bronchiectasis or lung fibrosis (termed *diffuse idiopathic pulmonary neuroendocrine cell hyperplasia* in the WHO system). In many cases these are hyperplastic. In other cases they are precursors to, or associated with, carcinoid tumors. They may be asymptomatic or associated with airway obstruction because of their relationship to the walls of small airways; Cushing's

FIG. 3.47. Multiple carcinoid tumorlets visible as small lung nodules.

syndrome is rarely associated. In occasional cases, they are visible as small lung nodules (Fig. 3-47). There is a distinct predominance in women.

SALIVARY GLAND TYPE TUMORS

Tumors referred to as "salivary gland type" because of histologic similarities to lesions originating in the salivary glands arise from mucous glands in the walls of the trachea and bronchi; they may also be termed "bronchial gland neoplasms." They are subdivided into several cell types; adenoid cystic carcinoma (cylindroma) and mucoepidermoid carcinoma are the most common. Bronchial gland tumors account for 0.1% to 0.2% of all lung and bronchial tumors and are one-tenth as common as carcinoid tumor.

Adenoid Cystic Carcinoma (Cylindroma)

Adenoid cystic carcinoma is the most common bronchial gland tumor, accounting for 75% of cases. The mean age at diagnosis is 50; it has not been associated with smoking.

Approximately 50% of adenoid cystic carcinomas originate in the main or lobar bronchi (Fig. 3-48), 40% originate in the trachea, and 10% present as peripheral lung nodules. Although adenoid cystic carcinoma is an uncommon neoplasm, it is responsible for as many as 30% to 35% of tracheal malignancies. Although carcinoid is much more common among central bronchial tumors, adenoid cystic carcinoma outnumbers carcinoid in the trachea by 20 to 1.

When it occurs in an endobronchial location, adenoid cystic carcinoma presents with symptoms and radiographic findings similar to carcinoid. The tumor usually protrudes into the airway lumen and may be polypoid or sessile.

When it is endotracheal, this lesion most commonly appears as a sessile mass, with obtuse angles where it contacts the tracheal wall; in some patients it is polypoid. It tends to originate from the posterior or posterolateral tracheal wall (see Figs. 22-5 and 22-6B in Chapter 22). Although CT can be helpful in assessing endotracheal adenoid cystic carcinoma,

FIG. 3.48. Adenoid cystic carcinoma. A polypoid lesion is visible in the right main bronchus (*large black arrow*). Thickening of the right upper lobe bronchial wall (*white arrow*) is due to local infiltration. Infiltration of the left main bronchus is associated with narrowing of its lumen (*small black arrow*).

it tends to underestimate the longitudinal extent of the tumor because of partial volume averaging and the tendency of adenoid cystic carcinoma to grow submucosally. CT, however, accurately demonstrates extratracheal extension of tumor, which is helpful in planning the surgical approach.

Adenoid cystic carcinoma has a much better prognosis than more common forms of lung carcinoma. However, it behaves in a more malignant fashion than carcinoid tumor, tends to be more infiltrative than carcinoid tumor (see Fig. 3-48), and metastasizes more frequently.

These tumors are treated using surgical excision but tend to recur locally. Recent advances in tracheal resection and carinal reconstruction have made many tracheal lesions resectable. The 5-year survival rate is about 75%.

Mucoepidermoid Carcinoma

Mucoepidermoid carcinoma is a rare tumor. The average age at diagnosis is 35 to 45 years. It usually occurs in the main or lobar bronchi; tracheal or peripheral lesions are uncommon. It tends to exhibit a more benign course than adenoid cystic carcinoma or carcinoid tumor, but it may be locally invasive. High-grade mucoepidermoid carcinoma has been reported to have a poor prognosis.

Presentation and radiographic findings are similar to those of adenoid cystic carcinoma. These tumors arise in the trachea or central bronchi and result in symptoms and radiographic findings of obstruction. Surgery is usually curative.

Bronchial Adenoma

True "bronchial adenomas" are rare. The most common cell type of bronchial adenoma is *mucous gland adenoma*. Rarer cell types include pleomorphic adenoma and oncocytoma.

These tumors are benign tumors originating from glands in the tracheal or bronchial wall. As with bronchial gland carcinomas, they are similar histologically to tumors arising in the salivary glands. Bronchial adenomas occur in patients of all ages. These tumors usually originate in the main, lobar, or segmental bronchi and are associated with findings of bronchial obstruction. Radiographically, they typically appear as smooth, sessile, or rounded endobronchial masses. Presentation as a solitary nodule is much less frequent. Excision is usually curative.

HAMARTOMA

Hamartoma is the most common mesenchymal tumor of the respiratory tract, and it accounts for more than 75% of benign lung tumors (Table 3-19). Hamartomas contain the various connective-tissue elements that are normally found in the lung and bronchi, but in a disorganized state. This tumor almost always contains cartilage and is sometimes referred to as *chondromatous hamartoma*. Also found in varying amounts are fat, fibrous tissue, smooth muscle, myxomatous tissue, and epithelial tissue. Hamartomas most likely originate within embryonic rests in the bronchial wall, but it has also been hypothesized that they derive from undifferentiated mesenchymal tissues and represent true neoplasms.

Hamartomas are most commonly diagnosed in patients older than 50 and are twice as common in men as in women. They are rare in children, and less than 10% occur in patients younger than 40. Prior to the advent of CT (which greatly assists in their preoperative diagnosis), hamartomas accounted for as many as 6% to 8% of resected lung nodules.

Despite their origin from bronchial tissues, only 5% to 15% of hamartomas present as an endobronchial mass (Fig. 3-49). In more than 85% of cases, hamartomas appear radiographically as a solitary pulmonary nodule. Peripheral hamartomas are usually 1 to 4 cm in diameter, well defined, sharply circumscribed, and often lobulated. Calcification of cartilage is reported to be visible on plain radiographs in approximately 30% of hamartomas, and the frequency of calcification increases with the tumor's size. Calcification is seen in less than 10% of hamartomas less than 3 cm in diameter but is present in 75% of those 5 cm or larger.

TABLE 3.19 Hamartoma

75% of benign lung tumors
Patients > 50 years of age
Twice as common in men
5%–15% endobronchial
≥85% present as solitary nodule
Usually 1–4 cm
Sharply circumscribed
Round or lobulated
Calcification in 25%
Popcorn calcification
Fat visible on CT in 60%
Slow growth

A

B

C

FIG. 3.49. Hamartoma with an endobronchial component. **A:** Lateral chest radiograph shows a well-defined hilar nodule (*arrows*). **B:** High-resolution CT with a lung window shows a sharply marginated lobulated nodule narrowing the right lower lobe bronchus (*arrow*). **C:** High-resolution with a soft-tissue window shows areas of fat attenuation (−80 HU; *arrows*), common in hamartoma.

Calcification of hamartomas can be stippled or conglomerate. Conglomerate or "popcorn" calcification is characteristic of hamartomas and is rarely seen with other lesions; it occurs because of calcification of nodules of cartilage (Fig. 3-50). Accumulations of fat can produce lucent or low-attenuation areas within the tumor, usually visible only on CT. Rarely cystic, air-filled hamartomas have been reported.

High-resolution CT is valuable in diagnosing pulmonary hamartoma. Nearly 65% of hamartomas may be diagnosed using high-resolution CT because of visible fat (see Figs. 3-49 and 3-51), either focal or diffuse (CT numbers ranging from −40 to −120 HU) or a combination of fat and calcium. Thin collimation (i.e., 1 mm) must be used to make the diagnosis of fat within a nodule; otherwise, volume averaging may simulate this appearance. A nodule

FIG. 3.50. Calcified hamartomas in two patients. **A:** Hamartoma (*arrow*) with focal calcification. The nodule is round and sharply defined. **B:** Hamartoma (*arrow*) with popcorn calcification. This appearance results from calcification of nodules of cartilage in the tumor.

containing fat has a very limited differential diagnosis; lipoid pneumonia is another but much less common cause of this finding. Pulmonary teratoma could also show fat, but this is extremely rare.

In most cases, hamartomas grow slowly, increasing in diameter from 0.5 to 5 mm/year (Fig. 3-52). Rapid growth can occur, however, causing hamartomas to be confused with lung carcinoma. Endobronchial lesions can be resected bronchoscopically unless infection has caused destruction of the distal lung. Needle biopsy can be diagnostic in some cases, but peripheral tumors may require excision for diagnosis.

RARE LUNG TUMORS

Mesenchymal Tumors

Except for hamartoma, mesenchymal tumors of the lung are rare. Benign mesenchymal tumors are much more common than malignant neoplasms.

Mesenchymal tumors may present as (1) an endobronchial lesion, often rounded or sessile, and associated with symptoms of bronchial obstruction or (2) a nodule or mass in the lung periphery, usually detected incidentally on chest radiographs or CT, or when malignant, associated with chest wall invasion.

Lipoma and Liposarcoma

Lipoma and liposarcoma originate in collections of fat found in the walls of cartilage-containing airways. Lipoma overlaps with fatty hamartoma; liposarcoma is rare. They may occur in patients of any age, usually ranging from 30 to 65, and nearly 90% occur in men.

Lipomas are most common in the main or lobar bronchi and typically are found in the bronchial lumen. Endobronchial lesions are usually oval, measuring several centimeters in length. They uncommonly occur in the peripheral lung. Symptoms and radiographic findings of bronchial obstruction are common, and obstructive pneumonitis and bronchiectasis are often present. Occasionally a lipoma extends in a dumbbell fashion to lie primarily outside the bronchus. CT can be diagnostic, showing uniform low attenuation indistinguishable from a fat-containing hamartoma.

Chondroma and Chondrosarcoma

True chondromas, containing only cartilage, are exceedingly rare, and their relationship to hamartomas is uncertain. They may occur as an endobronchial lesion or a well-defined solitary nodule. Calcification occurs in about 30%.

Pulmonary chondroma may occur as part of *Carney's triad.* This unusual entity is characterized by the combination of multiple pulmonary chondromas, gastric epithelioid leiomyosarcoma, and extraadrenal paraganglioma. In some cases, only two of the three manifestations are present. This syndrome is most common in young women less than 30; only 10% of cases occur in men.

Chondrosarcoma is rare. This tumor occurs much more commonly as a pulmonary mass lesion than as a mass within the trachea or bronchial lumen. In general, pulmonary lesions have a very poor prognosis.

Leiomyoma and Leiomyosarcoma

Leiomyoma is thought to arise from smooth muscle found in the walls of the bronchi or perhaps blood vessels. The average

FIG. 3.51. Hamartomas containing fat in three patients. Focal areas of low-attenuation fat are visible within the nodules (*arrows*). The nodules are rounded and sharply defined.

age at diagnosis is 50, but it occurs in patients ranging from 5 to 65; women are more frequently affected. Leiomyoma may occur as a lung nodule (slightly more common) or an endobronchial lesion. Pulmonary parenchymal leiomyomas are usually asymptomatic and detected incidentally. They appear radiographically as well-defined, lobulated, peripheral mass lesions and range up to 20 cm in diameter. Calcification is rare and cavitation does not occur. Endobronchial lesions usually occur in the main or lobar bronchi. Symptoms are common and often due to obstructive pneumonia.

In such patients, radiographic findings are usually limited to signs of airway obstruction. CT may show an endobronchial mass.

Leiomyosarcoma is more common than leiomyoma. Leiomyosarcoma is more common in men than women with a ratio of 2:1. Patients are usually symptomatic. Radiographs demonstrate a pulmonary mass in most cases, and in general tumors are larger than leiomyomas. Cavitation may occur. Endobronchial obstruction with atelectasis occurs in about a third of patients.

FIG. 3.52. Hamartoma with growth. **A:** Chest radiograph shows a well-defined upper lobe nodule measuring 1 cm. **B:** Radiograph 3 years later. The nodule now measures 2 cm in diameter. Several foci of calcification are visible within the nodule. The doubling time of this nodule is 1 year.

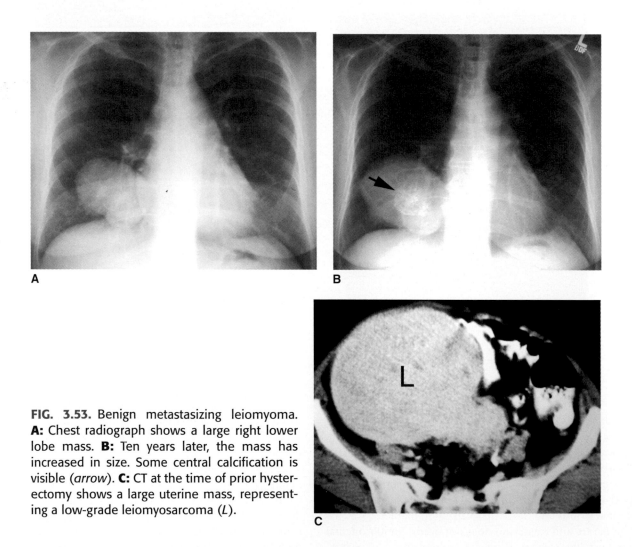

FIG. 3.53. Benign metastasizing leiomyoma. **A:** Chest radiograph shows a large right lower lobe mass. **B:** Ten years later, the mass has increased in size. Some central calcification is visible (*arrow*). **C:** CT at the time of prior hysterectomy shows a large uterine mass, representing a low-grade leiomyosarcoma (*L*).

Multiple pulmonary "leiomyomas" associated with smooth muscle tumors of the uterus in women ("benign metastasizing leiomyoma") represent pulmonary metastases from a low-grade uterine leiomyosarcoma. Single or multiple lung masses are usually seen. They may be quite large, may calcify, and grow slowly (Fig. 3-53).

Fibroma and Fibrosarcoma

Fibroma can involve the lung or tracheobronchial tree and is rare. Pulmonary parenchymal lesions are most common and are usually asymptomatic. Tracheal or bronchial lesions produce symptoms and signs of obstruction.

Fibrosarcomas, regardless of their location, are usually symptomatic. They more often appear as a nodule or mass rather than as an endobronchial lesion. Endobronchial lesions are most common in children and young adults, while pulmonary masses are found in patients of middle age. Pulmonary lesions are usually round and well defined, measuring up to 20 cm in diameter.

Malignant Fibrous Histiocytoma

Primary involvement of the lung is uncommon with this tumor. The average age at diagnosis is about 50. Most appear as smooth or lobulated lung masses.

Vascular Tumors

Vascular tumors of the lung and bronchi are rare. Although vessels are present within the tumors, they are solid masses and rarely exhibit significant opacification during angiography or CT.

Glomus tumor is derived from smooth muscle cells of the glomus body and consists of irregular vascular channels. It most often occurs as a polypoid mass arising from the tracheal or bronchial wall. Hemoptysis or bronchial obstruction may be present.

Hemangiopericytoma is characterized by profuse proliferation of capillaries surrounded by neoplastic accumulations of pericytes. Tumors tend to be peripheral, appearing as a well-defined solitary nodule or mass, and ranging in size from 2 to 15 cm. Hemangiopericytoma can be benign or malignant, and excision is the treatment of choice.

Epithelioid hemangioendothelioma is a rare multifocal pulmonary neoplasm. It is manifested by multiple well-defined lung nodules up to 2 cm in diameter, mimicking the appearance of metastases. Eighty percent of cases occur in women, often less than 40 years old. The tumors may be asymptomatic or associated with cough, hemoptysis, or systemic symptoms. This entity is thought to represent a low-grade sarcoma, and metastases may occur. Liver involvement may be associated, representing metastases or synchronous development in multiple sites.

Neural Tumors

Neurogenic tumors of the lung and tracheobronchial tree, both benign and malignant, are rare. They are thought to arise from sympathetic nerve fibers accompanying arterioles or bronchioles. Among benign tumors are neurofibroma, schwannoma, paraganglioma, meningioma, granular cell tumor (granular cell myoblastoma), and meningothelial-like nodules. Neurofibrosarcoma is less common. These most often present as well-defined solitary nodules within the lung parenchyma, but endobronchial lesions have been reported. Neurofibroma, schwannoma, and neurofibrosarcoma may be associated with neurofibromatosis, particularly when multiple.

Epithelial Tumors

Squamous Papilloma and Tracheobronchial Papillomatosis

Squamous papilloma represents an abnormal proliferation of stratified squamous or sometimes ciliated columnar epithelium forming a polypoid mass within the airway lumen. These lesions are supported by a core of fibrovascular tissue connecting them to the tracheal or bronchial wall. They are benign and of viral origin, caused by the human papillomavirus. Malignant change sometimes occurs.

Papilloma is the most common laryngeal tumor of childhood, and laryngeal papillomas occasionally occur in adults. Laryngeal lesions are often multiple and spread locally. In children, papillomas are successfully treated by surgical excision or regress at puberty. In 2% to 5% of patients,

FIG. 3.54. Tracheal papillomas. Small nodules (*arrows*) are visible arising from the tracheal wall.

FIG. 3.55. Tracheobronchial papillomatosis. Multiple cystic pulmonary lesions are present in the left lung (*arrows*).

however, the lesions spread distally to involve the tracheobronchial tree, a condition referred to as *tracheobronchial papillomatosis*; the trachea is almost always involved when distal spread occurs. Tracheobronchial spread is associated with instrumentation for resection of laryngeal lesions.

Involvement of the trachea often results in cough or hemoptysis. Hoarseness due to laryngeal lesions may also be present. In most cases, the lesions are multiple and small, ranging from a few millimeters to 1 cm in diameter, but they can be large, resulting in tracheal obstruction. Plain radiographs are rarely of value; CT is usually necessary for diagnosis (Fig. 3-54).

Extension of papillomas to the bronchi, bronchioles, and lung parenchyma is rare. The interval between the diagnosis of laryngeal lesions and bronchial spread ranges from 1 to more than 30 years. Although laryngeal lesions are most common in children younger than 5, the average age of patients with tumors involving the bronchial tree is 15. Bronchial obstruction results in wheezing, atelectasis, and recurrent pneumonia. Papillomas may be visible radiographically as nodular mass lesions within the lung, and they often cavitate. Eventually, cavitary lesions may progress to large thick- or thin-walled cysts. Nodules representing papillomas may be seen within cysts (Figs. 3-55 and 3-56).

A

B

C

FIG. 3.56. Tracheobronchial papillomatosis. **A,B:** Multiple thick- and thin-walled cavities, cysts, and nodules are visible bilaterally. A cystic lesion (*arrow*) contains a nodule. **C:** Progression of abnormalities with large masses indicates development of squamous cell carcinoma. A nodule of tumor (*arrow*) is visible within a fluid-filled cyst.

Bronchoscopic excision of tracheal or bronchial papillomas has been the treatment of choice, but the lesions recur following resection in more than 90% of patients. Tracheostomy may be required for associated laryngeal lesions that produce airway obstruction. Cystic pulmonary lesions are not usually associated with symptoms, and unless they are infected no treatment is necessary. In recent studies, interferon has been of some value in treatment. Malignant degeneration of pulmonary lesions may occur, leading to squamous cell carcinoma (see Fig. 3-56C).

Solitary papillomas occasionally occur in adults, usually middle-aged men, in the absence of prior laryngeal lesions. They are usually less than 1.5 cm in diameter and are most commonly found in a lobar or segmental bronchus. They may result in bronchial obstruction, and symptoms include cough and hemoptysis. Histology is identical to that found in papillomatosis.

Inflammatory Polyps

Inflammatory polyps of the tracheobronchial tree are characterized histologically by a loose connective-tissue core covered by normal bronchial epithelium; they lack the squamous overgrowth typical of papillomas and in general occur in older patients. These lesions may be polypoid or sessile and are larger than squamous papillomas. In most patients, polyps range from 0.5 to 2 cm in diameter (Fig. 3-57). Occasionally polyps are multiple, and findings

of bronchial obstruction are common. Recurrence following excision does not occur.

Pulmonary Adenomas

Tracheobronchial adenomas occurring as endobronchial lesions are reviewed above (see Salivary Gland Type Tumors). Adenomas arising in the lung periphery, derived from bronchiolar or alveolar epithelium and usually presenting as a lung nodule, include mucinous cystadenoma, papillary and alveolar adenoma, and sclerosing hemangioma.

Miscellaneous Tumors

Other tumors rarely occurring in the lung or bronchial tree include thymoma, teratoma, seminoma, endometriosis, and lymphangioma. With exception of teratoma, which may mimic mediastinal teratoma, their appearances are nonspecific.

SELECTED READING

Bepler G. Lung cancer epidemiology and genetics. J Thorac Imaging 1999; 14:228–234.

Dales RE, Stark RM, Raman S. Computed tomography to stage lung cancer: approaching a controversy using meta-analysis. Am Rev Respir Dis 1990; 141:1096–1101.

Detterbeck FC, Boffa DJ, Tanoue LT. The new lung cancer staging system. Chest 2009; 136:260–271.

Forster BB, Müller NL, Miller RR, et al. Neuroendocrine carcinomas of the lung: clinical, radiologic, and pathologic correlation. Radiology 1989; 170:441–445.

Glazer HS, Duncan MJ, Aronberg DJ, et al. Pleural and chest wall invasion in bronchogenic carcinoma: CT evaluation. Radiology 1985; 157: 191–194.

Glazer HS, Kaiser LR, Anderson DJ, et al. Indeterminate mediastinal invasion in bronchogenic carcinoma: CT evaluation. Radiology 1989; 173:37–42.

Heelan RT, Demas BE, Caravelli JF, et al. Superior sulcus tumors: CT and MR imaging. Radiology 1989; 170:637–641.

Kakinuma R, Ohmatsu H, Kaneko M, et al. Detection failures in spiral CT screening for lung cancer: analysis of CT findings. Radiology 1999; 212:61–66.

McLoud TC, Bourgouin PM, Greenberg RW, et al. Bronchogenic carcinoma: analysis of staging in the mediastinum with CT by correlative lymph node mapping and sampling. Radiology 1992; 182:319–323.

Mountain CF. Revisions in the international system for staging lung cancer. Chest 1997; 111:1710–1717.

Patel AM, Peters SG. Clinical manifestations of lung cancer. Mayo Clin Proc 1993; 68:273–277.

Pennes DR, Glazer GM, Wimbish KJ, et al. Chest wall invasion by lung cancer: limitations of CT evaluation. AJR Am J Roentgenol 1985; 144: 507–511.

Rami-Porta R, Crowley JJ, Goldstraw P. The revised TNM staging system for lung cancer. Ann Thorac Cardiovasc Surg 2009; 15:4–9.

Ratto GB, Piacenza G, Frola C, et al. Chest wall involvement by lung cancer: computed tomographic detection and results of operation. Ann Thorac Surg 1991; 51:182–188.

Rosado de Christenson ML, Abbott GF, Kirejczyk WM, et al. Thoracic carcinoids: radiologic-pathologic correlation. Radiographics 1999; 19: 707–736.

Salvatierra A, Baamonde C, Llamas JM, et al. Extrathoracic staging of bronchogenic carcinoma. Chest 1990; 97:1052–1058.

Scott IR, Müller NL, Miller RR, et al. Resectable stage III lung cancer: CT, surgical, and pathologic correlation. Radiology 1988; 166:75–79.

Siegelman SS, Khouri NF, Scott WW, et al. Pulmonary hamartoma: CT findings. Radiology 1986; 160:313–317.

FIG. 3.57. Inflammatory polyp. A polypoid lesion is visible in the left lower lobe bronchus (*arrow*).

Staples CA, Müller NL, Miller RR, et al. Mediastinal nodes in bronchogenic carcinoma: comparison between CT and mediastinoscopy. Radiology 1988; 167:367–372.

Travis WD. Pathology of lung cancer. Clin Chest Med 2002; 23:65–81.

Travis WD, Garg K, Franklin WA, et al. Evolving concepts in the pathology and computed tomography imaging of lung adenocarcinoma and bronchioloalveolar carcinoma. J Clin Oncol 2005; 23:3279–3287.

Webb WR, Gatsonis C, Zerhouni EA, et al. CT and MR imaging in staging non–small cell bronchogenic carcinoma: report of the Radiologic Diagnostic Oncology Group. Radiology 1991; 178:705–713.

Webb WR, Golden JA. Imaging strategies in the staging of lung cancer. Clin Chest Med 1991; 12:133–150.

White CS, Salis AI, Meyer CA. Missed lung cancer on chest radiography and computed tomography: imaging and medicolegal issues. J Thorac Imaging 1999; 14:63–68.

Whitesell PL, Drage CW. Occupational lung cancer. Mayo Clin Proc 1993; 68:183–188.

Zwiebel BR, Austin JHM, Grines MM. Bronchial carcinoid tumors: assessment with CT of location and intratumoral calcification in 31 patients. Radiology 1991; 179:483–486.

Zwirewich CV, Vedal S, Miller RR, Müller NL. Solitary pulmonary nodule: high-resolution CT and radiologic-pathologic correlation. Radiology 1991; 179:469–476.

Metastatic Tumor

W. RICHARD WEBB

T horacic structures commonly are involved in patients with metastatic neoplasm, and the chest is often the first site in which metastases are detected.

MECHANISMS OF SPREAD

Metastatic tumor may involve thoracic structures in several ways.

Direct extension from the primary tumor with secondary involvement of the lung, pleura, or mediastinal structures. This mode of spread is most common with thyroid tumors, esophageal carcinoma, thymoma and thymic malignancies, lymphoma, and malignant germ cell tumors.

Hematogenous spread of tumor emboli to pulmonary or bronchial arteries. This usually results in the presence of lung nodules and is most common with primary tumors that have a good vascular supply.

Lymphatic spread to involve the lung, pleura, or mediastinal lymph nodes. The lung may be diffusely involved by tumor following lymphatic or lymphangitic spread of cells from hematogenous metastases, hilar lymph node metastases, or upper abdominal tumors. Lymphatic spread of extrathoracic tumors to mediastinal lymph nodes also may occur via the thoracic duct, with retrograde involvement of hilar lymph nodes and the lung parenchyma. Tumors that commonly metastasize in this fashion include carcinomas of the breast, stomach, pancreas, prostate, cervix, and thyroid.

Spread within the pleural space due to pleural invasion from a local tumor (e.g., thymoma) or lung carcinoma.

Endobronchial spread of cells from an airway tumor. This mechanism of metastasis is uncommon. It is most common in patients with bronchioloalveolar carcinoma (Fig. 4-1) but may be seen with other cell types of lung cancer (Fig. 4-2). It is also thought to occur in patients with tracheobronchial papillomatosis (see Figs. 3-55 and 3-56 in Chapter 3).

MANIFESTATIONS OF METASTATIC TUMOR
Lung Nodules

Lung nodules are the most common thoracic manifestation of metastasis. In most cases they are hematogenous in origin (Table 4-1). They tend to predominate in the lung bases, which receive more blood flow than the upper lobes.

Nodules tend to be sharply marginated in most cases and round or lobulated in contour (Fig. 4-3). Poorly marginated nodules may be seen in the presence of surrounding hemorrhage or local invasion of the adjacent lung (Fig. 4-4). In some cases, individual metastases are seen to have a relationship to small vascular branches, suggesting a hematogenous origin. This is termed the "feeding vessel" sign (Fig. 4-5). Nodules may be small or large. Using computed tomography (CT), metastasis as small as 1 to 2 mm may be visible.

Cavitation of metastases is not as common as with primary lung carcinoma, but it occurs in about 5% of cases. It may be seen even with small nodules (Fig. 4-6). The likelihood of cavitation varies with histology. Cavitation is most common with squamous cell tumors and transitional cell tumors, but also may be seen in adenocarcinomas, particularly from the colon, and in some sarcomas.

Calcification of metastases occurs most commonly with osteogenic sarcoma, chondrosarcoma, synovial sarcoma, thyroid carcinoma, and mucinous adenocarcinoma

FIG. 4.1. Endobronchial spread of bronchioloalveolar carcinoma. Patchy areas of consolidation are visible. Centrilobular nodules (*arrows*) associated with bronchioloalveolar carcinoma are thought to be due to endobronchial spread.

117

A

B

FIG. 4.2. Endobronchial spread of squamous cell carcinoma. **A:** CT shows a cavitary mass closely associated with the right upper lobe bronchus. **B:** Years later, extensive bilateral nodular and cavitary masses are visible. Extensive endobronchial tumor was present.

(Fig. 4-7). Calcification may be dense, particularly with osteogenic sarcoma, mimicking a granuloma. Calcification may persist following successful chemotherapy despite resolution of the tumor.

CT is considerably more sensitive than plain radiographs in detecting lung nodules in patients with metastatic tumor, although the sensitivity of CT varies with slice thickness. The sensitivity of chest radiographs for detecting nodules in patients with lung metastases is about 40% to 45%, although this varies with the size of the nodules. Using spiral CT with 5-mm collimation, a sensitivity of more than 80% has been reported for detection of nodular metastases 5 mm or less in diameter; the sensitivity of CT in detecting metastases larger than 5 mm is 100%.

TABLE 4.1	Nodular Metastases

Hematogenous spread
Multiple nodules typically of different sizes
Basal predominance in size and number
Feeding vessel sign
Diffuse or "random" distribution
Poorly marginated nodules
    Hemorrhage or invasion
Small nodules
    Thyroid carcinoma
    Melanoma
    Adenocarcinoma
    Sarcomas
Cannonball metastases
    Renal cell carcinoma
    Testicular carcinoma
    Colon carcinoma
Cavitation
    Squamous cell
    Transitional cell
    Adenocarcioma (e.g., colon)
    Sarcomas
Calcification
    Osteogenic sarcoma
    Chondrosarcoma
    Synovial sarcoma
    Thyroid carcinoma
    Mucinous adenocarcinoma
Solitary metastases
    Colon carcinoma
    Renal cell carcinoma
    Testicular carcinoma
    Sarcomas
    Melanoma

FIG. 4.3. Metastatic salivary gland carcinoma with rounded and lobulated metastases. Nodules vary in size; this is typical with metastatic tumor and is less common with benign diseases.

FIG. 4.4. Metastases from choriocarcinoma. **A:** Chest radiograph shows multiple ill-defined lung nodules with a preponderance at the lung bases. **B:** CT shows rounded and lobulated nodules, many of which are surrounded by ground-glass opacity (i.e., the halo sign). This appearance results from hemorrhage and is common with choriocarcinoma and other vascular tumors. It also may reflect invasion of the adjacent lung.

On the other hand, lung nodules seen on CT in patients with a known tumor often represent something other than metastases. Granulomas, focal areas of infection, scarring, and intrapulmonary lymph nodes are all very common, and mimic metastases on CT. These are generally small, measuring a few mm in diameter. Nodules larger than a few mm, particularly when rounded and sharply defined, are more likely to represent metastatic tumor. If small nodules are seen on CT in a patient with a known tumor, obtaining a follow-up CT at 6 weeks to 3 months is appropriate. Nodules representing metastases typically show growth; benign nodules usually show no growth, decrease in size, or resolve.

Multiple Nodule

Nodular metastases usually are multiple. The nodules often vary in size, representing multiple episodes of tumor embolization or different growth rates (see Figs. 4-3, 4-4, and 4-8);

FIG. 4.5. The feeding vessel sign. Vascular supply of lung metastases (*arrows*) in a patient with bladder carcinoma is shown using a maximum-intensity projection image obtained with 1.25-mm slice thickness after contrast infusion.

FIG. 4.6. Cavitary nodule in metastatic transitional cell carcinoma. Even though the nodule is very small (*arrow*), a distinct cavity is visible.

A

B

FIG. 4.7. Ossified metastases secondary to osteogenic carcinoma. **A:** Chest radiograph shows dense nodules. **B:** CT shows dense calcification, which is typical of this tumor.

FIG. 4.8. Metastatic testicular carcinoma. Nodules vary in size and appear more numerous and larger at the lung bases. A basal preponderance is typical of metastases. Large nodular metastases are sometimes called "cannonball" metastases.

this appearance is less common with benign nodular disease, such as sarcoidosis. Occasionally, all of the nodular metastases are of the same size. When there are numerous nodules, they tend to be distributed throughout the lung (Fig. 4-9). When the metastases are few in number, they may be predominantly subpleural (see Fig. 4-4B).

On CT, numerous nodules tend to involve the lung in a diffuse fashion without regard for specific anatomic structures, a distribution termed "random" (see Figs. 4-3 and 4-9B). This pattern is described in detail in Chapter 10.

The size and number of nodules vary greatly. Nodules may be small (i.e., miliary) and very numerous (Fig. 4-10); this appearance often is seen with very vascular tumors (e.g., thyroid carcinoma, renal cell carcinoma, adenocarcinoma,

sarcomas) and presumably reflects a single massive shower of tumor emboli. Fewer, larger metastases also may be seen; when these are well defined, they are referred to as "cannonball metastases" (see Figs. 4-8 and 4-11). This type of metastasis is seen most commonly with tumors of the gastrointestinal or genitourinary tract.

Most patients (80% to 90%) with multiple metastases have a history of neoplasm. In some patients, however, there is no history of a primary tumor at the time of diagnosis; in others, the primary tumor may never be found.

Solitary Nodule

A metastatic tumor occasionally presents as a solitary nodule (Fig. 4-12). About 5% to 10% of solitary nodules represent solitary metastases. Solitary metastases are most common with carcinomas of the colon, kidney, and testis, and with sarcomas and melanoma. It must be emphasized that many patients who appear to have a solitary metastasis visible on chest radiograph are discovered to have multiple pulmonary nodules on CT, with one nodule being dominant.

A solitary metastasis is more likely to have a smooth margin than is primary lung carcinoma (see Fig. 4-12), but this finding on its own is not sufficient to permit a reliable distinction between primary and metastatic tumors. Solitary metastases may appear spiculated, and primary carcinomas may be smooth. A solitary metastasis is more likely when the tumor is located at the lung base; primary carcinoma is more common in the upper lobes.

A

B

FIG. 4.9. Metastatic adenocarcinoma. **A:** Chest radiograph shows numerous small, diffusely distributed nodules. Nodules appear more numerous and larger at the lung bases. **B:** CT shows a diffuse distribution of nodules. This pattern is termed "random," because it involves the lung randomly relative to lung structures. Some nodules typically are seen to involve the pleural surface with a random pattern.

FIG. 4.10. Metastatic thyroid carcinoma. Numerous small metastases are visible, distributed throughout the lung.

A

B

FIG. 4.11. Cannonball metastases in metastatic vaginal carcinoma. Frontal **(A)** and lateral **(B)** radiographs show several large, well-defined metastases.

FIG. 4.12. Solitary metastasis shown on CT at the lung base. No other nodules were visible. This nodule is sharply marginated. Biopsy showed the same cell type as the primary tumor.

TABLE 4.2 Lymphangitic Spread of Neoplasm
Results from:
Hematogenous metastasis with lymphatic invasion
Spread from hilar node metastases
Direct spread from upper abdominal tumors
Findings:
Interlobular septal thickening (i.e., Kerley's lines)
Thickening of the peribronchovascular interstitium
Thickening of the fissures
Perilymphatic nodules
Abnormalities asymmetric or unilateral in 50%
Common causes:
Breast carcinoma
Lung carcinoma
Stomach carcinwoma
Pancreas carcinoma
Prostate carcinoma
Cervical carcinoma
Thyroid carcinoma
Adenocarcinoma from an unknown site

In a patient with a known extrathoracic tumor and a solitary nodule detected radiographically, the likelihood that the nodule is a metastasis (as opposed to primary lung cancer) varies with the cell type of the primary tumor. Patients with carcinomas of the head and neck, bladder, breast, cervix, bile ducts, esophagus, ovary, prostate, or stomach are more likely to have primary lung carcinoma than lung metastasis (ratio, 8:1 for patients with head and neck cancers; 3:1 for patients with other types of cancer). Patients with carcinomas of the salivary glands, adrenal gland, colon, parotid gland, kidney, thyroid gland, thymus, or uterus have fairly even odds (ratio, 1:1). Patients with melanoma, sarcoma, or testicular carcinoma are more likely to have a solitary metastasis than a lung carcinoma (ratio, 2.5:1).

Lymphangitic Spread of Tumor

Lymphangitic spread of tumor refers to tumor growth in the lymphatic system of the lungs (Table 4-2). It occurs most commonly in patients with carcinomas of the breast, lung, stomach, pancreas, prostate, cervix, or thyroid, and in patients with metastatic adenocarcinoma from an unknown primary site; about 80% of cases are due to adenocarcinoma. It usually results from hematogenous spread to the lung, with subsequent interstitial and lymphatic invasion, but also can occur because of direct lymphatic spread of tumor from mediastinal and hilar lymph nodes. Symptoms of shortness of breath are common and can predate radiographic abnormalities.

The radiographic manifestations of pulmonary lymphangitic carcinomatosis include reticular or reticulonodular opacities, Kerley's lines, hilar and mediastinal lymphadenopathy, and pleural effusion (Fig. 4-13A and B). The appearance of unilateral or asymmetrical Kerley's lines is particularly suggestive. However, these findings are nonspecific. In some patients, the chest radiograph is normal.

On high-resolution CT (HRCT), lymphangitic spread of tumor typically shows (1) smooth thickening of the interlobular septa, (2) smooth thickening of the peribronchovascular interstitium surrounding vessels and bronchi in the perihilar lung (i.e., "peribronchial cuffing"), and (3) smooth subpleural interstitial thickening (i.e., thickening of the fissures; see Fig. 4-13C). Less often, nodular thickening of these structures is visible (Fig. 4-14). This pattern of nodules is termed "perilymphatic" (see Chapter 10).

In about 50% of patients, the abnormalities of lymphangitic spread appear focal, unilateral, or asymmetrical rather than diffuse on CT (see Fig. 4-13C). Hilar lymphadenopathy is visible on CT in only 50% of patients with lymphangitic spread. Mediastinal lymph node enlargement also can be seen. Lymph node enlargement can be symmetrical or asymmetrical. Pleural effusion is common.

Airway Metastases

Metastatic tumors may involve the tracheal or bronchial wall because of local spread from adjacent mediastinal structures (e.g., esophagus), lung, or lymph node metastases or because of hematogenous spread (Table 4-3). Oddly, involvement of the airway wall because of spread from other endobronchial tumors via the bronchial lumen is much less common; this pattern of metastasis occurs commonly with tracheobronchial papillomatosis (see Chapter 3).

Airway metastasis may present with symptoms or findings of airway obstruction and atelectasis (Fig. 4-15). If this occurs in the presence of multiple nodular metastases, the diagnosis is not difficult. However, if no other findings are

FIG. 4.13. Lymphangitic spread of breast carcinoma. **A:** Coned-down radiograph showing the right lower lobe demonstrates an abnormal reticular pattern and a right pleural effusion. **B:** Coned-down radiograph in another patient shows distinct Kerley's B lines. **C:** High-resolution CT in a patient with breast carcinoma. There is asymmetric lung involvement characterized by smooth interlobular septal thickening (*black arrows*) and thickening of the peribronchovascular inter-stitium surrounding vessels and bronchi in the perihilar lung (i.e., "peribronchial cuffing"; *white arrows*). Slight thickening of the left major fissure also is seen.

present, or if other findings include lymphangitic spread or hilar lymph node enlargement, it is difficult to distinguish between metastasis and primary lung cancer. In some patients, airway obstruction may be the first manifestation of the extrathoracic neoplasm.

Radiographs or CT may show a tapered narrowing of the airway lumen ("rat-tail" appearance), often due to local invasion, or a sessile or polypoid endobronchial mass (Fig. 4-16; see also Fig. 22-7 and 22-8 in Chapter 22), often due to hematogenous spread to the airway wall.

FIG. 4.14. Lymphangitic spread of thyroid carcinoma. High-resolution CT shows nodular thickening of interlobular septa (*small arrows*), the peribronchovascular interstitium (*large arrows*), and the left major fissure (*arrowhead*).

Airway metastases are most common in melanoma, thyroid carcinoma, renal cell carcinoma, testicular carcinoma, breast carcinoma, and sarcomas.

Vascular Metastases

Most tumor emboli associated with hematogenous metastasis are microscopic. In occasional patients, tumor emboli are large enough or numerous enough to result in symptoms or findings of vascular occlusion as a primary manifestation (Table 4-4). Vascular metastases may mimic pulmonary infarction (large tumor emboli) clinically and radiographically or pulmonary hypertension (large or numerous tumor emboli). Vascular metastases may occur with or without other findings of metastatic tumor.

Radiographic findings include (1) visible tumor emboli mimicking the appearance of pulmonary emboli on contrast-enhanced scans; (2) findings of pulmonary

TABLE 4.3 Airway Metastases

Result from
    Local spread from adjacent lung or lymph node metastases
    Hematogenous spread to bronchial wall
    Endobronchial spread
Mimics primary lung cancer
Bronchial narrowing or polypoid mass
Common causes:
    Melanoma
    Thyroid carcinoma
    Renal cell carcinoma
    Testicular carcinoma
    Breast carcinoma
    Sarcomas

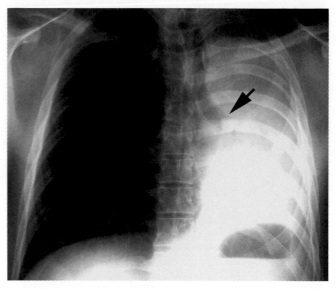

FIG. 4.15. Metastasis to the left main bronchus (*arrow*) from testicular carcinoma. There is obstruction of the left main bronchus with left lung atelectasis.

A

B

FIG. 4.16. Endobronchial metastases. **A:** Metastasis to the left main bronchus from a head and neck carcinoma. A polypoid mass is seen within the left main bronchus. **B:** Polypoid endobronchial mass in metastatic melanoma.

TABLE 4.4 Vascular Metastases

Large tumor emboli uncommon
Findings:
    Vascular filling defects mimicking pulmonary embolism
    Pulmonary infarction
    Beaded vessels
    Pulmonary artery dilatation
Common causes:
    Renal cell carcinoma
    Hepatoma
    Right atrial myxoma
    Angiosarcoma

TABLE 4.5 Lymph Node Metastases

Result from
    Spread via the thoracic duct
    Spread to lymph nodes from hematogenous
      lung metastases
Unilateral or bilateral
Sharply marginated node masses
Common causes:
    Head and neck tumors
    Thyroid carcinoma
    Renal cell carcinoma
    Testicular carcinoma
    Breast carcinoma
    Melanoma
Enhancing lymph node metastases, common causes:
    Thyroid carcinoma
    Renal cell carcinoma
    Testicular carcinoma
    Breast carcinoma
    Melanoma
Calcified lymph node metastases, common causes:
    Thyroid carcinoma
    Mucinous adenocarcinoma
    Sarcomas
Superior mediastinal lymph nodes, common causes:
    Head and neck tumor
    Thyroid carcinoma
Internal mammary lymph node metastases,
  common cause:
    Breast carcinoma
Posterior mediastinal lymph node metastases,
  common causes:
    Abdominal tumors
Paracardiac lymph node metastases, common causes:
    Colon carcinoma
    Lung carcinoma
    Ovarian carcinoma
    Breast carcinoma

infarction; (3) a nodular or beaded appearance of peripheral pulmonary arteries due to smaller tumor emboli; and (4) pulmonary artery dilatation due to large tumor emboli or pulmonary hypertension.

Large tumor emboli are most common with tumors resulting in invasion of large systemic veins or the right heart, most often renal cell carcinoma, hepatoma, right atrial myxoma, and angiosarcoma. Numerous small emboli resulting in pulmonary hypertension and cor pulmonale may occur with very vascular primary tumors. In addition to those listed, these include choriocarcinoma and adenocarcinoma.

Lymph Node Metastases

Metastases to mediastinal or hilar lymph nodes from extrathoracic malignancies are uncommon, occurring in less than 3% of cases. The extrathoracic tumors most likely to metastasize to the mediastinum and hila are carcinomas of the head and neck (including thyroid tumors), genitourinary tract (e.g., renal and testicular carcinoma), breast, and melanoma (Table 4-5). Enlarged lymph nodes may be unilateral or bilateral and symmetrical or asymmetrical. In distinction to hilar masses occurring in lung cancer, which may be quite irregular and ill-defined due to local invasion, hilar node enlargement in patients with metastases are often sharply marginated (Figs. 4-17 and 4-18).

Most metastatic tumors result in lymph node enlargement without distinguishing characteristics. However, enhancing nodes may be seen secondary to metastatic renal cell carcinoma, papillary thyroid carcinoma, lung cancer, sarcomas, melanoma, and some other tumors (Fig. 4-19). Calcified lymph node metastases are most typical of thyroid carcinoma, mucinous adenocarcinoma, and sarcomas. Calcification of treated metastases also may occur (Figs. 4-20 and 4-21). Necrotic, rim-enhancing, or low-attenuation lymph nodes also may be seen (Fig. 4-22); these are common in testicular carcinoma, renal cell carcinoma, breast cancer, and lung cancer.

The location of enlarged nodes sometimes is suggestive of the primary tumor site.

Superior mediastinal lymph node involvement suggests a head and neck tumor (see Fig. 4-18).

Posterior mediastinal or paravertebral lymph node enlargement suggests an abdominal location for the primary tumor (see Fig. 4-19) or tumors metastasizing via retroperitoneal lymph nodes, such as testicular carcinoma. Retrocrural lymph node enlargement often is an associated finding.

Internal mammary lymph node metastases are most like due to breast carcinoma (Fig. 4-23). They may be associated with paracardiac node enlargement.

Paracardiac lymph node enlargement may occur as a result of metastasis from abdominal or thoracic tumors, in approximately equal numbers; most common are carcinomas of the colon, lung, ovary, and breast (Figs. 4-24 and 4-25).

Pleural Metastases

The appearance of pleural metastases is discussed in detail in Chapter 26. Pleural metastasis may result from local spread,

FIG. 4.17. Hilar lymph node metastases from renal cell carcinoma. Well-defined, lobulated hilar masses are visible bilaterally.

hematogenous spread, or lymphatic spread. It is most common with adenocarcinoma (Table 4-6).

In patients with pleural metastases, plain films usually show pleural effusion or pleural thickening, which may be lobulated, nodular, or concentric (i.e., surrounding the lung). The presence of pleural effusion in patients with neoplasm is nonspecific; it may result from lymphatic obstruction (i.e.,

FIG. 4.19. Enhancing lymph node metastasis with metastatic paraganglioma. A left paraaortic lymph node (*arrow*) is densely enhancing.

lymphangitic spread of tumor, hilar or mediastinal node metastases, thoracic duct obstruction) rather than pleural metastases. CT may show pleural effusion with or without pleural thickening (see Fig. 4-24); pleural masses or nodular pleural thickening (see Fig. 4-25); or concentric pleural thickening. Nodular pleural thickening or pleural masses in a patient with known malignancy strongly suggests pleural metastasis.

Pneumothorax

Spontaneous pneumothorax may result from metastases involving the visceral pleural surface. The pleural metastases may appear necrotic or cavitary, or they may appear solid, with pneumothorax presumably resulting from other mechanisms of pleural disruption or airway obstruction with air trapping (Fig. 4-26). Pneumothorax is most typical of metastatic sarcoma, and may be the first symptom of metastasis.

FIG. 4.18. Mediastinal lymph node metastases from papillary thyroid carcinoma. Bilateral superior mediastinal and paratracheal masses are visible. The hila appear normal.

FIG. 4.20. Calcified lymph node metastasis in thyroid carcinoma. A faintly calcified and enlarged pretracheal lymph node (*arrow*) is visible. Lymph node calcification is characteristic of tumors that calcify at their primary site.

FIG. 4.21. Calcified lymph nodes following treatment of metastatic gastric cancer. Multiple densely calcified axillary and mediastinal nodes are visible.

FIG. 4.22. Necrotic lymph node in metastatic renal cell carcinoma. An enlarged pretracheal lymph node (*arrow*) shows a low-attenuation center and rim enhancement.

FIG. 4.23. Internal mammary lymph node metastasis in breast cancer. An enlarged node (*arrow*) is visible on the right.

FIG. 4.24. Paracardiac lymph node metastases in breast cancer. Enlarged right paracardiac lymph nodes (*arrows*) are visible. A malignant pleural effusion is also present. No pleural thickening is visible.

FIG. 4.25. Metastatic colon carcinoma with malignant effusion. Multiple pleural nodules (*white arrows*) are highly suggestive of metastases. Paracardiac lymph node enlargement (*black arrow*) is also present.

TABLE 4.6 Pleural Metastases
Result from
Local spread
Hematogenous spread
Lymphatic spread
Pleural effusion nonspecific
Findings suggesting neoplasm:
Nodular pleural thickening
Concentric pleural thickening

FIG. 4.26. Metastatic melanoma with pneumothorax. A solid-appearing metastasis (*arrow*) involving the visceral pleural surface of the left lung is associated with a pneumothorax. A large metastasis is also visible at the right apex.

KAPOSI'S SARCOMA

Kaposi's sarcoma (KS) is a tumor derived from primitive vascular tissues, occurring in (1) patients with AIDS, in whom lymph node and visceral organ involvement is common, and the prognosis is poor, and (2) in elderly individuals, in whom the disease primarily involves skin, and the prognosis is good. The former type is most common.

KS develops in about 15% to 20% of patients with AIDS (Table 4-7). KS is much more common among subjects who acquire AIDS through sexual contact. Almost all cases occur in homosexual or bisexual men, and KS occurs less frequently in intravenous drug users or patients exposed to HIV by different means. KS is associated with infection by KS-associated herpes virus (KSHV), also termed human herpes virus 8 (HHV-8).

Pulmonary involvement occurs in 20% to 50% of AIDS patients with KS, and usually, but not always, is preceded by cutaneous or visceral involvement. Endobronchial lesions detected at bronchoscopy tend to predict the presence of pulmonary disease. Pathologically, pulmonary involvement in KS is patchy, but it has a distinct relationship to the peribronchovascular interstitium in the perihilar regions and to the pleura.

TABLE 4.7 Kaposi's Sarcoma
Occurs in 15%–20% of AIDS patients
Caused by a herpes virus infection
Pulmonary involvement in 20%–50%
Usually preceded by cutaneous involvement
Airway lesions visible at bronchoscopy
Coarse reticular opacities at the lung bases
Ill-defined or spiculated (flame-shaped) nodules
Parahilar or peribronchovascular distribution
Interlobular septal thickening
Pleural effusion
Lymph node enlargement

A

B

FIG. 4.27. Radiographic appearances of KS in two AIDS patients. **A:** Coarse, ill-defined opacities, and consolidation are visible in the perihilar regions and lower lobes. This is typical of KS. Several nodules are also visible. **B:** Streaky opacities are visible in the lower lobes. Hilar lymph node enlargement is also visible.

Chest radiographs typically show bilateral, diffuse abnormalities characterized by the presence of (1) coarse reticular opacities or ill-defined consolidation in the perihilar regions or lower lobes (90% of cases; Fig. 4-27), (2) poorly defined nodules up to several centimeters in diameter (Fig. 4-28A), and (3) focal ill-defined areas of consolidation. A basal predominance of abnormalities is common, and the earliest abnormalities recognized often include thickening of the peribronchovascular interstitium at the lung bases (see Fig. 4-27). Kerley's lines may be seen. Pleural effusions,

FIG. 4.28. KS in an AIDS patient with a CD4 count of 41. **A:** Chest radiograph shows ill-defined nodular opacities and an increase in streaky opacity at the right base. **B:** CT with 5-mm slice thickness shows ill-defined and spiculated nodules (*arrows*). These are typical of the later stages of KS. **C:** CT with 5-mm slice thickness at a lower level shows involvement of the peribronchovascular regions (*arrows*) typical of KS. **D:** High-resolution CT shows spiculated nodules, peribronchovascular infiltration (*large arrow*), and interlobular septal thickening (*small arrows*). Areas of ground-glass opacity may represent associated pulmonary hemorrhage.

usually bilateral, are seen in 30% of cases. Hilar or mediastinal lymph node enlargement is apparent on the chest radiograph in approximately 10% of patients (see Fig. 4-27B). The chest radiographic appearance is somewhat analogous to that of lymphangitic spread of carcinoma.

Early CT findings include thickening of the peribronchovascular interstitium, particularly at the lung bases, mimicking the appearance of infectious AIDS-related airways disease. Typical CT features of KS in more advanced cases include (1) irregular and ill-defined or spiculated (flame-shaped) nodules, often predominating in the peribronchovascular regions (see Fig. 4-28B to D); (2) peribronchovascular interstitial thickening (see Fig. 4-27D); (3) interlobular septal thickening (see Fig. 4-27D); (4) pleural effusion; and (5) lymphadenopathy. Although a number of infections and tumors in AIDS patients may present radiographically with lung nodules, CT findings of irregular nodules, larger than 1 cm, with a perihilar distribution usually allow KS to be distinguished from other thoracic complications.

SELECTED READING

Aquino S. Imaging of metastatic disease to the thorax. Radiol Clin North Am 2005; 43:481–495.

Davis SD. CT evaluation for pulmonary metastases in patients with extrathoracic malignancy. Radiology 1991; 180:1–12.

Diederich S, Semik M, Lentschig MG, et al. Helical CT of pulmonary nodules in patients with extrathoracic malignancy: CT-surgical correlation. AJR Am J Roentgenol 1999; 172:353–360.

Edinburgh KJ, Jasmer RM, Huang L, et al. Multiple pulmonary nodules in AIDS: usefulness of CT in distinguishing among potential causes. Radiology 2000; 214:427–432.

Goldsmith SH, Bailey HD, Callahan EL, Beattie EJ. Pulmonary metastases from breast carcinoma. Arch Surg 1967; 94:483–488.

Gruden JF, Huang L, Webb WR, et al. AIDS-related Kaposi sarcoma of the lung: radiographic findings and staging system with bronchoscopic correlation. Radiology 1995; 195:545–552.

Hartman TE, Primack SL, Müller NL, Staples CA. Diagnosis of thoracic complications in AIDS: accuracy of CT. AJR Am J Roentgenol 1994; 162:547–553.

Janower ML, Blennerhasset JB. Lymphangitic spread of metastatic tumor to lung. Radiology 1971; 101:267–273.

Johkoh T, Ikezoe J, Tomiyama N, et al. CT findings in lymphangitic carcinomatosis of the lung: correlation with histologic findings and pulmonary function tests. AJR Am J Roentgenol 1992; 158:1217–1222.

McGuinness G, Gruden JF, Bhalla M, et al. AIDS-related airway disease. AJR Am J Roentgenol 1997; 168:67–77.

McLoud TC, Kalisher L, Stark P, Greene R. Intrathoracic lymph node metastases from extrathoracic neoplasms. AJR Am J Roentgenol 1978; 131:403–407.

Munden RF, Pugatch RD, Liptay MJ, et al. Small pulmonary lesions detected at CT: clinical importance. Radiology 1997; 202:105–110.

Munk PL, Müller NL, Miller RR, Ostrow DN. Pulmonary lymphangitic carcinomatosis: CT and pathologic findings. Radiology 1988; 166: 705–709.

Naidich DP, McGuinness G. Pulmonary manifestations of AIDS: CT and radiographic correlations. Radiol Clin North Am 1991; 29:999–1017.

Naidich DP, Tarras M, Garay SM, et al. Kaposi sarcoma: CT-radiographic correlation. Chest 1989; 96:723–728.

Peuchot M, Libshitz HI. Pulmonary metastatic disease: radiologic-surgical correlation. Radiology 1987; 164:719–722.

Quint LE, Park CH, Iannettoni MD. Solitary pulmonary nodules in patients with extrapulmonary neoplasms. Radiology 2000; 217:257–261.

Ren H, Hruban RH, Kuhlman JE, et al. Computed tomography of inflation-fixed lungs: the beaded septum sign of pulmonary metastases. J Comput Assist Tomogr 1989; 13:411–416.

Stein MG, Mayo J, Müller N, et al. Pulmonary lymphangitic spread of carcinoma: appearance on CT scans. Radiology 1987; 162:371–375.

Lymphoma and Lymphoproliferative Disease

W. RICHARD WEBB

Lymphoma accounts for about 4% of newly diagnosed malignancies and commonly involves the mediastinum, hila, and lung parenchyma.

Lymphomas are primary neoplasms of the lymphoreticular system and are classified in two main types: Hodgkin's disease (HD) and non-Hodgkin's lymphoma (NHL). Although HD is the less common of the two types, representing about 25% to 30% of cases, it is more common as a cause of mediastinal disease.

HODGKIN'S DISEASE

HD occurs at all ages, but its peak incidence is in the third and eighth decades; it accounts for about 0.5% to 1% of all newly diagnosed malignancies (Table 5-1). It is more prevalent in males, with a male-to-female ratio ranging from 1.4 to 1.9. Intrathoracic HD usually is associated with disease elsewhere; cervical lymph nodes are commonly involved. Constitutional symptoms may be present.

HD is characterized histologically by the presence of Reed-Sternberg cells. Four histologic types of HD are recognized in the Rye classification: nodular sclerosis (accounting for 50% to 80% of adult HD cases); lymphocyte predominance; mixed cellularity; and lymphocyte depletion.

HD has a predilection for thoracic involvement. Up to 85% of patients with HD have thoracic involvement at the time of diagnosis; nearly all of them have mediastinal lymph node enlargement.

Lymph Node Involvement

HD most often involves superior mediastinal (i.e., prevascular, paratracheal, and aortopulmonary) lymph nodes. These node groups are abnormal in as many as 85% of patients with HD and 98% of those with thoracic involvement (Figs. 5-1 and 5-2); if these nodes appear normal on computed tomography (CT), intrathoracic adenopathy is unlikely to represent HD.

Other sites of involvement in patients with thoracic disease are as follows: the hilar nodes, in about 35% of

patients; the subcarinal nodes, in about 25%; the paracardiac (cardiophrenic angle) lymph nodes, in 10%; the internal mammary nodes, in 5%; and the posterior mediastinal (i.e., paravertebral, paraaortic, and retrocrural) nodes, in 5% (see Figs. 5-2 and 5-3).

Multiple node groups are involved in 85% of those HD patients who have thoracic node involvement. Enlargement of a single node group can be seen in some patients with HD, but it is uncommon, occurring in only 15% of cases with node involvement. Anterior (prevascular) lymph nodes are most often involved as a single group (Fig. 5-4), and this appearance usually indicates the presence of nodular sclerosing HD.

On plain radiographs, anterior mediastinal lymph node enlargement may result in a unilateral or bilateral mediastinal abnormality (see Figs. 5-1A and 5-3A). Enlargement of paratracheal or aortopulmonary window nodes often results in a unilateral or asymmetrical abnormality. Because

---

TABLE 5.1 Hodgkin's Disease

Peak incidence in the third and eighth decades
Characterized by Reed-Sternberg cells
Nodular sclerosis cell type accounts for 50%–80% of adult cases
Staged using Ann Arbor system
Thoracic involvement in 85% of cases at diagnosis
Lymph node involvement in nearly all with thoracic involvement
    Superior mediastinal node enlargement in 98%
    Multiple node groups involved in 85%
    Nodes show low attenuation in 10%–20%
    Residual mediastinal masses common after treatment
    Calcification of lymph nodes common after treatment
Lung disease
    10% have lung involvement at diagnosis
    Nearly always associated with enlarged nodes
    Direct infiltration, lung nodules, or consolidation
    Air bronchograms and cavitation may be seen
    Lung recurrence may occur without enlarged nodes
Pleural effusion in 15%, usually due to lymphatic obstruction

FIG. 5.1. HD involving superior mediastinal lymph nodes. **A:** PA chest radiograph shows bilateral lobulated superior mediastinal masses (*arrows*). **B:** The lateral view shows an anterior mediastinal mass (*arrows*). **C:** Contrast-enhanced CT scan shows prevascular anterior mediastinal lymph node enlargement (*arrows*) and pretracheal lymph node enlargement (∗). Lymph node enlargement in these regions is typical of HD.

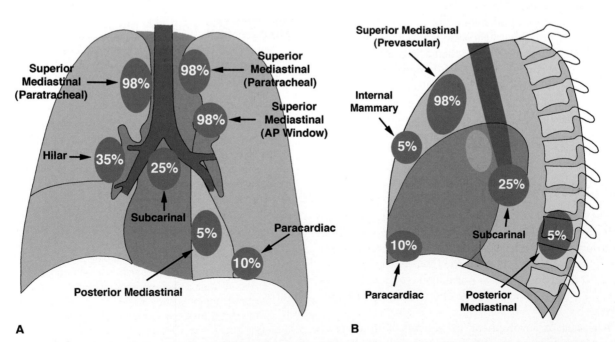

FIG. 5.2. Involvement of mediastinal lymph node groups in HD, illustrated as a percentage of patients with thoracic disease. Lymph node groups as shown on the PA (**A**) and lateral (**B**) radiographs.

FIG. 5.3. HD with involvement of multiple lymph node groups. **A:** PA chest radiograph shows superior mediastinal widening, hilar enlargement, and nodules in the left upper lobe. **B, C:** Large lymph nodes are visible in the prevascular anterior mediastinum (*A*), pretracheal space (*P*), aortopulmonary window (*W*), subcarinal space (*S*), and both hila (*H*). Some discrete lymph nodes are visible, but other enlarged node masses appear matted together, with fat planes between them being invisible. **D:** Paracardiac lymph node enlargement (*arrows*) is visible at a lower level on CT.

FIG. 5.4. Anterior mediastinal lymph node enlargement in nodular sclerosing HD. CT shows lymphadenopathy localized to the anterior mediastinum, which is typical of nodular sclerosing HD.

multiple lymph nodes are involved, mediastinal masses in HD often appear elongated or lobulated in contour. Roughly spherical masses also can be seen (Fig. 5-5). Poor definition of the mass can indicate invasion or extension into adjacent lung.

CT is advantageous in showing abnormalities of mediastinal lymph nodes in patients with HD. Although it is uncommon for CT to show evidence of mediastinal adenopathy if the chest radiograph is normal, in cases in which the radiograph shows lymph node enlargement, CT detects additional sites of adenopathy in many patients. Findings shown only on CT may change the treatment plan in as many as 10% of patients. CT is most helpful in diagnosing subcarinal, internal mammary, and aortopulmonary window node enlargement that is not visible on radiographs.

On CT, abnormal lymph nodes may appear well-defined and discrete (Fig. 5-6), may appear matted (with

FIG. 5.5. Large mediastinal mass in HD. **A:** The PA radiograph shows a large spherical mass projecting to the right, with a smaller left-sided component (*arrows*). **B:** The lateral view shows the mass to be anterior (*arrows*). **C:** At the level of the aortic arch, CT shows a large, rounded mass that largely involves the pretracheal mediastinum (*arrow*). The opacified brachiocephalic veins are displaced anteriorly. Discrete nodal masses are not visible; the mediastinum appears infiltrated by tumor, and no mediastinal fat is visible. **D:** At the level of the left pulmonary artery, CT reveals that the mass occupies the prevascular anterior mediastinum and the precarinal space. The superior vena cava is displaced anteriorly and is compressed. At this level the mass appears somewhat inhomogenous in attenuation. Discrete, enlarged lymph nodes are not seen. **E:** At the level of the right pulmonary artery, anterior mediastinal mass appears to represent thymic involvement.

A

B

FIG. 5.6. HD in a 9-year-old child. **A:** Chest radiograph shows bilateral superior mediastinal masses. **B:** On CT, multiple discrete, enlarged lymph nodes are visible in the middle and anterior mediastinum.

A

B

FIG. 5.7. Lymphoma with necrosis. **A:** Chest radiograph shows a large bilateral mediastinal mass and right pleural effusion, a portion of which is subpulmonic. **B:** Contrast-enhanced CT scan shows an anterior mediastinal mass containing an area of low attenuation (*arrows*). This finding is seen in 10% to 20% of patients with HD.

intervening fat planes poorly seen; see Fig. 5-3B and C), or may be associated with diffuse mediastinal infiltration (with individual lymph nodes being invisible; see Fig. 5-5C and D). Most often, enlarged lymph nodes are of homogeneous soft tissue attenuation, but in 10% to 20% of cases, lymph node masses show areas of low attenuation or necrosis following contrast enhancement (Fig. 5-7). Inhomogeneity without obvious necrosis also may be seen (see Fig. 5-5D). Invasion of mediastinal structures such as the superior vena cava, esophagus, or airways may occur.

Rarely, untreated patients show fine, stippled lymph node calcification. Lymph node calcification is much more common following treatment, with a stippled, confluent, or, less

often, "egg-shell" appearance (Fig. 5-8). Calcification usually occurs after radiation; calcification after chemotherapy is less common.

HD also has a predilection for involvement of the thymus in association with mediastinal lymph node enlargement. Thymic enlargement is seen in 30% to 40% of cases, but may be difficult to distinguish from an anterior mediastinal lymph node mass unless the normal thymic shape is preserved (see Figs. 5-5E and 5-9). In the presence of thymic involvement, a visible mediastinal mass can project to both sides of the mediastinum.

FIG. 5.8. Lymph node calcification following radiation treatment for HD. **A:** Coned-down lateral radiograph shows stippled calcification of enlarged anterior mediastinal lymph nodes (*arrows*), typical of radiated HD. Enlarged residual lymph nodes commonly are seen after treatment of HD. **B, C:** Focal calcifications of enlarged anterior mediastinal lymph nodes are shown on CT. Residual mediastinal lymph node masses following treatment of lymphoma are common, and most typical of nodular sclerosing HD.

FIG. 5.9. Thymic involvement in HD. The thymus is enlarged but maintains a normal shape (*arrows*).

HD is believed to be unifocal in origin, spreading to involve contiguous lymph nodes. It is unusual for HD to skip lymph node groups, and if nodes contiguous with the mediastinum, such as the lower neck or upper abdomen, are not involved by HD, it usually is not necessary to scan more distant regions, such as the pelvis.

However, in patients with mediastinal HD, scanning always should be extended to include the upper abdomen. Intra-abdominal paraaortic adenopathy can be found in 25% of patients with HD, and the spleen and liver are involved in 35% and 10% of patients, respectively.

The magnetic resonance imaging (MRI) appearance of lymph node masses in HD varies with the histology. In nodular sclerosing HD, large amounts of fibrous tissue typically are interlaced with malignant cells. Patients typically show a heterogeneous pattern with mixed high and low signal intensities on T2-weighted images. Low signal intensity areas on T2-weighted images are related to regions of fibrosis in the tumor, and high-intensity regions represent tumor tissue or cystic regions. HD also may demonstrate homogeneous high signal intensity similar to that of fat on T2-weighted images.

A   B

FIG. 5.10. Lung involvement in HD in the same patient shown in Figure 5-3. **A, B:** Large lobulated nodules are visible in the left lung. Some are associated with small bronchi or contain air bronchograms (*arrow*). Extensive mediastinal and hilar lymph node enlargement is present.

Lung Involvement

Lung involvement by HD is seen in 10% of patients at the time of presentation. It is almost always associated with mediastinal (and usually ipsilateral hilar) adenopathy (Fig. 5-10). A variety of manifestations of lung involvement may be seen, but the most common are (a) direct invasion of lung contiguous with abnormal nodes and (b) isolated single or multiple lung nodules, masses, or areas of consolidation. Direct invasion and the presence of nodules or masses occur with about equal frequency.

Direct extension from hilar or mediastinal nodes results in coarse linear or streaky opacities radiating outward into the lung, corresponding on CT to thickening of the peribronchovascular interstitium. Interlobular septal thickening may be associated. In some patients, the appearance may mimic that of lymphangitic spread of carcinoma.

Discrete, single or multiple, well-defined or ill-defined, large or small lung nodules or mass-like lesions, or localized areas of air-space consolidation associated with air bronchograms may be seen (Figs. 5-10 and 5-11). These can cavitate,

with thick or thin walls. Peripheral, subpleural masses are relatively common (Fig. 5-12).

HD occasionally involves bronchi with endobronchial masses or bronchial compression associated with atelectasis (Fig. 5-13).

In previously untreated patients, lung disease is uncommon in the absence of radiographically demonstrable lymph node enlargement; however, lung recurrence can be seen without node enlargement in patients with prior mediastinal radiation (see Fig. 5-11).

A

FIG. 5.11. Lung involvement in recurrent HD. Poorly defined nodules and areas of consolidation are visible. The large area of consolidation on the right contains a number of air bronchograms. There is no obvious lymph node enlargement.

B

FIG. 5.12. Peripheral lung nodule in HD. **A:** CT shows pretracheal and prevascular lymph node enlargement. **B:** A small, well-defined subpleural nodule is visible in the left lung. This was found at biopsy to represent HD.

A   **B**

FIG. 5.13. Endobronchial HD. **A:** The left lower lobe bronchus is narrowed (*arrow*) by a polypoid endobronchial mass. **B:** Endoscopic photograph showing the left upper lobe bronchus (*LUL*) and a polypoid mass (*white arrows*) filling the left lower lobe bronchus (*LLL*).

Pleural and Pericardial Effusion

Pleural effusion is present in about 15% of patients at diagnosis and usually reflects lymphatic or venous obstruction rather than pleural involvement by tumor (see Fig. 5-7). Effusions tend to resolve following local mediastinal or hilar radiation. However, about 20% to 25% of patients with HD who have effusion have CT findings of pleural or extrapleural tumor or lymph node enlargement. Pericardial effusion, present in 5% of patients, usually indicates direct involvement of the pericardium.

Chest Wall Involvement

Invasion of the chest wall contiguous with mediastinal or lung masses occurs in about 5% of cases. Tumor may involve ribs, sternum, or vertebral bodies and typically results in lytic bone destruction. Involvement of the skeleton because of dissemination often results in mixed lytic and blastic lesions (e.g., "ivory vertebra").

Staging

The Ann Arbor Staging Classification is used to describe the anatomic extent of the disease at the time of diagnosis and correlates well with prognosis (Table 5-2). Radiation is used for treatment of stages I and II. A combination of radiation and chemotherapy or chemotherapy alone is used in stages III and IV. There is a 75% to 80% cure rate for adult HD; in children, the cure rate is about 95%.

LYMPHOMA TREATMENT RESPONSE AND RELAPSE

Imaging studies commonly are obtained to judge the completeness of tumor response to treatment and to diagnose relapse.

Reduction of tumor bulk is always seen in patients with adequately treated tumor. Patients who show complete resolution of lymph node masses on CT usually are considered to have had a satisfactory response.

TABLE 5.2 Ann Arbor Staging Classification for Lymphoma

Stage[a]	Definition
I	Involvement of a single lymph node region (I) or a single extralymphatic organ or site (I_E)
II	Involvement of two or more lymph node regions on the same side of the diaphragm (II) or localized involvement of an extralymphatic organ or site and of one or more lymph node regions on the same side of the diaphragm (II_E)
III	Involvement of lymph node regions on both sides of the diaphragm (III), which may also be accompanied by involvement of the spleen (III_S) or by localized involvement of an extralymphatic organ or site (III_E) or both (III_{SE})
IV	Diffuse or disseminated involvement of one or more extralymphatic organs or tissues, with or without associated lymph node involvement

[a]The absence or presence of fever, night sweats, and/or unexplained loss of 10% or more of body weight in 6 months is denoted by the suffix A or B, respectively.

Residual mediastinal mass or lymph node enlargement often is seen in cured patients following treatment (see Figs. 5-8 and 5-14). This is particularly common in patients with treated nodular sclerosing HD; residual masses represent fibrous tissue components of the tumor itself, which change little with treatment, or post-treatment fibrosis. Residual mediastinal masses can be seen in as many as 88% of patients with HD and 40% of patients with NHL. In most patients, masses remain unchanged on follow-up. In some patients, residual masses continue to decrease in size or resolve over a period ranging from 3 to 11 months.

Most patients with thymic enlargement resulting from HD show a return to normal thymic size following treatment, although residual thymic enlargement may be seen in about 30% of cases.

Recurrent HD does not commonly involve previously irradiated (i.e., in field) intrathoracic lymph nodes. However, so-called "in-field recurrence" is seen in a small percentage of cases. Large masses and masses in the anterior mediastinum generally are considered to carry an increased risk of recurrence.

Common sites of recurrent HD include the upper mediastinum and lung, both seen in about half of cases with

A

B

C

FIG. 5.14. Residual mediastinal mass in HD. **A:** CT scan before treatment shows multiple enlarged mediastinal lymph nodes. **B:** CT performed 2 years after treatment shows a decrease in lymph node size, but lymph nodes remain enlarged. Persistent enlarged lymph nodes are common after treatment of HD. **C:** Chest radiograph taken at the same time as the CT scan shown in (**B**) shows widening of the superior mediastinum and prominence of the aortopulmonary window (*arrows*).

TABLE 5.3 Non-Hodgkin's Lymphoma

Diverse group of neoplasms
Specific tumor types classified by WHO
More common than HD
Mean age 55 years; more common than HD in children
Associated with immunodeficiency, HIV, immunosuppression
Prognosis related to cell type
Staging less important than with HD
Thoracic involvement in 40%–50%
Lymphadenopathy in 75% with thoracic disease
   Superior mediastinal lymph nodes involved in nearly all
   Involvement of a single node group common (40%)
   Posterior mediastinal lymph nodes relatively common
Lung involvement (30%) more common than with HD

recurrence. Lymph node recurrence also may involve paracardiac lymph nodes, which usually are excluded from the treatment field because of their close relation to the heart (to avoid radiation pericarditis). Lung recurrence usually is associated with central or peripheral lung nodules, masses, or areas of focal consolidation, any of which may show cavitation. Lung recurrence is uncommonly associated with visible lymph node enlargement on chest radiographs, although it is visible on CT in about half of cases. Pleural effusions or masses and chest wall involvement also are common.

A homogenous hypointense pattern on both T1- and T2-weighted MRI images is characteristic of residual fibrotic masses in cured patients. Approximately 80% of cases show this pattern within 6 to 8 weeks of treatment. A heterogeneous appearance on T2-weighted images is seen after treatment in about 20% of cases, with regions of high signal intensity representing areas of necrosis or inflammation, or, in some patients, residual tumor. Thus, a high relative intensity with T2 weighting indicates the need for biopsy, follow-up, or further imaging. Gallium-67 or positron emission tomographic (PET) imaging can help in distinguishing active tumor from residual benign masses.

NON-HODGKIN'S LYMPHOMA

The term *non-Hodgkin's lymphoma* refers to a diverse group of neoplasms, varying in histology, clinical presentation, radiologic findings, course, and prognosis (Table 5-3). NHL accounts for about 3% of malignancies in adults.

The National Cancer Institute Working Formulation originally classified NHL into low, intermediate, and high grades based on histology and prognosis. In 1994, the International Lymphoma Study Group developed a consensus list of lymphoid neoplasms, which was published as the Revised European-American Classification of Lymphoid Neoplasms (i.e., the REAL classification). A World Health Organization (WHO) classification of lymphoid malignancies has subsequently been developed, using an updated REAL classification. A large number of specific tumor types make up this classification and a distinction among cases as low, intermediate, or high grade is not generally employed. Nonetheless, these terms remain in use in describing NHL.

NHL usually occurs in older persons (40 to 70 years of age; mean, 55 years) than does HD. NHL also is more common than HD in children (Table 5-4).

The incidence of NHL is significantly higher in immunodeficient patients. NHL is associated with congenital immunodeficiency syndromes, human immunodeficiency virus (HIV) infection, and immunosuppressive therapy. These tumors differ somewhat from those that occur spontaneously in immunocompetent patients: they usually are polyclonal rather than monoclonal and usually involve extranodal sites (e.g., central nervous system, lung, gastrointestinal tract).

Thoracic involvement is about half as common as with HD, occurring in 40% to 50% of cases.

Lymph Node Involvement

As with HD, mediastinal lymph node involvement is the most common thoracic abnormality in patients with NHL. It is present in more than 75% of patients with intrathoracic

TABLE 5.4 Comparison of HD and NHL

	HD	NHL
Incidence	0.5%–1% malignancies	3% malignancies
Age at presentation	Peaks in third and eighth decades	Peaks at age 40–70 years; more common than HD in children
Thoracic involvement	85% of cases	40–50% of cases
Node involvement		
Mediastinal nodes	Nearly all cases with thoracic involvement	75% of cases with thoracic involvement
Multiple node groups	85% of patients with lymph node disease	60% of patients with lymph node disease
Single node group	15% of patients with lymph node disease	40% of patients with lymph node disease
Superior mediastinal nodes	98% of cases with thoracic lymph node enlargement	75% of cases with thoracic lymph node enlargement
Posterior mediastinal nodes	5% of cases with thoracic lymph node enlargement	20% of cases with thoracic lymph node enlargement
Skips lymph node groups	Uncommon	Common
Lung involvement	10% of cases	30% of cases
Staging	Important (Ann Arbor classification)	Less important (histology more valuable)

FIG. 5.15. Involvement of mediastinal lymph node groups in NHL, as a percentage of patients with thoracic disease. Lymph node groups as seen on the PA (**A**) and lateral (**B**) radiographs.

disease. Enlargement of pretracheal or anterior mediastinal (superior mediastinal) lymph nodes is the abnormality seen most often; 75% of patients with an intrathoracic abnormality (and 35% of all cases) have prevascular or pretracheal node involvement (Figs. 5-15 and 5-16). Subcarinal lymph node enlargement is present in about 30% of patients with an intrathoracic abnormality (15% of all cases; Fig. 5-17). Other sites of lymph node enlargement (expressed as a percentage of patients with intrathoracic disease) include the hila (20%); posterior mediastinal paraaortic, paravertebral, and retrocrural nodes (20%); and paracardiac nodes (10%).

The pattern of lymph node disease is different than that seen in HD. Involvement of a single node group is much more common in patients with NHL (see Figs. 5-17 and 5-18); 40% of patients with NHL and thoracic involvement have involvement of only one node group, whereas this is seen in only 15% of patients with HD. In addition, the involvement of posterior mediastinal nodal groups is relatively more common with NHL than with HD; posterior lymph node masses often are contiguous with upper abdominal node enlargement (see Fig. 5-17).

Enlarged lymph nodes or mediastinal masses may appear low in attenuation due to necrosis, or may be cystic (Figs. 5-19 and 5-20). Calcification of nodes or masses is rare.

As with HD, CT is more sensitive than chest radiographs in detecting lymph node enlargement in patients with NHL. It is most helpful in detecting subcarinal, posterior mediastinal, and paracardiac lymph nodes.

On MRI, lymph node masses in NHL appear homogeneous on T1-weighted images. They may demonstrate homogeneous high signal intensity similar to that of fat on T2-weighted images, because tumors may be composed almost entirely of malignant cells without significant

FIG. 5.16. Mediastinal lymph node enlargement with NHL. Bulky lymphadenopathy is seen in the prevascular mediastinum with compression of the superior vena cava. Enlarged lymph nodes also are seen in the precarinal region. Nearly 75% of patients with NHL and an intrathoracic abnormality have prevascular or pretracheal node involvement.

FIG. 5.17. Subcarinal and retrocrural lymph node enlargement with NHL. **A:** Subcarinal and paraesophageal lymph node enlargement is visible (*arrow*). **B:** At a lower level, retrocrural lymph node enlargement (*arrow*) also is seen. **C:** Multiple enlarged paraaortic lymph nodes (*arrows*) are visible in the upper abdomen.

FIG. 5.18. Anterior mediastinal lymph node enlargement with NHL. **A:** Left mediastinal mass is visible on the PA radiograph. Elevation of the left hemidiaphragm may reflect left diaphragmatic paralysis related to invasion or compression of the left phrenic nerve. **B:** Lymphadenopathy is limited to the prevascular mediastinum (*arrow*). Involvement of a single lymph node group is much more common in patients with NHL than in those with HD.

FIG. 5.19. NHL with a low-attenuation anterior mediastinal mass. The mass appears cystic due to necrosis. Bilateral pleural effusions also are present.

A

B

C

FIG. 5.20. MRI in a patient with mediastinal NHL. **A, B:** A large anterior mediastinal mass is visible on T1-weighted coronal images. With this technique, the mass appears homogeneous in intensity **C:** An axial T1-weighted, gadolinium-enhanced, fat-saturated image shows enhancement of the large anterior mediastinal tumor. An irregular area of low intensity represents necrosis.

fibrous tissue. However, areas of necrosis may be seen on T2-weighted images or with contrast enhancement (see Fig. 5-20).

Extranodal Disease

Extranodal involvement is much more common with NHL than it is with HD. Extranodal disease seen in patients with a thoracic abnormality includes lung involvement in 30% of patients, pleural effusion or mass in 45% of patients, pericardial effusion or mass in 15% of patients, and chest wall involvement in 10% of patients.

Lung involvement may appear as discrete nodules or masses (Fig. 5-21), air-space consolidation, infiltration contiguous with enlarged lymph nodes or masses (Fig. 5-22), or interstitial thickening resembling lymphangitic spread of carcinoma (Fig. 5-23). In some patients lung infiltration may be rapid, mimicking pneumonia. Bronchial narrowing or obstruction may occur because of compression by hilar mass (Fig. 5-24A) or bronchial involvement by tumor (see Fig. 5-24B).

As with HD, pleural effusion most likely reflects lymphatic obstruction. Pleural effusion may be associated with gross pleural or extrapleural (chest wall) tumor (Fig. 5-25).

FIG. 5.21. Lung involvement with NHL. HRCT in the prone position shows focal masses. This appearance is common when the lung is involved.

FIG. 5.22. Lung infiltration contiguous with mediastinal mass. **A:** Chest radiograph shows opacification of the left hemithorax. **B:** Enhanced CT shows invasion of the lung (*arrows*) adjacent to a large mediastinal mass. Bilateral pleural effusions also are present.

FIG. 5.23. Lymphangitic spread of NHL. **A:** HRCT at a soft-tissue window shows enlarged mediastinal lymph nodes. **B:** HRCT shows diffuse lung infiltration with interlobular septal thickening and some nodularity closely mimicking the appearance of lymphangitic spread of carcinoma.

FIG. 5.24. Airway abnormalities in NHL. **A:** Bilateral hilar masses with bronchial obstruction and atelectasis. The masses (*arrows*) appear lower in attenuation than the collapsed lung. **B:** Airway involvement by NHL in a patient with AIDS. There is irregular narrowing of the left bronchi because of tumor involvement of the bronchial wall.

A

B

C

FIG. 5.25. NHL with pleural effusion and pleural and extrapleural tumor. **A:** Chest radiograph shows a right superior mediastinal mass and a large right pleural effusion. **B:** CT shows a large mass (*M*) posterior to the trachea and associated pleural or extrapleural masses (*arrows*). **C:** At a lower level, a large pleural effusion is visible, with extensive infiltration of the parietal pleura or chest wall by tumor (*black arrows*). A localized chest wall mass with rib destruction also is visible (*white arrows*).

Staging

In about 20% of patients with intrathoracic disease, CT shows abnormalities that are not recognized on plain radiographs. CT also shows more extensive intrathoracic disease in 75% of patients with abnormal chest radiographs. However, precise anatomic staging usually is less important in patients with NHL than in patients with HD. With HD, the anatomic extent of the tumor strongly predicts outcome; with NHL, the histopathologic classification is more predictive.

Patients with aggressive NHL usually are treated with chemotherapy regardless of their anatomic stage, as are the majority of patients with low-grade lymphoma. The use of primary radiotherapy usually is limited to the 20% to 25% of patients with low-grade NHL who are stage I or II at diagnosis (about 20% to 25%). In patients thought to have stage I or II low-grade NHL, CT is appropriate for determining whether intrathoracic disease is present and, if localized, in helping to plan the course of radiation; in patients with intermediate- or high-grade NHL or stage III or IV disease, CT assessment of disease extent has little role.

In contrast to HD, NHL is assumed to be multifocal in origin. The abdomen, pelvis, and neck must be scanned in patients with NHL, because noncontiguous spread is common. Abdominal involvement is more common than in patients with HD, and a variety of findings may be present: intra-abdominal paraaortic adenopathy is found in about 50% of patients with NHL (see Fig. 5-17C), the spleen is involved in 40% of patients, and the liver in 15% of patients. CT of the abdomen and pelvis results in an upgrading of the clinical stage in about 30% of patients with NHL and may detect unsuspected active disease in 40% of patients thought to be in remission.

Specific Types of NHL

Primary Pulmonary Lymphoma

Pulmonary NHL is considered to be primary to the lung if it shows no evidence of extrathoracic dissemination for at least 3 months after the initial diagnosis (Table 5-5). Less than 1% of pulmonary lymphomas are primary. Primary pulmonary lymphoma is generally classified as a MALToma (B-cell lymphoma) or more aggressive high-grade lymphoma.

TABLE 5.5 Primary Pulmonary NHL

No evidence of extrathoracic dissemination for at least
  3 months
<1% incidence of pulmonary lymphomas
Low-grade (MALToma)
Arises from MALT
Solitary nodule or focal consolidation
Multiple nodules or areas of consolidation
Air bronchograms in 50%
Lymph node enlargement in 5%–30%
Good prognosis
High-grade (non-MALT)
Solitary or multiple nodules
Air bronchograms common
Multifocal consolidation

A

B

FIG. 5.26. High-grade primary pulmonary NHL. A: HRCT shows multiple lung nodules and masses, some containing air bronchograms or arising in relation to bronchi. **B:** HRCT with a tissue window shows mildly enlarged mediastinal lymph nodes (*arrows*).

MALToma

MALToma (low-grade B-cell lymphoma) accounts for 75% to 80% of primary pulmonary lymphomas. These are derived from mucosa-associated lymphoid tissue (MALT), hence the term *MALToma* or *MALT lymphoma*, which commonly is used to describe this entity. These tumors are indolent, and patients with primary pulmonary B-cell lymphoma of MALT have a good prognosis. These tumors are thought to arise because of chronic antigenic stimulation associated with smoking, autoimmune disease, or infection.

The most common radiologic manifestation of primary B-cell lymphoma of MALT is a solitary nodule or a focal area of consolidation, ranging in size from a few centimeters to an entire lobe. Multiple nodules or multifocal areas of consolidation also may be present. Air bronchograms are visible in 50% of cases. The parenchymal abnormalities typically show an indolent course with slow growth over months or years. On CT, the single or multiple masses or areas of consolidation may appear primarily peribronchial in location. Pleural effusion is present in approximately 10% of cases, usually in association with evidence of parenchymal involvement. Lymphadenopathy is evident radiographically in 5% to 30% of cases at presentation.

High-Grade (non-MALT) Lymphoma

High-grade (non-MALT) lymphoma is variable in histology. Some tumors occur in patients who have acquired immunodeficiency syndrome (AIDS) or organ transplants (posttransplant lymphoproliferative disorder). The most common radiographic presentation consists of solitary or multiple nodules (Fig. 5-26). As with MALToma, air bronchograms may be visible. Lymph node enlargement may be present. Other manifestations include bilateral consolidation or a diffuse reticulonodular pattern.

Primary Mediastinal Lymphoma

NHL may occur primarily in the mediastinum. The most common cell types presenting in this fashion are lymphoblastic

lymphoma and large cell lymphoma (Table 5-6). These resemble the appearance of mediastinal HD.

Lymphoblastic Lymphoma

Lymphoblastic lymphoma accounts for about 60% of primary mediastinal NHL. If bone marrow and hematologic

TABLE 5.6 Primary Mediastinal NHL

Lymphoblastic lymphoma
60% of primary mediastinal NHL
Termed *lymphoblastic leukemia* if bone marrow and hematologic abnormalities predominate
Children or young adults
Large anterior mediastinal mass
Primary mediastinal large cell lymphoma
Resembles HD
Median age 35 years
Large anterior mediastinal mass

A
B

FIG. 5.27. Lymphoblastic lymphoma in a 14-year-old patient. **A:** Chest radiograph shows a left mediastinal mass (*arrow*). **B:** CT shows an anterior mediastinal mass (*arrows*) that probably represents thymic enlargement. This appearance in a young patient is typical.

involvement are predominant features of this disease, it is termed *lymphoblastic leukemia*. Most patients are children or young adults. A large mediastinal mass representing thymic or lymph node enlargement typically is present; anterior mediastinal lymph nodes are commonly involved (Fig. 5-27). Presenting symptoms usually are related to compression of mediastinal structures.

Primary Mediastinal Large Cell Lymphoma

Primary mediastinal large cell lymphoma is thought to arise from thymic medullary B cells. This entity is difficult to distinguish from HD, both clinically and radiographically. Affected patients usually are younger than other patients with NHL, with a median age of 35 years. A large, lobulated, anterior mediastinal mass averaging 10 cm in diameter is the predominant finding in nearly all patients (Fig. 5-28).

Lymph node enlargement also may be seen in the subcarinal space and posterior mediastinum, but is less common. Low-attenuation areas of necrosis within the mass are seen in almost half of cases; calcification is uncommon. Pleural and pericardial effusions are present in about one third of cases.

AIDS-related Lymphoma

Lymphoma has an incidence of about 2% to 5% in patients with AIDS. In 90% of these patients, it is a B-cell NHL. AIDS-related lymphoma (ARL) typically is characterized by advanced clinical stage, high histologic grade, frequent post-treatment relapse, and poor survival. It originates predominantly in extranodal locations and often involves multiple sites, including bone marrow, central nervous system, lung, liver, and bowel. ARL is associated with advanced AIDS and low CD4 counts.

A
B

FIG. 5.28. Primary mediastinal large cell lymphoma in a 36-year-old man. **A:** Chest radiograph shows mediastinal widening. **B:** CT shows a large inhomogeneous anterior mediastinal mass with regions of low attenuation that probably are due to necrosis.

TABLE 5.7 AIDS-related Lymphoma

High histologic grade and poor survival
Thoracic involvement in 20%–40%
Multiple nodules or masses most common, usually
  well-defined
Cavitation in some
Consolidation or reticular opacities
Lymph node enlargement in 30%–50%, usually in those
  with dissemination
Pulmonary ARL often unassociated with lymph node
  enlargement

Thoracic involvement is present in 20% to 40% of patients with ARL (Table 5-7). Primary pulmonary ARL accounts for only 10% to 15% of cases.

Multiple pulmonary nodules and masses, ranging in size from 1 to 5 cm, are seen most commonly on radiographs or CT (Fig. 5-29). The nodules are usually well-defined. Cavitation may be present but is not common. Localized consolidation, mass lesions, or reticular opacities also may be seen. Mediastinal lymph node enlargement (30% to 50% of cases) is more common in patients with lung involvement associated with disseminated ARL than it is in patients with

A

B

FIG. 5.29. AIDS-related lymphoma. A: A typical appearance of an ARL is that of multiple well-defined nodules, without visible lymph node enlargement. **B:** In another patient with AIDS, a large mass represents pulmonary lymphoma.

FIG. 5.30. Waldenström's macroglobulinemia. CT shows hilar and mediastinal lymph node enlargement (*large arrows*), pleural effusion, and pleural or extrapleural tumor (*small arrows*).

primary or localized pulmonary ARL. Pleural effusion is common, usually in combination with multiple nodules.

Waldenström's Macroglobulinemia

Waldenström's macroglobulinemia is an uncommon form of lymphoma characterized by malignant lymphoma plasmacytoid cells and a monoclonal IgM gammopathy. Bone marrow infiltration, hepatosplenomegaly, and peripheral lymph node enlargement are common manifestations. Lung or mediastinal involvement is very uncommon. Radiographs or CT may show lung consolidation or interstitial infiltration, mediastinal lymph node enlargement, or pleural effusion (Fig. 5-30).

Mycosis Fungoides

Mycosis fungoides is a T-cell lymphoma that primarily affects the skin. Dissemination (Sézary's syndrome) commonly is associated with lung involvement. Radiographic findings are similar to those of other lymphomas and include lung nodules, infiltration of the perihilar peribronchovascular interstitium, areas of lung consolidation, diffuse interstitial infiltration, pleural effusion, and hilar or mediastinal lymph node enlargement.

Plasmacytoma

Plasmacytoma is a focal neoplastic proliferation of plasma cells unassociated with a generalized plasma cell disorder, such as multiple myeloma. Plasmacytoma usually originates in bone, resulting in an expansile osteolytic lesion; extramedullary plasmacytoma, which arises in soft tissues, is much less common. Radiologic manifestations of extramedullary plasmacytoma include a tracheal or endobronchial mass or pulmonary nodules or mass lesions. Plasma cell tumor associated with myeloma can show similar findings.

TABLE 5.8 Pulmonary Lymphoproliferative Diseases

Focal lymphoid hyperplasia
Benign focal lesion
Formerly termed pseudolymphoma
Solitary nodule or a focal consolidation
Multiple nodules less common
Air bronchograms
No lymph node enlargement

Lymphocytic interstitial pneumonia
Benign
Diffuse interstitial infiltrate
Sjögren's syndrome and AIDS
Ground-glass opacity
Consolidation
Poorly defined centrilobular nodules
Small well-defined nodules
Interlobular septal thickening
Cystic air spaces

Angioimmunoblastic lymphadenopathy
Intrathoracic lymph node enlargement in 50%
Interstitial lung involvement in 35%
May progress to lymphoma
Fever and weight loss
Hepatomegaly and splenomegaly
Polyclonal hypergammopathy

Posttransplantation lymphoproliferative disorder
Bone marrow or solid organ transplantation
Occurs in the first year after transplantation
Ranges from benign to lymphoma
Associated with Epstein-Barr virus infection
85% show single or multiple lung nodules
5%–25% lymph node enlargement

Lymphomatoid granulomatosis
Angiocentric, angiodestructive lesions
May progress to lymphoma
Associated with Epstein-Barr virus
Lung commonly involved
Mimics Wegener's granulomatosis
　Bilateral, poorly defined nodules or masses
　Basal predominance
　Cavitation

LYMPHOPROLIFERATIVE DISEASES

In addition to HD and the NHLs, pulmonary lymphoproliferative diseases represent a spectrum of focal and diffuse lung abnormalities associated with either a benign or malignant course (Table 5-8). As with MALToma, described earlier, many of these diseases are related to abnormal proliferation of submucosal lymphoid follicles distributed along distal bronchi and bronchioles, termed *mucosa-associated lymphoid tissue* (MALT). Proliferations of MALT may be either hyperplastic or neoplastic. Polyclonal cellular proliferations usually are hyperplastic and benign, whereas most monoclonal cellular proliferations are malignant. However, in some cases both hyperplasia and neoplasia may be present, and

many lymphoproliferative diseases at least have malignant potential.

Focal Lymphoid Hyperplasia

Focal lymphoid hyperplasia is an uncommon benign condition characterized histologically by localized proliferation of benign mononuclear cells consisting of a mixture of polyclonal lymphocytes, plasma cells, and histiocytes. It has been referred to as a "pseudolymphoma." The most frequently seen radiologic manifestation of focal lymphoid hyperplasia is a solitary nodule or a focal area of consolidation, but multiple nodules may be seen. The nodules or nodular areas of consolidation usually measure several centimeters in diameter and contain air bronchograms (Fig. 5-31). There is no

A

B

FIG. 5.31. Focal lymphoid hyperplasia in a patient with Sjögren's syndrome. **A:** Chest radiograph shows multiple nodular opacities. **B:** CT shows multiple ill-defined nodules, many of which contain air bronchograms.

associated lymphadenopathy. It may occur in association with Sjögren's syndrome.

Lymphoid Interstitial Pneumonia

Lymphoid (lymphocytic) interstitial pneumonia (LIP) may be classified as a benign lymphoproliferative disorder or an interstitial pneumonia (see Chapter 13). It is characterized histologically by a diffuse interstitial infiltrate of mononuclear cells consisting predominantly of lymphocytes and plasma cells. LIP often occurs in association with Sjögren's syndrome or AIDS. In patients with AIDS, LIP usually occurs in children (Fig. 5-32); most other patients with LIP are adults (mean age, 50 years). The main clinical symptoms are cough and dyspnea.

The radiographic findings consist of a reticular or reticulonodular pattern involving mainly the lower lung zones. Less common abnormalities include a nodular pattern or air-space consolidation. On high-resolution CT (HRCT) typical findings include diffuse or patchy areas of ground-glass opacity or consolidation; poorly defined centrilobular nodules; small, well-defined nodules (see Fig. 5-32); and cystic air spaces (typical in Sjögren's syndrome; see Chapter 14).

FIG. 5.32. Lymphoid (lymphocytic) interstitial pneumonia. An 11-year-old child with AIDS shows multiple small nodules and a focal area of consolidation.

The appearance also may mimic lymphangitic spread of carcinoma, with interlobular septal thickening and nodules.

Angioimmunoblastic Lymphadenopathy

Angioimmunoblastic lymphadenopathy (AILD) is an uncommon systemic disease that commonly results in intrathoracic lymph node enlargement. In some cases, the lung and pleura also are involved. Histologically, abnormal lymph nodes show a proliferation of vessels and infiltration by a heterogeneous population of lymphocytes, plasma cells, and immunoblasts. An association with drug treatment suggests that a hypersensitivity reaction also may be involved in the development of AILD. Progression to malignant lymphoma may occur, a condition termed *AILD-like T-cell lymphoma*. Patients usually are over 50 years of age. Constitutional symptoms are typical, with fever and weight loss; other findings include hepatomegaly, splenomegaly, rash, generalized lymph node enlargement, polyclonal hypergammopathy, and Coombs'-positive anemia. The clinical course is variable, with three distinct patterns identified thus far. Fifty percent of patients have rapid progression to death, 25% have prolonged survival with corticosteroid and antineoplastic treatment, and 25% have prolonged survival without treatment.

The radiographic appearance of AILD is similar to that of lymphoma. Approximately 50% of cases show extensive mediastinal and hilar lymph node enlargement, and 35% of cases show lung involvement. Interstitial infiltration in the lower lobes associated with septal thickening or patchy consolidation is typical. Pleural effusion may be present. Enlarged lymph nodes may be seen to enhance if CT with contrast infusion is used.

Posttransplantation Lymphoproliferative Disorder

Several histologic patterns of lymphocyte proliferation, known collectively as *posttransplantation lymphoproliferative disorder* (PTLD), can occur after bone marrow or solid organ transplantation. The histologic patterns range from benign hyperplastic proliferation of lymphocytes to malignant lymphoma.

Most cases of PTLD have been associated with Epstein-Barr virus infection. PTLD affects up to 10% of transplant recipients. Most patients present in the first year after transplantation. PTLD can manifest as localized or disseminated disease and has a predilection for extranodal involvement. Lung involvement may occur as part of multiorgan disease or in isolation.

In 85% of cases, radiographs and CT show single or multiple pulmonary nodules, which may be small or large (0.3 to 5 cm) and well- or ill defined (Fig. 5-33). Other findings include patchy or focal consolidation or ground-glass opacity, a predominantly peribronchial and subpleural or diffuse distribution of parenchymal abnormalities, and hilar or mediastinal lymphadenopathy (5% to 25%). Pleural effusion may be present.

A   **B**

FIG. 5.33. Posttransplantation lymphoproliferative disorder. **A:** Lateral radiograph shows a nodule (*arrows*) in the posterior lower lobe. **B:** CT shows two irregular and poorly margin-ated nodules (*arrows*).

Lymphomatoid Granulomatosis

The term *lymphomatoid granulomatosis* refers to a group of angiocentric, angiodestructive abnormalities characterized by a lymphoid infiltrate and a variable degree of cellular aty-pia. Three grades are thought to exist, based on the degree of cytologic abnormalities and necrosis and their response to treatment. Progression to histologically overt lymphoma may occur. B cells appear to constitute the primary neoplas-tic proliferation in patients with lymphomatoid granuloma-tosis, although an exuberant T-cell reaction also is present. Epstein-Barr virus has been detected in most cases. The lung is the primary site of disease, although other organs—in-cluding skin, brain, kidneys, and heart—may be involved.

Radiographic and CT findings consist primarily of bilat-eral, poorly defined nodular lesions, ranging from 0.5 to 8 cm in diameter, with a basal predominance. Lesions may progress rapidly and cavitate, mimicking Wegener's granulo-matosis. Pleural effusion may be present.

LEUKEMIA

Leukemia may result in lymph node enlargement, lung infil-tration, or pleural abnormalities (Table 5-9).

Mediastinal Abnormalities

Mediastinal lymph nodes commonly are involved in patients with chronic lymphocytic leukemia (CLL) and acute lym-phoblastic leukemia (ALL) (see section on "Lymphoblastic lymphoma" earlier in this chapter). CLL typically occurs in adults older than 60 years; ALL is more common in children than in adults.

Mediastinal lymph node enlargement is visible radio-graphically in about 25% of patients with CLL (Fig. 5-34) and 10% to 20% of patients with ALL, although it is more common at autopsy, being present in more than half of cases. Hilar lymph node enlargement also may be seen but is less common. CLL typically presents with painless lymph node enlargement or hepatosplenomegaly; these abnormalities

TABLE 5.9 Leukemia
Mediastinal lymph node enlargement
25% of CLL
Chronic, slowly progressive
10%–20% of ALL
Large symptomatic anterior mediastinal mass
Acute lymphoblastic lymphoma
5% of acute or chronic myelogenous leukemia
Granulocytic sarcoma (chloroma)
Lung abnormalities
20%–40% lung infiltration at autopsy
Radiographic and CT abnormalities seldom due to leukemia alone
Pneumonia, hemorrhage, drug reactions, edema
Pulmonary leukostasis
Acute myelogenous leukemia
WBC count usually >200,000/mm³
Pulmonary edema

A   **B**

FIG. 5.34. Mediastinal lymph node enlargement in CLL. Enlarged lymph nodes are visible in the prevascular space and internal mammary chain (*arrows* in **A**) and subcarinal space (*arrow* in **B**). A left pleural effusion, which may reflect lymphatic obstruction, also is present.

may be chronic and slowly progressive over a period of years. ALL may present with a large, symptomatic anterior mediastinal mass (see Fig. 5-27).

In patients with acute or chronic myelogenous leukemia, masses of malignant myeloid precursor cells may be found in an extramedullary location, including lymph nodes; these masses are termed *granulocytic sarcoma* or *chloroma* (because of their green color). Granulocytic sarcoma occurs in about 5% of adults and 15% of children with myelogenous leukemia; the thorax is involved uncommonly. In about 50% of cases with thoracic involvement, it involves the mediastinum, either as a focal mass, lymph node enlargement, or generalized widening (Fig. 5-35). Less common sites of involvement include the lungs, pleura, the pericardium, and the hila.

Lung Abnormalities

Pulmonary infiltration is evident at autopsy in 20% to 40% of patients with leukemia. Radiographic findings of pulmonary leukemic infiltration consist of bilateral reticulation that resembles interstitial edema or lymphangitic carcinomatosis. HRCT abnormalities consist of interlobular septal thickening and thickening of the peribronchovascular interstitium.

However, pulmonary abnormalities seen on radiographs or CT in patients with leukemia seldom are due to leukemic infiltration alone. In almost all patients, lung abnormalities are due to pneumonia, hemorrhage, drug-induced lung damage, or pulmonary edema.

Dyspnea in patients with leukemia is sometimes related to *pulmonary leukostasis*. Leukostasis is most common in acute

A   **B**

FIG. 5.35. Chronic granulocytic leukemia with the involvement of mediastinal lymph nodes, so-called granulocytic sarcoma or "chloroma." **A:** Chest radiograph shows a lobulated mediastinal mass (*arrows*). **B:** CT shows extensive lymph node enlargement in the pretracheal and prevascular mediastinum.

FIG. 5.36. Pulmonary leukostasis. A patient with acute leukemia, high white cell count, and leukostasis shows patchy areas of consolidation in the peripheral lung. These usually represent pulmonary edema.

FIG. 5.37. CLL with extrapleural involvement and pleural effusion. A number of masses (*arrows*) appear to be associated with the sternum and ribs. A left pleural effusion also is present. This appearance is similar to that in Figures 5-25 and 5-30.

myelogenous leukemia, and it occurs in patients with very high white blood cell counts (usually over 200,000/mm³). Symptoms result from vascular obstruction (in the lungs and other organs) by leukemic cells. Little, if any, invasion of the pulmonary interstitium occurs in patients with pulmonary leukostasis, and chest radiographs are often normal. In some cases, however, air-space consolidation is visible radiographically due to pulmonary edema (Fig. 5-36). Edema may be due to increased capillary permeability related to the presence of numerous white cells or cardiac failure related to coronary artery leukostasis. Leukostasis is considered an oncologic emergency.

Pleural Disease

As with lymphoma, pleural effusion may reflect lymphatic obstruction (see Fig. 5-34) or pleural involvement by tumor (Fig. 5-37).

SELECTED READING

Aquino SL, Chen MY, Kuo WT, Chiles C. The CT appearance of pleural and extrapleural disease in lymphoma. Clin Radiol 1999; 54:647–650.

Au V, Leung AN. Radiologic manifestations of lymphoma in the thorax. AJR Am J Roentgenol 1997; 168:93–98.

Bae YA, Lee KS. Cross-sectional evaluation of thoracic lymphoma. Radiol Clin North Am. 2008; 46:253–264.

Blunt DM, Padley SP. Radiographic manifestations of AIDS related lymphoma in the thorax. Clin Radiol 1995; 50:607–612.

Bragg DG, Colby TV, Ward JH. New concepts in the non-Hodgkin lymphomas: radiologic implications. Radiology 1986; 159:289–304.

Bragg DG, Chor PJ, Murray KA, Kjeldsberg CR. Lymphoproliferative disorders of the lung: histopathology, clinical manifestations, and imaging features. AJR Am J Roentgenol 1994; 163:273–281.

Carignan S, Staples CA, Müller NL. Intrathoracic lymphoproliferative disorders in the immunocompromised patient: CT findings. Radiology 1995; 197:53–58.

Castellino RA. Hodgkin disease: practical concepts for the diagnostic radiologist. Radiology 1986; 157:305–310.

Castellino RA. The non-Hodgkin lymphomas: practical concepts for the diagnostic radiologist. Radiology 1991; 178:315–321.

Castellino RA, Blank N, Hoppe RT, Cho C. Hodgkin disease: contributions of chest CT in the initial staging evaluation. Radiology 1986; 160: 603–605.

Castellino RA, Hilton S, O'Brien JP, Portlock CS. Non-Hodgkin lymphoma: contribution of chest CT in the initial staging evaluation. Radiology 1996; 199:129–132.

Cobby M, Whipp E, Bullimore J, et al. CT appearances of relapse of lymphoma in the lung. Clin Radiol 1990; 41:232–238.

Collins J, Müller NL, Leung AN, et al. Epstein-Barr virus–associated lymphoproliferative disease of the lung: CT and histologic findings. Radiology 1998; 208:749–759.

Costello P, Mauch P. Radiographic features of recurrent intrathoracic Hodgkin's disease following radiation therapy. AJR Am J Roentgenol 1979; 133:201–206.

Do KH, Lee JS, Seo JB, et al. Pulmonary parenchymal involvement of low-grade lymphoproliferative disorders. J Comput Assist Tomogr 2005; 29:825–830.

Dodd G, Ledesma-Medina J, Baron RL, Fuhrman CR. Posttransplant lymphoproliferative disorder: intrathoracic manifestations. Radiology 1992; 184:65–69.

Eisner MD, Kaplan LD, Herndier B, Stulbarg MS. The pulmonary manifestations of AIDS-related non-Hodgkin's lymphoma. Chest 1996; 110:729–736.

Filly R, Blank N, Castellino R. Radiographic distribution of intrathoracic disease in previously untreated patients with Hodgkin's disease and non-Hodgkin's lymphoma. Radiology 1976; 120:277.

Gibson M, Hansell DM. Lymphocytic disorders of the chest: pathology and imaging. Clin Radiol 1998; 53:469–480.

Harris NL, Jaffe ES, Stein H, et al. A revised European-American classification of lymphoid neoplasms: a proposal from the International Lymphoma Study Group. Blood 1994; 84:1361–1392.

Harris NL, Jaffe ES, Diebold J, et al. The World Health Organization classification of neoplastic diseases of the hematopoietic and lymphoid tissues. Report of the Clinical Advisory Committee meeting, Airlie House, Virginia, November, 1997. Ann Oncol 1999; 10:1419–1432.

Heyneman LE, Johkoh T, Ward S, et al. Pulmonary leukemic infiltrates: high-resolution CT findings in 10 patients. AJR Am J Roentgenol 2000; 174:517–521.

Jochelson M, Mauch P, Balikian J, et al. The significance of the residual mediastinal mass in treated Hodgkin's disease. J Clin Oncol 1985; 3:637–640.

Johkoh T, Müller NL, Pickford HA, et al. Lymphocytic interstitial pneumonia: thin-section CT findings in 22 patients. Radiology 1999; 212:567–572.

Kim HJ, Lee S-H, Park J, et al. Primary pulmonary non-hodgkin lymphoma. Jpn J Clin Oncol 2004; 34:510–514.

Knisely BL, Mastey LA, Mergo PJ, et al. Pulmonary mucosa-associated lymphoid tissue lymphoma: CT and pathologic findings. AJR Am J Roentgenol 1999; 172:1321–1326.

Koss MN. Pulmonary lymphoid disorders. Semin Diagn Pathol 1995; 12:158–171.

Lee DK, Im JG, Lee KS, et al. B-cell lymphoma of bronchus-associated lymphoid tissue (BALT): CT features in 10 patients. J Comput Assist Tomogr 2000; 24:30–34.

Lee KS, Kim Y, Primack SL. Imaging of pulmonary lymphomas. AJR Am J Roentgenol 1997; 168:339–345.

Lee WK, Duddalwar VA, Rouse HC, et al. Extranodal lymphoma in the thorax: cross-sectional imaging findings. Clin Radiol 2009; 64:542–549.

Limpert J, MacMahon H, Variakojis D. Angioimmunoblastic lymphadenopathy: clinical and radiological features. Radiology 1984; 152:27–30.

Lu P. Staging and classification of lymphoma. Semin Nucl Med. 2005; 35:160–164.

O'Donnell PG, Jackson SA, Tung KT, et al. Radiological appearances of lymphomas arising from mucosa-associated lymphoid tissue (MALT) in the lung. Clin Radiol 1998; 53:258–263.

Okada F, Ando Y, Kondo Y, et al. Thoracic CT findings of adult T-cell leukemia or lymphoma. AJR Am J Roentgenol 2004; 182:761–767.

Rappaport DC, Chamberlain DW, Shepherd FA, Hutcheon MA. Lymphoproliferative disorders after lung transplantation: imaging features. Radiology 1998; 206:519–524.

Shaffer K, Smith D, Kirn D, et al. Primary mediastinal large–B-cell lymphoma: radiologic findings at presentation. AJR 1996; 167:425–430.

Sider L, Weiss AJ, Smith MD, et al. Varied appearance of AIDS-related lymphoma in the chest. Radiology 1989; 171:629–632.

Takasugi JE, Godwin JD, Marglin SI, Petersdorf SH. Intrathoracic granulocytic sarcomas. J Thorac Imaging 1996; 11:223–230.

Tateishi U, Muller NL, Johkoh T, et al. Primary mediastinal lymphoma: characteristic features of the various histological subtypes on CT. J Comput Assist Tomogr 2004; 28:782–789.

Thompson GP, Utz JP, Rosenow EC, et al. Pulmonary lymphoproliferative disorders. Mayo Clin Proc 1993; 68:804–817.

Zinzani PL. Lymphoma: diagnosis, staging, natural history, and treatment strategies. Semin Oncol 2005; 32:4–10.

The Pulmonary Hila

W. RICHARD WEBB

CHEST RADIOGRAPHS

In most cases, plain films are adequate for identifying large hilar masses. Small masses can be more difficult to detect because of variation in the radiographic appearances of the normal hila.

Nonetheless, careful evaluation of the hila on chest radiographs can often yield significant diagnostic information. Abnormalities may present as a change in hilar size or density, bronchial wall thickening or narrowing of the bronchial lumen, or an alteration in the hilar contours.

Normal Hilar Contours

Frontal Radiograph

On a frontal (posteroanterior [PA] or anteroposterior [AP]) radiograph, the hilar shadows primarily represent the silhouettes of the hilar pulmonary arteries. The left pulmonary artery is situated higher than the right, and consequently the left hilum appears higher than the right in 97% of cases; in the remainder, they are at the same level.

Right Hilum

The superior portion of the right hilum is made up of the medially located truncus anterior, the artery supplying most of the upper lobe, and the right superior pulmonary vein, which forms the lateral margin of the upper hilum (Fig. 6-1). The anterior segment bronchus of the right upper lobe (RUL) is visible in 80% of patients as a 4- to 5-mm ring shadow in the lateral aspect of the hilum, accompanied by an artery of similar size. The RUL bronchus is sometimes visible.

The lower aspect of the right hilum is made up of the interlobar or descending pulmonary artery laterally and the bronchus intermedius medially. The pulmonary artery should measure 16 mm or less in thickness lateral to the bronchus (approximately the diameter of a dime) in men and 15 mm or less in women. The interlobar artery tapers inferiorly as it branches, with its lateral aspect appearing straight or slightly convex. Branches of the interlobar artery and segmental bronchi may be seen in the inferior

hilum. Occasionally the lower part of the interlobar artery appears rounded, mimicking a mass or enlarged lymph node. This is most commonly seen when lung volumes are low.

A shallow concave angle is formed at the point where the superior pulmonary vein crosses the interlobar pulmonary artery. This is termed the *hilar angle* (Fig. 6-1).

The right inferior pulmonary vein is located inferior and medial to the hilum, and does not contribute significantly to the hilar silhouette.

Left Hilum

The left pulmonary artery passes above the left main and upper lobe bronchus, gives off small upper lobe branches, and descends posterior and lateral to the left upper lobe (LUL) bronchus and lower lobe bronchus. The superior hilar shadow is made up of the superior aspect of the left pulmonary artery, superior pulmonary vein, and small arterial branches (Fig. 6-2). The anterior segmental bronchus of the LUL may be seen in the lateral hilum at this level. As on the right, the interlobar pulmonary artery tapers caudally, but it is less clearly seen and more difficult to measure than the right pulmonary artery. The left inferior pulmonary vein contributes little to the hilar shadow.

Lateral Radiograph

The right and left hilar shadows are superimposed on the lateral radiograph, but specific parts of the right and left hila can be seen (Figs. 6-3 and 6-4). Identification of the hilar bronchi should be the first step in analysis of the hila on lateral films.

Right Hilum

The location of the tracheal carina and therefore the origins of the main bronchi can be determined by following the tracheal air column inferiorly. The carina is located at the point the air column begins to taper (Fig. 6-3B).

Below this level, a thin line, termed the *intermediate stem line*, is at least partially visible in 95% of patients (see Fig. 6-3). This line may be 5 cm or more in length and

A

B

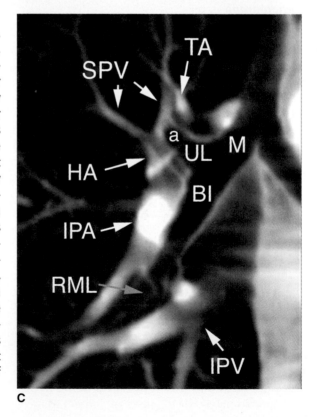

C

FIG. 6.1. Normal right hilum. **A:** Plain radiograph. The large bronchi (*M*, right main bronchus; *UL*, right upper lobe bronchus; *BI*, bronchus intermedius) are visible in the medial hilum. The anterior segment bronchus (*a*) is visible as a ring shadow lateral to the pulmonary arteries. Visible vascular structures include the apical branch of the truncus anterior (*TA*) in the medial superior hilum, and the superior pulmonary vein (*SPV*) in the lateral aspect of the superior hilum. The interlobar pulmonary artery (*IPA*) forms the lateral aspect of the inferior hilum and should measure 16 mm or less in men and 15 mm or less in women. A concavity is visible in the lateral hilum at the point the superior pulmonary vein crosses the interlobar pulmonary artery. This is termed the hilar angle (*HA*). **B, C:** Coronal CT reformations through the right hilum in two patients. In addition to the structures visible in **A,** the right middle lobe bronchus (*RML*) is visible inferiorly. The inferior pulmonary vein (*IPV*) lies medial and below the hilar shadow and is difficult to recognize on the chest radiograph because of the heart shadow.

measures up to 3 mm in thickness. It corresponds superiorly to the posterior wall of the right main bronchus and more inferiorly to the posterior wall of the bronchus intermedius. The RUL bronchus is visible in 50% of patients as a rounded lucency anterior to the upper aspect of the intermediate stem line, but it is seldom seen well.

The anterior wall of the bronchus intermedius is visible as an edge, outlined by the right pulmonary artery and superior

A   **B**

FIG. 6.2. Normal left hilum. **A:** PA radiograph. **B:** Coronal CT reformation. *MB*, left main bronchus; *LUL*, left upper lobe bronchus; *LL*, left lower lobe bronchus. The anterior segment bronchus (*a*) is visible as a ring shadow lateral to the main pulmonary artery, overlying the superior trunk of the left upper lobe bronchus. The left pulmonary artery (*LPA*) is visible as an oval opacity above the main and left upper lobe bronchus. The apical branch of the left pulmonary artery (*PA*) arises from the superior aspect of the pulmonary artery and as on the right is located medially. The superior pulmonary vein (*SPV*) forms the lateral aspect of the superior hilum. The interlobar pulmonary artery (*IPA*) forms the lateral aspect of the inferior hilum. The inferior pulmonary vein (*IPV*) may be visible inferiorly.

pulmonary vein. In combination, these vessels create an oval shadow making up the anterior portion of the hilar silhouette. The right middle lobe bronchus is sometimes seen curving anteriorly below the inferior edge of this oval shadow. In 15% of individuals, the anterior wall of the RLL bronchus is visible below this level as a thin straight line, 1 to 2 cm long.

Left Hilum

Below the carina, the left main bronchus is superimposed on the right main bronchus (see Fig. 6-4). A well-defined rounded lucency representing the horizontal portion of the distal left main bronchus and LUL (LM/LUL) bronchus is visible in 80% of subjects several centimeters below the carina. This lucency is more clearly seen, is larger, and is better defined than the rounded lucency representing the RUL bronchus because vessels surround much of its circumference. Localizing the LM/LUL bronchus is an important first step in identifying left hilar structures on the lateral radiograph. Because the left main bronchus is longer than the right, the LM/LUL bronchus is seen at a lower level than the RUL bronchus.

The anterior wall of the left lower lobe (LLL) bronchus is visible below the lucency of the LM/LUL bronchus as a

thin curved line, concave anteriorly, in about 45% of cases. It arises tangential to the anterior wall of the LM/LUL bronchus.

The left pulmonary artery forms a comma-shaped opacity seen above the lucency of the LM/LUL bronchus and then passing posterior to it. Thus, while the right hilar vasculature largely accounts for the soft tissue in the anterior aspect of the combined hilar silhouette, the left pulmonary artery primarily accounts for its posterior aspect.

Plain Film Diagnosis of Hilar Mass or Lymphadenopathy

Frontal Radiograph

On a frontal radiograph, patients with a hilar mass or lymph node enlargement may show one of several findings:

- Hilar enlargement (Fig. 6-5A)
- A focal mass (see Fig. 6-5B)
- Increase in hilar density (see Fig. 6-5C)
- Hilar lobulation (see Fig. 6-5D)
- Convexity of the hilar angle (see Fig. 6-5E)

(text continues on page 161)

FIG. 6.3. Lateral chest radiograph; normal right hilar anatomy **A:** Diagram of right hilar structures. Anterior is to the left and posterior to the right. Right hilar structures appear dark and left hilar structures are dimmed. *RUL*, right upper lobe bronchus; *BI*, bronchus intermedius; *RML*, right middle lobe bronchus; *RLL*, right lower lobe bronchus; *ISL*, intermediate stem line; *PWBI*, posterior wall of bronchus intermedius. The interlobar right pulmonary artery (*RPA*) results in an oval shadow anterior to the BI. The superior pulmonary vein (*SPV*), along with the truncus anterior, forms the superior part of the vascular shadow anterior to the bronchi. The inferior pulmonary veins (*IPV*) are inferior. Left hilar structures are described in Figure 6-4A. **B:** Lateral radiograph showing right hilar anatomy. The trachea (*T*) is visible superiorly. The point at which the tracheal air column narrows (*large white arrow*) is the carina; the main and lobar bronchi are seen below this level. The right upper lobe bronchus (*RUL*) may be seen as a rounded lucency within the superior hilar shadow, slightly below the carina. Below the RUL, the bronchus intermedius (*BI*) is visible to the level of its bifurcation. The intermediate stem line or posterior wall of the bronchus intermedius is often visible as a thin white line (*small white arrows*). The oval shadow of the right hilar arteries and veins (*black arrows; AV*) is visible anterior to the bronchus intermedius. **C:** Lateral radiograph showing right hilar anatomy in a patient with left pneumonectomy. Only right hilar structures are visible. The trachea (*T*) is visible superiorly. Visible are the right upper lobe bronchus (*RUL*), intermediate stem line (posterior wall of the bronchus intermedius) (*white arrows*), right middle lobe bronchus (*RML*), superior segmental bronchus of the right lower lobe (*SS RLL*), and the anterior wall of the right lower lobe bronchus (*arrows; RLL*). Below the RUL, the bronchus intermedius (*BI*) is visible to the level of its bifurcation. The oval shadow of the right hilar arteries and veins (*AV*) is visible anterior to the bronchus intermedius, and the inferior pulmonary veins (*V*) are located inferiorly. **D:** CT reformation through the right hilum. *RUL*, right upper lobe bronchus; *white arrows*, intermediate stem line (posterior wall of the bronchus intermedius); *RML*, right middle lobe bronchus; *SS RLL*, superior segment bronchus of the right lower lobe; *RLL*, anterior wall of the right lower lobe bronchus; *AV*, right hilar arteries and veins; *V*, inferior pulmonary veins.

FIG. 6.4. Lateral chest radiograph; normal left hilar anatomy **A:** Diagram of hilar anatomy. Left hilar structures appear dark and right hilar structures are dimmed. *LMB*, left main bronchus; *M/U*, lucency of the left main and left upper lobe bronchus; *LLL*, left lower lobe bronchus; *LPA*, left pulmonary artery; *IPV*, inferior pulmonary veins; *SPV*, superior pulmonary vein. For right hilar structures see Figure 6-3A. **B:** Lateral radiograph showing left hilar anatomy; this is the same radiograph as in Figure 6-3B. The trachea (*T*) is visible superiorly. The horizontal portion of the left main and left upper lobe bronchus (*LM/UL*) results in an easily seen oval lucency. Above this level and superimposed on the bronchus intermedius, the main portion of the left main bronchus may be seen. The anterior wall of the left lower lobe bronchus (*LLL*) is visible below the *LM/UL* as a thin white line and typically appears concave anteriorly. *PA*, pulmonary artery. **C:** Lateral radiograph showing left hilar anatomy in a patient with a right pneumonectomy. Only left hilar structures are visible. The trachea (*T*) is visible superiorly. The oval lucency of the horizontal portion of the left main and left upper lobe bronchus (*LM/UL*) is easily seen. Below this level, the anterior wall of the left lower lobe (*LLL*) bronchus is visible as a thin white line, concave anteriorly. The left pulmonary artery (*PA*) is situated above and behind the LMB (*black arrows*). The left superior pulmonary veins (*SPV*) are visible anterior and superior to the LMB, and the inferior pulmonary veins (*IPV*) are located inferiorly. **D:** CT reformation through the left hilum. LMB, left main and left upper lobe bronchus; LLL, anterior wall of the left lower lobe bronchus; PA, left pulmonary artery; IPV, inferior pulmonary veins.

FIG. 6.5. Radiographic findings in hilar mass or lymph node enlargement. **A:** Hilar enlargement in a patient with lymph node enlargement due to metastatic renal cell carcinoma. The right hilum (*arrows*) is markedly enlarged and is rounded in contour, without its normal "vascular" shape. **B:** Focal hilar mass in bronchogenic carcinoma. A single, poorly marginated mass (*arrows*) obscures the upper left hilum. This appearance is typical of lung cancer originating in the hilum. **C:** Increase in hilar density due to right hilar carcinoma. The right hilum appears denser than the left. This is often due to mass or enlarged nodes anterior or posterior to the hilum. The right hilum is also enlarged, with a subtle convexity in the hilar angle. **D:** Hilar lobulation due to sarcoidosis. The hila have distinct lobulated contours (*arrows*) typical of lymph node enlargement. Node calcification is also seen. **E:** Convexity of the hilar angle in a patient with Castleman's disease involving the right hilum. A mass (*arrow*) is visible in the region of the hilar angle. The mass projects lateral to the anterior segment bronchus (*a*) of the upper lobe.

Hilar enlargement is often present in patients with hilar lymph node abnormalities (see Fig. 6-5A) or hilar mass (see Fig. 6-5B); it may be unilateral or bilateral. In the large majority of normal patients, the hila appear equal in size on frontal radiographs; comparison of the two hila is helpful in patients with a unilateral abnormality. Measurement of the width of the right hilum lateral to the bronchus intermedius may also be valuable in diagnosis; as indicated above, this measurement should be 16 mm or less in men and 15 mm or less in women.

Masses sometimes produce a unilateral increase in the hilar density on frontal radiographs (see Fig. 6-5A and C). This generally results when a mass or lymph node enlargement is located in the anterior or posterior hilum and is superimposed on the hilar shadow. In some patients, an increase in hilar density may be the only visible abnormality on the frontal radiograph; in such cases, the mass is often better seen on the lateral radiograph.

Hilar mass results in a focal alteration of the normal hilar contours. Lymph node enlargement may result in a focal abnormality or a more generalized lobulated appearance (see Fig. 6-5A and D). A common site for lymph node enlargement in the right hilum is the normally concave hilar angle; a convexity in this region is abnormal (see Fig. 6-5E).

The normal hila look vascular. The hilar shadows, primarily representing the pulmonary arteries, taper gradually with vessels arising from their periphery. Enlargement of a pulmonary artery results in increased hilar size and density, but the hilum retains its "vascular" appearance (Fig. 6-6). The appearance of pulmonary vessels converging on the lateral aspect of the hilum is termed the "hilum convergence" sign and is indicative of vascular dilatation as the cause of hilar enlargement. The hilar angle typically retains its normal concave appearance.

Enlargement of hilar arteries is most typical of pulmonary hypertension. In addition to hilar enlargement, patients with pulmonary hypertension often show abnormal prominence of the main pulmonary artery on the PA radiograph and the main pulmonary artery and right ventricle on the lateral view. Pulmonic stenosis results in enlargement of the main and left pulmonary artery, while the right pulmonary artery usually appears normal in size.

Bronchial narrowing and obstruction associated with a hilar mass are usually difficult to diagnose on plain radiographs unless associated abnormalities such as mucous plugging, atelectasis, or obstructive pneumonia are visible (see Chapter 3).

Lateral Radiograph

Enlargement of the oval and comma-shaped shadows of the right and left pulmonary arteries indicates pulmonary artery dilatation (see Fig. 6-6B). As on the frontal radiograph, increased hilar size, focal mass, lobulation of hilar contours, or

A   B

FIG. 6.6. Hilar enlargement in pulmonary hypertension. **A:** Enlargement of a pulmonary artery results in increased hilar size and density, but the hilum retains its "vascular" appearance. Vessels (*small arrows*) may be seen arising from the edges of the hilar shadow, the so-called hilum convergence sign, indicating the presence of vascular enlargement. The hilar angle (*large arrow*) remains concave. The main pulmonary artery (*PA*) is also enlarged. **B:** Lateral view. Although increased in size, the right (*RPA*) and left (*LPA*) pulmonary arteries retain their shape. Small branches arising from the edges of the arteries (*arrows*) result in the hilum convergence sign. (*Figure continues.*)

C

D

FIG. 6.6. *(Continued.)* **C, D:** CT shows enlargement of the main pulmonary artery (*PA*), right (*RPA*) and left (*LPA*) pulmonary arteries, and the interlobar and middle lobe branches (*arrows*).

alternation in the normal oval and comma-shaped shadows can indicate a hilar mass or lymph node enlargement.

Attention to several specific regions visible on the lateral radiograph may also be helpful in diagnosis, including the posterior wall of the bronchus intermedius (PWBI), the inferior hilar window, and the RUL bronchus (sign).

Posterior Wall of the Bronchus Intermedius

The PWBI is seen as a vertical or slightly oblique line or stripe in about 95% of patients (see Fig. 6-3). At its upper extent, the PWBI is contiguous with the posterior wall of the right main bronchus, forming the intermediate stem line described

above. This stripe is normally 0.5 to 3 mm thick. Thickening of this stripe may be seen in patients with neoplasm involving the hilum (Fig. 6-7), hilar adenopathy, interstitial pulmonary edema (Fig. 6-8), or interstitial thickening of various causes. Obliteration of the posterior bronchial wall and the presence of soft-tissue opacity behind it are virtually diagnostic of a mass in the hilum or adjacent lung.

Inferior Hilar Window

On the lateral radiograph, the oval soft-tissue shadow representing the right hilar vessels is visible in the anterior aspect of the silhouette of the superimposed hila, while the

A

B

FIG. 6.7. Thickening of the posterior wall of the bronchus intermedius in right hilar carcinoma. **A:** Lateral chest radiograph shows marked thickening of the posterior wall of the bronchus intermedius (*arrows*). **B:** CT in this patient shows a right hilar mass (*M*) with infiltration and thickening of the posterior bronchial wall (*arrows*).

A   **B**

FIG. 6.8. Thickening of the posterior wall of the bronchus intermedius in pulmonary edema. **A:** A patient with longstanding renal failure shows a normal posterior bronchial wall (*arrows*). **B:** When the patient is in pulmonary edema, the posterior bronchial wall appears thickened (*arrows*).

comma-shaped left pulmonary artery occupies its superior and posterior aspect. The inferior hilar shadow contains no large vessels and consequently is termed the inferior hilar window (IHW). The IHW corresponds to an avascular region anterior to both lower lobe bronchi. It appears as a roughly triangular lucency in the anterior and inferior hilar shadow (Figs. 6-9).

In normal subjects, the inferior hilum appears radiolucent, and the composite hilar silhouette appears as an incomplete oval. The presence of a soft-tissue opacity of more than 1 cm in the IHW is more than 90% accurate in diagnosing a hilar mass or adenopathy in this region. In abnormals, the addition of an opacity in the inferior hilum (IHW) results in the appearance of a complete oval shadow on lateral radiographs

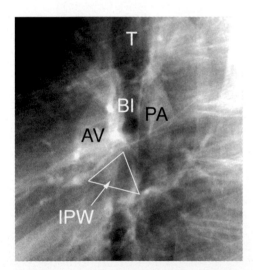

FIG. 6.9. The inferior hilar window. Lateral view. This image is the same as that in Figures 6-3B and 6-4B. The right hilar vessels (*AV*) occupy the anterior part of the hilar shadow. The left pulmonary artery (*PA*) is visible posteriorly and superiorly. The inferior hilar window is a roughly triangular lucency (*IPW*) in the anterior and inferior hilar shadow, below these major vascular branches. It represents an avascular region anterior to both lower lobe bronchi. *T*, trachea; *BI*, bronchus intermedius.

FIG. 6.10. Lymph node enlargement in sarcoidosis, with filling in of the inferior hilar window. Enlarged lymph nodes in the inferior hilar window (*large arrow*), when added to the shadows of the pulmonary arteries, result in a complete oval shadow on the lateral view (*small arrows*). This differs from the normal incomplete oval.

FIG. 6.11. Lymph node enlargement in sarcoidosis, with filling in of the inferior hilar window. **A:** PA chest radiograph shows subtle hilar lobulation. **B:** Lateral view shows lobulation of the hilar contours with filling in of the inferior hilar window (*arrow*). The hilar silhouette forms a complete oval. **C:** CT shows lymph node enlargement in the anterior inferior hila, in the space anterior to the lower lobe bronchi. **D:** CT reformation through the right hilum shows lymph node enlargement in the inferior hilar window (*large arrow*), inferior to the right hilar artery and vein *(RAV). RUL*, right upper lobe bronchus; *BI*, bronchus intermedius.

(Figs. 6-10 and 6-11). The side of the mass may be difficult to determine, although the frontal radiograph may help. Also, if a lower lobe bronchus is visible as a linear shadow, the mass must be on the opposite side.

Right Upper Lobe Bronchus (Sign)

Below the tracheal carina, two rounded radiolucencies are commonly seen, one above the other, in line with the tracheal air column and overlying the hilar bronchi. The lower of the two lucencies represents the horizontal portion of the left main and upper lobe bronchus. The upper lucency represents the RUL bronchus (see Fig. 6-3). It is usually less well seen, as it is not surrounded by vascular structures.

If the RUL bronchus is sharply margined throughout its circumference (and more importantly if this represents a change compared to prior radiographs), hilar mass or adenopathy (surrounding and outlining the bronchus) is likely present (see Fig. 6-12). This sign can also be helpful in distinguishing hilar vascular enlargement (which does not result in this sign) from hilar node enlargement.

FIG. 6.12. Right upper lobe bronchus sign in lung cancer. **A:** Lateral radiograph shows the right upper lobe bronchus (*RUL*) as a lucency surrounded by mass (*arrows*). Thickening of the posterior wall of the bronchus intermedius is also visible. **B:** CT shows a large mass (*arrows*) surrounding the upper lobe bronchus.

CT OF THE HILA

The pulmonary hila are complex structures containing the lobar and segmental bronchi, pulmonary arteries and veins, bronchial arteries and veins, soft tissue, and lymph nodes. The appearances of bronchi, vessels, and nodes and their consistent relationships at different hilar levels allow for reliable identification of these structures. Identification of specific bronchi is the first step in analysis of the hila. Bronchi are quite consistent in their branching pattern (Fig. 6-13).

CT of the Hilar Bronchi

Using a spiral CT technique and a slice thickness of 5 mm or less, all segmental bronchi should be visible. Their appearance depends on their orientation.

Bronchi oriented in or near the scan plane, and therefore seen along their axes as tubular structures, include the RUL bronchus (including both the anterior and posterior segmental bronchi), the LUL bronchus (including the anterior segmental bronchus), a portion of the middle lobe bronchus, and the superior segmental bronchi of both lower lobes.

Bronchi having a vertical course are seen in cross section and appear as circular lucencies. These include the apical segmental bronchus of the RUL, the apical-posterior segmental bronchus of the LUL, and proximal portions of both lower lobe bronchi (below the takeoff of the superior segmental bronchi), and the medial and posterior basal lower lobe segments.

The most difficult bronchi to visualize clearly are those oriented obliquely relative to the scan plane, including the superior and inferior lingular bronchi, the lateral and medial segmental bronchi of the middle lobe, and the anterior and

FIG. 6.13. Normal bronchial anatomy. **A:** Anatomy of bronchial segments as shown on a PA chest radiograph. **B:** Levels of CT slices shown in Figures 6-14 to 6-22.

FIG. 6.14. Apical segment bronchus right upper lobe. The bronchus (*A*) is visible as a ring shadow at a level near the carina. A vessel of similar size and shape medial to the bronchus represents the artery to the apical segment. A vein characteristically lies lateral to the bronchus.

lateral basal lower lobe segments. Such bronchi appear elliptical on CT.

Right Bronchial Anatomy

The right main bronchus is relatively short, dividing into the RUL bronchus and bronchus intermedius. Often the carina, right main bronchus, and RUL bronchus are visible on a single scan.

Right Upper Lobe Bronchus

The RUL bronchus is always found at or just below the carina. The RUL bronchus courses laterally for 1 to 2 cm before

dividing into its three segmental branches (apical, anterior, and posterior; Figs. 6-14 and 6-15A). Characteristically, the posterior wall of the RUL bronchus is sharply outlined by lung and is seen as a thin line (see Fig. 6-15A). The upper limit of normal for thickness of the posterior wall of the RUL bronchus is 3 to 5 mm. However, the posterior part of the arch of the azygos vein can result in apparent bronchial wall thickening.

The precise branching pattern of the RUL bronchus is variable, primarily due to variation in the site of origin of the apical segmental bronchus.

Apical Segment

The apical segmental bronchus of the RUL is visible above the RUL bronchus itself, usually at or near the level of the distal trachea (see Fig. 6-14). It is seen in cross section as a circular lucency.

Anterior and Posterior Segments

The anterior and posterior segmental bronchi arise as a Y-shaped bifurcation of the RUL bronchus (see Fig. 6-15A). The anterior segment bronchus almost always lies in the plane of scan and is more easily seen. The posterior segmental bronchus may have a similar appearance but often angles slightly cephalad from its origin and is usually visible at progressively higher levels as it courses posteriorly.

In many patients a trifurcation of the RUL bronchus is present, with the origin of the apical segment bronchus seen as a rounded area of lucency superimposed on the distal

A

B

FIG. 6.15. Right upper lobe bronchus; apical posterior segment bronchus of left upper lobe. **A:** Lung window. On the right side, slightly below the carina, the right upper lobe bronchus (*UL*) is visible along its axis. Its posterior wall is visible as a thin white line. It branches in a Y shape into its anterior (*Ant*) and posterior (*P*) segments. On the left side, the apical posterior segment bronchus (*AP*) is visible as a ring shadow. **B:** Soft-tissue window scan following contrast enhancement. On the right, the truncus anterior (*TA*) lies anterior to the right upper lobe bronchus and appears similar in size to the main bronchus seen on the same scan. A vein lies between the anterior and posterior segmental bronchi (V in A.). On the left, the left pulmonary artery (*LPA*) is posterior. The artery supplying the anterior segment (*AS*) of the left upper lobe is located medial to the apical posterior segment bronchus. The superior pulmonary vein (*SPV*) is anterior and medial to the anterior segment artery.

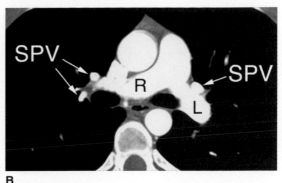

A   **B**

FIG. 6.16. Bronchus intermedius; anterior segment left upper lobe. **A:** On the right, the bronchus intermedius (*BI*) is visible as an oval lucency. Its posterior wall is sharply outlined by lung and appears a few millimeters thick. On the left, the anterior segment bronchus (*Ant*) of the left upper lobe is seen arising from the anterior aspect of the superior bronchial trunk (*ST*) of the left upper lobe. **B:** On the right, the right pulmonary artery (*R*) is visible medial to the bronchus, with the interlobar pulmonary artery passing anterior to the BI. Two branches of the superior pulmonary vein (*SPV*) are visible anterior and lateral to the artery and bronchus. Normal lymph nodes are visible lateral to the pulmonary artery and medial to the SPV. On the left, the left pulmonary artery (*L*) is posterior. The SPV is anterior and medial to the superior trunk.

portion of the RUL bronchus, at or just above the origins of the anterior and posterior segments. Major anatomic variants are unusual. Most frequent is tracheal bronchus, described in Chapter 1.

Bronchus Intermedius

The bronchus intermedius is 3 to 4 cm long, beginning at the level of the RUL bronchus. It gives rise to the middle lobe and lower lobe bronchi inferiorly. Because of its length, it is seen on a number of adjacent scans (Figs. 6-16 to 6-18).

The bronchus intermedius appears round or oval in cross section. The posterior wall of the bronchus intermedius is in contact with the superior segment of the RLL and is sharply outlined. It should appear thin and of uniform thickness, usually measuring no more than 3 mm. A portion of the medial bronchial wall also may be outlined by lung.

An anomalous bronchus termed the accessory cardiac bronchus may arise from the medial bronchus intermedius or lower lobe bronchus, extending medially toward the heart. It supplies a small area of aerated lung or rudimentary (nonaerated) lung tissue (see Fig. 1-3 in Chapter 1).

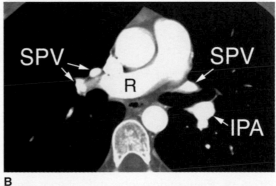

A   **B**

FIG. 6.17. Bronchus intermedius; left main bronchus and upper aspect of the left upper lobe bronchus. **A:** On the right, the bronchus intermedius (*BI*) appears as an oval lucency. On the left, the posterior wall of the left main bronchus (*LM*) is visible as a thin stripe, the left retrobronchial stripe (*RBS*). The superior aspect of the left upper lobe bronchus (*UL*) is visible, giving rise laterally to the superior trunk (*ST*) of the left upper lobe. The posterior wall of the left upper lobe bronchus is slightly concave at this level. **B:** On the right, the anatomy of hilar vessels is similar to Figure 6-16B. The right pulmonary artery is medial, the interlobar pulmonary artery is anterior to the bronchus, and the superior pulmonary vein (*SPV*) branches are visible anterior and lateral to the artery and bronchus. On the left, the interlobar left pulmonary artery (*IPA*) produces a large convexity in the posterior hilum, and the superior pulmonary vein (*SPV*) results in an anterior convexity.

A   B

FIG. 6.18. Bronchus intermedius; lower aspect of the left upper lobe bronchus and lingular bronchus. **A:** On the right, the bronchus intermedius (*BI*) appears as an oval lucency. On the left, the left retrobronchial stripe (*RBS*) is again seen. The inferior aspect of the left upper lobe bronchus (*UL*) is visible, giving rise laterally to the lingular branch (*Lin*) of the left upper lobe. **B:** On the right, the interlobar pulmonary artery (*IPA*) passes anterior and lateral to the BI. Branches to the superior segment of the lower lobe are directed posteriorly. The combination of the IPA and superior segment branches resembles an elephant's head. The SPV is visible anteriorly. On the left, the left IPA is seen in cross section and lies posterolateral to the lingular bronchus. It is round or oval. The SPV passes anterior and medial to the bronchi to enter the left atrium.

Right Middle Lobe Bronchus

The middle lobe bronchus arises from the anterolateral wall of the bronchus intermedius and extends anteriorly at an angle of about 45 degrees. The origin of the middle lobe bronchus also marks the point of origin of the RLL bronchus (Fig. 6-19A). A thin carina may be seen separating the origins of the right middle lobe (RML) and RLL bronchi. The middle lobe bronchus lies oblique to the scan plane and appears as an oval lucency. Only a short segment of the RML bronchus

may be visible on any one scan, depending on its orientation, the scan thickness, and the degree of volume averaging.

Medial and Lateral Segments

The middle lobe bronchus extends for about 1 to 2 cm before dividing into its medial and lateral segmental branches. Because of its orientation, the main portion of the RML bronchus and the medial and lateral segments are often seen at a level 1 to 2 cm below the origin of the RML bronchus (Fig. 6-20A).

A   B

FIG. 6.19. Right middle lobe and superior segment right lower lobe; lingular bronchus and superior segment left lower lobe. **A:** On the right, the origin of the right middle lobe bronchus (*RML*) is visible. Posterior to it is the lower lobe bronchus (*L*) and the superior segment of the lower lobe (*Sup*). A thin carina separates the middle and lower lobe bronchi. On the left, the lingular bronchus (*Lin*), lower lobe bronchus (*L*), and superior segment of the lower lobe (*Sup*) have a similar appearance to the right-sided bronchi. **B:** On the right, the lower lobe pulmonary artery (*LL*) lies lateral to the lateral borders of both the middle and lower lobe bronchi. The lower lobe artery at this point is oriented perpendicular to the scan plane and is thus seen in cross section as an elliptical structure. The right middle lobe artery (*RML*) is seen as an anterior branch. The right superior pulmonary vein (*SPV*) passes anterior and medial to the middle and lower lobe bronchi. On the left, the lower lobe artery (*LL*) lies lateral to the lower lobe bronchus. The lingular artery (*Lin*) is anterior.

A   B

FIG. 6.20. Right middle lobe and its segments; basal lower lobe trunks. **A:** On the right, the right middle lobe bronchus (*RML*) and its medial (*MS*) and lateral segments (*LS*) are visible. The truncus basalis (*TB*) or basal lower lobe trunk is visible on both sides. The anterior wall of the left TB is outlined by lung. **B:** On the right, the lower lobe pulmonary artery (*LL*) lies lateral to the lateral border of the lower lobe bronchus. The right middle lobe artery (*RML*) is seen as an anterior branch. The right inferior pulmonary vein lies medial to the lower lobe bronchus. On the left, the lower lobe artery (*LL*) has a lobulated appearance as it begins to divide. Inferior pulmonary vein branches (*IPV*) are medial and posterior.

In 60% of cases, the middle lobe bronchus divides into medial and lateral segmental branches of equal size. In most of the remaining cases, the medial segmental bronchus appears larger. Although both middle lobe segmental bronchi are directed inferiorly, the lateral segmental bronchus lies closer to the scan plane and is imaged over a greater distance on each scan.

Right Lower Lobe Bronchus

The undivided lower lobe bronchus is very short. Near its origin, it gives rise to the superior segmental bronchus (see Fig. 6-19A). Distal to the origin of the superior segment, the basal bronchial trunk continues for a short distance (see Fig. 6-20A) before dividing into the four basal segmental branches of the RLL: the medial, anterior, lateral, and posterior segments (Fig. 6-21A).

Superior Segment

The superior segmental bronchus of the RLL bronchus may arise at the same level as or slightly caudal to the origin of the RML bronchus (see Fig. 6-19A). In some cases, the superior segmental bronchus arises at a level cephalad to the origin of the RML bronchus.

The superior segmental bronchus, which is about 1 cm in length, arises from the posterior wall of the RLL bronchus and courses posteriorly and laterally within the scan plane (see Fig. 6-19A). Lung often outlines the medial aspect of the superior segment bronchus.

A   B

FIG. 6.21. Basal segments of the right lower lobe. **A:** On the right, the four basal segments are visible. In a counter-clockwise direction, these are the medial basal (*M*), anterior basal (*A*), lateral basal (*L*), and posterior basal (*P*), spelling MALP. On the left, two branches of the truncus basalis are visible at this level. **B:** On both sides, the segmental arteries (*Seg*) lie posterolateral to the proximal portions of the basilar segmental bronchi. The inferior pulmonary vein (*IPV*) passes posterior to the lower lobe bronchi and arteries before entering into the lower portion of the left atrium.

Truncus Basalis and Basal Segments

Below the origin of the superior segmental bronchus, the lower lobe bronchus continues for about 5 to 10 mm as the truncus basalis or basal bronchial trunk, visible as a circular lucency (see Fig. 6-20A). The anterior wall of the truncus basalis is commonly outlined by lung.

The basal segments have a typical orientation of M-A-L-P, beginning medially and anteriorly and proceeding counterclockwise (see Fig. 6-21A). The medial basal segmental bronchus usually arises as the first branch of the basal trunk, lying just anterior to the inferior pulmonary vein. Although variable in appearance, the anterior, lateral, and posterior basilar bronchi may all be identified because of their positions relative to one another and because they each course toward the segments they supply. In general, the medial and posterior segmental bronchi are imaged more nearly in cross section than the anterior and lateral, which are more obliquely oriented (see Figs. 6-21A and 6-22A). Anatomic variation in the origins of these segments is common.

Left Bronchial Anatomy

The left main bronchus is much longer than the right and is typically seen on three or four contiguous 5-mm slices below the carina (see Figs. 6-13 and 6-15 to 6-17). It divides into left upper and lower lobe branches.

Left Upper Lobe Bronchus

The LUL bronchus is 2 to 3 cm long (see Figs. 6-17 and 6-18). In about 75% of patients, the LUL branches into a superior trunk and the lingular bronchus. The superior trunk is about 1 cm in length, giving rise to the anterior and apical-posterior segmental bronchi (Figs. 6-16 to 6-18). In 25% of cases, the LUL bronchus trifurcates into the apical-posterior segment bronchus, anterior segment bronchus, and lingular bronchus.

At the level of the superior aspect of the LUL bronchus, its posterior wall is smooth and slightly concave (see Fig. 6-17A). At this level, the origin of the apical-posterior segmental bronchus, or the superior bronchial trunk that gives rise to the apical posterior and anterior segmental bronchi, can be recognized as a rounded area of increased lucency superimposed on the distal portion of the LUL bronchus.

In 90% of cases, the superior segment of the LLL abuts the posterior wall of the left main or upper lobe bronchus, outlining the *left retrobronchial stripe* (see Figs. 6-17A and 6-18A). The bronchial wall should appear similar in thickness to the posterior bronchus intermedius.

Apical-posterior and Anterior Segments

The anterior segment bronchus of the LUL bronchus is usually visible above the level of the LUL bronchus itself (see Fig. 6-16A). It lies roughly in the plane of scan and is oriented almost directly anteriorly; it is usually visible over several centimeters. It is the only LUL branch that has this course.

The apical-posterior segment bronchus is visible as a circular lucency at and above the origin of the anterior segment bronchus (see Fig. 6-15A). If a bronchus is seen in cross section below the anterior segment and above the LUL bronchus, it represents the short superior bronchial trunk; although similar in appearance to the apical-posterior segment and following the same course, it is larger.

Lingular Bronchus

The lingular bronchus arises from the undersurface of the distal portion of the LUL bronchus and courses obliquely downward, as does the RML bronchus (see Fig. 6-18A). It usually appears elliptical in shape. The origin of the lingular bronchus may be identified as a lucency superimposed on the distal portion of the LUL bronchus. The origin of the lingular bronchus may be distinguished from the origin of the anterior segmental bronchus of the LUL bronchus by noting

FIG. 6.22. Basal segments of the left lower lobe. **A:** On the left, the three basal segments are visible. In a clockwise direction, these are the anteromedial basal (*AM*), lateral basal (*L*), and posterior basal (*P*). The four basal segments are again visible on the right. **B:** On both sides, the segmental arteries (*Seg*) lie posterolateral to the proximal portions of the basilar segmental bronchi. The inferior pulmonary vein (*IPV*) passes posterior and medial to the lower lobe bronchi.

its relationship to the inferior aspect of the upper lobe bronchus, or by identifying a thin carina or spur that is usually seen between the lingular bronchus and the LLL bronchus.

Superior and Inferior Lingular Segments

The lingular bronchus extends anteriorly and inferiorly for 2 to 3 cm before dividing into its superior and inferior segmental branches. The superior segmental bronchus of the lingula is directed more laterally than the inferior segment and lies closer to the scan plane, analogous to the pattern of branching of the medial and lateral segments of the right middle lobe.

Left Lower Lobe Bronchus

The LLL bronchus usually conforms to the same general branching pattern as the RLL bronchus, although only three basal segments are generally present: the anteromedial, lateral, and posterior.

Superior Segment

The superior segmental bronchus of the LLL bronchus arises within 1 cm of the origin of the LLL bronchus and is identical in shape and configuration to the superior segment bronchus on the right side (see Fig. 6-19A).

Truncus Basalis and Basal Segments

The truncus basalis, the lower lobe bronchus giving rise to the basal lower lobe segments, is visible below the origin of the superior segment for a distance of 1 to 2 cm (see Fig. 6-20A). It is generally longer than the truncus basalis on the right. As on the right, the anterior wall of the basal trunk may be outlined by lung.

The basilar segmental bronchi are almost mirror images of the RLL basilar bronchi, except that on the left side the medial and anterior basilar bronchi characteristically originate together as a common trunk (see Fig. 6-22A). Again, the key to the identification of the basal segments is to note the general configuration and position of these bronchi as they course to their corresponding segments. In a clockwise fashion, the relative positions of the bronchi are M-A (in this case named anteromedial)-L-P.

CT of the Hilar Vessels

Bronchi serve as an anatomic framework for the hila. Hilar vessels have a consistent relationship to bronchi, and identifying hilar bronchi is the first step to analyzing the hila. Despite some variation in the branching of segmental hilar arteries, most can be identified by noting their close association with specific segmental bronchi, by following their courses on sequential images, and by determining their sites of origin.

Evaluation of the vascular structures of the hila is simplified by the recognition of specific levels relative to the bronchi (see Figs. 6-15 to 6-22). At these levels, the hila have characteristic silhouettes.

Right side:

- Tracheal carina and apical segmental bronchus of the RUL
- RUL bronchus
- Bronchus intermedius
- Middle lobe bronchus
- Lower lobe basilar segmental bronchi

Left side:

- Apical posterior and anterior segmental bronchi of the LUL
- LUL bronchus
- Lingular bronchus
- Lower lobe basilar segmental bronchi

Vascular Anatomy of the Right Hilum

Tracheal Carina and Apical Segmental Bronchus Level

At or near the level of the carina, a branch or branches of the truncus anterior supplying the apical segment of the RUL and a branch or branches of the right superior pulmonary vein draining the apical segment are visible in cross section, adjacent to the apical segmental bronchus. Typically, the apical segmental artery lies medial to the bronchus and the veins lie lateral to it (see Fig. 6-14).

Right Upper Lobe Bronchus Level

At the level of the RUL bronchus, the undivided truncus anterior is usually identifiable (see Fig. 6-15B). This large vessel is the first major branch of the right main pulmonary artery, arising within the pericardium, and characteristically lies just anterior to the RUL bronchus. As a rule of thumb, the truncus anterior usually appears similar in size and shape to the right main bronchus seen at the same level.

Typically, a large branch of the right superior pulmonary vein, the posterior vein, lies within the angle formed by the bifurcation of the RUL bronchus into anterior and posterior segmental bronchi (see Fig. 6-15A). Anterior and medial to the truncus anterior, a small convexity is frequently visible touching the mediastinum, representing another RUL vein, the apical-anterior vein, which is often identifiable without the injection of contrast agent.

Bronchus Intermedius Level

On scans showing the bronchus intermedius, the interlobar pulmonary artery lies anterior and lateral to the bronchus (see Figs. 6-16 to 6-18). The right superior pulmonary vein lies anterior to the right interlobar pulmonary artery.

Frequently, two veins are visible in this location; these should not be mistaken for lymph node enlargement. Infrequently, a small vein branch draining a portion of the posterior segment of the upper lobe passes posterior to the bronchus intermedius; it can be seen to pass medially at successively lower levels to join the inferior pulmonary vein.

Once the interlobar pulmonary artery reaches the lateral border of the bronchus intermedius and enters the major fissure, the artery often resembles an elephant's head (the main portion of the artery) and trunk (the superior segment artery; see Fig. 6-18).

Middle Lobe Bronchus Level

At the level of the origin of the middle lobe bronchus, the lower lobe pulmonary artery lies immediately lateral to the lateral borders of both the middle and lower lobe bronchi, and the right middle lobe artery parallels the RML bronchus (see Figs. 6-19 and 6-20). The lower lobe artery at this point is oriented perpendicular to the scan plane and is thus seen in cross section as an elliptical structure.

The right superior pulmonary vein passes anterior and medial to the middle and lower lobe bronchi and can be seen entering the upper portion of the left atrium. The middle lobe vein is sometimes seen joining the superior pulmonary vein at this level.

Level of the Basal Segmental Bronchi of the Right Lower Lobe

Below the level of the origin of the middle lobe bronchus, the lower lobe pulmonary artery often bifurcates into two short trunks, which in turn divide into the four basilar segmental pulmonary arteries. These have a characteristic, rounded configuration, lying posterolateral to the proximal portions of the basilar segmental bronchi (see Figs. 6-21 and 6-22). Unlike the basilar pulmonary arteries, which are imaged in cross section, the inferior pulmonary veins are oriented in the transverse plane. They join to form the inferior pulmonary vein, which passes posterior to the lower lobe bronchi and arteries before entering into the lower portion of the left atrium.

Vascular Anatomy of the Left Hilum

On the left side, although characteristic relationships between vessels and airways are also present, there is far more anatomic variation than on the right.

Level of the Apical-posterior and Anterior Segments of the Left Upper Lobe

The apical-posterior segmental bronchus and associated arteries and veins have a similar appearance to the right apical segmental bronchus and associated vessels. The artery supplying the anterior segment of the LUL is seen medial to the anterior segment bronchus (see Fig. 6-15).

Left Upper Lobe Bronchus Level

At the level of the left upper bronchus, the interlobar left pulmonary artery produces a large convexity in the posterior hilum, and the superior pulmonary vein results in an anterior convexity, medial to the ascending bronchial trunk or anterior segmental bronchus, if visible (see Fig. 6-17).

Lingular Bronchus Level

The lingular bronchus is usually visible at a level near the undersurface of the LUL bronchus. The appearance of the hilar vessels at this level is analogous to that of the right hilum at the level of the middle lobe bronchus. The left interlobar pulmonary artery is seen in cross section and lies lateral to the lower lobe bronchi, posterolateral to the lingular bronchus, and anterolateral to the superior segmental bronchus (see Fig. 6-18). It is round or oval. The superior pulmonary vein passes anterior and medial to the bronchi to enter the left atrium.

Level of the Basilar Segmental Bronchi of the Left Lower Lobe

At the level of the basilar segmental bronchi, the anatomy of the inferior portion of the left hilum is nearly a mirror image of that on the right (see Figs. 6-21 and 6-22). Branches of the pulmonary artery to the LLL lie lateral and posterior to the LLL basilar bronchi. The left inferior pulmonary vein passes anterolateral to descending aorta and posterior to the bronchi and arteries to enter the left atrium.

CT of the Hilar Lymph Nodes

The use of contrast enhancement usually allows the accurate differentiation of hilar lymph nodes from normal vessels. Hilar lymph nodes are not located randomly but are found in consistent locations. The most important groups are described below in relation to bronchial anatomy.

Right Upper Lobe Bronchus and Left Pulmonary Artery Level

Lymph nodes are common adjacent to the segmental branches of the RUL bronchus but tend to be small (Fig. 6-23). Lymph nodes are commonly seen both medial and lateral to the left pulmonary artery. Lateral nodes are medial to the superior bronchial trunk. These may be mistaken for pulmonary embolism.

Bronchus Intermedius and Left Upper Lobe Bronchus Level

On the right, slightly below the RUL bronchus, lateral to the bifurcation of the main pulmonary artery, anterolateral to the bronchus intermedius, and medial to superior pulmonary vein branches, it is very common in normal subjects to see a

FIG. 6.23. Lymph node groups, level of the right upper lobe bronchus and left pulmonary artery. **A:** Diagram of common node groups. *LPA*, left pulmonary artery; *Seg Br*, segment bronchus; *Art*, artery. **B:** Enlarged lymph nodes (*arrows*) in these groups in a patient with non-Hodgkin's lymphoma. **C.** Calcified lymph nodes (*arrows*) at this level in sarcoidosis.

large area of unenhanced soft tissue comprising small nodes and fat (see Figs. 6-16B and 6-24). This can range up to 1.5 cm in diameter in some normals. Nodes in this region represent part of the "lymphatic sump" of the right lung. They can be easily mistaken for a hilar mass or thrombus in the right pulmonary artery. Lymph nodes tend to be medial and lateral to the posterior wall of the bronchus intermedius but not immediately posterior to it. Lymph nodes in this region are in the hilar angle.

At the level of the upper portion of the LUL bronchus, a rim of soft tissue largely representing normal nodes is always seen between the posterior bronchial wall and the pulmonary artery. Lymph nodes are common adjacent to the retrobronchial stripe but are not normally seen.

Right Middle Lobe Bronchus and Lingular Level

At the level of the right middle lobe bronchus and node group, lymph nodes are commonly seen (70%) lateral to the origin of the middle lobe or lower lobe bronchi and medial to the interlobar pulmonary artery (Fig. 6-25). These can be more than 5 mm in some normal patients. Normal lymph nodes having a similar appearance are

also commonly seen on the left, in relation to the lingular bronchus.

Level of the Lower Lobe Bronchi and the Inferior Hilar Window

At the level of the lower lobe bronchial segments, most nodes are interposed between bronchi and pulmonary arteries (Fig. 6-26). Lymph nodes anterior to the truncus basalis and basal lower lobe bronchi are also commonly present, visible in about 15% to 20% of normals. These nodes lie within the region termed the inferior hilar window.

Normal Hilar Lymph Node Size

In most regions, normal nodes measure only a few millimeters in size as shown on CT, with a short axis diameter of 3 mm or less. In three locations described above, however, larger conglomerates of nodes and soft tissue are often visible. These three regions are found at the levels of (1) the bronchus intermedius and bifurcation of the right pulmonary artery, (2) the right middle lobe bronchus, and (3) the LUL and lingular and bronchus. In only the first of these, however, can

FIG. 6.24. Lymph node groups, level of the bronchus intermedius and left upper lobe bronchus. **A:** Diagram of common node groups. *Pulm,* pulmonary; *RBS,* retrobronchial stripe; *PA,* pulmonary artery. **B:** Enlarged lymph nodes (*arrows*) in these groups in a patient with non-Hodgkin's lymphoma. **C:** Calcified lymph nodes (*arrows*) at this level in sarcoidosis.

soft tissue exceeding 1 cm in least diameter be seen. Except in this one region, it would seem appropriate to use a least node diameter of 10 mm as the upper limit of normal.

CT DIAGNOSIS OF HILAR ABNORMALITIES

Bronchial Abnormalities

Generally speaking, scans viewed with a lung window setting (−700/1,000 HU) are best for identifying normal bronchi and detecting bronchial abnormalities but may overestimate the degree of bronchial narrowing. Also, a normal bronchus slightly out of the plane of scan and being volume-averaged with adjacent soft tissue can appear narrowed on lung window scans. A soft-tissue window is often best for looking at narrowed or obstructed bronchi and associated mass or lymph node enlargement. A wide lung window (−600/1,500 HU) is a good compromise, providing information about bronchi and soft-tissue masses.

Thin-collimation scans or high-resolution CT, particularly with spiral acquisition, can be of great value in identifying bronchial abnormalities. Although the use of 3D reconstruction techniques may be of some value in the diagnosis of bronchial lesions, their advantage appears to be minimal compared to careful review of the transaxial images and 2D multiplanar reconstructions.

Accurate indicators of bronchial pathology include bronchial wall thickening, endobronchial mass, bronchial obstruction, and narrowing of the bronchial lumen. Other findings that may indicate the presence of a bronchial abnormality include mucous plugging, air trapping, atelectasis, or obstructive pneumonia. The differential diagnosis of an endobronchial mass or bronchial obstruction is listed in Table 3-11 in Chapter 3.

Bronchial Wall Thickening

Bronchial wall thickening is most easily assessed for bronchi partially outlined by lung. Specific bronchi assessed in this manner include the right main bronchus, RUL bronchus, bronchus intermedius, and left main and upper lobe bronchus (left retrobronchial stripe). Smooth bronchial wall thickening can be due to inflammation or tumor infiltration, while a localized or lobulated thickening usually indicates localized tumor infiltration or lymph node enlargement.

Right Main and Right Upper Lobe Bronchus

The posterior walls of the RML and RUL bronchi are sharply outlined by lung in normal subjects and should appear quite thin. Generalized thickening suggests tumor infiltration (see Fig. 6-12B).

A

B

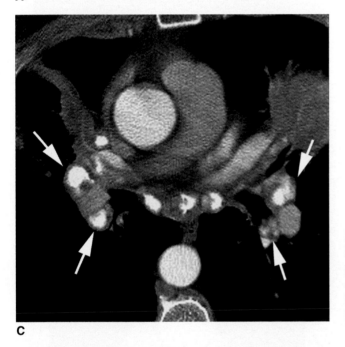

C

FIG. 6.25. Lymph node groups, level of the right middle lobe and lingular bronchi. **A:** Diagram of common node groups. *Pulm*, pulmonary; *Art*, artery; *PA*, pulmonary artery; *Seg*, segment. **B:** Enlarged lymph nodes (*arrows*) in these groups in a patient with sarcoidosis. **C:** Calcified lymph nodes (*arrows*) at this level in sarcoidosis.

Posterior Wall of the Bronchus Intermedius

On CT, the PWBI is visible in all patients. Its upper extent is clearly definable by, and is contiguous with, the origin of the RUL bronchus. The inferior extent of the PWBI is obscured by a branch of the inferior pulmonary vein crossing behind the bronchus to enter the left atrium. This usually occurs at the level of the origin of the superior segmental bronchus of the RLL. Thickening or nodularity of the PWBI can be seen with tumor infiltration (see Fig. 6-7B), most commonly by bronchogenic carcinoma, or lymph node enlargement. Slight thickening may be seen in patients with pulmonary edema or interstitial lung disease. Obliteration of the posterior bronchial wall and the presence of soft-tissue densities behind it are virtually diagnostic of a mass in the hilum or adjacent lung.

Left Retrobronchial Stripe

The left posterior bronchial wall is outlined by lung only at the level of the LUL bronchus. On CT, in approximately 90% of subjects, lung sharply outlines the posterior wall of the left main or upper lobe bronchus, medial to the descending pulmonary artery, termed the left retrobronchial stripe (see Fig. 6-17). Thickening of the left retrobronchial stripe,

FIG. 6.26. Lymph node groups, level of the lower lobe bronchi. **A:** Diagram of common node groups. *Pulm*, pulmonary; *Art*, artery; *Br*, bronchus; *Seg*, segment. **B:** Enlarged lymph nodes (*arrows*) in a patient with sarcoidosis. The left-sided lymph nodes are in the region of the inferior hilar window. **C:** Calcified lymph nodes (*arrows*) at this level in sarcoidosis.

as seen on CT, indicates lymph node enlargement or bronchial wall thickening, analogous to thickening of the PWBI on the right (Fig. 6-27). In 10% of normal individuals, lung does not contact the bronchial wall because the descending pulmonary artery is positioned medially, contacting the lateral aorta.

Endobronchial Lesions and Bronchial Obstruction

Endobronchial lesions are sometimes diagnosed because a lesion is visible within the bronchus or focal bronchial obstruction is present in the absence of hilar mass. The differential diagnosis of an endobronchial lesion includes primary malignant and benign bronchial tumors, metastases, lymphoma, stricture, granulomas (infectious or noninfectious), foreign body, broncholith, and mucus (see Table 3-11 in Chapter 3).

Caveats: In patients with a hilar mass, it is difficult to distinguish bronchial compression and obstruction from an endobronchial mass. Endobronchial abnormalities that are primarily mucosal can be missed using CT.

FIG. 6.27. Thickening of the left retrobronchial stripe due to metastatic nasopharyngeal carcinoma. Lymph node enlargement posterior to the left upper lobe bronchus (*arrow*) results in thickening of this stripe. Left hilar and subcarinal lymph node enlargement is also seen.

Narrowing of the Bronchial Lumen

Bronchial narrowing in the absence of obstruction may be caused by an infiltrating tumor, inflammation, stricture, or bronchomalacia. Carcinoma often produces a gradual or tapered bronchial narrowing, a so-called rat-tail appearance, because of bronchial wall infiltration by tumor (see Fig. 3-17 in Chapter 3). The presence of an associated mass is important in the differential diagnosis and strongly suggests carcinoma. It is important to look at adjacent scans to confirm that the apparent bronchial narrowing does not reflect an oblique bronchial course or volume averaging.

Vascular Abnormalities

CT is very useful in the diagnosis of pulmonary vascular abnormalities. Pulmonary embolism is discussed in Chapter 27.

Pulmonary Artery

Involvement of the pulmonary artery is common in patients with bronchogenic carcinoma involving the hilum. Usually artery narrowing or obstruction occurs. Rarely a false aneurysm is seen in relation to the tumor (Fig. 6-28).

Increased Artery Size

A variety of conditions may result in pulmonary artery enlargement (Table 6-1). Most common is pulmonary hypertension with dilatation of the main and hilar pulmonary arteries (see Fig. 6-6). In normal subjects, the main pulmonary artery measures 22 to 36 mm in diameter. Dilatation of the main pulmonary artery (more than 35 mm) correlates with the presence of pulmonary hypertension. The main

TABLE 6.1 Pulmonary Artery Enlargement
Pulmonary hypertension
Left-to-right shunt
Pulmonary embolism
Pulmonic stenosis
Absent pulmonary valve
Pulmonary artery sarcoma
Pulmonary artery aneurysm
Mycotic
Catheter-related complication
Takayasu's arteritis
Williams syndrome
Prenatal varicella
Pulmonary hypertension
Behcet's syndrome

pulmonary artery may also be considered dilated if it appears larger than the adjacent ascending aorta on CT. Pulmonary artery dilatation also occurs with left-to-right shunt.

Enlargement of a hilar pulmonary artery may occur because of pulmonary embolism. This generally reflects the presence of a large clot impacted in the artery, but pulmonary hypertension associated with the embolus also may contribute to this appearance.

Enlargement of the main and left pulmonary arteries is seen in patients with pulmonic stenosis or absent pulmonary valve. The pulmonary outflow tract usually appears dilated as well. The right pulmonary artery usually appears normal.

Pulmonary artery sarcoma is a rare neoplasm resulting in an intravascular mass. This may result in dilatation of the main, right, or left pulmonary arteries.

Pulmonary artery aneurysms are rarely seen (Fig. 6-29); they may be (1) mycotic in origin; (2) due to catheter-related complications; (3) associated with multiple pulmonary artery stenoses or coarctations in patients with Takayasu's arteritis, Williams syndrome, and prenatal varicella; (4) associated with pulmonary hypertension; or (5) associated with Behcet's syndrome.

Decreased Artery Size

Decrease in size of a hilar pulmonary artery has a variety of causes (Table 6-2). It may represent artery or lung hypoplasia, proximal interruption of the pulmonary artery, or conditions resulting in decreased lung perfusion such as chronic pulmonary embolism (Fig. 6-30), chronic collapse, severe unilateral fibrosis or lung destruction, or Swyer–James syndrome. In some patients, enlargement of bronchial arteries is seen on the side of decreased perfusion (see Fig. 6-30). These are best seen with thin slices and rapid contrast infusion.

Pulmonary Veins

Pulmonary vein abnormalities are uncommon. Pulmonary vein dilatation (i.e., vein varices) occurring in association

FIG. 6.28. False aneurysm in bronchogenic carcinoma. A right hilar carcinoma results in right upper lobe collapse. The right hilar mass is associated with pooling of contrast in a false aneurysm (*arrow*).

B

FIG. 6.29. Pulmonary artery aneurysm in pulmonary hypertension. **A:** Chest radiograph shows enlargement of the main pulmonary artery (*arrow*) due to pulmonary hypertension. A focal lesion is visible overlying the inferior hilum. **B:** Contrast-enhanced CT shows a focal aneurysm (*arrow*) of a segmental pulmonary artery.

with chronic elevation of left atrial pressure and anomalous pulmonary vein drainage are most common (see Fig. 9-47 in Chapter 9). In patients with lung cancer or metastatic neoplasm, tumor may invade the pulmonary vein, appearing as a filling defect on contrast-enhanced scans.

TABLE 6.2 Decreased Pulmonary Artery Size
Hypoplastic lung
Scimitar syndrome
Proximal interruption of the pulmonary artery
Pulmonary embolism
Atelectasis
Swyer–James syndrome
Ipsilateral lung disease

Hilar Lymph Node Enlargement and Hilar Masses

There is some value in attempting to distinguish hilar lymph node enlargement from hilar mass, although this is not always possible.

Hilar Lymph Node Enlargement

Hilar lymph node enlargement may be suggested if abnormal soft tissue is localized to node-bearing regions, particularly if more than one node group is involved (see Figs. 6-23 to 6-27). Nodes usually appear well defined, smooth, and rounded. Except at the level of the bronchus intermedius, nodes larger than 1 cm may be considered pathologic. Nodes larger than 5 mm are usually abnormal, but these are commonly seen and are likely to be hyperplastic. Very large hilar nodes may result in smooth bronchial compression.

The presence of hilar lymph node enlargement, depending on the clinical situation, suggests hilar metastases from bronchogenic carcinoma, metastatic carcinoma, lymphoma, sarcoidosis, or infection. The differential diagnosis of hilar lymph node enlargement depends on whether it is unilateral or bilateral (Table 6-3).

FIG. 6.30. Decreased size of pulmonary artery in chronic pulmonary embolism. The right interlobar pulmonary artery is markedly reduced in size (*large arrow*). Bronchial arteries (*small arrows*) are enlarged.

TABLE 6.3	Unilateral and Bilateral Lymph Node Enlargement

Unilateral
Bronchogenic carcinoma
Lymph node metastases
    Head and neck
    Thyroid carcinoma
    Melanoma
    Renal
    Testicular
    Breast
Lymphoma
Tuberculosis
Histoplasmosis
Coccidioidomycosis
Bacterial infection
Viral infection
Bilateral
Sarcoid or berylliosis
Silicosis
Amyloidosis
Collagen-vascular diseases
Lymphoma
Lymph node metastases

Hilar Masses

Hilar masses usually are localized to one region, appear irregular in contour, and are often associated with an endobronchial mass or bronchial obstruction (Fig. 6-31). The presence of a mass suggests bronchogenic carcinoma or other primary tumor and makes lymph node diseases less likely. In patients with a hilar mass and bronchial obstruction, collapse or consolidation of distal lung can obscure the margins of the mass, making it more difficult to diagnose.

Common Causes of Hilar Node Enlargement or Mass

Bronchogenic Carcinoma

The most common cause of hilar mass or lymph node enlargement is bronchogenic carcinoma. The hilar mass can appear irregular because of local infiltration of the lung parenchyma (see Figs. 6-5B, 6-7B, 6-28, and 6-31). In patients with tumors arising centrally (usually squamous cell carcinoma or small cell carcinoma), bronchial abnormalities are commonly visible on CT. When the carcinoma arises in the peripheral lung and the hila is abnormal because of node metastases, the hilar mass or masses may be smoother and more sharply defined than when the hilar mass represents the primary tumor. However, this distinction is not always easily made. Patients with a central mass and bronchial obstruction often show peripheral parenchymal abnormalities.

In patients with hilar node metastases, a bronchial abnormality seen on CT usually reflects external compression by the enlarged hilar nodes, but bronchial invasion may also be present. Hilar node metastases are present at surgery in up to 40% of patients with lung cancer.

A

B

FIG. 6.31. Right hilar mass in small cell carcinoma. **A:** A large, ill-defined hilar enlargement is visible on the chest radiograph. This is more typical of hilar mass than lymph node enlargement. **B:** CT shows a large localized right hilar mass associated with obstruction of the right middle lobe bronchus and infiltration of adjacent lung.

Other Primary Bronchial Tumors

Other primary bronchial tumors may be associated with a hilar mass. The most common of these is carcinoid tumor. This malignant tumor arises from the main, lobar, or segmental bronchi in 80% of cases. It tends to be slow-growing and locally invasive. A well-defined endobronchial mass is typical, but a large exobronchial, hilar mass is sometimes seen. Carcinoid tumors are very vascular and often enhance following contrast infusion. Carcinoid tumors occasionally calcify. Adenoid cystic carcinoma (cylindroma) can result in a similar appearance.

Benign bronchial tumors, such as fibroma, chondroma, or lipoma, usually appear focal and endobronchial on CT, rather than infiltrative, and do not commonly produce an exobronchial mass. Obstruction is the primary finding on CT. They are relatively rare.

Lymphoma

Hilar adenopathy is present in 25% of patients with Hodg-kin's and 10% of patients with non-Hodgkin's lymphoma (see Figs. 6-23B and 6-24B). Hilar involvement is usually asymmetrical. Multiple nodes in the hilum or mediastinum are usually involved. Endobronchial lesions can also be seen, or bronchi may be compressed by enlarged nodes, but this is much less common than with lung cancer. There are no specific features of the hilar abnormality seen in patients with lymphoma that allow a definite diagnosis.

Metastases

Metastases to hilar lymph nodes from an extrathoracic primary tumor are not uncommon. Hilar node metastases may be unilateral or bilateral (see Fig. 6-5A). Endobronchial metastases can also be seen without there being hilar node metastases; these may appear to be focal and endobronchial or infiltrative. Head and neck carcinomas, thyroid carcinoma, genitourinary tumors (particularly renal cell and testicular carcinoma), melanoma, and breast carcinomas are most commonly responsible for hilar or endobronchial metastases.

Inflammatory Disease

Unilateral or bilateral hilar lymphadenopathy can be seen in a number of infectious or inflammatory conditions. Primary tuberculosis usually causes unilateral hilar adenopathy (Fig. 6-32), and the presence of low-attenuation nodes on

A

B

C

FIG. 6.32. Tuberculosis in an AIDS patient resulting in hilar and mediastinal lymph node enlargement. **A:** PA chest radiograph shows a right hilar mass (*large arrow*) and right paratracheal mediastinal lymph node enlargement (*small arrow*). **B:** Lateral view shows enlarged lymph nodes (*arrows*) in the inferior hilar window. **C:** CT shows lymph node enlargement (*arrows*) in the inferior hilum.

contrast-enhanced scans strongly suggests this diagnosis. Fungal infections, most notably histoplasmosis and coc-cidioidomycosis, cause unilateral or bilateral adenopathy. Sarcoidosis causes smooth, lobulated, bilateral, and symmetrical adenopathy in most patients (see Figs. 6-5D, 6-10, 6-11, and 6-23C).

SELECTED READING

Bankier AA, Fleischmann D, Mallek R, et al. Bronchial wall thickness: appropriate window settings for thin-section CT and radiologic-anatomic correlation. Radiology 1996; 199:831–836.

Friedman PJ. Practical radiology of the hila and mediastinum. Postgrad Radiol 1981; 1:269–304.

Jardin M, Remy J. Segmental bronchovascular anatomy of the lower lobes: CT analysis. AJR Am J Roentgenol 1986; 147:457–468.

Lang EV, Friedman PJ. The anterior wall stripe of the left lower lobe bronchus on the lateral chest radiograph: CT correlative study. AJR Am J Roentgenol 1990; 154:33–39.

McGuinness G, Naidich DP, Garay SM, et al. Accessory cardiac bronchus: computed tomographic features and clinical significance. Radiology 1993; 189:563–566.

Müller NL, Webb WR. Radiographic imaging of the pulmonary hila. Invest Radiol 1985; 20:661–671.

Naidich DP, Khouri NF, Scott WJ, et al. Computed tomography of the pulmonary hila, 1: normal anatomy. J Comput Assist Tomogr 1981; 5: 459–467.

Naidich DP, Khouri NF, Stitik FP, et al. Computed tomography of the pulmonary hila. 2. Abnormal anatomy. J Comput Assist Tomogr 1981; 5:468–475.

Naidich DP, Stitik FP, Khouri NF, et al. Computed tomography of the bronchi. 2. Pathology. J Comput Assist Tomogr 1980; 4:754–762.

Naidich DP, Terry PB, Stitik FP, Siegelman SS. Computed tomography of the bronchi. 1. Normal anatomy. J Comput Assist Tomogr 1980; 4:746–753.

Naidich DP, Zinn WL, Ettenger NA, et al. Basilar segmental bronchi: thin-section CT evaluation. Radiology 1988; 169:11–16.

Ng CS, Wells AU, Padley SP. A CT sign of chronic pulmonary arterial hypertension: the ratio of main pulmonary artery to aortic diameter. J Thorac Imaging 1999; 14:270–278.

Park CK, Webb WR, Klein JS. Inferior hilar window. Radiology 1991; 178:163–168.

Proto AV, Speckman JM. The left lateral radiograph of the chest. Med Radiogr Photogr 1979; 55:30–74.

Quint LE, Whyte RI, Kazerooni EA, et al. Stenosis of the central airways: evaluation by using helical CT with multiplanar reconstructions. Radiology 1995; 194:871–877.

Remy-Jardin M, Duyck P, Remy J, et al. Hilar lymph nodes: identification with spiral CT and histologic correlation. Radiology 1995; 196:387–394.

Remy-Jardin M, Remy J, Artaud D, et al. Volume rendering of the tracheobronchial tree: clinical evaluation of bronchographic images. Radiology 1998; 208:761–770.

Schnur MJ, Winkler B, Austin JHM. Thickening of the posterior wall of the bronchus intermedius: a sign on lateral chest radiographs of congestive heart failure, lymph node enlargement, and neoplastic infiltration. Radiology 1981; 139:551–559.

Sone S, Higashihara T, Morimoto S, et al. CT anatomy of hilar lymphadenopathy. AJR Am J Roentgenol 1983; 140:887–892.

Vix VA, Klatte EC. The lateral chest radiograph in the diagnosis of hilar and mediastinal masses. Radiology 1970; 96:307–316.

Webb WR. Radiologic imaging of the pulmonary hila. Postgrad Radiol 1986; 6:145–168.

Webb WR, Gamsu G. Computed tomography of the left retrobronchial stripe. J Comput Assist Tomogr 1983; 7:65–69.

Webb WR, Gamsu G, Glazer G. Computed tomography of the abnormal pulmonary hilum. J Comput Assist Tomogr 1981; 5:485–490.

Webb WR, Glazer G, Gamsu G. Computed tomography of the normal pulmonary hilum. J Comput Assist Tomogr 1981; 5:476–484.

Webb WR, Hirji M, Gamsu G. Posterior wall of the bronchus intermedius: radiographic-CT correlation. AJR Am J Roentgenol 1984; 142: 907–911.

The Normal Mediastinum

W. RICHARD WEBB

T he mediastinum is defined as the tissue compartment located between the two lungs, posterior to the sternum, anterior to the vertebral column, and extending from the thoracic inlet to the diaphragm.

CT ANATOMY

The aorta and its branches, the great veins, the pulmonary arteries, and the trachea and main bronchi serve as reliable guides to localizing other important mediastinal structures. As an aid to understanding regional anatomy, the mediastinum can be divided into four compartments, respectively, from superior to inferior: (a) the supraaortic or superior mediastinum; (b) the region of the aortic arch and aortopulmonary window (APW); (c) the pulmonary arteries, subcarinal space, and azygoesophageal recess; and (d) the heart and paracardiac mediastinum.

Supraaortic (Superior) Mediastinum

Just below the thoracic inlet (Fig. 7-1A,B), the mediastinum is relatively narrow from anterior to posterior. The trachea is centrally located.

The *esophagus* lies posterior to the trachea but can be displaced to the left (more common) or right. It is often collapsed and appears as a flattened structure of soft-tissue attenuation. Small amounts of air or fluid may be seen in its lumen.

Other than the trachea and esophagus, the great arterial branches of the aorta and the brachiocephalic veins are the most apparent normal structures at this level. The *brachiocephalic veins* are the most anterior and lateral vessels visible, lying immediately behind the clavicular heads. Although they vary in size, their positions are relatively constant.

The *right brachiocephalic vein* has a nearly vertical course throughout its length. The *left brachiocephalic vein* is longer and courses horizontally as it crosses the mediastinum (see Fig. 7-1B). The precise cephalocaudal location of this vein is quite variable; although it is most frequently visible at this level, the horizontal portion of the left brachiocephalic vein also can be seen at the level of the aortic arch.

The innominate, subclavian, and carotid arteries lie posterior to the veins and adjacent to the anterior and lateral walls of the trachea. These can be reliably identified by their consistent positions. The *innominate (brachiocephalic) artery* is located in close proximity to the anterior tracheal wall, near its midline or slightly to the right of midline in most normals; it is the most variable of all the great arteries. The *left common carotid artery* lies to the left and slightly posterior to the innominate artery; generally it has the smallest diameter of the three major arterial branches. The *left subclavian artery* is a relatively posterior structure throughout most of its course, lying to the left of the trachea or slightly posterior to its midline. The lateral border of the left subclavian artery typically indents the mediastinal surface of the left upper lobe. Small vascular branches, particularly the internal mammary veins and vertebral arteries, are often seen in this part of the mediastinum.

In some patients, the *thyroid gland* extends into the superior mediastinum, and the right and left thyroid lobes may be visible on each side of the trachea. On CT, the thyroid can be distinguished from other tissues or masses because of its iodine content; its attenuation is greater than that of soft tissue.

Aortic Arch and Aortopulmonary Window

While the supraaortic region largely contains arterial and venous branches of the aorta and vena cava, this compartment contains the undivided mediastinal great vessels, the aorta and superior vena cava, and also several important mediastinal spaces and lymph node groups (Figs. 7-2 to 7-4).

The *aortic arch* has a characteristic but variable appearance (see Fig. 7-2A). The anterior aspect of the arch is located anterior and to the right of the trachea, with the arch passing to the left and posteriorly. The posterior arch usually lies anterior and lateral to the spine. The aortic arch tapers slightly along its length, from anterior to posterior.

The position of the anterior and posterior aspects of the arch can vary in the presence of atherosclerosis and aortic tortuosity; typically the anterior arch is located more anteriorly and to the right in patients with a tortuous aorta, while the posterior aorta lies more laterally and posteriorly, in a position to the left of the spine.

At this level, the *superior vena cava* is visible anterior and to the right of the trachea, usually being elliptical in shape (see Fig. 7-2A).

A   **B**

FIG. 7.1. Normal CT anatomy. Supraaortic mediastinum. **A:** *M*, manubrium; *c*, clavicular head; *T*, trachea; *Esoph*, esophagus; *BCV*, brachiocephalic vein; *IA*, innominate artery; *LCA*, left carotid artery; *LSA*, left subclavian artery. **B:** *T*, trachea; *RBCV*, right brachiocephalic vein; *LBCV*, left brachiocephalic vein; *IA*, innominate artery; *LCA*, left carotid artery; *LSA*, left subclavian artery.

The *esophagus* appears the same as at higher levels, being posterior to the trachea but variable in position. Often it lies somewhat to the left of the tracheal midline (see Fig. 7-2A).

The *aortic arch* on the left, the superior vena cava and mediastinal pleura on the right, and the trachea posteriorly serve to define a somewhat triangular space called the *pretracheal space* (see Fig. 7-2A and B). This fat-filled space contains mediastinal lymph nodes in the pretracheal or anterior paratracheal chain. Other mediastinal node groups are closely related to this group both spatially and in regard to lymphatic drainage. It is common to see a few normal-sized lymph nodes in the pretracheal space.

Anterior to the great vessels (aorta and superior vena cava) at this level is another triangular space called the *prevascular space* (see Figs. 7-2 and 7-3). The apex of this triangular space represents the "anterior junction line" (see Figs. 7-2A, and 7-3A and B). This compartment, which is anterior mediastinal, primarily contains thymus (described in detail below), lymph nodes, and fat (see Figs. 7-2 and 7-3). The mediastinal pleural reflections bordering the prevascular space may be concave or convex laterally, although a marked convexity suggests anterior mediastinal mass or thymic enlargement.

At a level slightly below the aortic arch, the ascending aorta and descending aorta are visible as separate structures

A   **B**

FIG. 7.2. Normal CT anatomy. Aortic arch level. **A:** Contrast-enhanced CT at a lower level in the same patient as in Figure 7-1. *T*, trachea; *Es*, esophagus; *A*, aortic arch; *SVC*, superior vena cava; *Azyg*, azygos arch; *Prevasc*, prevascular space containing thymus; *Pretr*, pretracheal space. **B:** Unenhanced high-resolution CT. *T*, trachea; *A*, aortic arch; *SVC*, superior vena cava; *Prevasc*, prevascular space; *Pretrach*, pretracheal space containing normal lymph nodes; *Prevsc*, prevascular space containing thymus replaced by fat.

A   **B**   **C**

FIG. 7.3. Normal CT anatomy. Aortopulmonary window level. **A:** Contrast-enhanced CT at a lower level in the same patient as in Figures 7-1 and 7-2A. *MBr,* main bronchi at the level of the carina; *AA,* ascending aorta; *DA,* descending aorta; *SVC,* superior vena cava; *AAA,* anterior azygos arch; *PAA,* posterior azygos arch; *Prevasc,* prevascular space containing thymus; *APW,* aortopulmonary window with volume averaging of superior aspect of the left pulmonary artery. **B:** Lung window scan, same level as (**A**). The tracheal carina (*carina*) is visible. The apex of the triangular prevascular space represents the anterior junction line (*white arrows*). The mediastinal pleural reflections bordering the prevascular space are concave laterally. **C:** Unenhanced high-resolution CT at a lower level in the same patient as in Figure 7-2B. *A,* ascending aorta; *SVC,* superior vena cava; *PVS,* prevascular space containing thymus replaced by fat; *Pretrach Space,* pretracheal space containing normal lymph nodes; *APW,* aortopulmonary window containing normal lymph nodes; *LA,* ligamentum arteriosum.

(Fig. 7-3A and C). The average diameter of the proximal ascending aorta averages 3.6 cm (range, 2.4 to 4.7 cm), the ascending aorta just below the arch 3.5 cm (range, 2.2 to 4.6 cm), the proximal descending aorta 2.6 cm (range, 1.6 to 3.7 cm), the mid-descending aorta 2.5 cm (range, 1.6 to 3.7 cm), and the distal descending aorta 2.4 cm (range, 1.4 to 3.3 cm).

At or near this level, the *trachea* bifurcates into the *right and left main bronchi.* Near the carina, the trachea commonly assumes a somewhat triangular shape (see Fig. 7-2A). The carina is usually visible on CT (see Fig. 7-3A and B).

On the right side, the *azygos arch* arises from the posterior wall of the superior vena cava, passes over the right main bronchus, and continues posteriorly along the mediastinum to lie to the right and anterior to the spine (see Figs. 7-2A and 7-3A). Below the level of the azygos arch, the *azygos vein* is consistently seen in this position. The azygos arch is often visible on one or two adjacent slices and sometimes appears nodular. However, its characteristic location is usually sufficient to allow its correct identification. When the azygos arch is visible, it marginates the right border of the pretracheal space.

The *APW* is located on the left side of the mediastinum, caudal to the aortic arch but cephalic to the main pulmonary artery (see Fig. 7-3A and C). The APW contains fat, lymph nodes, the recurrent laryngeal nerve, and the ligamentum

arteriosum; the latter two are usually invisible. In some patients, the APW is not well seen, with the main pulmonary artery lying immediately below the aortic arch.

The *superior pericardial recess*, containing a small amount of pericardial fluid, is often visible in the pretracheal space immediately behind the ascending aorta (see Fig. 7-4A). Although it is sometimes confused with a lymph node, its typical location, contact with the aortic wall, oval or crescentic shape, and relatively low (water) attenuation allow it to be distinguished from an abnormality. The anterior recess of the pericardial space is sometimes seen anterior to the aortic arch, ascending aorta, and pulmonary artery (see Fig. 7-4B).

Pulmonary Arteries, Subcarinal Space, and Azygoesophageal Recess

At or near the level of the tracheal carina or main bronchi, the *main pulmonary artery* divides into its right and left branches (Fig. 7-5A to C). The *left pulmonary artery* is somewhat higher than the right, usually being seen 1 cm above it, and appears as the continuation of the main pulmonary artery, directed posterolaterally and to the left (see Fig. 7-5A and B). The *right pulmonary artery* arises at nearly a right angle to the main and left pulmonary and crosses the mediastinum from left to right, anterior to the carina or main

FIG. 7.4. Normal superior pericardial recess. Unenhanced CT. **A:** The superior pericardial recess (*arrows*) is visible posterior to the ascending aorta (*AA*) in the precarinal space. **B:** At a lower level, the anterior reflection of the superior pericardial recess (*arrow*) is visible in the groove between the ascending aorta (*AA*) and main pulmonary artery (*P*).

bronchi (see Fig. 7-5B and C). The right pulmonary artery limits the most caudal extent of the pretracheal space and the anterior aspect of the subcarinal space.

The *azygos vein* parallels the esophagus along the right side of the mediastinum and laterally contacts the medial pleural reflections of the right lower lobe, defining the posterior border of the azygoesophageal recess (see Fig. 7-5A to C). On the left side, the *hemiazygos vein* parallels the descending aorta, lying posterior to it (see Fig. 7-5A to C); it is not always visible. The hemiazygos vein generally drains into the azygos vein via a branch that crosses the midline behind the aorta, near the level of the T8 vertebral body. This branch is sometimes seen on CT in normal individuals.

The *subcarinal space* is the region of the mediastinum immediately below the carina, marginated laterally by the main bronchi. It contains a number of lymph nodes and is closely related to the esophagus (see Fig. 7-5B and D).

Below the level of the tracheal carina and azygos arch, the medial aspect of the right lung contacts the mediastinum in close apposition to the azygos vein, esophagus, and subcarinal space. This region of the mediastinum is called the *azygoesophageal recess* (see Fig. 7-5C and D). The contour of the azygoesophageal recess is concave laterally in the large majority of normal subjects; a convexity in this region should be regarded as suspicious of mass and the scan examined closely for a pathologic process. However, a convexity in this region may also be produced by a prominent normal esophagus or azygos vein and is particularly common in patients with a narrow mediastinum and in children.

Normal nodes are commonly visible in the subcarinal space, being larger than normal nodes in other parts of the mediastinum and up to 1.5 cm in short-axis diameter (see Fig. 7-5D). The esophagus usually is seen immediately posterior to the subcarinal space, and distinguishing nodes and esophagus may be difficult unless the esophagus contains air or contrast material, or its course is traced on adjacent scans.

Heart and Paracardiac Mediastinum

At the level of the heart, the prevascular mediastinum becomes thin or is obliterated by the heart contacting the anterior chest wall (Fig. 7-6). Little soft tissue is visible anterior and lateral to the cardiac chambers and origins of the main pulmonary artery and aorta. However, posterior to the heart, the azygoesophageal recess remains visible to the level of the diaphragm. As at higher levels, the contour of the azygoesophageal recess is concave laterally, closely opposed to the esophagus and azygos vein. Posterior to the descending aorta, fat, the hemiazygos vein and small lymph nodes occupy the left paravertebral space. The right paravertebral space is considerably thinner or invisible.

PLAIN RADIOGRAPHIC ANATOMY

On frontal (posteroanterior [PA] or anteroposterior [AP]) chest films, five important mediastinal structures should be easily identified (Fig. 7-7). In addition to their intrinsic importance in diagnosis, these structures serve to anchor a number of important mediastinal stripes, lines, and interfaces and orient the observer to specific mediastinal regions and compartments that are important in diagnosis. These structures are as follows:

- Trachea, tracheal carina, and main bronchi
- Aortic arch
- Main pulmonary artery
- Azygos vein
- Heart and its chambers

FIG. 7.5. Normal CT anatomy. Level of the pulmonary arteries, subcarinal space, and azygoesophageal recess. **A:** Contrast-enhanced CT at a lower level in the same patient as in Figures 7-1, 7-2A, and 7-3A. *rb*, right main bronchus; *lb*, left main bronchus; *AA*, ascending aorta; *DA*, descending aorta; *SVC*, superior vena cava; *azygos*, azygos vein; *Eo*, esophagus; *Prevasc*, prevascular space containing thymus; *LP*, left pulmonary artery. **B:** Contrast-enhanced CT slightly below level shown in (**A**). *AA*, ascending aorta; *P*, main pulmonary artery; *LP*, left pulmonary artery; *RP*, right pulmonary artery; *DA*, descending aorta; *SVC*, superior vena cava; *Prevasc*, prevascular space containing thymus; *Subcar space*, subcarinal space. **C:** Contrast-enhanced CT slightly below level shown in (**B**). *AA*, ascending aorta; *P*, main pulmonary artery; *RP*, right pulmonary artery; *DA*, descending aorta; *SVC*, superior vena cava; *Az*, azygos vein; *Hemiaz*, hemiazygos vein; *AER*, azygoesophageal recess. **D:** Unenhanced high-resolution CT at a lower level in the same patient as (**B**) and (**C**). *A*, ascending aorta; *PA*, main pulmonary artery; *RPA*, right pulmonary artery; *PVS*, prevascular space containing thymus replaced by fat; *SPR*, anterior superior pericardial recess; *SCS*, subcarinal space containing normal lymph nodes; *AER*, azygoesophageal recess; *Az*, azygos, vein; *Es*, esophagus.

Trachea, Tracheal Carina, and Main Bronchi

The trachea extends from the inferior aspect of the cricoid cartilage to the tracheal carina. It is 10 to 12 cm in length in most individuals. It is divided into extrathoracic and intrathoracic portions at the point it passes posterior to the manubrium (see Fig. 7-7).

The trachea may appear to have a slightly serrated wall because of indentations on the tracheal air column adjacent to the tracheal rings. On the lateral view, serration is seen only along the anterior tracheal wall, as the posterior wall lacks cartilage. Calcification of tracheal cartilages is common in older patients, particularly women. Slight tracheal narrowing with an indentation on the left aortic wall is often seen at the level of the aortic arch.

The tracheal carina is visible at the bifurcation of the trachea into right and left main bronchi. The carina is usually seen

CARDIOPHRENIC ANGLES (RIGHT AND LEFT)

Location: Junction of the anterior hemidiaphragms with the right and left heart borders

Anatomy: Inferior extent of the anterior mediastinum, containing fat and lymph nodes

Appearance: Usually concave laterally on both sides; may be convex in the presence of increased mediastinal fat

Visibility: Very common

Significance: Convexity or mass may be seen in the presence of (1) large mediastinal fat pad, (2) lipoma, (3) pericardial cyst, (4) enlarged epicardiac lymph nodes, (5) thymic neoplasm or other anterior mediastinal mass, or (6) Morgagni hernia

A

B

C

FIG. 7.9. Cardiophrenic angles. **A:** PA chest radiograph. The costophrenic angles (*CPA*) are seen at the junction of the anterior hemidiaphragms with the right and left heart borders. **B:** CT in the same patient at the level of the costophrenic angles. These represent contact of the lung with the fat-filled anterior mediastinum (*arrows*) anterior to the heart and liver. **C:** Coronal reformation in the same patient shows the concave costophrenic angles (*arrows*).

RIGHT PARATRACHEAL STRIPE

Location:	Linear region of contact between the right lung and the right tracheal wall, below the thoracic inlet and above the azygos arch
Anatomy:	Tracheal wall, a thin layer of mediastinal fat, two layers of pleura (visceral and parietal)
Appearance:	A line or stripe, up to 4-mm thick in normal individuals, seen below the clavicles and blending with the superior aspect of the azygos arch
Visibility:	Common, reported to be visible in up to 95% of normal individuals
Significance:	Thickening (i.e., more than 4 mm) may be due to (1) tracheal wall abnormalities such as tumor or inflammatory disease; (2) pleural thickening or effusion adjacent to the trachea; (3) enlargement of pretracheal lymph nodes; (thickening of the paratracheal stripe occurs in about 30% of patients with pretracheal lymph node enlargement); or (4) mediastinal infiltration (e.g., hemorrhage, infection, neoplasm)

A

B

C

FIG. 7.10. Right paratracheal stripe. **A:** PA chest radiograph. The right paratracheal stripe (*RPS*) is a few millimeters thick and is seen from the level of the thoracic inlet to the azygos arch. **B:** CT shows lung contacting the trachea (*T*), forming the right paratracheal stripe (*RPS*). **C:** Coronal reformation in the same patient shows the right paratracheal stripe (*RPS*), trachea (*T*), and azygos arch.

SUPERIOR VENA CAVA INTERFACE

Location/anatomy:	Interface between the right lung and the right superior mediastinum, above the azygos arch and below the thoracic inlet, lateral to the superior vena cava and right brachiocephalic vein
Appearance:	An interface between lung and mediastinum, slightly concave laterally, above the azygos arch and below the medial right clavicle
Visibility:	Seen in almost all patients
Significance:	Lateral convexity of the superior vena cava interface and increased density of the shadow of the superior vena cava may be seen with (1) dilatation of the superior vena cava (due to deep inspiration or Mueller maneuver [physiologic dilatation], supine position, pregnancy, increased blood volume, increased central venous pressure); (2) lymph node enlargement in the pretracheal space, (3) mediastinal mass, (4) mediastinal infiltration (blood, infection, tumor), or (5) a pleural abnormality

A

B

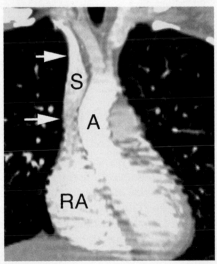

C

FIG. 7.11. Superior vena cava interface. **A:** PA chest radiograph. The right edge of the superior vena cava (*SVC*) is outlined by lung, forming an interface that is slightly concave laterally. It is seen from the thoracic inlet to the level of the azygos arch. **B:** CT in the same patient shows lung contacting the lateral wall of the superior vena cava (*S*). This edge (*arrow*) forms the superior vena cava interface. **C:** Coronal reformation in the same patient shows the superior vena cava interface (*arrows*). *S*, superior vena cava; *A*, aorta; *RA*, right atrium.

LEFT PARATRACHEAL STRIPE OR INTERFACE

Location:	Linear region of contact between the left lung and the left tracheal wall and adjacent mediastinal soft tissues, below the thoracic inlet and above the aorta
Anatomy:	Tracheal wall, mediastinal fat, two layers of pleura (visceral and parietal)
Appearance:	A line or stripe of variable thickness seen below the clavicles and above the aortic arch
Visibility:	Uncommonly visible as a thin stripe; in 90%, the left subclavian or carotid artery and mediastinal fat are interposed between the left tracheal wall and aerated lung; what is often perceived as the lateral aspect of the "left paratracheal stripe" usually represents the interface of left subclavian artery or mediastinal fat with lung
Significance:	Thickening is difficult to diagnose because of variability in appearance

FIG. 7.12. Left paratracheal stripe. **A:** PA chest radiograph. The left paratracheal stripe (*LPS*) represents the linear region of contact between the left lung and the left tracheal wall or adjacent mediastinal soft tissues, below the thoracic inlet and above the aorta. It is usually much thicker than the right paratracheal stripe. **B:** CT in the same patient shows lung contacting the lateral wall of the left mediastinum anterior to the left subclavian artery (*subclav artery*). Mediastinal soft tissues along with left tracheal wall make up the left paratracheal stripe (*LPS*). **C:** Coronal reformation in the same patient shows the left paratracheal stripe above the aorta (*A*). **D:** CT in a different patient shows a thin left paratracheal stripe corresponding to the left tracheal wall. It is anterior to the left subclavian artery (*subclav artery*).

LEFT SUBCLAVIAN ARTERY INTERFACE

Location:	Interface between the left lung and the left superior mediastinum, above the aorta and below the thoracic inlet
Anatomy:	Pleura outlining the lateral aspect of the left subclavian artery or adjacent mediastinal fat
Appearance:	An interface, usually concave laterally, extending from the shadow of the aortic arch to the level of the medial left clavicle
Visibility:	Common
Significance:	Convexity of this interface indicates (1) subclavian artery dilatation or tortuosity, (2) mediastinal mass or lymph node enlargement, or (3) paramediastinal pleural abnormality

A

C

B

FIG. 7.13. Left subclavian artery interface. **A:** PA chest radiograph. Contact of the left lung with the left subclavian artery above the aortic arch results in an interface (*LSA*), concave laterally, extending superiorly to the thoracic inlet. It is somewhat lateral to the left paratracheal stripe and more concave. **B:** CT in the same patient shows lung contacting the lateral wall of the left subclavian artery (*LSA*). **C:** Coronal reformation in the same patient shows the left subclavian artery above the aorta (*A*). It results in a concave edge.

C

D

FIG. 7.16. (*Continued.*) **C:** Radiograph in another patient shows enlargement of the left superior intercostal vein (*LSIV*). It serves as a collateral pathway. **D:** CT in the same patient as (**C**) shows enlargement of the left superior intercostal vein (*arrows*).

LEFT SUPERIOR INTERCOSTAL VEIN	
Appearance:	A small round or triangular shadow ("aortic nipple") less than 5 mm in diameter
Visibility:	Uncommon; less than 5% of normal subjects
Significance:	Dilatation typically occurs as a result of collateral flow through this vein to the hemiazygos and azygos systems; most commonly due to obstruction of the superior vena cava or left brachiocephalic vein

AORTOPULMONARY WINDOW	
Location:	Aortopulmonary window (APW) is outlined by the left lung between the aortic arch and the left pulmonary artery
Anatomy:	Lateral boundary of the APW is the parietal pleura forming the visible interface; the medial boundary of the APW is the ligamentum arteriosum; the APW largely contains fat and lymph nodes

A   **B**

FIG. 7.17. Aortopulmonary window. **A:** The aortopulmonary window (*APW*) represents a concave interface between the aorta (*Ao*) and main pulmonary artery (*Pa*). **B:** CT in the same patient shows fat in the aortopulmonary window (*APW*), under the aortic arch (*A*). (*Figure continues.*)

B   C

FIG. 7.20. (*Continued.*) **B:** CT shows the preaortic recess (*arrow*) outlined by lung, anterior to the aorta (*A*). **C:** Coronal reformation in the same patient shows the preaortic recess (*large arrows*). Its contour is similar to that of the azygoesophageal recess on the right (*small arrows*). *A,* aortic arch; *V,* left pulmonary veins.

	PREAORTIC RECESS
Variant:	If air is present in the esophagus, a stripe is commonly visible representing the left esophageal wall; this is referred to as the *left inferior esophageal (or pleuroesophageal) stripe*; it is most commonly seen immediately under the aortic arch
Visibility:	Uncommon
Significance:	Most useful in diagnosing esophageal or aortic lesions; a lateral convexity in the inferior portion of this line is common with hiatal hernia in association with convexity in the inferior azygoesophageal recess

PARAVERTEBRAL STRIPES (LEFT AND RIGHT)

Location: Linear regions of contact between the posterior lower lobes and the paravertebral soft tissues adjacent to the spine

Anatomy: Pleural reflections over paravertebral fat, lymph nodes, and vessels; on the left, the pleural reflection is posterior to the descending aorta and closely related to the hemiazygos vein

Appearance: Left paravertebral stripe:

1. Commonly visible below the aortic arch, although in obese individuals it may be seen above the arch because of increased paravertebral fat
2. Inferiorly visible below the level of the diaphragmatic dome, merging with the shadow of the diaphragmatic crus
3. Parallels the spine; often seen halfway between the spine and lateral margin of the aorta
4. Usually thin

Right paravertebral stripe:

1. Thinner and less often seen than the left paravertebral stripe
2. Visible only adjacent to the lower thoracic spine
3. Inferiorly, it merges with the shadow of the diaphragmatic crus

A

FIG. 7.21. Paravertebral stripes. **A:** PA chest radiograph. The paravertebral stripes (*arrows*) represent the linear regions of contact between the posterior lower lobes and the paravertebral soft tissues adjacent to the spine. They parallel the spine. On the left, this stripe is seen medial to the descending aorta. The left paravertebral stripe is usually better seen and seen over a longer course than the right. (*Figure continues.*)

B   C

FIG. 7.21. (*Continued.*) **B:** CT in the same patient shows the left (*LPVS*) and right (*RPVS*) paravertebral stripes (*arrows*) outlined by lung, lateral to the vertebral body (*V*). The LPVS is thicker and located posterior to the descending aorta (*A*) and medial to its lateral edge. **C:** Coronal reformation in the same patient shows the right (*small arrows*) and left paravertebral stripes (*large arrows*). Their edges parallel the edges of the vertebral column (*V*). Intercostal arteries and veins are visible within soft tissue of the paravertebral stripes.

PARAVERTEBRAL STRIPES (LEFT AND RIGHT)

Caveats:	Left stripe increases in thickness with aortic tortuosity or supine position; right stripe increases in thickness in patients with osteophytes
Significance:	Increased in thickness with (1) pleural effusion; (2) lymph node enlargement; (3) vertebral abnormalities (fracture, infection, neoplasm); (4) posterior mediastinal masses; (5) hemiazygos vein enlargement (left stripe); or (6) azygos vein enlargement (right stripe)

RETROSTERNAL STRIPE

Location:	The linear region of contact between the anterior lungs and the retrosternal soft tissues
Anatomy:	Retrosternal fat anterior to the lungs associated with the internal mammary lymph nodes and vessels
Appearance:	A smooth stripe of soft tissue, up to 7 mm in thickness in normal individuals, seen posterior to the sternum; inferiorly, the thickness of this stripe increases significantly in relation to the cardiac incisura and is variable in appearance; superiorly, the thickness increases in relation to the brachiocephalic veins and is variable

A   B

FIG. 7.22. Retrosternal stripe. **A:** Lateral radiograph in the same patient as shown in Figure 7-21. The retrosternal stripe is a linear region of contact between the anterior lungs and the retrosternal soft tissues and is visible as a thin line of soft tissue behind the sternum. **B:** CT in the same patient shows soft tissue posterior to the sternum (*s*) forming an interface with the anterior lung (*large arrows*). The retrosternal stripe may also reflect contact of anterior lung with the region of the internal mammary vessels (*small arrows*) or nodes. (*Figure continues.*)

C

D

FIG. 7.22. (*Continued.*) **C:** Sagittal reformation in the same patient shows a very thin retrosternal stripe (*arrows*) posterior to the sternum (*S*). *A*, ascending aorta; *P*, main pulmonary artery. **D:** Sagittal reformation in a more lateral location in the same patient shows a wavy contour of the soft-tissue stripe (*white arrows*). This contour is typically seen with slight rotation. The wavy contour is related to the ribs or costal cartilage. The internal mammary artery (*black arrows*) is visible.

	RETROSTERNAL STRIPE
Caveat:	Slight rotation may project the right or left anterior chest wall posterior to the sternum, mimicking increased thickness of the retrosternal stripe; look for the location of the anterior ribs and costal cartilage before diagnosing an apparent thickening of the retrosternal stripe; a wavy contour of the soft tissue stripe (related to the ribs) often indicates it is due to rotation
Visibility:	Common
Significance:	Increases in thickness with (1) internal mammary lymph node enlargement, (2) tortuosity of internal mammary arteries (e.g., coarctation), (3) post-median sternotomy, or (4) sternal lesions

	RETROSTERNAL CLEAR SPACE
Synonym:	Anterior clear space
Location:	Region posterior to the sternum; anterior and superior to the heart, main pulmonary artery, and ascending aorta; and anterior to the trachea and superior vena cava
Anatomy:	This space corresponds to the prevascular space seen on CT, largely representing thymus and retrosternal tissues
Appearance:	An area of lucency anterior to the heart and great vessels; the anterior margins of the heart and great vessels may or may not be clearly seen

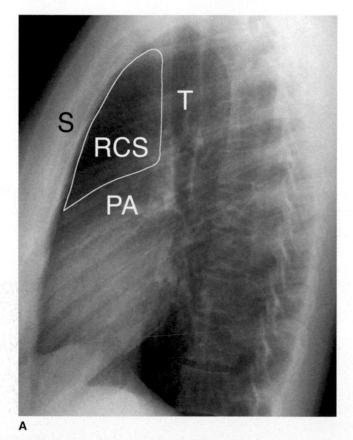

A

FIG. 7.23. Retrosternal clear space. **A:** Lateral radiograph shows an area of relative lucency (*RCS*) posterior to the sternum (*S*), superior to the main pulmonary artery (*PA*), and anterior to the trachea (*T*). (*Figure continues.*)

FIG. 7.23. (*Continued.*) **B:** Sagittal reformation in the same patient to the right of midline shows this area of lucency (∗) posterior to costal cartilage (*C*), anterior to the superior vena cava (*S*), and anterior and superior to the right atrium (*RA*). **C:** Sagittal reformation in the same patient to the left of midline shows the retrosternal lucency (∗) posterior to the costal cartilage (*C*), anterior to the aortic arch (*A*) and main pulmonary artery (*P*).

RETROSTERNAL CLEAR SPACE	
Caveat:	In patients with a large amount of prevascular fat, lucency may be minimal
Visibility:	Common
Significance:	Increase in depth and lucency with emphysema; decrease in depth with right ventricular or main pulmonary artery dilatation; decrease in lucency in patients with anterior mediastinal mass

POSTERIOR TRACHEAL BAND OR STRIPE

Location: Linear region corresponding to the posterior tracheal wall and sometimes esophagus; below the thoracic inlet and above the tracheal bifurcation

Anatomy: Posterior tracheal wall, a small amount of mediastinal fat, and (variably) one or both esophageal walls, outlined posteriorly by air in lung or the esophageal lumen and outlined anteriorly by air in the tracheal lumen

Appearance: Variable appearance because of variable anatomy:

1. Posterior tracheal wall only: visible as a very thin line
2. Posterior tracheal wall, esophagus with or without air in the esophageal lumen: a thicker stripe or band

May be seen for the entire length of the trachea; because of variable anatomy, may measure 1- to 6-mm thick in normal individuals

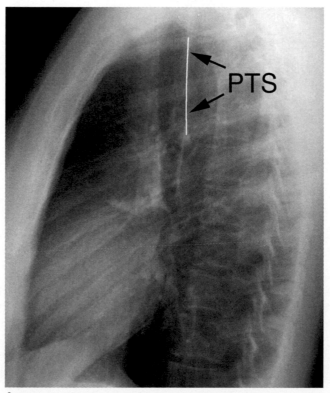

A

FIG. 7.24. Posterior tracheal stripe. **A:** Lateral radiograph. The posterior tracheal stripe (*PTS*) is a linear opacity corresponding to the posterior tracheal wall and sometimes the esophagus, seen below the thoracic inlet and above the tracheal bifurcation. It is of variable thickness. (*Figure continues.*)

FIG. 7.24. (*Continued.*) **B:** CT in the same patient shows lung contacting posterior tracheal wall, outlining the posterior tracheal stripe (*PTS*). *T*, trachea; *esoph*, esophagus. **C:** Sagittal reformation in the same patient shows lung outlining the posterior wall of the trachea (*T*), forming the posterior tracheal stripe.

POSTERIOR TRACHEAL BAND OR STRIPE	
Variant:	If the stripe also includes anterior esophageal wall (with air in the esophageal lumen) or the entire esophagus, it is termed the posterior tracheoesophageal stripe
Visibility:	Common
Significance:	Variability in thickness limits usefulness; increased thickness usually indicates (1) esophageal carcinoma, (2) much less often, tracheal wall thickening, or (3) focal thickening with aberrant subclavian artery

RETROTRACHEAL TRIANGLE

Location:	Region posterior to the trachea, anterior to the spine, and above the posterior aortic arch
Anatomy:	Primarily esophagus with associated lymph nodes; it corresponds to the region of the posterior junction line seen on the frontal film
Appearance:	A relatively lucent region marginated anteriorly by the posterior tracheal stripe and posteriorly by the spine
Visibility:	Common
Significance:	Increased attenuation in this space most common with (1) esophageal lesions, (2) lymph node enlargement, (3) thyroid mass, (4) aberrant subclavian artery, (5) aneurysm, (6) bronchogenic cyst

FIG. 7.25. Retrotracheal triangle. **A:** Lateral radiograph. The retrotracheal triangle (*RTT*) a relatively lucent region marginated anteriorly by the posterior tracheal stripe and posteriorly by the spine. **B:** CT in the same patient. The retrotracheal triangle corresponds to the region of the posterior junction line seen on the PA radiograph and reflects a narrowing of the mediastinum (*arrow*) behind the trachea (*T*) and left subclavian artery (*subclav*), and in relation to the esophagus (*esoph*). **C:** Sagittal reformation in the same patient shows the lucent retrotracheal triangle (*), posterior to the trachea (*T*), anterior to the vertebral column (*V*), and above the aortic arch (*A*).

SELECTED READING

Aronberg DJ, Glazer HS, Madsen K, Sagel SS. Normal thoracic aortic diameters by computed tomography. J Comput Assist Tomogr 1984; 8:247–250.

Aronberg DJ, Peterson RR, Glazer HS, Sagel SS. The superior sinus of the pericardium: CT appearance. Radiology 1984; 153:489–492.

Baron RL, Lee JK, Sagel SS, Peterson RR. Computed tomography of the normal thymus. Radiology 1982; 142:121–125.

Blank N, Castellino RA. Patterns of pleural reflections of the left superior mediastinum. Normal anatomy and distortions produced by adenopathy. Radiology 1972; 102:585–589.

Breatnach E, Abbott GC, Fraser RG. Dimensions of the normal human trachea. AJR Am J Roentgenol 1984; 141:903.

de Geer G, Webb WR, Gamsu G. Normal thymus: assessment with MR and CT. Radiology 1986; 158:313–317.

Friedmand AC, Chambers E, Sprayregen S. The normal and abnormal left superior intercostal vein. AJR Am J Roentgenol 1978; 131:599–602.

Gamsu G, Webb WR. Computed tomography of the trachea and mainstem bronchi. Semin Roentgenol 1983; 18:51–60.

Genereux GP. The posterior pleural reflections. AJR Am J Roentgenol 1983; 141:141–149.

Glazer GM, Gross BH, Quint LE, et al. Normal mediastinal lymph nodes: number and size according to American Thoracic Society mapping. AJR Am J Roentgenol 1985; 144:261–265.

Heitzman ER, Lane EJ, Hammack DB, Rimmler LJ. Radiological evaluation of the aortic-pulmonic window. Radiology 1975; 116:513–518.

Heitzman ER, Scrivani JV, Martino J, Moro J. The azygos vein and its pleural reflections. I. Normal roentgen anatomy. Radiology 1971; 101:249–258.

Kiyono K, Sone S, Sakai F, et al. The number and size of normal mediastinal lymph nodes: a postmortem study. AJR Am J Roentgenol 1988; 150:771–776.

Landay MJ. Anterior clear space: how clear? How often? How come? Radiology 1994; 192:165–169.

Milne EN, Pistolesi M, Miniati M, Giuntini C. The vascular pedicle of the heart and the vena azygos. Part I: The normal subject. Radiology 1984; 152:1–8.

Palayew MJ. The tracheo-esophageal stripe and the posterior tracheal band. Radiology 1979; 132:11–13.

Proto AV. Mediastinal anatomy: emphasis on conventional images with anatomic and computed tomographic correlations. J Thorac Imaging 1987; 2:1–48.

Savoca CJ, Austin JH, Goldberg HI. The right paratracheal stripe. Radiology 1977; 122:295–301.

Smathers RL, Buschi AJ, Pope TL, et al. The azygos arch: normal and pathologic CT appearance. AJR Am J Roentgenol 1982; 139:477–483.

The Mediastinum: Mediastinal Masses

W. RICHARD WEBB

DIAGNOSIS OF MEDIASTINAL MASS

Although radiographs can show recognizable abnormalities in many patients with mediastinal pathology, they are limited in their sensitivity and ability to delineate the extent of mediastinal abnormalities and their relationship to specific mediastinal structures. Computed tomography (CT) is indispensable in the radiographic assessment of the mediastinum.

CT techniques vary somewhat according to the specific indications for the study and the type of scanner used. In patients with a suspected mediastinal mass, an appropriate CT protocol would be as follows:

- Scan at full inspiration
- Supine position
- 1.25- to 5-mm slice thickness
- Infusion of contrast agent at a rate of 3 to 5 mL/s

The differential diagnosis of a mediastinal mass on CT is usually based on several findings:

1. Location (anterior, middle, posterior mediastinum, or specific mediastinal compartments, such as aortopulmonary window) or the identification of the specific structure from which it is arising
2. Nature
   a. Solitary lesion
   b. Multifocal (i.e., lymph nodes)
   c. Diffuse mediastinal involvement
3. Attenuation
   a. Fat
   b. Fluid
   c. Soft tissue
   d. Calcification
   e. Opacification following administration of contrast agents

MEDIASTINAL COMPARTMENTS

Anatomically, the mediastinum is divided into four compartments: anterior, middle, posterior, and superior. These divisions do not necessarily correspond to those generally used for the interpretation of radiographs or CT

Anatomic Divisions

Anterior

Extent: anterior to the pericardium, posterior to the sternum

Contents: fat, lymph vessels, and nodes

Middle

Extent: posterior to the anterior mediastinum, anterior to the posterior mediastinum; defined by its contents

Contents: the heart, pericardium, ascending aorta, superior vena cava, azygos arch, tracheal bifurcation, right and left pulmonary arteries and veins

Posterior

Extent: anterior to the spine, posterior to the heart and pericardium

Contents: descending aorta, azygos vein, superior intercostal vein, thoracic duct, esophagus, vagus nerves

Superior

Extent: below the root of the neck, above the pericardium

Contents: trachea, esophagus, thymus, and great vessels

Plain Radiographic Divisions

To allow an easier localization of mediastinal abnormalities on plain radiographs, the boundaries of the anterior, middle, and posterior mediastinal compartments were redefined by Felson. In this classification, the superior mediastinum is not considered to be distinct and its structures are assigned to the anterior, middle, or posterior compartment based on easily recognizable anatomic features (Fig. 8-1).

A more detailed analysis of the plain film, and localization of mediastinal abnormalities, may be based on identification of specific mediastinal lines, stripes, interfaces, and spaces, listed below and described in Chapter 7.

Anterior

Extent: posterior to the sternum, anterior to a line drawn along the anterior tracheal wall in the upper mediastinum and the posterior border of the heart in the lower mediastinum

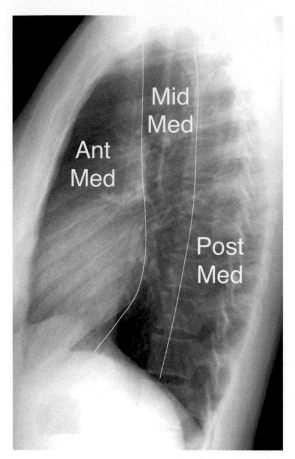

FIG. 8.1. Lateral chest radiograph showing Felson's mediastinal divisions. The anterior mediastinum (*Ant Med*) lies posterior to the sternum and anterior to a line drawn along the anterior tracheal wall in the upper mediastinum and the posterior border of the heart in the lower mediastinum. The posterior mediastinum (*Post Med*) lies posterior to a line 1 cm behind the anterior margin of the vertebral column and anterior to the chest wall. The middle mediastinum (*Mid Med*) lies between these.

Contents: thymus, heart, ascending aorta and great vessels, anterior portion of the main pulmonary artery, pericardium, fat, lymph vessels, nodes

Corresponding plain film features: anterior junction line, cardiophrenic angles, retrosternal stripe, retrosternal space

Middle

Extent: between the anterior compartment in front and the posterior compartment behind

Contents: the trachea and main bronchi, superior vena cava, mid portion of the aortic arch, azygos arch, lymph nodes, esophagus, descending aorta (sometimes)

Corresponding plain film features: right and left paratracheal stripes, superior vena cava interface, aortopulmonary window, left subclavian artery interface, azygoesophageal recess, preaortic interface

Posterior

Extent: posterior to a line 1 cm behind the anterior margin of the vertebral column, anterior to the chest wall

Contents: vertebral bodies, paravertebral tissues, descending aorta (sometimes), posterior azygos vein, hemiazygos vein, lymph nodes

Corresponding plain film features: paravertebral stripes

CT Divisions

On CT, it is most appropriate to base the differential diagnosis of a mediastinal mass on a direct observation of the tissue or structure from which the mass is arising (e.g., lymph nodes, veins and arteries, thymus, thyroid, trachea, esophagus, vertebral column). If this is not possible, then localizing the mass to specific regions of the mediastinum (e.g., prevascular space, pretracheal space, subcarinal space, aortopulmonary window, anterior cardiophrenic angle, paraspinal region) is valuable in differential diagnosis and more specific than considering only the anterior, middle, and posterior divisions (Table 8-1). The normal appearances of these regions are described in Chapter 7.

THE NORMAL THYMUS

The thymus has two lobes, the right and the left, which are fused superiorly near the thyroid gland and smoothly molded to the anterior aspect of the great vessels and anterior heart. It occupies the *thyropericardic space*. The thymus is rarely found in an ectopic location, usually the neck. The left thymic lobe usually is larger than the right.

The thymus weighs an average of about 25 g at birth and increases progressively to reach a maximum weight of approximately 35 to 50 g at puberty. The thymus begins to involute after puberty, and this process continues for a period of 5 to 15 years. During thymic involution, thymic follicles atrophy and are progressively replaced by fat. The relative proportion of fat to thymic tissue increases progressively until after age 60. At this age, little thymic tissue remains.

Plain Radiographs

In adults, the thymus is usually invisible on chest radiographs. In children, the thymus may be quite prominent, mimicking a mass (Fig. 8-2). However, radiographic findings may help in the correct identification of the thymus in children.

The thymus may project to one or both sides of the mediastinum, showing a sharply marginated undersurface, having the appearance of a sail (the "thymic sail" sign). The edge of the thymus may have a wavy appearance because of indentation by the anterior ribs or costal cartilage (the "thymic wave" sign).

Computed Tomography

In children, the normal thymus fills the prevascular space, draping itself over the great vessels and cardiac margins

TABLE 8.1   Differential Diagnosis of Mediastinal Masses Based on Common Sites of Origin

Anterior mediastinum (prevascular space)
  Thymic masses
    Hyperplasia
    Thymoma
    Thymic carcinoma
    Thymic neuroendocrine tumor
    Thymolipoma
    Thymic cyst
    Thymic lymphoma and metastases
  Germ cell tumors
    Teratoma
    Seminoma
    Nonseminomatous germ cell tumors
  Thyroid abnormalities (goiter and neoplasm)
  Parathyroid tumor or hyperplasia
  Lymph node masses (particularly Hodgkin's lymphoma)
  Vascular abnormalities (aorta and great vessels)
  Mesenchymal abnormalities (e.g., lipomatosis, lipoma)
  Foregut cyst
  Lymphangioma and hemangioma
Anterior mediastinum (cardiophrenic angle)
  Lymph node masses (particularly lymphoma and metastases)
  Pericardial cyst
  Morgagni hernia
  Thymic masses
  Germ cell tumors
Middle mediastinum (pretracheal space)
  Lymph node masses
    Lung carcinoma
    Sarcoidosis
    Lymphoma (particularly Hodgkin's disease)
    Metastases
    Infections (e.g., tuberculosis)
  Foregut cyst
  Tracheal tumor
  Mesenchymal masses (e.g., lipomatosis, lipoma)
  Thyroid abnormalities
  Vascular abnormalities (aorta and great vessels)
  Lymphangioma and hemangioma
Middle mediastinum (aortopulmonary window)
  Lymph node masses
    Lung carcinoma

    Sarcoidosis
    Lymphoma
    Metastases
    Infections (e.g., tuberculosis)
  Mesenchymal masses (e.g., lipomatosis, lipoma)
  Vascular abnormalities (aorta or pulmonary artery)
  Chemodectoma
  Foregut cyst
Middle mediastinum (subcarinal space and
  azygoesophageal recess)
  Lymph node masses
    Lung carcinoma
    Sarcoidosis
    Lymphoma
    Metastases
    Infections (e.g., tuberculosis)
  Foregut cyst
  Dilated azygos vein
  Esophageal masses
  Varices
  Hernia
Posterior mediastinum (paravertebral region)
  Neurogenic tumor
    Nerve sheath tumors
    Sympathetic ganglia tumors
    Paraganglioma
  Foregut cyst
  Meningocele
  Extramedullary hematopoiesis
  Pseudocyst
  Thoracic spine abnormalities
  Hernias
  Esophageal masses
  Varices
  Mesenchymal masses (e.g., lipomatosis, lipoma)
  Lymph node masses
    Lymphoma (particularly non-Hodgkin's)
    Metastases
  Dilated azygos or hemiazygos vein
  Hernia
  Lymphangioma and hemangioma
  Thymic mass or germ cell tumor

(see Fig. 8-2B and C). Cephalad, the thymus extends above the innominate vein (see Fig. 8-2D). In infancy, the thymus is commonly seen to the level of the pulmonary arteries or below, but its inferior extent decreases with age.

In infants and young children, the thymus appears quadrilateral on CT. As the child grows, the thymus assumes a more triangular shape, often appearing arrowhead shaped or bilobed, with each of the two thymic lobes contacting the mediastinal pleura. Its margins are sharp, smooth, and convex in infants (see Fig. 8-2B) and often become straight in older children. Each lobe usually measures 1 to 2 cm in thickness (perpendicular to the pleura), but this is variable.

On unenhanced CT, the thymus has approximately the same attenuation as muscle. In young subjects, the mean attenuation of the thymus is 36 HU; the thymus shows homogeneous enhancement of 20 to 30 HU after bolus contrast injection.

From puberty to the age of about 25 years, the thymus appears triangular or bilobed, usually outlined by mediastinal fat (Fig. 8-3). The left lobe is usually larger, being seen lateral to the aortic arch; the right lobe may be inconspicuous. Typically, the lateral borders of the thymus are flat or concave where they contact the pleura; uncommonly they are slightly convex. Its attenuation is usually less than that of muscle because of fatty replacement.

FIG. 8.2. Prominent normal thymus mimicking mass in a 1-year-old. **A:** PA chest radiograph shows an apparent right mediastinal mass representing thymus (*T*). A slight wavy contour laterally is an example of the thymic wave sign. **B:** CT shows a prominent normal thymus (*T*) in the prevascular space. Both the right lobe (*RL*) and left lobe (*LL*) are visible. **C:** The right (*RL*) and left lobes (*LL*) lie lateral to the heart. **D:** T1-weighted coronal MRI showing intermediate-intensity thymus (*T*), with some tissue extending above the innominate vein into the base of the neck (∗). Inferiorly, the thymus extends below the pulmonary artery (*P*). *A*, aortic arch.

FIG. 8.3. Normal thymus in a 21-year-old patient. The thymus occupies the prevascular space and appears triangular and of soft tissue attenuation, the left lobe (*LL*) being larger than the right (*RL*).

Over the age of 25 years, the thymus is no longer recognizable as a soft-tissue structure on CT because of progressive fatty involution. The thymus appears to be composed primarily of fat, containing islands or wisps of soft tissue (Fig. 8-4). The rapidity and degree of thymic involution are variable, and occasionally, the thymus is still recognized as a discrete structure at the age of 40. With complete thymic involution, the anterior mediastinum appears to be entirely filled with fat; this fat represents the thymic remnant and may have a CT density slightly higher than that of subcutaneous fat.

Thymic Measurement

Thymic size can be quantitated using its length (measured in the cephalocaudal dimension), width (measured in the transverse dimension), and thickness (usually measured

FIG. 8.4. Normal thymus in a 51-year-old patient. The thymus (*arrows*) appears to be composed primarily of fat, containing islands or wisps of soft tissue. The left thymic lobe extends more posteriorly than the right.

FIG. 8.5. Thymic lymphoid follicular hyperplasia. A focal mass (*arrow*) in the prevascular space represented follicular hyperplasia. Its appearance is nonspecific and cannot be distinguished from thymoma.

perpendicular to the pleura). On CT, the average thickness of the thymus is 1.4 cm in children aged 5 years or less. The maximum normal thickness is 1.8 cm in patients under 20 and 1.3 cm in older adults.

Magnetic Resonance Imaging

On magnetic resonance imaging (MRI), the normal thymus characteristically appears homogeneous and of intermediate signal intensity on T1-weighted images, being less intense than surrounding mediastinal fat, but of greater intensity than muscle (see Fig. 8-2D). However, because of progressive involution, the appearance of the thymus is dependent on the age of the patient. In patients over 30 years of age, differentiation between the thymus and adjacent mediastinal fat may be difficult because of thymic involution. The T2 relaxation times of the thymus are similar to fat at all ages.

THYMIC LYMPHOID FOLLICULAR HYPERPLASIA

The term thymic lymphoid follicular hyperplasia (LFH) is used to describe a condition characterized by the presence of hyperplastic lymphoid germinal centers in the thymic medulla, associated with a lymphocytic and plasma cell infiltrate. The presence of LFH is commonly associated with myasthenia gravis, connective tissue disease, pure red blood

cell hypoplasia, and infection with HIV; it may also be seen in some normal young subjects.

Plain radiographs are usually normal. On CT, patients with LFH can have a normal-appearing thymus (45%), an enlarged thymus with a normal shape (35%), or a focal thymic mass (20%) (Fig. 8-5).

THYMIC HYPERPLASIA AND REBOUND

Thymic hyperplasia, as distinguished from LFH, is defined by an increase in size of the thymus associated with an otherwise normal gross and histologic appearance. It may be associated with hyperthyroidism (Graves' disease; Fig. 8-6), sarcoidosis, red blood cell aplasia, and other entities. It most commonly is seen in association with recovery from chemotherapy, stress, or burns, a phenomenon known as thymic rebound (described below).

Chest radiographs in adults are usually normal. In children, thymic enlargement may be seen. CT demonstrates increased thickness of the thymic lobes but an otherwise normal-appearing thymus.

Thymic Rebound

The thymus involutes during periods of stress (e.g., illness, burns, chemotherapy) and may decrease significantly in size, depending on the age of the patient and the severity and duration of the stress. This is most marked in children, but it has also been observed in young adults (Fig. 8-7). A decrease in

FIG. 8.6. Thymic hyperplasia in Graves' disease. **A:** Chest radiograph in a 40-year-old woman shows mediastinal widening (*arrows*). **B, C:** CT shows enlargement of the thymus (*T*) in the prevascular space. The left thymic lobe is largest.

FIG. 8.7. Thymic rebound in a 10-year-old patient following chemotherapy for lymphoma. The thymus (*T*) is enlarged.

thymic volume of more than 40% may be seen. The thymus generally regrows to its original size within several months of the stressful episode. It may also exhibit "rebound" or growth to a size significantly larger than its original size; an increase in thymic volume of 50% in comparison to baseline may be seen. Thymic enlargement may be observed shortly after the stressful episode or from 1 to 9 months afterward. In children and young adults, the incidence of thymic rebound following chemotherapy is 10% to 25%.

Increased thymic size may be seen on plain radiographs, particularly in children, but thymic rebound is detected with greater frequency when CT is used. In patients being treated for an extrathoracic malignancy, the appearance of thymic rebound should not pose a diagnostic problem; however, in patients with lymphoma, distinction from recurrent mediastinal tumor may be difficult. The presence of lymph node enlargement in association with thymic enlargement should suggest recurrent tumor, while isolated thymic enlargement should suggest thymic rebound. On MR, patients with thymic hyperplasia or thymic rebound may show enlargement of the thymus, but its signal intensity is the same as for normal thymus.

THYMIC MASSES

A number of masses arise in relation to the thymus. Thymic masses and tumors include thymic epithelial tumors (thymoma and thymic carcinoma), thymic neuroendocrine tumors, thymic cyst, thymolipoma, and lymphoma. Overall, they account for 20% to 25% of primary mediastinal tumors.

Thymoma

The term *thymoma* should only be used to describe neoplasms originating from thymic epithelium, although these tumors also contain a variable number of lymphocytes. Thymoma is the most common primary thymic tumor. It accounts for about 15% to 20% of primary mediastinal masses (Table 8-2).

TABLE 8.2 Thymoma

Originates from thymic epithelium
Most common thymic tumor
15%–20% of mediastinal masses
Most common in patients 50–60 years old
Myasthenia gravis in 30%–50%
10%–30% of patients with myasthenia have thymoma
Classified based on behavior as invasive (30%) or
  noninvasive (70%)
Classified histologically (WHO) as thymic epithelial tumor
  types A, AB, B1-3
WHO classifications associated with likelyhood of invasion
  and survival (A best, B3 worst)
Metastases outside thorax in 3%–5%
Radiographic findings
  Sharply marginated, smooth or lobulated
  Usually project to one side of the mediastinum
  Retrosternal clear space or costophrenic angles
CT findings
  Focal or lobulated mass
  Homogeneous or cystic, may calcify
  Invasion difficult to diagnose with certainty

Thymomas are rare before age 20 and are most common in patients aged 50 to 60 years. No distinct sex predominance is present. Patients may be asymptomatic, but 20% to 30% have symptoms related to compression of mediastinal structures. Myasthenia gravis develops in 30% to 50% of patients with a thymoma. Hematologic abnormalities are also associated with thymoma and include pure red blood cell aplasia and hypogammaglobulinemia. Approximately 10% to 30% of patients with myasthenia or red cell aplasia have a thymoma. Autoimmune and collagen-vascular diseases such as systemic lupus erythematosus, rheumatoid arthritis, Graves' disease, and inflammatory bowel disease may also be associated with thymoma.

Thymomas are usually encapsulated and round or lobular in shape. They may contain areas of calcification, necrosis, cysts, or hemorrhage. Thymomas appear benign histologically. If a thymic epithelial tumor appears malignant on histologic examination, it is termed *thymic carcinoma* rather than thymoma.

Most thymomas are slow-growing and behave in a benign fashion. However, about 30% are locally aggressive and invasive, or recur following excision. Invasive thymomas infiltrate the tumor capsule and adjacent structures, including the pericardium, pleura, superior vena cava, great vessels, airways, and heart, and may cross the diaphragm to involve the retroperitoneum. Spread to involve one pleural cavity can result in a typical appearance of multiple lenticular pleural implants occurring in the absence of pleural effusion. Thymoma rarely (3% to 5%) metastasizes outside the thorax.

Although various systems for the classification of thymic epithelilal tumors have been proposed, the simplest, and that in general use, consists of three groups based on a combination of histologic features and behavior. These are *noninvasive thymoma* (benign histology and without invasion), *invasive thymoma* (benign histology with invasion), and *thymic carcinoma* (malignant histology).

Recently, the World Health Organization (WHO) proposed a detailed histologic classification of thymomas. In the WHO system, thymomas are divided into two groups (type A and B) depending on whether the neoplastic epithelial cells and their nuclei are spindle- or oval-shaped (type A), or have a dendritic or epithelioid appearance (type B); type AB tumors have mixed features. Type B tumors are further divided into three subtypes (B1-B3) according to the proportional increase in their epithelial component and the presence of atypical cells. All types of thymic carcinoma are classified as type C. The WHO classification of thymic epithelial tumors has been shown to correlate significantly with tumor stage at diagnosis and prognosis. Types A, AB, and B1 thymoma are less likely to be invasive or recur after surgery and are associated with a greater likelihood of complete resection and a better survival than types B2 and B3 (Table 8-3). A detailed knowledge of this classification system is not necessary, but pathology reports in patients with thymoma often use this classification.

Thymomas can be staged at the time of surgery, based on the presence and extent of invasion:

Stage I: tumor capsule is intact
Stage II: invasion of the tumor capsule, surrounding fat, or mediastinal pleura
Stage III: invasion of surrounding organs
Stage IVa: pleural or pericardial implants
Stage IVb: hematogenous or lymphogenous metastases

Resection is usually indicated, sometimes in association with radiation, or radiation or chemotherapy for stages II and III. Although invasive thymomas may recur, they tend to grow slowly, and prolonged survival is usually possible. The 5-year survival rate for noninvasive thymoma is 75% to 90%; for invasive thymoma, the 5-year survival rate is 50% to 60%.

TABLE 8.3 WHO Classification of Thymoma Associated With Likelihood of Invasion and Survival

WHO Type	Percent With Invasion (%)	20-year Survival (%)
A	11	100
AB	42	87
B1	47	91
B2	69	59
B3	85	36

(Modified from **Okumura M, Ohta M, Tateyama H, et al.** The World Health Organization histologic classification system reflects the oncologic behavior of thymoma: a clinical study of 273 patients. Cancer 2002; 94:624–632.)

Plain Radiographs

Most thymomas arise near the junction of the heart and great vessels, although they may be seen superiorly to the level of the clavicles and inferiorly to the level of the costophrenic angles. Their distribution on the frontal radiograph may be likened to an upside-down horseshoe embracing the heart. They may be subtle or invisible on chest radiographs.

In most cases, thymomas appear sharply marginated, smooth or lobulated in contour, and usually project to one side of the mediastinum (Figs. 8-8A and 8-9A). They typically range in size from 5 to 10 cm in diameter when visible on radiographs and may obscure the right or left heart border, depending on their location and size. Dense calcification may be seen throughout the mass or in its periphery.

On lateral radiographs, a thymoma may result in a distinct opacity in the inferior aspect of the retrosternal clear space, the relatively lucent triangular region posterior to the sternum and anterior to the aortic arch, main pulmonary artery, and heart (see Figs. 8-8B and 8-9B). However, lack of lucency in this space or poor definition or obscuration of the anterior margin of the ascending aorta or pulmonary artery may be normal findings. A mass overlying the heart and region of the cardiophrenic angle may be seen, although this can be mimicked by fat pads and the normal cardiac incisura of the left lung.

Invasive and noninvasive thymomas cannot usually be distinguished on plain radiographs; however, pleural involvement with invasive thymoma occasionally results in pleural thickening, nodularity, or pleural effusion.

FIG. 8.8. Thymoma, invasive. **A:** PA chest radiograph shows prominence of the right mediastinum (*arrows*) due to a thymoma (*T*). **B:** On the lateral radiograph, an opacity (*T*) is visible in the inferior aspect of the retrosternal clear space, with a well-defined edge inferiorly (*arrows*). **C:** CT shows a homogeneous soft-tissue mass in the prevascular space. No fat plane is seen separating the thymoma (*T*) from the ascending aorta. Pericardial invasion was found at surgery. This was WHO type B1.

A

B

C

FIG. 8.9. Cystic thymoma, noninvasive. **A:** PA chest radiograph shows a large thymoma (*T, arrows*), obscuring the right heart border, extending into the right cardiophrenic angle. **B:** On the lateral radiograph, the thymoma (*T*) is visible overlying the heart shadow (*arrows*). **C:** CT shows a cystic (fluid attenuation) mass in the right cardiophrenic angle. The mass shows dense calcification, including calcification of its capsule. A noninvasive cystic thymoma was found at surgery.

Computed Tomography

In nearly all cases, thymomas occur in the prevascular space and displace the great vessels (aorta and its branches, superior vena cava and its branches, and main pulmonary artery) posteriorly (see Figs. 8-8C and 8-9C).

Thymoma or other thymic neoplasm may be distinguished from thymic hyperplasia if enlargement of the thymus is grossly asymmetric, if the thymus has a lobular contour, or if a focal rounded lesion is visible (Fig. 8-10). However, follicular thymic hyperplasia can result in a focal thymic mass up to 5 cm in diameter (see Fig. 8-5).

Approximately 80% of thymomas occur at the base of the heart, as shown on CT (see Figs. 8-8C and 8-9C). They usually appear as masses that are sharply demarcated and oval, round, or lobulated and do not conform to the normal shape of the thymus (see Figs. 8-8C, 8-9C, and 8-10).

Most often the tumor grows asymmetrically to one side of the mediastinum. Because ectopic thymic tissue in the neck is found in up to 20% of subjects, thymoma can occur in the neck or at the thoracic inlet, thus mimicking a thyroid mass (Fig. 8-11). Thymoma rarely occurs in the posterior mediastinum.

Thymomas usually appear homogeneous in attenuation with or without contrast injection (see Figs. 8-8C and 8-10). However, some large thymomas appear cystic (see Fig. 8-9C) or contain areas of necrosis. Calcification may occur in the capsule (see Fig. 8-9C) or within the tumor (see Figs. 8-10B and 8-12).

It is often difficult to distinguish invasive and noninvasive thymomas on CT. The presence of clearly defined fat planes between the tumor and adjacent mediastinal structures suggests the absence of extensive local invasion (Fig. 8-13), but

A   B

FIG. 8.10. Invasive thymoma with calcification in a patient with myasthenia gravis. **A:** CT shows a lobulated mass (*T*) in the prevascular space, typical of thymoma. Medially, the mass invades mediastinal fat (*large arrow*). A small pleural nodule (*small arrow*) is also seen, resulting from pleural invasion. Compression of the superior vena cava is also present. **B:** At a lower level, calcification is visible.

limited invasion cannot be excluded. Also, obliteration of fat planes between the tumor and mediastinal structures suggests the possibility of invasion, but this finding cannot be relied upon (see Fig. 8-8C). Findings highly suggestive of invasion include pericardial thickening contiguous with the tumor, pleural thickening, nodules, or effusion (see Figs. 8-10A, 8-12, and 8-14), encasement of mediastinal structures, fat infiltration (see Fig. 8-10A), and an irregular interface between the tumor and lung. Invasive thymomas may extend to involve the posterior mediastinum and by contiguity, the retroperitoneum. Consequently, it has been recommended that CT staging of thymoma include the upper abdomen.

Myasthenia gravis is commonly associated with thymic pathology (see Fig. 8-10). Sixty-five percent of patients with

myasthenia gravis have thymic hyperplasia, and 10% to 30% have thymoma. In patients with myasthenia, a normal-appearing thymus on CT may be associated with normal histology or focal lymphoid hyperplasia; an enlarged but otherwise normal-appearing thymus indicates focal lymphoid hyperplasia; and a focal nodule or mass may represent focal lymphoid hyperplasia or thymoma.

Magnetic Resonance

The role of MR in diagnosing thymic masses is limited. On MR, thymomas typically have a low signal intensity on T1-weighted images, which increases with T2 weighting; they may appear homogeneous in intensity or inhomogeneous

A   B

FIG. 8.11. Cervical thymoma. **A:** CT through the neck shows a left neck mass (*arrow*), mimicking thyroid enlargement. **B:** The mass (*arrow*) extends into the upper mediastinum. This was a non-invasive thymoma, WHO type A.

FIG. 8.12. Invasive thymoma with calcification. CT shows a lobulated thymoma with multiple calcifications. The presence of pleural effusion strongly suggests invasion.

with or without cystic components, or may show nodules or lobules of tumor separated by relatively low-intensity septations. MR has proven valuable in identifying the presence or absence of vascular invasion in patients with thymoma, especially in patients to whom intravenous contrast cannot be administered.

Thymic Carcinoma

Thymic carcinoma, like thymoma, arises from thymic epithelial cells, but it is much less common. Thymic carcinoma accounts for about 20% of thymic epithelial tumors (Table 8-4). Unlike thymoma, thymic carcinoma can be diagnosed as malignant on the basis of histologic criteria; however, the specific histologic pattern is variable. In the WHO classification of thymic epithelial tumors, thymic carcinoma is type C.

This tumor is aggressive and more likely to result in distant metastases than invasive thymoma. Although distant metastases are found in only about 5% of patients with invasive thymoma, they are present at diagnosis in 50% to 65% of patients with thymic carcinoma. Frequent sites of metastasis include the lungs, liver, brain, and bone. It has a poor prognosis, with a 5-year survival rate of 30%. Average age at presentation is 50 years.

Symptoms are usually attributable to the mediastinal mass. Invasion of mediastinal structures is common, and superior vena cava syndrome may be present. Although paraneoplastic syndromes such as myasthenia gravis, pure red cell aplasia, and hypogammaglobulinemia are common with thymoma, they are rare with thymic carcinoma.

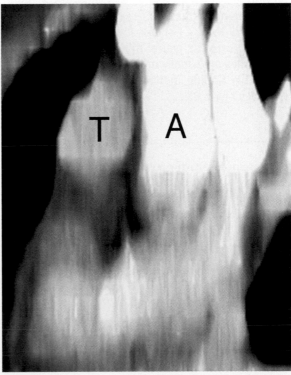

A

B

FIG. 8.13. Noninvasive thymoma. **A:** CT shows a homogeneous thymoma (*T*) separated from the aorta (*A*) and pulmonary artery (*P*) by a layer of fat. **B:** Oblique sagittal reconstruction shows separation of the thymoma (*T*) from the ascending aorta (*A*).

FIG. 8.14. Invasive thymoma with pleural metastases. **A:** PA chest radiograph shows a mass at the left cardiophrenic angle (*arrows*). **B:** CT shows a homogeneous rounded mass (*T*) representing thymoma. **C:** At a lower level, CT shows focal pleural thickening or nodules (*arrows*), typical of pleural metastases. Pleural nodules are usually unassociated with pleural effusion. This finding indicates invasion. This thymoma was WHO type B3.

Thymic carcinoma usually results in a mass 5 to 15 cm in diameter, with or without areas of low attenuation (Fig. 8-15). Calcification may be present (see Fig. 8-15) but is uncommon. Thymic carcinoma cannot be distinguished from thymoma on CT, although the presence of enlarged lymph nodes distinct from the primary tumor, distant metastases, and irregular tumor margins are all more common with carcinoma. Thymic carcinoma is less likely than thymoma to result in pleural implants.

On MR, thymic carcinoma appears higher in signal intensity than muscle on T1-weighted MR images, with an increase in signal on T2-weighted images. Heterogeneous signal may reflect the presence of necrosis, cystic regions within the tumor, or hemorrhage. Thymoma appears to have a greater tendency to show a multinodular appearance on MR than does thymic carcinoma.

Thymic Neuroendocrine Tumor

Thymic neuroendocrine tumors are believed to arise from thymic cells of neural crest origin (amine precursor uptake and decarboxylase cells; APUD); They may be

TABLE 8.4 Thymic Carcinoma

Originates from thymic epithelium
20% of thymic epithelial tumors
Average age 50
Unlike thymoma, appears malignant histologically
Classified histologically (WHO) as thymic epithelial tumor type C
Invasion common, distant metastases in 50%–65%
Myasthenia rare
Appearance indistinguishable from thymoma unless metastases are visible

A   B

FIG. 8.15. Thymic carcinoma. **A:** A large mass is visible in the prevascular space. It is lobulated and poorly marginated. **B:** At a lower level, calcifications are visible within the mass. An enlarged lymph node (*arrow*) adjacent to the mass suggests thymic carcinoma or invasive thymoma as the diagnosis.

classified as carcinoid tumor, atypical carcinoid, or small cell neuroendocrine carcinoma, depending on their histologic characteristics and in order of increasing malignancy. The biologic behavior of these tumors shows a direct relation to their degree of differentiation, but each of these tumor types behaves in an aggressive and malignant fashion, with a tendency for local recurrence or distant metastases following resection (Table 8-5). Average age at presentation is 45 years; men are more commonly involved.

Most patients present with symptoms related to compression of mediastinal structures. Approximately 25% to 40% of patients have Cushing's syndrome as a result of tumor secretion of adrenocorticotrophic hormone. Nearly

20% of cases have been associated with multiple endocrine neoplasia (MEN) syndromes I (more common) and II.

Although dense contrast enhancement may be seen on CT in some cases, neuroendocrine tumor does not differ significantly from thymoma in its radiographic or CT appearance (Fig. 8-16). In some patients, a mediastinal mass is not visible on CT despite the presence of endocrine abnormalities. MR findings are nonspecific and identical to those of thymoma.

This tumor is more aggressive than thymoma, and superior vena cava obstruction is much more common with thymic neuroendocrine tumor than with thymoma. The 5-year survival rate is about 65%. Mediastinal lymph node or distant metastases may be present.

Thymolipoma

Thymolipoma is a rare, benign, well-encapsulated thymic tumor consisting primarily of fat but also containing variable amounts of thymic tissue; it can arise within the thymus or be connected to the thymus by a pedicle. Eighty percent of patients present in the first four decades. It accounts for less than 5% of thymic tumors (Table 8-6).

In most cases, thymolipoma is unaccompanied by symptoms and is detected incidentally on chest radiographs. It is often large, averaging nearly 20 cm in diameter at diagnosis,

TABLE 8.5   Thymic Neuroendocrine Tumor

Classified as carcinoid, atypical carcinoid, or small cell neuroendocrine carcinoma in order of increasing malignancy
Originates from neural crest cells (APUDoma)
Average age 45
Usually malignant
Cushing's syndrome in 25%–40%
MEN in 20%
Mimics thymoma radiographically
Dense enhancement possibly seen on CT

A   B

FIG. 8.16. Thymic carcinoid tumor in a patient with Cushing's syndrome. **A:** A prevascular space mass (*arrows*) shows significant enhancement following contrast infusion. This may be seen in carcinoid tumor. **B:** Lung window scans showed pulmonary metastases (*arrow*).

and it may project into both hemithoraces. Because of its fatty content and pliability, thymolipoma tends to drape over the heart, extending inferiorly into the cardiophrenic angles, but may not obscure the cardiac margin (Fig. 8-17A). It can simulate cardiac enlargement, lower lobe collapse, or elevation of a hemidiaphragm. There is no known association with myasthenia gravis.

On CT, thymolipoma may appear to be predominantly fat but usually appears to contain wisps, whorls, or small nodules of soft tissue in combination with fat (see Fig. 8-17B). Uncommonly, it appears to be primarily of soft-tissue attenuation. In all cases, CT shows a connection between the mass and the thymic bed.

As would be expected from its fat content, MR shows areas of high signal intensity on T1-weighted spin-echo images, similar to the intensity of subcutaneous fat, with areas of intermediate signal intensity reflecting the presence of soft tissue. Despite attaining a large size, thymolipomas do not invade surrounding structures. However, some compression

of mediastinal structures is visible in half of cases. They do not recur following resection.

Thymic Cyst

Thymic cysts are uncommon. They can be either congenital or acquired. Congenital thymic cysts are rare; acquired thymic cysts have been reported following radiation therapy, in association with thymic tumors, and following thoracotomy. Their attenuation is usually that of water but can be higher or lower depending on the presence of hemorrhage or fat.

One should be cautious in making the diagnosis of thymic cyst; cystic regions can be seen in a variety of thymic tumors, including thymoma and lymphoma. CT can suggest the diagnosis of thymic cyst if the lesion (a) appears thin-walled; (b) is unassociated with a mass lesion; (c) contains fluid with a density close to that of water; and (d) remains unopacified following contrast infusion. Calcification of the cyst wall can also be seen. MR characteristics are similar to those of other cystic lesions.

Thymic Lymphoma and Metastases

Hodgkin's disease (HD) has a predilection for the involvement of the thymus in conjunction with the involvement of mediastinal lymph nodes. Thymic enlargement may be seen in 30% of patients with intrathoracic HD. Non-Hodgkin's lymphoma (NHL) less commonly involves the thymus.

TABLE 8.6 Thymolipoma
Consists of fat and thymic tissue
5% of thymic tumors
Benign
Often young patients
Usually asymptomatic
Large droopy mediastinal mass containing fat and strands of tissue

A   B

FIG. 8.17. Thymolipoma. **A:** PA chest radiograph shows a mass (*white arrow*) in the right cardio-phrenic angle. The right heart border remains faintly visible (*black arrows*), a finding that reflects the fatty nature of the mass. **B:** CT shows the mass (*arrows*) to be in the anterior mediastinum. It is composed of fat and strands of soft tissue.

Thymic lymphoma usually results in homogeneous thymic enlargement (Fig. 8-18). However, lobulation or a nodular appearance is seen in some patients, and cystic areas of necrosis are visible on CT in 20% of adults. Calcification uncommonly occurs in the absence of radiation or chemotherapy. Although its appearance is nonspecific, the combination of a thymic mass with mass or lymph node enlargement in other areas of the mediastinum is suggestive of this diagnosis. On MR, thymic lymphoma shows low intensity on T1-weighted images, with a variable change on T2-weighted images.

Metastatic tumors, particularly lung and breast carcinomas, can also involve the thymus. Involvement of mediastinal lymph nodes is also typically present. CT and MRI appearances of thymic metastases are nonspecific.

GERM CELL TUMORS

Germ cell tumors account for about 10% of primary mediastinal masses and arise from primitive germ cells that have arrested their embryologic migration in the mediastinum, frequently within the thymus. They are most common in the anterior mediastinum; only about 5% originate in the posterior mediastinum. Most germ cell tumors present during the second to fourth decades of life.

Germ cell tumors include benign and malignant teratoma, seminoma, embryonal carcinoma, endodermal sinus (yolk sac) tumor, choriocarcinoma, and mixed cell types.

Overall, more than 80% of germ cell tumors are benign, with the large majority of these being benign teratomas. Although the sex distribution of benign germ cell tumors is about equal, there is a strong preponderance of males among patients with malignant germ cell tumors. Among patients with malignant tumors, seminoma is most common, representing about 30% of cases, with embryonal carcinoma and malignant teratoma each responsible for about 10%, and choriocarcinoma and endodermal sinus

FIG. 8.18. Thymic enlargement in Hodgkin's disease. The thymus (*arrows*) is homogeneously enlarged.

tumor responsible for about 5% each; the remainder of malignancies, approximately 40% of cases, represent mixed tumors.

Benign tumors are often asymptomatic, while malignant tumors are more likely to cause symptoms. Confirmation that these lesions are primary to the mediastinum requires that there be no evidence of a testicular or retroperitoneal tumor.

Teratoma

Teratomas contain elements of all germinal layers. They are classified as mature, cystic (dermoid cyst), immature, and malignant (Table 8-7).

Mature teratomas are most common and are composed of well-differentiated tissues, with ectodermal elements such as skin and hair predominating, but they also contain cartilage, fat, and muscle. They are benign. They constitute 60% to 75% of mediastinal germ cell tumors. Sex incidence is equal, and they most commonly occur in children and young adults. They do not usually result in symptoms unless large.

Dermoid cysts are said to contain elements of only the ectodermal layer of germ cells, specifically skin and its appendages, but small rests of endodermal and mesodermal cells are often present; they are benign. Dermoid cysts are also referred to as *mature cystic teratoma*.

Immature teratomas contain less well-developed tissues more typical of those present during fetal development; in infancy or early childhood, these tumors often have a benign

TABLE 8.7 Teratoma
Contains elements of all germinal layers
Mature teratomas (contain mature tissues)
Benign
60%–75% of mediastinal germ cell tumors
Occur in children and young adults
Dermoid cyst
Immature teratomas (contain immature tissue)
Often have benign course in infants or young children
Often aggressive and malignant in adults
Malignant teratoma (contains frankly malignant tissues)
Poor prognosis
Usually men
Anterior mediastinal mass; posterior in 5%
Smooth, rounded, or lobulated mass
Mature teratoma
Well defined, smooth, cystic
Teeth and bone rare
Fluid in 90%; fat in 75%; calcification in 50%
Immature or malignant teratoma
Nodular or poorly defined
Fat in 40%
Compression or invasion of mediastinal structures
Enhancing capsule

course, while in adults they usually behave in an aggressive and malignant fashion.

Malignant teratomas contain frankly malignant tissues in addition to immature or mature tissues and have a very poor prognosis; they are seen almost exclusively in men.

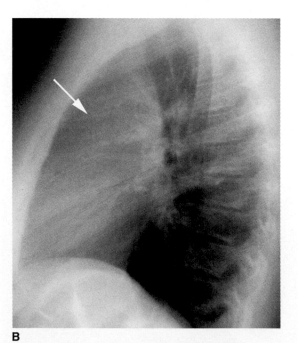

A   B

FIG. 8.19. Mature mediastinal teratoma. **A:** PA chest radiograph shows a smooth, sharply marginated left mediastinal mass (*arrows*). It obscures the left heart border, indicating its anterior location. **B:** Lateral view shows increased density of the retrosternal clear space (*arrow*), but a discrete mass is not visible.

Plain Radiographs

Plain radiographs usually show an anterior mediastinal mass projecting to one side of the mediastinum (Fig. 8-19). Their distribution is similar to that of thymoma. Middle mediastinal or posterior masses are occasionally seen. Teratoma appears as a smooth, rounded, or lobulated mass. Mature teratoma is typically well defined and often large at diagnosis, averaging 8 to 10 cm in diameter. Calcification is visible in about 20% of mature teratomas. Teeth and bone are diagnostic but rarely seen.

Computed Tomography

Teratomas are usually found in the prevascular space, although 5% occur in the posterior mediastinum. Regardless of their histology, CT often shows a combination of fluid-filled cysts, fat, soft tissue, and areas of calcification (Fig. 8-20). Calcification is visible in about 50% of cases, being focal or rimlike or rarely representing teeth or bone. In patients with mature teratoma, 90% contain fluid and 75% contain fat. Common combinations include fluid, soft tissue, fat, and calcium (40% of cases); fluid, soft tissue, and fat (25% of cases); and fluid and soft tissue (15% of cases). A fat-fluid level within the mass is diagnostic and is present in about 10% of cases. The fluid within cystic parts of the tumors may vary in attenuation. Teratomas are typically encapsulated and well demarcated. Rim enhancement can be seen.

Various CT findings can help in differentiating benign and malignant lesions. Benign lesions are typically well defined, smooth, and cystic, and 90% contain fat. Malignant teratomas are nodular or poorly defined, they are more likely to appear solid, and a smaller proportion (40%) contains fat. Malignant teratoma has a greater tendency to compress surrounding structures. Following contrast infusion, malignant teratoma can show a thick enhancing capsule.

A

B

C

FIG. 8.20. Appearance of mediastinal teratoma. **A:** Mature teratoma in an adult appears as a large mass compressing right cardiac structures. It contains calcifications, areas of fat (*arrow*), and cystic or soft-tissue regions. **B:** Mixed mature and immature teratoma in a young man with Kleinfelter's syndrome appears heterogeneous in attenuation, with areas of fat, calcification, soft tissue and fluid-filled cysts. **C:** Cystic teratoma in a 12-year-old boy shows fluid attenuation with a localized collection of fat.

MR can show various appearances, depending on the composition of the tumor. They commonly contain fat, which is intense on T1-weighted images, and cystic areas, which are low in intensity on T1-weighted images but increase with T2 weighting.

Seminoma

Seminoma occurs almost entirely in men, with a mean age at presentation of 29 years. It is the most common malignant mediastinal germ cell tumor, accounting for 30% of cases (Table 8-8).

Plain radiographs typically show a large, lobulated, anterior mediastinal mass projecting to one or both sides of the

TABLE 8.8	Seminoma

30% of germ cell tumors
Mean age 29
Large, lobulated, anterior mediastinal mass
Homogeneous in attenuation
Good prognosis; 5-year survival rate 50%–75%

mediastinum and often obscuring a portion of the heart border (Fig. 8-21). On CT, primary mediastinal seminomas present as large, smooth or lobulated, homogeneous soft-tissue masses, although small areas of low attenuation can be seen. Obliteration of fat planes is common, and pleural

A   **B**   **C**   **D**

FIG. 8.21. Mediastinal seminoma. A: PA radiograph shows a large, lobulated mediastinal mass (*arrows*) obscuring the right heart border. A right pleural effusion is also visible. **B:** Lateral view shows a large anterior mediastinal mass (*arrows*). **C, D:** CT shows a large, relatively homogeneous mass in the prevascular space, displacing mediastinal structures to the left. A pleural effusion is associated.

TABLE 8.9	Nonseminomatous Germ Cell Tumor

Cell types
  Embryonal carcinoma
  Endodermal sinus (yolk sac) tumor
  Choriocarcinoma
  Mixed types
Large, lobulated, anterior mediastinal mass
Inhomogeneous in attenuation
Long-term survival 45%–80%

or pericardial effusion may be present. Seminomas are very radiosensitive, and the 5-year survival rate is 50% to 75%.

Nonseminomatous Germ Cell Tumors

Nonseminomatous germ cell tumors, namely embryonal carcinoma, endodermal sinus (yolk sac) tumor, choriocarcinoma, and mixed types, are often grouped together because of their relative infrequency, similar appearance, and aggressive behavior (Table 8-9). In recent years, there have been significant advances in the treatment of non-seminomatous germ cell tumors. With the introduction of cisplatin-based chemotherapeutic regimens, the likelihood of long-term survival has risen from 10% or less to 45% to

80%. Surgery is reserved for those patients with radiologic evidence of persistent masses and may improve survival.

Plain radiographs show large, lobulated, anterior mediastinal masses. They may be ill defined or associated with pleural effusion because of local invasion of lung and pleura.

On CT, these tumors often show heterogeneous opacity, including ill-defined areas of low attenuation secondary to necrosis and hemorrhage or cystic areas (Fig. 8-22). They often appear infiltrative, with obliteration of fat planes, and may be spiculated. Calcification may be seen. MR findings also reflect the inhomogeneous nature of these lesions.

THYROID GLAND AND THYROID ENLARGEMENT

The thyroid gland is located in close approximation to the thoracic inlet, and thyroid enlargement is commonly associated with extension into the mediastinum. Multinodular goiter is the most common condition in which a mediastinal thyroid abnormality is detected; carcinoma and thyroiditis are relatively rare causes.

Intrathoracic extension of thyroid lesions is common, representing nearly 10% of mediastinal masses resected at thoracotomy (Table 8-10). Such lesions are almost

A

B

C

FIG. 8.22. Nonseminomatous (mixed) germ cell tumor in a 23-year-old man. **A, B:** CT shows a large, heterogeneous mass in the prevascular space, with densely enhancing vessels within it. Cystic areas are visible within the tumor. **C:** Coronal reconstruction shows the large heterogenous anterior mediastinal mass.

TABLE 8.10 Mediastinal Thyroid Mass

10% of mediastinal masses
Almost always connected to cervical thyroid
Anterior in 75%–90%; posterior in 10%–25%
Masses high in attenuation on CT; densely enhance with contrast
Cystic or inhomogeneous
Punctate calcifications
Distinguishing goiter and carcinoma difficult

always connected to the thyroid, being seen in the superior mediastinum. Truly ectopic mediastinal thyroid tissue, not showing a connection to the thyroid gland, is uncommon.

Thyroid masses are most often anterior in location. In 75% to 90% of cases, an enlarged thyroid extends into the thyropericardiac space anterior to the subclavian and innominate vessels. Posterior mediastinal goiters constitute approximately 10% to 25% of cases. Presumably arising from the posterolateral portion of the gland, posterior goiters descend behind the brachiocephalic vessels and are most commonly found on the right side, in close proximity to the trachea. Less often, thyroid tissue extends between the esophagus and trachea or posterior to the esophagus.

Plain Radiographs

Mediastinal thyroid abnormalities typically present as a sharply marginated, superior mediastinal mass, causing tracheal narrowing or displacement of the trachea to the contralateral side. The mass usually appears poorly marginated above the level of the clavicles (Fig. 8-23A).

Computed Tomography

The appearance of normal thyroid tissue is characteristic. On noncontrast scans, thyroid tissue is high in attenuation relative to adjacent soft tissues because of its high iodine content. Normal thyroid tissue measures around 100 HU, although in hypothyroid patients, thyroid attenuation is only slightly greater than that of soft tissue. Following the administration of contrast, thyroid tissue significantly enhances (see Figs. 8-23B and 8-24).

Recognizing that a mediastinal mass originates from the thyroid gland depends on (a) demonstration of a communication with the cervical portion of the thyroid gland on contiguous slices (see Fig. 8-24); (b) high attenuation of at least a portion of the mass; (c) marked enhancement after contrast injection (see Figs. 8-24 and 8-25); and (d) prolonged enhancement (more than 2 minutes). Mediastinal thyroid masses commonly appear inhomogeneous and cystic (see Figs. 8-23B and 8-25) on CT. Curvilinear, punctate, or ringlike calcifications can also be seen. The appearance of thyroid masses is usually nonspecific. Differentiation of goiter and thyroid carcinoma is difficult unless associated lymph node metastases are seen.

Magnetic Resonance

Characteristically, on T1-weighted images, the signal intensity of the normal thyroid is equal to or slightly greater than that seen in the adjacent sternocleidomastoid muscle; on T2-weighted scans, the signal intensity of the thyroid gland is significantly greater (Fig. 8-26). Most focal pathologic processes, including adenomas, cysts, and cancer, are

A

B

FIG. 8.23. Cystic cervical and mediastinal goiter. **A:** Chest radiograph shows displacement of the trachea to the right (*arrow*) and poorly defined superior mediastinal widening at the level of the thoracic inlet. **B:** CT shows an enhancing multicystic mass (*arrows*) at the level of the thoracic inlet. The trachea (*T*) is displaced to the right and slightly narrowed.

FIG. 8.24. Mediastinal goiter. **A:** An enhancing mass is visible in the right paratracheal mediastinum (*arrow*). **B:** At a higher level, this mass is seen to arise from the inferior pole of the right thyroid lobe (*arrow*). The thyroid also densely enhances.

easily identified on T2-weighted sequences because of their markedly prolonged T2 values. Multinodular goiter has inhomogeneous signal characteristics.

PARATHYROID ADENOMA

Four parathyroid glands are usually present. The upper pair is typically located dorsal to the superior poles of the thyroid gland, while the lower pair lies just below the lower thyroid poles. However, the precise location of glands may vary, and the lower pair is most variable in location. Most parathyroid adenomas are found in the lower group of parathyroid glands.

FIG. 8.25. Large cystic goiter. A large mass (*arrows*) at the thoracic inlet has a densely enhancing rim and a cystic center. The trachea is displaced to the right and narrowed. The mass protrudes anteriorly into the suprasternal notch.

Approximately 10% of parathyroid glands are ectopic (Table 8-11). About 60% of these are located in the anterior mediastinum; 30% are embedded within the thyroid tissue; and 10% are found in the posterior-superior mediastinum, in the region of the tracheoesophageal groove. Anterior mediastinal parathyroid glands are thought to result from islands of parathyroid tissue that are carried into the anterior mediastinum by the descending thymus during embryologic development. Anterior mediastinal parathyroid adenomas are intimately associated with the thymus.

Primary hyperparathyroidism results from a solitary adenoma in approximately 85% of cases. Other causes include diffuse hyperplasia (10%), multiple adenomas (5%), and rarely carcinoma (1%). Various studies are available for detecting parathyroid abnormalities. These include high-resolution ultrasonography, radionuclide imaging using thallium or sestamibi, high-resolution contrast-enhanced CT, MRI, and selective venous catheterization.

Normal parathyroid glands cannot be identified on CT. Parathyroid adenomas and hyperplastic glands are usually small but vary in size from 0.3 to 3 cm; rarely are they large enough to be detected on plain radiographs. When visible on CT, they usually appear homogeneous in density. Rarely, parathyroid adenomas appear calcified. No CT criteria reliably differentiate an adenoma from hyperplasia or carcinoma.

In patients with primary hyperparathyroidism, surgical neck exploration with resection of parathyroid tissues is curative in about 90% to 95% of cases. As a consequence, imaging is not generally performed prior to surgery. However, the persistence of hyperparathyroidism following surgical resection of the cervical glands suggests the presence of an ectopic parathyroid adenoma or ectopic hyperfunctioning gland. Forty to fifty percent of these patients will have mediastinal parathyroid glands. In the anterior mediastinum, ectopic

A   **B**

FIG. 8.26. MR of goiter. **A:** T1-weighted image shows a left thyroid mass to be slightly more intense than strap muscles. The trachea (*T*) is displaced to the right. **B:** With T2 weighting, the mass is more intense than muscle. *T*, trachea.

adenoma is usually found in the expected location of the thymus and may be indistinguishable from a small thymic remnant, small thymoma, or small lymph node (Fig. 8-27). Parathyroid adenomas are rarely found in the aortopulmonary window.

Similar to thyroid adenomas, most parathyroid adenomas, hyperplastic glands, and carcinomas appear intense on T2-weighted images, increasing significantly in intensity compared to T1-weighted images. Enhancement following gadolinium infusion is typical, and fat-suppression images can be valuable.

MEDIASTINAL LYMPH NODES AND LYMPH NODE MASSES

On average, more than 60 mediastinal lymph nodes are found at autopsy. Almost 80% of mediastinal lymph nodes are located in relation to the trachea and main bronchi and serve to drain the lungs.

Mediastinal lymph node abnormalities can be seen in any part of the mediastinum, although they most commonly involve middle mediastinal regions such as the pretracheal space, aortopulmonary window, and subcarinal space. Their detection and diagnosis are important in the evaluation of a number of thoracic diseases, including bronchogenic carcinoma, lymphoma, and granulomatous diseases. The

FIG. 8.27. Anterior mediastinal parathyroid adenoma on T1-weighted MRI in a patient with persistent hyperparathyroidism after parathyroid surgery. A small mass (*arrow*) is visible anterior to the ascending aorta (*A*) and main pulmonary artery (*P*), in the region of the thymus.

TABLE 8.11 Mediastinal Parathyroid Mass

10% of parathyroid glands are ectopic
  60% in the anterior mediastinum
  10% in the posterior-superior mediastinum
Adenoma and hyperplastic gland usually small
Mediastinal parathyroid gland or adenoma present in
  40%–50% of patients with persistent hyperparathyroidism
  after surgery

assessment of mediastinal lymph nodes in patients with bronchogenic carcinoma is discussed in detail in Chapter 3.

Mediastinal lymph nodes are generally classified by location, and most descriptive systems are based on Rouvière's classification of lymph node groups. Thoracic lymph nodes are usually grouped into parietal and visceral, depending on their location and drainage. The parietal lymph nodes lie outside the parietal pleura, primarily drain structures of the chest wall, and are classified as internal mammary, diaphragmatic, paracardiac, and intercostal. Visceral node groups are located within the mediastinum or are related to the lung hila, and include intrapulmonary, bronchopulmonary, tracheobronchial, paratracheal, paraesophageal, and anterior mediastinal lymph nodes.

Lymph Node Groups

The following classification is based on a modification of well-recognized anatomic descriptions of lymphatic anatomy, although some terms have been modified to be consistent with current usage and emphasize the localization of lymph nodes on imaging studies.

Lymph nodes are considered in anterior, tracheobronchial, and posterior node groups, generally corresponding to the plain radiographic divisions of anterior, middle, and posterior mediastinum.

Anterior Lymph Nodes

Internal mammary lymph nodes are located in a retrosternal position, in the anterior intercostal spaces, near the internal mammary artery and veins; they are considered to be part of the parietal lymph node group. They drain the anterior chest wall, anterior diaphragm, and medial breasts and freely communicate with prevascular lymph nodes and paracardiac or diaphragmatic lymph nodes. They are most often enlarged as a result of lymphoma or metastatic breast cancer (Figs. 8-28A and B, and 8-29A and B).

FIG. 8.28. Internal mammary and paracardiac lymph node enlargement. **A:** Lateral plain radiograph in a patient with non-Hodgkin's lymphoma shows thickening of the retrosternal stripe (*arrows*). **B:** CT shows enlargement of internal mammary lymph nodes (*arrows*) bilaterally, in association with involvement of the thymus (*T*) in the anterior mediastinum, left axillary lymph node enlargement, and pleural effusions. **C:** At a lower level, a right paracardiac lymph node (*arrow*) is also enlarged.

FIG. 8.29. Internal mammary and paracardiac lymph node enlargement. **A:** Lateral plain radiograph in a patient with non-Hodgkin's lymphoma shows lobulation of the retrosternal stripe (*arrows*). **B:** CT shows enlargement of an internal mammary lymph node (*arrow*), in association with the internal mammary vessels. **C:** At a lower level, a group of enlarged paracardiac lymph nodes (*arrows*) is also visible.

Prevascular lymph nodes lie anterior to the aorta and in relation to the great vessels. These nodes drain most anterior mediastinal structures, including the pericardium, thymus, thyroid, pleura, and the anterior hila. They represent visceral nodes. They communicate with the internal mammary chain of nodes anteriorly and paratracheal and aortopulmonary lymph nodes posteriorly. They may be involved in a variety of diseases, notably lymphoma (see Figs. 5-3 and 5-4 in Chapter 5) and granulomatous diseases, but their involvement in lung cancer is relatively uncommon.

Paracardiac or cardiophrenic angle lymph nodes lie anterior to or lateral to the heart and pericardium, on the surface of the diaphragm. They communicate with the lower internal mammary chain and drain the lower intercostal spaces, pericardium, diaphragm, and liver. As with internal mammary nodes, paracardiac nodes are most commonly enlarged in patients with lymphoma (see Fig. 8-28C) and metastatic carcinoma, particularly breast cancer. Paracardiac lymph nodes correspond to the anterior (prepericardiac) and middle (juxtaphrenic) subgroups of the diaphragmatic parietal lymph node group. Prepericardiac

nodes are located posterior to the xiphoid process and slightly lateral to it. Juxtaphrenic lymph nodes are situated adjacent to the pericardium, where the phrenic nerves meet the diaphragm. From a clinical standpoint, there is little reason to distinguish between them.

Tracheobronchial Lymph Nodes

Tracheobronchial lymph nodes generally serve to drain the lungs. Lung diseases (e.g., lung cancer, sarcoidosis, tuberculosis, fungal infections) that secondarily involve lymph nodes typically involve the tracheobronchial lymph nodes. Tracheobronchial lymph nodes are subdivided into a number of important node groups, which are all closely related.

Paratracheal nodes lie anterior to, and on either side of, the trachea, thus occupying the pretracheal (or anterior paratracheal) space (Figs. 8-30 and 8-31). Retrotracheal nodes may also be seen. The most inferior node in this region is the so-called azygos node, medial to the azygos arch. These nodes form the final pathway of lymphatic drainage from most of both lungs, excepting the left upper lobe. Because of this,

A

B

FIG. 8.30. Paratracheal lymph node enlargement in metastatic carcinoma. **A:** Chest radiographs show abnormal convexity of the right superior mediastinum (*arrows*). The right paratracheal stripe and the normal contour of the superior vena cava are not visible. **B:** CT shows lymph node enlargement in the pretracheal space (*arrow*), corresponding to paratracheal lymph nodes. The superior vena cava is displaced laterally and anteriorly, and the normal right paratracheal stripe is obscured by the large nodes.

they are commonly abnormal regardless of the location of lung disease.

Aortopulmonary nodes are grouped by Rouvière with prevascular nodes, but because they serve the same function on the left as paratracheal nodes on the right and freely communicate with paratracheal nodes, it is most appropriate

FIG. 8.31. Paratracheal and aortopulmonary window lymph node enlargement in non-Hodgkin's lymphoma. Enlarged nodes in the pretracheal space (*large arrow*) and aortopulmonary window (*small arrow*) are visible.

to group them together. They lie in the aortopulmonary window, lateral to the left main bronchus and between the aorta and pulmonary artery. The left upper lobe drains via this node group.

Peribronchial nodes surround the main bronchi on each side and lie between the main bronchi in the subcarinal space. These drain the lungs. *Bronchopulmonary nodes* are located distal to the main bronchi and are usually considered to be hilar.

Subcarinal nodes represent peribronchial nodes lying between the main bronchi in the subcarinal space (Fig. 8-32). These nodes drain the inferior hila and lower lobes on both the right and left and communicate in turn with the right paratracheal chain.

Posterior Lymph Nodes

Paraesophageal and inferior pulmonary ligament nodes are associated with the esophagus and descending aorta and lie medial to the inferior pulmonary ligament (Fig. 8-33A and B). They represent visceral nodes and drain the medial lower lobes, esophagus, pericardium, and posterior diaphragm. On the right, they are impossible to distinguish from subcarinal nodes unless they are near the diaphragm.

Intercostal and paravertebral lymph nodes are found in the posterior intercostal spaces and adjacent to thoracic vertebral bodies (see Fig. 8-33B and C). These drain the posterior

A   B

FIG. 8.32. Subcarinal lymph node enlargement in chronic lymphocytic leukemia. **A:** Chest radiographs show an abnormal convexity in the region of the azygoesophageal recess (*arrows*), corresponding to subcarinal lymph node enlargement. **B:** CT shows abnormally enlarged subcarinal lymph nodes (*arrows*).

pleura, chest wall, and spine and communicate with other posterior mediastinal lymph nodes.

Retrocrural lymph nodes lie posterior to the diaphragmatic crura (Fig. 8-34). They communicate with lumbar nodes and posterior mediastinal lymph nodes, drain the diaphragm and liver, and represent the posterior group of diaphragmatic parietal lymph nodes.

Lymph Node Stations

In the 1970s, the American Joint Committee on Cancer (AJCC) and the Union Internationale Contre le Cancer (UICC) introduced a numeric system for localization of intrathoracic lymph nodes for the purpose of lung cancer staging. Lymph nodes were described relative to regions in the mediastinum termed "lymph node stations" (Table 8-12). The AJCC/UICC node mapping system was modified in 1983 by the American Thoracic Society (ATS) to more precisely define anatomic and CT criteria for each station, and the ATS classification system has been in common usage since then (Fig. 8-35).

In 1997, the AJCC/UICC published a further revision intended to be a compromise between the AJCC and ATS classifications (Fig. 8-36). A detailed knowledge of lymph node stations is not necessary in clinical practice, but a passing familiarity with this classification is encouraged. Figures 8-35 and 8-36 and Table 8-12 may be used for reference and provide a comparison of ATS and AJCC/UICC criteria.

In the 2009 modification of the TNM Staging System for lung cancer (TNM7) by the International Association for the Study of Lung Cancer (IASLC) International Staging Committee and accepted by the AJCC/UICC, a simplification of this numerical system of lymph node stations into nodal zones has been recommended for the purposes of lung cancer staging. These include only four mediastinal zones (upper zone, aortopulmonary zone, subcarinal zone, lower zone) and two hilar zones (hilar/interlobar and peripheral zones) (Table 8-13). In an analysis of the survival of lung cancer patients with nodal metastases, a consideration of specific lymph node stations was found to be of little value.

(*text continues on page 247*)

FIG. 8.33. Paraesophageal and paravertebral lymph node enlargement in metastatic carcinoma. **A:** An enlarged lymph node (*arrow*) is visible in the right paraesophageal region. Pleural effusions are also seen. **B:** At a lower level, paraesophageal and paraaortic lymph nodes (*large arrows*) and paravertebral lymph nodes (*small arrows*) are enlarged. **C:** At a level below (**B**), enlarged paravertebral lymph nodes (*arrows*) are visible. They are higher in attenuation than the pleural fluid.

FIG. 8.34. Retrocrural lymph node enlargement in lymphoma. Enlarged nodes (*arrows*) are visible in a retrocrural, paraaortic location.

TABLE 8.12 Comparison of ATS and AJCC/UICC Lymph Node Stations

Node Group	ATS Node Station	ATS Designation	ATS Anatomic Criteria	AJCC/UICC Station	AJCC/UICC Designation	AJCC/UICC Anatomic Criteria
Paratracheal				1	Highest mediastinal	Cranial to the superior aspect of L brachiocephalic vein
Paratracheal	2R	R upper paratracheal	R of the tracheal midline, between the lung apex and the caudal margin of the innominate artery (or for radiologists, the superior aspect of the aortic arch as with 2L)	2	Upper paratracheal	Below station 1 and cranial to superior aspect of the aortic arch
	2L	L upper paratracheal	L of the tracheal midline, between the lung apex and the superior aortic arch			
Prevascular				3	Prevascular	Anterior to the great vessel branches and cranial to aortic arch
Paraesophageal					Retrotracheal	Posterior to the trachea and cranial to the inferior aspect of azygos arch
Paratracheal	4R	R lower paratracheal	R of the tracheal midline, below 2R and above the azygos arch	4R	R lower paratracheal	R of tracheal midline, below 2, and cranial to the RUL bronchus (this equals ATS 4R + 10R)
	4L	L lower paratracheal	L of the tracheal midline, below 2L, cephalad to the carina, and medial to the ligamentum arteriosum	4L	L lower paratracheal	L of the tracheal midline, below 2, and cranial to the LUL bronchus (this equals ATS 4L + 10L)
Aortopulmonary	5	Aortopulmonary	Subaortic and paraaortic nodes lateral to the ligamentum arteriosum, aorta, or LPA, proximal to the first branch of the LPA	5	Subaortic or aortopulmonary	Lateral to the ligamentum arteriosum, aorta, or LPA, proximal to the first branch of the LPA within the mediastinal pleural envelope
Prevascular	6	Anterior	Anterior to aortic arch or innominate artery (including some pretracheal and preaortic nodes)	6	Paraaortic (ascending aortic or phrenic)	Anterior and lateral to the ascending aorta and the aortic arch and innominate artery, caudal to the superior aspect of aortic arch
Subcarinal	7	Subcarinal	Caudal to the carina but not associated with the lower lobe bronchi or arteries within the lung	7	Subcarinal	Caudal to the carina but not associated with the lower lobe bronchi or pulmonary arteries within the lung
Paraesophageal	8	Paraesophageal	Dorsal to the posterior wall of trachea and on either side of the esophagus (not subcarinal nodes)	8	Paraesophageal	Adjacent to the wall of the esophagus and to the right of left of esophagus
Inferior pulmonary ligament	9	R or L pulmonary ligament	In relation to right or left inferior pulmonary ligaments	9	Pulmonary ligament	Within the pulmonary ligament, including those in the posterior wall and lower part of the inferior pulmonary vein
Peribronchial (hilar)	10R	Tracheobronchial	R of the tracheal midline, caudal to 4R and above the origin of the RUL bronchus	10R	R hilar	Caudal to the superior RUL bronchus, adjacent to the R main bronchus or proximal bronchus intermedius
	10L	Peribronchial	L of the tracheal midline, between the carina and the LUL bronchus, medial to the ligamentum arteriosum	10L	R hilar	Caudal to the superior LUL bronchus, adjacent to L main bronchus
Bronchopulmonary (hilar)	11	Intrapulmonary	Nodes removed at pneumonectomy or distal to the mainstem bronchi or secondary carina (includes interlobar, lobar, and segmental nodes)	11	Interlobar	Between lobar bronchi and adjacent to proximal lobar bronchi
Lobar	12		May be determined postthoracotomy	12	Lobar	Adjacent to distal lobar bronchi
Segmental	13		May be determined postthoracotomy	13	Segmental	Adjacent to segmental bronchi
				14	Subsegmental	Adjacent to subsegmental bronchi

L, left; R, right; LPA, left pulmonary artery; LUL, left upper lobe; RUL, right upper lobe.

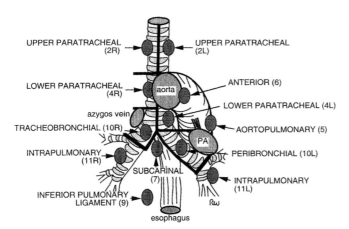

FIG. 8.35. ATS lymph node stations.

Diagnosis of Lymph Node Enlargement

Radiographs

Normal lymph nodes are not visible on chest radiographs. Abnormally enlarged nodes may be recognized because of distortion of normal mediastinal contours or abnormalities of mediastinal lines, interfaces, or spaces (Table 8-14).

Enlarged right paratracheal (pretracheal lymph) nodes usually result in an abnormal convexity of the superior vena cava interface or thickening of the right paratracheal stripe (see Fig. 8-30A). Inferiorly, right paratracheal nodes are contiguous with the right tracheobronchial nodes, recognizable when enlarged as a convexity in the region of the azygos arch.

Enlarged left paratracheal lymph nodes are not commonly visible on chest radiographs but may result in an convexity in the region of the left paratracheal stripe or in relation to the left subclavian artery interface, above the aortic arch.

Enlargement of aortopulmonary nodes results in a convexity of the aortopulmonary window.

Enlarged subcarinal lymph nodes result in a convexity in the region of the superior aspect of the azygoesophageal recess (see Fig. 8-32A). Paraesophageal lymph node enlargement also may result in an abnormal convexity in the azygoesophageal recess or an abnormality of the retrotracheal band on the lateral film.

Computed Tomography

On CT, lymph nodes are generally visible as round, elliptical, or triangular; discrete and surrounded by mediastinal fat; and of soft-tissue attenuation (see Figs. 8-28 to 8-34). The node hilum is sometimes seen to contain a small quantity of fat.

A

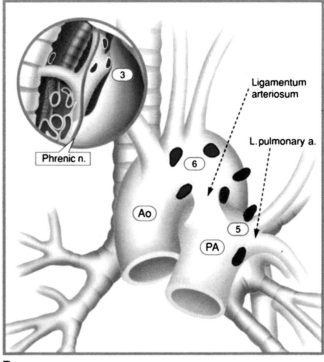

B

FIG. 8.36. American Joint Committee on Cancer/Union Internationale Contre le Cancer lymph node stations. **A, B:** (From **Mountain CF, Dresler CM**. Regional lymph node classification for lung cancer staging. Chest 1997; 111:1718–1723.)

FIG. 8.45. Lymph node enlargement and calcification in sarcoidosis. **A:** Coronal reconstruction shows symmetric mediastinal and hilar involvement with sarcoidosis (i.e., the 1-2-3-4 pattern). The lymph nodes are densely calcified. *Pre,* pretracheal; *APW,* aortopulmonary window; *H,* hilar; *Sc,* subcarinal; *A,* aorta; *T,* trachea. **B:** Calcified pretracheal (*Pre*) and aortopulmonary window (*APW*) nodes in the same patient. **C:** Calcified precarinal and hilar nodes. **D:** Calcified subcarinal (*Sc*) and hilar nodes (*arrows*). Areas of consolidation represent atelectasis due to bronchial narrowing by nodes.

associated with large localized masses as is lymphoma. Lymph node calcification is visible on CT in 25% to 50% of cases (see Fig. 8-45). As on chest radiographs, it may appear hazy or dense or have a stippled or eggshell appearance. Rarely,

TABLE 8.20 Sarcoidosis: Frequency of Enlarged Nodes Seen on Chest Radiograph and CT by Lymph Node Group in Patients with Enlarged Nodes

Node Group	Radiograph (%)	CT (%)
Hilar	85–95	90
Right paratracheal	75	100
Aortopulmonary window	50–75	90
Subcarinal	20	65
Anterior mediastinal	10–15	50
Posterior mediastinal	<5	15

nodes appear necrotic or low in attenuation or enhancing on contrast-enhanced scans.

A variety of patterns of pulmonary involvement, from small nodules to large ill-defined masses or pulmonary fibrosis, can also be seen in patients with sarcoidosis (see Chapter 15). It is common to see typical features of sarcoid lung involvement on high-resolution CT without lymph node enlargement being visible.

INFECTIONS

A variety of infectious agents can cause mediastinal lymph node enlargement during the acute phase of disease. These include tuberculosis, a number of fungal infections including histoplasmosis and coccidioidomycosis, bacterial infections, and viral infections. Typically, there are symptoms and signs of acute infection and chest radiographs show evidence of lung disease, although this is not always the case. In patients with prior granulomatous infection, lymph node calcification is common, with such nodes appearing normal in size or enlarged.

Tuberculosis

Hilar and mediastinal lymph node enlargement is commonly seen on plain radiographs and CT in patients with active tuberculosis (Table 8-21), although it is more frequently seen in children than adults.

Lymph node enlargement is usually present on the side of lung disease (Fig. 8-46A), but involvement of contralateral nodes is sometimes present. Although the presence of lymphadenopathy on chest radiographs in the absence of visible lung disease is unusual in tuberculosis, this is not always the case (see Fig. 8-46B).

Right-sided adenopathy usually predominates, and specifically, right paratracheal lymph node enlargement is most common (see Fig. 8-46A and B). Bilateral hilar lymph node enlargement is much less common than in sarcoidosis.

In patients with active tuberculosis, nodes larger than 2 cm in diameter commonly show central areas of low attenuation on contrast-enhanced CT, with peripheral rim enhancement (see Fig. 8-46C). The areas of relative low attenuation are not of water density, but range from about 40 to 60 HU; they are usually visible only on contrast-enhanced scans. Areas of low attenuation involving the mediastinum with obliteration of mediastinal fat represent tuberculous mediastinitis or a cold abscess. Rim-enhancing lymph nodes have also been reported in nearly 85% of AIDS patients with tuberculosis.

Three patterns of lymph node enlargement have been reported on MR in patients with tuberculosis, correlating with clinical symptoms and pathologic findings and paralleling the expected CT findings in such patients. In patients with necrosis and active TB, nodes are inhomogeneous with marked peripheral enhancement after injection of contrast material. Nodes with granulomatous inflammation,

A

B

C

FIG. 8.46. Lymph node enlargement in tuberculosis. **A:** Primary tuberculosis with right lung consolidation, right hilar lymph node enlargement (*black arrow*), and right paratracheal lymph node enlargement manifested by widening of the right paratracheal stripe (*white arrow*). **B:** Tuberculosis in AIDS with right hilar and right paratracheal lymph node enlargement (*arrows*). **C:** Tuberculosis with a low-attenuation, rim-enhancing subcarinal lymph node mass (*arrow*).

TABLE 8.21	Lymph Node Enlargement in Patients with Active Tuberculosis Shown on CT	
Site	ATS Designation	% Abnormal
Right paratracheal	2R	80
Left paratracheal	2L	5
Right paratracheal	4R	85
Left paratracheal	4L	10
Right tracheo-bronchial	10R	65
Subcarinal	7	50
Aortopulmonary	5	35
Right hilar	11R	30
Left hilar	11L	10

FIG. 8.53. Bronchogenic cyst. **A:** A large subcarinal mass (*arrows*) is visible on chest radiograph. **B:** Unenhanced CT shows a large subcarinal bronchogenic cyst (*C, white arrows*), appearing slightly less dense than soft tissue. Focal calcification of the cyst wall is visible (*black arrow*). **C:** Coronal T1-weighted MRI shows a large subcarinal cyst. Signal from the cyst (*C*) is due to its protein content. **D:** Transaxial T2-weighted, fat-saturated image shows high signal intensity. This is typical. *C*, cyst.

Large bronchogenic cysts may be associated with symptoms because of compression of adjacent structures such as the trachea and carina, mediastinal vessels, and left atrium. Small, asymptomatic cysts can be followed. However, enlargement over years is typical, and rapid enlargement associated with pain can indicate hemorrhage or infection. Because of their tendency to enlarge, surgical management has been traditional. Recently, percutaneous and transbronchial needle aspiration has also been used for the diagnosis and treatment of bronchogenic and esophageal duplication cysts.

Esophageal Duplication Cyst

Esophageal duplication cysts are lined by gastrointestinal tract mucosa and are often connected to the esophagus; unlike bronchogenic cysts, they do not contain cartilage. Sixty percent are found in the lower middle or posterior mediastinum, adjacent to the esophagus, and are sometimes found within its wall. Their appearance on plain radiographs, CT, and MRI is indistinguishable from that of bronchogenic cysts, except for their paraesophageal location (Fig. 8-54). Rarely, the cyst wall calcifies.

Neurenteric Cyst

Neurenteric cyst is rare. It occurs in the posterior mediastinum and is connected to the meninges within the spinal canal through a midline defect in one or more vertebral bodies. They are composed of both neural and gastrointestinal elements, including gastric, salivary gland, adrenal, pancreatic, and intestinal tissues. A connection with the esophagus is often present. The appearance of neurenteric cyst on CT is the same as that of other duplication cysts, but the presence of a vertebral abnormality can point to the diagnosis (Fig. 8-55); vertebral anomalies (e.g., hemivertebrae or butterfly vertebrae) or scoliosis is present in about half of cases. The cysts rarely contain air, because of communication with

A   **B**

FIG. 8.54. Esophageal duplication cyst. **A:** Coronal MR shows a paraesophageal cyst (*arrow*). **B:** Transaxial T2-weighted, fat-saturated image shows high signal intensity typical of cyst (*arrow*). The cyst is paraesophageal in location.

the esophagus. They frequently cause pain and are generally diagnosed at a young age.

Pericardial Cyst

Pericardial cyst reflects a defect in the embryogenesis of the coelomic cavity. The wall of a pericardial cyst is composed of connective tissue and a single layer of mesothelial cells. Most patients are asymptomatic.

FIG. 8.55. Neurenteric cyst. A low-attenuation paravertebral cystic lesion (*arrow*) is associated with scoliosis.

On plain radiographs, pericardial cysts are smooth and sharply marginated (Fig. 8-56A). Approximately 90% of pericardial cysts contact the diaphragm, with 65% occurring in the right cardiophrenic angle and 25% in the left cardiophrenic angle. In this location, they sometimes are seen to extend into the major fissure, having a lenticular shape on lateral chest films. Ten percent of pericardial cysts do not touch the diaphragm and are seen at higher levels, contiguous with the proximal aorta or pulmonary arteries.

On CT, they appear sharply marginated and their attenuation is usually similar to that of water (see Fig. 8-56B); however, pericardial cysts with high CT numbers are occasionally seen. When occurring within the upper mediastinum, they may be seen to have a relationship to the superior pericardial recesses. Pericardial cysts are not always round; they may assume different shapes when studied at different times. On MRI, pericardial cysts containing serous fluid appear less intense than muscle on T1-weighted images.

Mediastinal Pseudocyst

Pancreatic pseudocyst represents an encapsulated collection of pancreatic secretions, blood, and necrotic material. Mediastinal extension of a pancreatic pseudocyst is rare but can occur via the aortic hiatus or esophageal hiatus or through a defect in the diaphragm. Symptoms are generally those of pancreatitis.

Plain radiographs may show a retrocardiac mediastinal mass. CT shows a cystic and low-attenuation mass in the posterior mediastinum or adjacent thoracic cavity, associated with compression or displacement of the esophagus or splaying of the diaphragmatic crura. Mediastinal pseudocysts are commonly located under and posterior to the heart, anterior

A **B**

FIG. 8.56. Pericardial cyst. **A:** Chest radiograph shows a mass in the right cardio-phrenic angle (*arrow*). **B:** CT shows a low-attenuation cyst (*arrow*) contacting the pericardium.

to the aorta and esophagus, and medial to the inferior vena cava. The fluid can be of water attenuation or greater, depending on the presence of blood or infection. An abdominal fluid collection is common but not invariably present.

Other Cystic Lesions

Cystic or fluid-filled mediastinal lesions may represent congenital cysts or cystic masses (Table 8-25). Differentiation of an uncomplicated congenital cyst from other cystic encapsulated lesions, such as abscess, chronic hematoma, cystic lymphangioma or hemangioma, cystic teratoma, or other cystic tumor relies on the clinical presentation, findings on correlative radiographic studies, and the location and CT appearance of the cyst. Abscess, hematoma, and cys-

TABLE 8.25 Cystic, Low-attenuation, or Fluid-filled Masses

Congenital or acquired cysts (bronchogenic, esophageal, neurenteric, pericardial, and thymic)
Necrotic or cystic neoplasms (germ cell tumors, cystic thymoma, lymphoma)
Necrotic lymph nodes
Cystic lymphangioma (hygroma)
Thoracic meningocele
Mediastinal abscess
Mediastinal hematoma
Mediastinal pseudocyst
Cystic goiter
Dilated, fluid-filled esophagus
Pericardial fluid collections

tic tumors commonly demonstrate thick or irregular walls, septations, and mixed-density fluids. Cystic masses in the anterior mediastinum rarely represent a congenital cyst and are more likely related to the presence of a cystic tumor or a thymic cyst. Anterior or lateral meningocele may closely resemble a congenital cyst, but careful examination of adjacent sections should demonstrate the intraspinal connection of the mass through the neural foramen.

VASCULAR TUMORS

Lymphangioma and Cystic Hygroma

Lymphangiomas are rare benign lesions of lymphatic origin and represent 1% to 5% of mediastinal tumors; most are present at birth and are detected in the first 2 years of life (Table 8-26). Patients may be asymptomatic, but compression of mediastinal structures can result in chest pain, cough, or dyspnea. Because of a tendency for local growth, surgery is recommended. Lymphangioma can be seen in adults, with or without a history of incomplete resection as a child.

Lymphangiomas are most common in the neck (75%) and axilla (20%). Although 10% of cervical lymphangiomas extend into the mediastinum, less than 5% of lymphangiomas are limited to the mediastinum. In adults, it is more common for lymphangioma to be localized to the mediastinum.

Lymphangiomas are classified as capillary, cavernous, or cystic (hygroma), depending on the size of the lymph channels they contain. Cystic lymphangioma is most common, accounting for more than 60% cases of lymphangioma in adults (Fig. 8-57). Cystic lymphangioma may be either

TABLE 8.26 Lymphangioma

1%–5% of mediastinal tumors
Usually present in childhood
Compression of mediastinal structures
Most common in neck (75%) and axilla (20%)
10% of cervical masses extend into mediastinum
5% limited to mediastinum
Classified as capillary, cavernous, or cystic (hygroma)
Unilocular or multilocular cystic masses
Contain serous or chylous fluid
May contain fat and enhancing vessels

unilocular or multilocular and can contain either serous or chylous fluid; thin septations within the mass are sometimes seen. In adults, lymphangiomas are most common in the anterior (25% to 35%) or superior (15% to 35%) mediastinum but are also seen in the middle (20% to 25%) and posterior (15% to 30%) mediastinum. They can be quite large, ranging up to 30 cm in diameter.

On plain radiographs, a focal mass in the upper mediastinum may be visible or diffuse mediastinal widening may be seen (Fig. 8-58). An increase in cervical soft tissues may be associated.

On CT, the attenuation of lymphangiomas is usually homogeneous and near to that of water (see Fig. 8-57), but they can be of higher attenuation or variably composed of a combination of fluid, solid tissue, and fat (see Fig. 8-58); calcification is rare. Although they are usually well circumscribed and localized, they may appear to envelop mediastinal structures. Lymphangioma may be associated with vascular malformations that are easily identifiable following the administration of intravenous contrast. Simple lymphangiomas and hemangiomas composed of capillary-sized, thin-walled channels may appear as solid masses. On MR,

FIG. 8.57. Cystic lymphangioma (hygroma). A low-attenuation lesion (*arrow*) is visible in the superior mediastinum.

heterogeneous signal intensity is typical, with increased signal on T2-weighted images reflecting their fluid content (see Fig. 8-58).

Hemangioma

Hemangiomas are rare benign vascular tumors, accounting for less than 0.5% of mediastinal masses. They are composed of large interconnecting vascular channels with regions of thrombosis and varying amounts of interposed stroma, such as fat and fibrous tissue. Tumors are categorized according to the size and nature of their vascular spaces as capillary, cavernous, or venous; cavernous hemangiomas make up about 75% of cases. They are well defined and rarely are invasive.

Mediastinal hemangiomas are most common in young patients; about 75% present before the age of 35. One third to one half of cases are asymptomatic, but some patients present with symptoms of compression of mediastinal structures. Occasional cases are associated with peripheral hemangiomas or Osler-Weber-Rendu syndrome.

Hemangiomas most commonly arise in the anterior mediastinum (45% to 70% of cases) and posterior mediastinum (20% to 35% of cases). Extension into the neck may occur (7%). Masses may appear well marginated on CT (70%), inseparable from adjacent mediastinal structures (21%), or diffusely infiltrative (7%). Apparent infiltration may or may not predict unresectability.

On CT, tumors are often heterogeneous in attenuation on unenhanced scans, and fat is occasionally seen within them. Heterogeneous enhancement is typical following contrast infusion but is not always present. Enhancement may be dense, multifocal, or diffuse, and central or peripheral. Opacified vascular channels can be seen within the mass, with rapid enhancement similar to that of normal mediastinal vessels. Phleboliths, thought to be pathognomonic, are visible in up to 10% of cases on plain radiographs. On CT, punctate calcifications or phleboliths are visible in 10% to 20% (Fig. 8-59). Dilated mediastinal vessels may be associated with the mass (Fig. 8-59).

Other Vascular Lesions

Other mediastinal lesions may be associated with significant enhancement following contrast infusion (Table 8-27).

ESOPHAGUS

At successive levels in the mediastinum, the esophagus is in intimate contact anteriorly with the posterior or posterolateral trachea, the left mainstem bronchus, and the left atrium. The esophagus lies between the aorta on the left and the azygos vein on the right. Intraluminal air or a small amount of fluid is common and a normal finding with CT. Evaluation of esophageal disease is limited if the esophagus is incompletely distended.

FIG. 8.58. Lymphangioma in a young boy. **A:** Chest radiograph shows a mass (*arrows*) involving the left superior mediastinum, obscuring the left heart border. **B:** Contrast-enhanced CT shows a multicystic mass containing enhancing vessels (*arrow*). **C:** Transaxial T1-weighted image shows a large cystic mass with a fluid-fluid level (*arrow*). **D:** Transaxial T2-weighted image shows a complex cystic mass. The fluid-fluid level is visible (*arrow*).

CT has several distinct indications in patients with suspected esophageal disease. It is indicated (1) to evaluate and stage patients with esophageal carcinoma and to provide a means for assessing response to therapy and resultant complications, (2) to evaluate and characterize esophageal contour abnormalities detected at esophagography, and their relationship to intrinsic or extrinsic masses, and (3) to evaluate patients with suspected esophageal perforation and to assess the extent of pleural and mediastinal fluid collections.

Esophageal Carcinoma

Esophageal carcinoma represents approximately 10% of all cancers of the gastrointestinal tract. Excluding adenocarcinomas of gastric origin with secondary esophageal involvement, 90% to 95% of esophageal tumors are squamous cell carcinoma. These tumors usually present in an advanced stage, with 5-year survival rates varying between 3% and 20%. This poor prognosis results from rapid submucosal extension of the tumor and early transmural invasion. This

A   B

FIG. 8.59. Mediastinal hemangioma. **A:** A large mass (*arrow*) in the subcarinal space contains phleboliths. **B:** At a higher level, the superior vena cava (*large arrow*) and azygos vein (*small arrow*) are dilated. Dilated veins are visible in the mediastinum, posterior to the superior vena cava.

leads to early spread to regional and distal lymphatics as well as the liver, adrenals, and lung. Esophageal carcinoma often presents with symptoms of obstruction, and incidental detection with plain radiographs or CT is unusual.

Plain radiographs show some abnormality in about half of patients with esophageal carcinoma, including an abnormal convexity of the azygoesophageal recess (25%), mediastinal widening (20%), a retrotracheal mass (15%) or thickening of the posterior tracheal band (10%), and tracheal displacement (10%).

The CT manifestations of esophageal carcinoma include (1) narrowing of the esophageal lumen or dilatation due to obstruction; (2) thickening of the esophageal wall, either symmetrical or asymmetrical; (3) loss of periesophageal fat planes, with or without evidence of invasion of surrounding organs; and (4) periesophageal adenopathy. Wall thickening must be distinguished from idiopathic muscular hypertrophy of the esophagus.

TABLE 8.27 Enhancing Masses

Mediastinal thyroid glands or masses
Ectopic parathyroid glands or masses
Carcinoid tumors
Lymphangioma
Hemangioma
Paraganglioma
Castleman's disease

Mesenchymal Tumors

Benign tumors of the esophagus, arising from components of the esophageal wall, include leiomyoma, fibroma, and lipoma. Unlike esophageal carcinoma, these tumors may be detected incidentally as a mediastinal mass in asymptomatic patients. Leiomyoma is most common and predominates in the middle and lower esophagus. An abnormality in the subcarinal space or involving the azygoesophageal recess may be seen (Fig. 8-60). On lateral radiographs, an abnormality of the posterior tracheal band may be seen.

Esophageal Dilatation

Esophageal dilatation may result from obstructing tumors, stricture, or achalasia. Achalasia or strictures secondary to scleroderma are usually associated with the greatest degree of esophageal dilatation. An increase in air or fluid in the esophageal lumen and retained ingested material are common findings.

With marked esophageal dilatation, or megaesophagus, the esophagus usually projects to the right of the mediastinum, with a marked abnormality of the azygoesophageal recess seen on the chest radiograph (Fig. 8-61A). The left wall of the dilated distal esophagus is often visible in a left retrocardiac location. The trachea may be displaced forward if the upper esophagus is dilated, and there may be thickening of the posterior tracheal band or filling in of the retrotracheal triangle.

FIG. 8.62 Paraesophageal varices appearing as a mediastinal mass in a patient with hepatitis B and portal hypertension. **A:** Scout view shows a convex right posterior mediastinal mass (*arrows*). **B:** CT shows very large paraesophageal varices (*arrows*). The air-filled esophagus is also visible.

Many cases of mediastinitis occur after median sternotomy. In subjects having CT after an uncomplicated sternotomy, findings can closely mimic the appearance of mediastinitis. More than 75% of patients having median sternotomy show retrosternal fluid collections, air, hematoma, or a combination of these in the early postoperative period. After 2 weeks, these abnormalities should largely resolve, although some abnormal findings may persist for up to 3 weeks.

FIG. 8.63 Mediastinitis secondary to esophageal perforation. **A:** The mediastinum is widened (*white arrows*) and streaky pneumomediastinum is visible (*black arrows*). Air extends into the neck. **B:** CT shows mediastinal widening, increased attenuation of mediastinal fat, and pneumomediastinum.

PARASPINAL ABNORMALITIES

A wide variety of pathologic processes may involve the paraspinal regions. Most frequently, paraspinal masses are neural in origin, including neurogenic tumors, neurenteric cyst, and anterior or lateral thoracic meningocele, or are related to the spine. Infections involving the spine may lead to the development of paraspinal abscess. In addition, lymphoma and other causes of lymph node enlargement may result in abnormalities in this region; paraspinal lymph nodes freely communicate with lymph nodes in the upper abdomen, and contiguous involvement is common. Since the mediastinum communicates with the retroperitoneal space via the esophageal hiatus, aortic hiatus, and other defects in the diaphragm, diseases can spread between the abdomen and thorax by direct extension; inflammatory masses such as pancreatic pseudocysts can involve the paraspinal mediastinal regions. Rare entities such as extramedullary hematopoiesis, primary myelolipomas of the mediastinum, benign hemangioendotheliomas, aggressive fibromatosis, and fibrosing mediastinitis have been reported in the paravertebral regions.

NEUROGENIC TUMORS

Neurogenic tumors account for about 10% to 20% of primary mediastinal masses in adults and 30% to 35% of mediastinal tumors in children. Seventy-five percent of posterior mediastinal masses are neurogenic tumors. Tumors may arise from peripheral nerves and nerve sheath (neurofibroma, schwannoma, malignant peripheral nerve sheath tumors) or sympathetic ganglia (ganglioneuroma, ganglioneuroblastoma, neuroblastoma). The most common cell types are schwannoma (35%), ganglioneuroma (25%), neuroblastoma (15% to 20%), ganglioneuroblastomas (7% to 15%), and neurofibroma (5% to 10%), but the incidence varies with the patient's age. Eighty percent are benign.

Nearly 85% of neurogenic tumors in children are of ganglionic origin, while in adults more than 75% are nerve sheath tumors. Specifically, schwannoma and neurofibroma are more common in adults, while ganglioneuroblastoma and neuroblastoma are more common in children. The mean age at diagnosis is about 5 years for neuroblastoma, 10 years for ganglioneuroblastoma, 20 years for ganglioneuroma, 30 years for neurofibroma, and 40 years for schwannoma.

Neurogenic tumors occurring in the superior mediastinum commonly show a finding termed the "cervicothoracic sign" on plain radiographs. The sign is said to be present if a mediastinal mass shows a sharply marginated border, outlined by lung, above the level of the clavicles. Only posterior mediastinal masses show this finding. Above the level of the clavicles, anterior and middle mediastinal masses enter the neck and are no longer outlined by lung (i.e., they no longer have a sharply marginated border).

Peripheral Nerve Sheath Tumors

Nerve sheath tumors include neurilemmoma (schwannoma), neurofibroma, and neurogenic sarcoma (malignant schwannoma) (Table 8-28). Schwannomas are composed of spindle cells densely packed together (Antoni A pattern) or organized more loosely in association with a myxoid stroma (Antoni B pattern); areas of infarction are common. Neurofibromas are also variable in appearance, consisting of spindle cells, a loose myxoid matrix, neurofibrils, and collagen.

On plain radiographs, nerve sheath tumors typically appear as sharply marginated round, elliptical, or lobulated paravertebral masses, although they may be well seen only on the frontal radiograph (Figs. 8-64, 8-65A,B, 8-66A,B, and 8-67A). They tend to be limited to one or two interspaces in length but in some patients can be large. Associated rib or vertebral deformity or enlargement of a neural foramen is visible in about 50% of cases (see Fig. 8-64). Nerve sheath tumors may also be seen in the middle or anterior mediastinum, occurring in relation to the vagus, phrenic, or recurrent laryngeal nerves, or along the courses of intercostal nerves (Figs. 8-68 to 8-71).

On CT, nerve sheath tumors typically appear as well-marginated, smooth, rounded or elliptical masses (see Figs. 8-65C, 8-66C,D, and 8-67B). Enlargement of neural foramina is better shown on CT than on plain films (see Fig. 8-67B). In over 70% of cases, peripheral nerve or nerve sheath tumors appear to be lower in attenuation than chest wall muscle (see Figs. 8-66C and 8-68A); in the remainder, they are of soft-tissue attenuation. Low-density areas within nerve sheath tumors can be due to the presence of (1) lipid-rich Schwann cells; (2) adipocytes; (3) perineural adipose tissue entrapped by plexiform neurofibromas; or (4) cystic spaces in the tumor. Variable enhancement of the tumor may be seen following contrast infusion; peripheral enhancement is common (Figs. 8-66D and 8-67B). Small areas of calcification are seen in 5% to 10% of cases. Extension into the spinal canal is present in 10% and is best demonstrated with MRI (Fig. 8-67B to D).

Neurofibromas may be associated with von Recklinghausen's disease, which can result in vertebral abnormalities including kyphoscoliosis, scalloped vertebrae, and lateral meningocele. More than one third of patients with

TABLE 8.28 Peripheral Nerve Sheath Tumors

Neurilemmoma (schwannoma), neurofibroma, and neurogenic sarcoma
Most common in adults
Round, elliptical, or lobulated paravertebral mass
Often one or two interspaces in length
Rib or vertebral abnormalities in 50%
Lower attenuation than muscle in 70%
One third of patients with neurofibromas have neurofibromatosis
Plexiform neurofibroma: extensive fusiform or infiltrating mass

FIG. 8.67. Schwannoma. **A:** PA chest radiograph shows a well-defined, rounded retrocardiac mediastinal mass. **B:** CT shows a left paravertebral mass with heterogeneous peripheral enhancement. The mass entends into the left neural foramen (*arrows*), which is enlarged in comparison to the right. **C:** T1-weighted MRI shows extension into the neural foramen (*arrow*) to better advantage. **D:** T2-weighted MRI also shows extension into the neural foramen (*arrow*). The mass has heterogenous signal intensity.

Malignant nerve sheath tumors, termed malignant schwannoma, neurogenic sarcoma, or neurofibrosarcoma, are relatively uncommon but represent up to 15% of nerve sheath tumors. Malignant nerve sheath tumors tend to be large, infiltrating, irregular in contour, and inhomogeneous in attenuation, although these findings are not sufficiently reliable for diagnosis. Both benign and malignant lesions may be symptomatic, rendering attempts at clinical differentiation of limited utility. Calcification and some degree of contrast opacification may be present with either benign or malignant tumors.

Tumors Originating From Sympathetic Ganglia

In children, 80% of posterior mediastinal masses are derived from sympathetic ganglia. Included in this group are ganglioneuroma, ganglioneuroblastoma, and neuroblastoma (Table 8-29).

A

B

C

FIG. 8.68. Extensive (plexiform) neurofibromas in neurofibromatosis. **A:** CT shows multiple neurofibromas (*arrows*) in the subcutaneous tissues, along the courses of mediastinal and intercostal nerves, and in a paravertebral location. The masses appear low in attenuation on CT, measuring 15 HU. Enlargement of the left neural foramen is visible, contiguous with a left paravertebral neurofibroma. **B:** T1-weighted MRI of the lower neck and upper mediastinum shows numerous neurofibromas along the courses of cervical and mediastinal (*arrows*) nerves. **C:** Contrast-enhanced MRI shows irregular enhancement. The centers of some lesions appear low in intensity.

Ganglioneuroma, a benign tumor made up of Schwann cells, collagen, and ganglion cells, is a common neoplasm in teenagers and young adults. On plain radiographs, this tumor often appears as an oblong or sausage-shaped mass in a paravertebral location; it tends to be longer than nerve sheath tumors occurring in a similar location. Ganglioneuroma cannot be distinguished from schwannoma or neurofibroma on the basis of its CT appearance. Calcification is seen in about 20% of cases, and vertebral abnormalities may be seen. On MRI, ganglioneuroma may appear homogenous in intensity on T1-weighted and T2-weighted images or may show a unique whorled appearance of layers of varying intensity.

Approximately 15% of *neuroblastomas* arise in the mediastinum, and almost all are located posteriorly (Fig. 8-72). Mediastinal neuroblastoma is seen almost exclusively in young children under the age of 5 years. It is malignant and may present with a wide variety of signs and symptoms including chest pain, fever, malaise, anemia, Horner's syndrome, and extremity weakness. On CT, neuroblastomas appear as soft-tissue attenuation masses, but up to 40% contain speckled or curvilinear calcifications (see Fig. 8-72C). They are most common in the paravertebral regions and may extend superiorly and inferiorly for several centimeters. Neuroblastoma often shows inhomogeneous enhancement following contrast injection. CT and MR may be used to help determine the presence and extent of mediastinal or vertebral column invasion (see Fig. 8-72D). Invasion of the extradural spinal canal is common, even in the absence of neurologic signs and symptoms. On T2-weighted images, neuroblastoma appears intense (see Fig. 8-72D). MR has the advantage of allowing tumor and surrounding soft tissues to be distinguished more readily than on CT and is more accurate in the recognition of bone marrow involvement. Neuroblastoma may extend

A

B

FIG. 8.69. Neurofibromatosis with paravertebral and intercostal neurofibromas. **A, B:** Multiple paravertebral and intercostal neurofibromas are visible (*arrows*). They appear slightly lower in attenuation than muscle.

from a primary site in the abdomen into the thorax. Most commonly, this occurs by direct invasion through the retrocrural space and into the lower paravertebral regions, often on both sides. In the rare instance of adult neuroblastoma, differentiation from lymphoma may be difficult.

Ganglioneuroblastoma is found in somewhat older children than neuroblastoma and is less common. Ganglioneuroblastomas are regarded by some as partially matured

FIG. 8.70. Plexiform neurofibromas in neurofibromatosis. Mediastinal widening (*large arrows*) reflects the presence of multiple, infiltrative neurofibromas along the courses of mediastinal nerves. Extensive intercostal neurofibromas (*small arrows*) mimic the appearance of pleural thickening.

malignant neuroblastomas and are somewhat intermediate in histology between neuroblastoma and ganglioneuroma. Their imaging characteristics are indistinguishable from neuroblastoma. They can present as either a large, smooth spherical mass or a small, elongated sausage-shaped mass.

Paraganglioma

Paraganglioma (chemodectoma) is a rare tumor originating from neuroectodermal cells located in relation to the autonomic nervous system, especially in the region of the aortopulmonary window (Fig. 8-73) and the posterior mediastinum; it has also been identified within the atria. It accounts for less than 5% of thoracic neurogenic tumors.

Radiographs usually show a well-defined, round or elliptical mass indistinguishable from other neurogenic tumors. It has a predilection for the midthoracic region. On unenhanced CT, paraganglioma has no characteristic features. However, scanning with contrast infusion shows dense enhancement (see Fig. 8-40B).

Patients may be asymptomatic, with the tumor being detected incidentally. About half of patients with paravertebral paraganglioma have symptoms of catecholamine secretion by the tumor or associated tumors in other locations, but catecholamine secretion is rare in patients with aortopulmonary window tumors. Compression of mediastinal structures may also result in symptoms.

Identification of hormonally active lesions has been greatly aided recently by use of 131-I metaiodobenzylguanidine scintigraphy, which localizes catecholamine-producing tumors, including neuroblastoma and neuroendocrine tumor. Octreotide scintigraphy is also useful in localization of these lesions.

FIG. 8.71. Multiple neurofibromas in neurofibromatosis. **A:** CT shows multiple mediastinal and intercostal neurofibromas (*arrows*). **B:** Coronal MRI shows multiple paravertebral neurofibromas.

Approximately 10% of paragangliomas are malignant or invasive. Paravertebral paragangliomas are more easily resectable than aortopulmonary window tumors and have a better prognosis. Local recurrence is common following surgery in patients with aortopulmonary paraganglioma.

ANTERIOR OR LATERAL THORACIC MENINGOCELE

This entity represents anomalous herniation of the spinal meninges through an intervertebral foramen or a defect in the vertebral body. In many patients, this abnormality is associated with neurofibromatosis; most are detected in adults. Meningoceles are described as lateral or anterior, depending on their relationship to the spine. They are slightly more common on the right side.

On chest radiographs, meningoceles commonly result in a sharply marginated paravertebral soft-tissue mass associated with scoliosis or rib and vertebral anomalies at the same level (Fig. 8-74A). When scoliosis is present, meningoceles typically occur at the apex of a convex curve. On CT they appear low in attenuation, as they contain cerebrospinal fluid (see Fig. 8-74B). MRI is diagnostic (see Fig. 8-74C to E), as is filling of the meningocele with contrast on CT myelography.

TABLE 8.29 Tumors Derived from Sympathetic Ganglia

Ganglioneuroma, ganglioneuroblastoma, and neuroblastoma
20% of posterior masses in children
Oblong or sausage-shaped paravertebral mass
Calcification in 20%

EXTRAMEDULLARY HEMATOPOIESIS

Extramedullary hematopoiesis can result in paravertebral masses in patients with severe anemia caused by inadequate production or excessive destruction of blood cells. It can be seen in the presence of thalassemia, hereditary spherocytosis, and sickle cell anemia. These masses are of unknown origin but may arise from herniations of vertebral or rib marrow through small cortical defects, or may arise from lymph nodes or elements of the reticuloendothelial system.

Lobulated paravertebral masses, usually multiple and bilateral and caudad to the sixth thoracic vertebra, are typically seen (Fig. 8-75). They appear well marginated. On CT, the paravertebral masses are of homogeneous soft-tissue attenuation (30 to 65 HU) or may show areas of fat attenuation (−50 HU), which may increase in extent after treatment.

The diagnosis can be suggested by the presence of paravertebral masses in a patient with chronic anemia and skeletal abnormalities visible on radiographs or CT findings suggesting a bone marrow abnormality. Coarsening of the trabecular pattern, rib expansion, and periosteal new bone may be seen. Although not always present, splenomegaly may also be visible.

ABNORMALITIES OF THE THORACIC SPINE

Tumors either primary or malignant, infectious spondylitis, or vertebral fracture with associated hemorrhage can produce a paravertebral mass. Frequently, the abnormality is bilateral and fusiform, allowing it to be distinguished from solitary masses such as a neurogenic tumor. Associated abnormalities of the vertebral bodies or discs assist in diagnosis and should be sought.

FIG. 8.72. Mediastinal neuroblastoma in a 16-month-old child. PA (**A**) and lateral (**B**) chest radio-graphs show a large superior, posterior mediastinal mass. **C:** CT shows a large paravertebral, posterior mediastinal mass containing small areas of calcification (*arrows*). **D:** T2-weighted MRI shows a large mass in the posterior mediastinum. The tumor extends into the spinal canal through a neural foramen (*white arrow*), displacing the spinal cord to the right (*black arrow*).

FIG. 8.73. Paraganglioma (chemodectoma). Chest radiograph shows a mass (*arrows*) in the aortopulmonary window.

A

B

C

D

FIG. 8.74. Lateral thoracic meningocele in neurofibromatosis. **A:** PA chest radiograph shows large right and small left mediastinal masses (*arrows*). Scoliosis and rib deformities are present. **B:** CT shows the large right and small left mediastinal masses. They are low in attenuation. The vertebral body is abnormal in appearance and the neural foramina (*arrows*) are enlarged. **C:** Coronal MRI shows the right and left meningoceles (*arrows*) and associated scoliosis. **D:** T1-weighted MRI shows low intensity typical of fluid. **E:** T2-weighted MRI shows high intensity.

E

FIG. 8.75. Extrathoracic hematopoiesis. CT in a patient with thalassemia major. Paravertebral masses (*arrows*) reflect hematopoietic tissue. Ribs and vertebral bodies are expanded and show an abnormal trabecular pattern, typical of severe anemia.

SELECTED READING

Agrons GA, Rosado-de-Christenson ML, Kirejczyk WM, et al. Pulmonary inflammatory pseudotumor: radiologic features. Radiology 1998; 206:511–518.

Ahn JM, Lee KS, Goo JM, et al. Predicting the histology of anterior mediastinal masses: comparison of chest radiography and CT. J Thorac Imaging 1996; 11:265–271.

Armstrong EA, Harwood-Nash DCF, Ritz CR, et al. CT of neuroblastomas and ganglioneuromas in children. AJR Am J Roentgenol 1982; 139:571–576.

Balthazar EJ, Naidich DP, Megibow AJ, et al. CT evaluation of esophageal varices. AJR Am J Roentgenol 1987; 148:131–135.

Bashist B, Ellis K, Gold RP. Computed tomography of intrathoracic goiters. AJR Am J Roentgenol 1983; 140:455–460.

Bourgouin PM, Shepard JO, Moore EH, et al. Plexiform neurofibromatosis of the mediastinum: CT appearance. AJR Am J Roentgenol 1988; 151:461–463.

Bragg DG, Chor PJ, Murray KA, et al. Lymphoproliferative disorders of the lung: histopathology, clinical manifestations, and imaging features. AJR Am J Roentgenol 1994; 163:273–281.

Brown LR, Aughenbaugh GL. Masses of the anterior mediastinum: CT and MR imaging. AJR Am J Roentgenol 1991; 157:1171–1180.

Cakir O, Topal U, Bayram AS, Tolunay S. Sarcomas: rare primary malignant tumors of the thorax. Diagn Interv Radiol 2005; 11:23–27.

Castellino RA, Blank N, Hoppe RT, Cho C. Hodgkin disease: contributions of chest CT in the initial staging evaluation. Radiology 1986; 160:603–605.

Castellino RA, Hilton S, O'Brien JP, Portlock CS. Non-Hodgkin lymphoma: contribution of chest CT in the initial staging evaluation. Radiology 1996; 199:129–132.

Cohen LA, Schwartz AM, Rockoff SD. Benign schwannomas: pathologic basis for CT inhomogeneities. AJR Am J Roentgenol 1986; 147:141–143.

de Geer G, Webb WR, Gamsu G. Normal thymus: assessment with MR and CT. Radiology 1986; 158:313–317.

Detterbeck FC, Boffa DJ, Tanoue LT. The new lung cancer staging system. Chest 2009; 136:260–271.

Do YS, Im JG, Lee BH, et al. CT findings in malignant tumors of thymic epithelium. J Comput Assist Tomogr 1995; 19:192–197.

Drucker EA, McLoud TC, Dedrick CG, et al. Mediastinal paraganglioma: radiologic evaluation of an unusual vascular tumor. AJR Am J Roentgenol 1987; 148:521–522.

Filly R, Blank N, Castellino R. Radiographic distribution of intrathoracic disease in previously untreated patients with Hodgkin's disease and non-Hodgkin's lymphoma. Radiology 1976; 120:277.

Fitch SJ, Tonkin ILD, Tonkin AK. Imaging of foregut duplication cysts. Radiographics 1986; 6:189–201.

Freundlich IM, McGavran MH. Abnormalities of the thymus. J Thorac Imaging 1996; 58–65.

Gal AA, Kornstein MJ, Cohen C, et al. Neuroendocrine tumors of the thymus: a clinicopathological and prognostic study. Ann Thorac Surg 2001; 72:1179–1182.

Glazer GM, Gross BH, Quint LE, et al. Normal mediastinal lymph nodes: number and size according to American Thoracic Society mapping. AJR Am J Roentgenol 1985; 144:261–265.

Glazer HS, Molina PL, Siege MJ, Sagel SS. Pictorial essay. Low-attenuation mediastinal masses on CT. AJR Am J Roentgenol 1989; 152:1173–1177.

Glazer HS, Siege MJ, Sagel SS. Pictorial essay. High-attenuation mediastinal masses on unenhanced CT. AJR Am J Roentgenol 1991; 156:45–50.

Glazer HS, Wick MR, Anderson DJ, et al. CT of fatty thoracic masses. AJR Am J Roentgenol 1992; 159:1181–1187.

Hoeffel C, Floquet J, Regent D, et al. Periesophageal mediastinal fibromatosis. Abdom Imaging 2000; 25:235–238.

Hoffman OA, Gillespie DJ, Aughenbaugh GL, Brown LR. Primary mediastinal neoplasms (other than thymoma). Mayo Clin Proc 1993; 68:880–891.

Jolles H, Henry DA, Roberson JP, et al. Mediastinitis following median sternotomy: CT findings. Radiology 1996; 201:463–466.

Kang YS, Rosen K, Clark OH, Higgins CB. Localization of abnormal parathyroid glands of the mediastinum with MR imaging. Radiology 1993; 189:137–141.

Kawashima A, Fishman EK, Kuhlman JE, Nixon MS. CT of posterior mediastinal masses. Radiographics 1991; 11:1045–1067.

Kim DJ, Yang WI, Choi SS, et al. Prognostic and clinical relevance of the world health organization schema for the classification of thymic epithelial tumors: a clinicopathologic study of 108 patients and literature review. Chest 2005; 127:755–761.

Kirchner SG, Heller RM, Smith CW. Pancreatic pseudocyst of the mediastinum. Radiology 1977; 123:37–42.

Kirks DR, McCormick VD, Greenspan RH. Pulmonary sarcoidosis: roentgenographic analysis of 150 patients. AJR Am J Roentgenol 1973; 117:777–786.

Kirsch CFE, Webb EM, Webb WR. Multicentric Castleman's disease and POEMS syndrome: CT findings. J Thorac Imaging 1997; 12:75–77.

Kiyono K, Sone S, Sakai F, et al. The number and size of normal mediastinal lymph nodes: a postmortem study. AJR Am J Roentgenol 1988; 150:771–776.

Kushihashi T, Munechika H, Motoya H, et al. CT and MR findings in tuberculous mediastinitis. J Comput Assist Tomogr 1995; 19:379–382.

Lee KS, Im JG, Han CH, et al. Malignant primary germ cell tumors of the mediastinum: CT features. AJR Am J Roentgenol 1989; 153:947–951.

Long JA, Doppman JL, Nienhuis AW. Computed tomographic studies of thoracic extramedullary hematopoiesis. J Comput Assist Tomogr 1980; 4:67–70.

McAdams HP, Rosado de Christenson ML, Moran CA. Mediastinal hemangioma: radiographic and CT features in 4 patients. Radiology 1994; 193:399–402.

McLoud TC, Kalisher L, Stark P, Greene R. Intrathoracic lymph node metastases from extrathoracic neoplasms. AJR Am J Roentgenol 1978; 131:403–407.

Miyake H, Shiga M, Takaki H, et al. Mediastinal lymphangiomas in adults: CT findings. J Thorac Imaging 1996; 11:83–85.

Moeller KH, Rosado-de-Christenson ML, Templeton PA. Mediastinal mature teratoma: imaging features. AJR Am J Roentgenol 1997; 169:985–990.

Moon WK, Im JG, In KY, et al. Mediastinal tuberculous lymphandenitis: MR imaging appearance with clinicopathologic correlation. AJR Am J Roentgenol 1996; 166:21–25.

Moon WK, Im JG, Kim JS, et al. Mediastinal Castleman's disease: CT findings. J Comput Assist Tomogr 1994; 18:43–46.

Mountain CF, Dresler CM. Regional lymph node classification for lung cancer staging. Chest 1997; 111:1718–1723.

Müller NL, Webb WR, Gamsu G. Paratracheal lymphadenopathy: radiographic findings and correlation with CT. Radiology 1985; 156:761–765.

Müller NL, Webb WR, Gamsu G. Subcarinal lymph node enlargement: Radiographic findings and CT correlation. AJR Am J Roentgenol 1985; 145:15–19.

Nicolaou S, Müller NL, Li DK, Oger JJ. Thymus in myasthenia gravis: comparison of CT and pathologic findings and clinical outcome after thymectomy. Radiology 1996; 20:471–474.

Okumura M, Ohta M, Tateyama H, et al. The World Health Organization histologic classification system reflects the oncologic behavior of thymoma: a clinical study of 273 patients. Cancer 2002; 94:624–632.

Patil SN, Levin DL. Distribution of thoracic lymphadenopathy in sarcoidosis using computed tomography. J Thorac Imaging 1999; 14:114–117.

Rami-Porta R, Crowley JJ, Goldstraw P. The revised TNM staging system for lung cancer. Ann Thorac Cardiovasc Surg 2009; 15:4–9.

Reed JC, Hallet KK, Feigin DS. Neural tumors of the thorax: subject review from the AFIP. Radiology 1978; 126:9–17.

Reed JC, Sobonya RE. Morphologic analysis of foregut cysts in the thorax. AJR Am J Roentgenol 1974; 120:851–860.

Rosado de Christenson ML, Pugatch RD, Moran CA, Galobardes J. Thymolipoma: analysis of 27 cases. Radiology 1994; 193:121–126.

Rosado de Christenson ML, Templeton PA, Moran CA. Mediastinal germ-cell tumors: radiologic and pathologic correlation. Radiographics 1992; 12:1013–1030.

Rossi SE, McAdams HP, Rosado-de-Christenson ML, et al. Fibrosing mediastinitis. Radiographics 2001; 21:737–757.

Sakai F, Sone S, Kiyono K, et al. Intrathoracic neurogenic tumors: MR-pathologic correlation. AJR Am J Roentgenol 1992; 159:279–283.

Sherrick AD, Brown LR, Harms GF, Myers JL. Radiographic findings of fibrosing mediastinitis. Chest 1994; 106:484–489.

Spector JA, Willis DN, Ginsburg HB. Paraganglioma (pheochromocytoma) of the posterior mediastinum: a case report and review of the literature. J Pediatr Surg 2003; 38:1114–1116.

Strollo DC, Rosado-de-Christenson ML. Primary mediastinal malignant germ cell neoplasms: imaging features. Chest Surg Clin N Am 2002; 12:645–658.

Tomiyama N, Johkoh T, Mihara N, et al. Using the World Health Organization Classification of thymic epithelial neoplasms to describe CT findings. AJR Am J Roentgenol 2002; 179:881–886.

Solitary and Multiple Nodules, Masses, Cavities, and Cysts

W. RICHARD WEBB

The radiographic assessment of patients with solitary or multiple lung nodules, masses, or cavities is a common clinical problem. A primary or metastatic tumor usually is the first consideration in patients with these findings. However, many other diseases or abnormalities may present with focal lung abnormalities. Some have specific appearances that may suggest the correct diagnosis or limit the differential diagnosis.

THE SOLITARY PULMONARY NODULE

A solitary pulmonary nodule (SPN) usually is defined as a focal opacity, visible on chest radiographs or computed tomography (CT), which fits the following criteria:

1. It is relatively well-defined.
2. It is surrounded, at least partially, by lung.
3. It is roughly spherical in shape.
4. It is 3 cm or less in diameter (Fig. 9-1).

Lesions larger than 3 cm in diameter usually are referred to using the term "mass." This cutoff also is used to distinguish a T1 carcinoma (3 cm or less in diameter) from a T2 carcinoma (more than 3 cm).

Clinical Evaluation

Clinical and historical information is helpful in the differential diagnosis of a solitary lung nodule. Important considerations that increase the likelihood of cancer include a history of smoking, age over 40, occupational exposures (e.g., asbestos), lung fibrosis, coexisting chronic obstructive pulmonary disease (COPD) and emphysema, and a family history of lung cancer. Risk factors for cancer are reviewed in Chapter 3.

Recent travel history, a positive skin test for tuberculosis (TB) or fungus, or the presence of other diseases (e.g., rheumatoid arthritis) increases the likelihood of a benign SPN. In a patient younger than 30 years of age, cancer is very uncommon as a cause of SPN.

An SPN found in a patient with a history of extrathoracic malignancy may be a metastasis, a primary lung carcinoma, or an insignificant benign lesion. Certain tumors have a propensity to metastasize as SPNs. Among patients with an SPN, those with a history of melanoma, sarcoma, or testicular carcinoma are more than twice as likely to have a solitary metastasis than a bronchogenic carcinoma. On the other hand, patients with an SPN who have a history of carcinoma of the head and neck, bladder, breast, cervix, bile ducts, esophagus, ovary, prostate, or stomach are more than three times as likely to have primary bronchogenic carcinoma than lung metastasis. In patients with other types of tumors, the relative likelihood of metastasis and lung cancer is about equal.

Radiographic Evaluation

The differential diagnosis of an SPN is extensive (Table 9-1). In patients with an SPN, plain films and CT are used to determine the nodule's (1) morphologic characteristics, (2) density or attenuation (i.e., calcium, fat, or contrast enhancement), and (3) growth rate.

Morphologic Characteristics

Using plain radiographs or CT, an SPN sometimes may be diagnosed as a specific lesion based on its appearance. Some such lesions include mucous plug, arteriovenous fistula, rounded atelectasis, mycetoma, and focal pleural lesions. These are described later in this chapter.

Much more often, radiographic studies are used to assess less specific morphologic characteristics that suggest that an SPN is likely malignant or likely benign.

Size

The likelihood of malignancy in a nodule or mass is directly related to its size (Table 9-2). The likelihood of cancer is about 35% for a nodule ranging from 0.5 to 1.0 cm in diameter, 50% for an SPN 1.0 to 2.0 cm in diameter, and more than 85% for an SPN more than 2.0 cm in diameter (see Fig. 9-1). It should be kept in mind, however, that even a very small lesion can represent a carcinoma.

One or more small lung nodules are exceedingly common as an incidental finding on CT scans, and the large majority represent benign lesions such as granuloma or

A   B

FIG. 9.1. Right upper lobe nodule representing an adenocarcinoma. **A:** Chest radiograph shows a right upper lobe nodule (*arrow*). This lesion is classified as a nodule because it is relatively well-defined, at least partially surrounded by lung, roughly spherical in shape, and 3 cm or less in diameter. Because the nodule exceeds 2 cm in diameter, it is very likely malignant. **B:** CT shows the edge of the nodule to be ill defined and lobulated, and a pleural tail (*arrow*) extends to the pleural surface.

TABLE 9.1 Differential Diagnosis of an SPN or Mass

Congenital Lesions and Normal Variants
Arteriovenous fistula
Bronchogenic cyst
Congenital cystic adenomatoid malformation
Intrapulmonary lymph node
Mucoid impaction (bronchial atresia)
Pulmonary vein varix
Sequestration

Malignant Neoplasms
Carcinoma
Lymphoma
Lymphoproliferative disease
Metastatic neoplasm
Sarcoma (e.g., chondrosarcoma, liposarcoma, fibrosarcoma)

Benign Neoplasms and Neoplasm-like Conditions
Endometrioma
Hamartoma
Lymphoproliferative disease
Miscellaneous benign tumors
   Mesenchymal tumors (e.g., chondroma, lipoma, fibroma)
   Epithelial tumors (e.g., atypical adenomatous
     hyperplasia, mucous gland adenoma)
   Vascular tumors

Infection and Parasites
Aspergillosis, angioinvasive
Dirofilaria immitis (dog heartworm)
Echinococcus
Focal (round) pneumonia
Granulomatous infection or granuloma
   Tuberculosis
   Nontuberculous mycobacteria (e.g., *Mycobacterium
    avium-intracellulare* complex)
   Coccidioidomycosis

   Histoplasmosis
   Cryptococcus
Lung abscess
Mycetoma (aspergilloma)
Pulmonary gangrene
Septic embolism

Inflammatory (Noninfectious)
Churg-Strauss syndrome
Focal organizing pneumonia
Rheumatoid nodule
Sarcoidosis
Wegener's granulomatosis

Airways and Inhalational Disease
Mucoid impaction (mucous plug)
   Asthma
   Allergic bronchopulmonary aspergillosis
   Bronchial atresia
   Bronchiectasis
   Cystic fibrosis
Conglomerate mass or progressive massive fibrosis
   (e.g., silicosis)
Lipoid pneumonia

Vascular Lesions
Arteriovenous fistula
Hematoma
Infarction
Pulmonary artery aneurysm
Pulmonary vein varix
Septic embolism

Idiopathic and Miscellaneous
Amyloidosis
Fluid-filled bulla
Round atelectasis

TABLE 9.2 Likelihood of Malignancy Related to Nodule Diameter

Diameter (cm)	Malignancy Rate (%)
<1	35
1–2	50
2–3	80
>3	97

intrapulmonary lymph node. Follow-up CT is the only practical method of evaluating their significance.

Location

About two thirds of lung cancers occur in the upper lobes, and the right upper lobe is most commonly involved (see Fig. 9-1). Sixty percent of cancers presenting as an SPN on chest radiographs are seen in the lung periphery; only 10% are visible in the medial third of the lung.

A metastatic tumor presenting as an SPN tends to be located in the subpleural or outer third of the lung. Two thirds of metastatic lesions occur in the lower lobes.

Edge Appearance

Although plain radiographs do not allow the edge of a lung nodule or mass to be assessed with the precision of CT, cancers can appear to be ill defined, irregular in contour, spiculated, or lobulated on plain films (see Fig. 9-1).

FIG. 9.2. Adenocarcinoma with a spiculated margin seen on CT. Two pleural tails (*arrows*) extend to the pleural surface. This appearance has been termed *corona radiata* or *corona maligna*. The surface of the nodule is lobulated and shows notches, both of which are findings indicating malignancy. Several lucencies within the nodule represent air bronchograms of areas of pseudocavitation, typical findings in adenocarcinoma and BAC.

FIG. 9.3. Smooth, sharply marginated, rounded nodule representing a granuloma. Its appearance (*arrow*) is typical of a benign lesion. Its small size also makes malignancy less likely.

On CT, malignant nodules are much more likely to have an ill-defined, irregular, lobulated, or spiculated margin (see Figs. 9-1B and 9-2). Benign lesions tend to have a smooth, sharply defined edge (Figs. 9-3 and 9-4; Table 9-3). Nearly 90% of nodules with an irregular or spiculated edge are malignant; only 20% of nodules with a smooth, sharp margin are malignant. Malignancies that tend to have a sharp and smooth edge include metastases (Fig. 9-5) and carcinoid tumors (see Fig. 3-44 in Chapter 3).

The terms *corona radiate* and *corona maligna* have been used to describe the appearance of spiculation associated with a nodule or mass (see Figs. 9-2 and 9-6). Particularly in patients with adenocarcinoma and bronchioloalveolar carcinoma (BAC), this appearance reflects the presence of fibrosis surrounding the tumor, although tumor invasion of the adjacent lung also may be present. The fibrosis usually reflects a desmoplastic reaction rather than preexisting lung fibrosis. Spiculation is less common with large cell carcinoma than other cell types that present as a solitary nodule or mass.

In addition, carcinomas can show the presence of a *pleural tail sign*, in which a thin linear opacity is seen extending from the edge of a lung nodule to the pleural surface (see Figs. 9-1B, 9-2, and 9-6). This tail, which can be from a few millimeters to a few centimeters in length, often is seen in association with spiculation. As with spiculation, it reflects the presence of fibrosis and often is associated with a dimpling of the visceral pleura. In patients with lung cancer, a pleural tail sign most often is associated with adenocarcinoma or BAC; it uncommonly indicates the presence of a large cell carcinoma. The pleural tail sign also can be seen in

A   B

FIG. 9.4. Hamartoma presenting as a sharply defined, round nodule. **A:** Chest radiograph shows a round nodule (*arrows*) in the right upper lobe. **B:** CT shows the nodule (*arrow*) to be rounded in shape and sharply marginated. Slight lobulation may be seen with hamartomas.

association with benign lung nodules, which are associated with fibrosis, including various granulomatous diseases. The presence of a spiculated contour is more suggestive of malignancy than a pleural tail.

The *halo sign*, a halo of ground-glass opacity surrounding a lung nodule, may be seen in some patients with an SPN. It is commonly present in leukemic patients with angioinvasive aspergillosis (Fig. 9-7) but also can be seen in patients with other infections (see Fig. 9-35C) and in some tumors, particularly adenocarcinoma or BAC (Fig. 9-8; Table 9-4). The histologic nature of the halo varies with the disease. In patients with invasive aspergillosis, the halo sign represents hemorrhage; in patients with carcinoma, it reflects the presence of lepidic spread of tumor.

TABLE 9.3 Edge Appearances and Common Diagnoses

Sharply marginated
Granuloma
Hamartoma or benign tumor
Carcinoid tumor
Metastasis
Spiculated (corona radiata) or pleural tail
Bronchioloalveolar carcinoma
Carcinoma
Granuloma or focal scarring

FIG. 9.5. Solitary metastasis from a head and neck carcinoma. A left upper lobe nodule (*arrow*) is smooth and sharply defined on CT. This appearance is common with metastases.

FIG. 9.6. Adenocarcinoma. HRCT shows an irregular, spiculated nodule with multiple pleural tails. Air bronchograms are visible within the nodule.

Shape

Lung carcinomas tend to be irregular in shape, lobulated, or notched (see Figs. 9-1, 9-2, and 9-6) but uncommonly have concave margins. Granulomas often are round (see

FIG. 9.7. Halo sign in invasive aspergillosis. HRCT in a young patient with leukemia and granulocytopenia shows a dense left lower lobe nodule surrounded by a halo (*arrows*) of ground-glass opacity. In patients with invasive aspergillosis, the halo represents hemorrhage surrounding a septic infarction.

FIG. 9.8. Halo sign in BAC. HRCT shows a dense central nodule surrounded by a halo (*arrows*). In BAC, the halo represents the presence of lepidic tumor growth.

Fig. 9-3). Hamartomas and metastases may be round, oval, or lobulated (see Figs. 9-4 and 9-5). Scars or areas of atelectasis or scarring may appear linear or angular. A number of other benign lesions (e.g., AVM, mucous plugs) may be identified by their characteristic shapes.

Air Bronchograms and Pseudocavitation

On HRCT, air bronchograms commonly are seen in cancers presenting as an SPN (25% to 65% of cases; see Figs. 9-2 and 9-6). This finding is most typical of adenocarcinoma or BAC. Air bronchograms are much less common in benign lesions but have a variety of causes, such as focal pneumonia, infarction, round atelectasis, or conglomerate masses in patients with silicosis or sarcoidosis (Table 9-5). An appearance mimicking the presence of air bronchograms may be seen in patients with developing mycetoma; the apparent air bronchograms

TABLE 9.4   Causes of the Halo Sign

Fungi: invasive aspergillosis, candidiasis, coccidioidomycosis
Bacteria: tuberculosis, *Nocardia, Legionella*
Viruses: cytomegalovirus, herpes
Pneumocystis jiroveci (*P. carinii*)
Organizing pneumonia
Wegener's granulomatosis
Infarct
Metastatic tumor
Kaposi's sarcoma
Bronchioloalveolar carcinoma
Adenocarcinoma

TABLE 9.5 Causes of Air Bronchograms in SPNs

Adenocarcinoma
Bronchioloalveolar carcinoma
Conglomerate mass (e.g., silicosis, sarcoidosis)
Focal pneumonia
Infarction
Rounded atelectasis
Bronchiolitis obliterans with organizing pneumonia
Lymphoma
Lymphoproliferative diseases
Mycetoma (may mimic an air bronchogram)

represent air-filled spaces between fronds of fungus. Small bronchi seen in relation to lung cancers often appear abnormal, being narrowed, obstructed, or irregular in contour.

In addition to air bronchograms, small bubbly lucencies may be seen in cancers (see Fig. 9-2). These may represent air bronchograms, small air-filled cystic areas in the tumor (so-called pseudocavitation), or small cavities. They have the same significance as air bronchograms.

Cavitation

By general agreement, a cyst is an air-filled lesion that has a smooth and uniform wall 3 mm or less in thickness. The term *cavity* usually is used to describe a lesion with a thicker or more irregular wall or a lesion that has *cavitated* (i.e., evolved by developing an air-filled space, regardless of how thick the wall is). Thus, a thin-walled lesion may be either a cyst or a cavity, whereas a thick-walled or irregular lesion is a cavity. An exception to this rule is an infected cyst: surrounding lung inflammation may result in a thick "wall."

Cavitation occurs in about 10% of cancers, most commonly in patients with squamous cell carcinoma (Fig. 9-9A and B; see also Figs. 3-4 and 3-26 in Chapter 3). Approximately 80% of cavitary lung cancers are squamous cell carcinomas. Cavitation of large cell carcinoma and adenocarcinoma also occurs (see Fig. 9-9C); small cell carcinoma rarely cavitates.

Although a long list of abnormalities may be associated with cysts or cavities, described in Table 9-6 and in detail below, for practical purposes, radiographic evaluation is directed at determining the likelihood of malignancy. Cavitary malignant lesions tend to have a thick, nodular wall (see Fig. 9-9B and C; see also Figs. 3-4 and 3-26 in Chapter 3); benign lesions often have a thin, smooth wall (Fig. 9-10). The thickness of the wall of a cavity serves as an indicator of its likelihood of being malignant. Nearly 85% of cavities with a wall measuring more than 15 mm in its thickest portion are malignant (see Fig. 9-9B). If the thickest part of the wall is less than 5 mm, 95% are benign (see Fig. 9-10). Seventy-five

A

B

C

FIG. 9.9. Cavitary carcinoma. **A:** Plain radiograph showing a cavitary left lung mass that represents a squamous cell carcinoma. **B:** Cavitary squamous cell carcinoma shown at two levels. The wall of the cavity is irregular, with several thick nodular regions (*white arrow*). The cavity contains an air-fluid level (*black arrows*). This is uncommon in malignancy and may represent hemorrhage or infection. **C:** Cavitary adenocarcinoma shown on HRCT in six contiguous scans. The nodule contains an irregular cavity; is irregular and lobulated in shape, notched, and spiculated; and is associated with pleural tails. It also contains several air bronchograms.

TABLE 9.6 Causes of a Cyst or Cavity (Solitary or Multiple)

Amyloidosis—solitary or multiple
Aspergillosis, angioinvasive—usually multiple
Aspergillosis, semi-invasive—usually solitary
Bronchogenic cyst—usually single
Bulla—solitary or multiple
Carcinoma
Congenital cystic adenomatoid malformation—solitary, but often multiloculated
Conglomerate mass or progressive massive fibrosis—often bilateral
Cystic bronchiectasis—usually multiple
Cystic lung disease (e.g., histiocytosis, lymphangiomyomatosis)—multiple
Echinococcus—solitary or multiple
Endometrioma
Granulomatous infection
  Tuberculosis
  Nontuberculous mycobacteria (e.g., *Mycobacterium avium-intracellulare* complex)
  Coccidioidomycosis
  Histoplasmosis
  Cryptococcus
Hematoma—solitary or multiple
Intralobar sequestration—may be lucent, cystic, or multicystic
Lung abscess—solitary or multiple
Lymphoma—solitary or multiple
Metastatic neoplasm—usually multiple
Mycetoma—aspergilloma
Papillomatosis—usually multiple
Paragonimiasis—usually multiple
Pneumatocele—solitary or multiple
Pulmonary gangrene—usually solitary
Pulmonary laceration—traumatic
Rheumatoid nodule—usually multiple
Sarcoidosis—usually multiple
Sarcoma—solitary
Septic embolism—usually multiple
Wegener's granulomatosis—usually multiple

FIG. 9.10. CT scan of a lung abscess. The wall is thin and smooth, measuring less than 5 mm in thickness. An air-fluid level is visible.

percent of cavities with a wall 5 to 15 mm in thickness are benign. If the thickest part of the cavity wall measures 1 mm or less, malignancy is rare. However, thin-walled cystic lesions may rarely be seen with BAC or metastases.

Lung cancer resulting in bronchial obstruction also can be associated with an abscess in the distal lung, mimicking a cavitary carcinoma. In addition, lung cancer sometimes can arise in a bulla or cyst or be associated with a preexisting cavity. In such a case, focal thickening of the cyst or cavity wall or fluid within the cyst may be the only findings suggesting this diagnosis.

Air-crescent Sign

In some patients with a cavitary nodule or lung cyst, a mass or nodule may be present within the cavity. Air outlining or capping the superior aspect of the mass results in a crescent-shaped collection of air, termed the "air-crescent" sign. The most likely cause of this appearance is aspergilloma (mycetoma), but the differential diagnosis includes other entities as well (Table 9-7). Gravitational shift of the intracavity mass strongly suggests mycetoma and excludes carcinoma.

Air-fluid Level

The presence of an air-fluid level in a patient with a cavitary SPN tends to indicate a benign lesion, particularly lung abscess (see Fig. 9-10). Any infected cystic or cavitary lesion may be associated with an air-fluid level. An air-fluid level is

TABLE 9.7 Causes of the Air-crescent Sign

Aspergilloma (mycetoma)
Angioinvasive aspergillosis with septic infarction
Carcinoma arising in a cyst
Cavitary carcinoma
Clot in a cyst or cavity
Echinococcus
Mucous plug in cystic bronchiectasis
Papillomatosis
Pulmonary gangrene
Rasmussen aneurysm (mycotic pulmonary artery aneurysm in a tubercular cavity)

FIG. 9.11. Tuberculosis. A right upper lobe nodule is associated with satellites (*arrows*). This appearance is most typical of a benign process but sometimes is seen with carcinoma.

FIG. 9.12. Metastatic nasopharyngeal carcinoma. Multiple nodules (*arrows*) are associated with a feeding vessel.

uncommon in a cavitary carcinoma but may be seen in the presence of hemorrhage or superinfection (see Fig. 9-9B).

Satellite Nodules

Satellite nodules are small nodules seen adjacent to a larger nodule or mass. They tend to predict a benign lesion (Fig. 9-11). Satellites are most common with granulomatous diseases and infections such as TB (Table 9-8). Only a small percentage of carcinomas are associated with satellite nodules. In patients with sarcoidosis, the presence of satellite nodules has been termed the "galaxy" sign.

Feeding Vessel Sign

The "feeding vessel" sign is present if a small pulmonary artery is seen leading directly to a nodule (Fig. 9-12). This appearance is most common with metastasis, infarct, and arteriovenous fistula. It is less common with primary lung carcinomas or benign lesions such as granuloma.

Attenuation

A lung nodule usually is examined using volumetric HRCT to determine its attenuation before contrast injection. Because of volume averaging, unless an SPN is grossly calcified, CT with thick collimation (5 mm) usually cannot be used to determine its attenuation accurately. Most cancers appear to be of soft tissue attenuation.

Ground-glass Opacity

With thin collimation, some nodules appear to be of ground-glass opacity. Many focal opacities of ground-glass opacity are inflammatory and resolve on follow-up. However, BAC may present as a nodule entirely of ground-glass opacity, and a high degree of suspicion should be maintained (Fig. 9-13). Follow-up of such a lesion is appropriate.

Calcification or High Attenuation

The presence of calcium in an SPN increases its chances of being benign (Table 9-9). Diagnosing a small nodule as calcified on chest radiographs is somewhat subjective and subject to error. However, if a nodule a few millimeters in diameter is easily seen on radiographs, it probably is calcified.

TABLE 9.8	**Causes of Satellite Nodules**

Tuberculosis
Nontuberculous mycobacterial infection
Bacterial infections with endobronchial spread
Fungal infections
Sarcoid
Conglomerate masses (silicosis, coal worker's
 pneumoconiosis, talcosis)
Bronchioloalveolar carcinoma
Adenocarcinoma

FIG. 9.13. Bronchioloalveolar carcinoma. A spiculated nodule (*arrows*) is visible on CT with 3-mm slice thickness. The nodule is of ground-glass opacity. This appearance may be seen with BAC.

CT is more sensitive and accurate in diagnosing calcification. Volumetric HRCT images usually should be obtained through a lung nodule to look for calcium. HRCT demonstrates calcification in about 25% of benign SPNs that do not appear calcified on plain radiographs.

The pattern of calcification is important in determining its diagnostic significance. Generally, the following four patterns of calcification can be used to predict the presence of a benign lesion with sufficient accuracy to allow appropriate management (Fig. 9-14):

TABLE 9.9 Causes of Calcification or High Attenuation in an SPN

Amyloidosis—dense or stippled
Carcinoid tumor—punctuate, eccentric
Carcinoma—punctuate, eccentric
Conglomerate mass—multiple foci
Dirofilaria immitis
Granuloma—diffuse, central, concentric
Hamartoma or chondroma—popcorn, central
Mucoid impaction in allergic bronchopulmonary aspergillosis or bronchial atresia
Metastases—diffuse, punctuate
Talcosis—secondary to talc not calcium
Amiodarone toxicity—due to iodine content

FIG. 9.14. Benign patterns of calcification. With rare exceptions, these indicate the presence of a benign lesion.

1. Homogeneous calcification (Fig. 9-15)
2. Dense central (bull's-eye) calcification (Fig. 9-16)
3. Concentric rings of calcium ("target" calcification; Fig. 9-17)
4. Conglomerate foci of calcification involving a large part of the nodule ("popcorn" calcification; Fig. 9-18)

A

B

FIG. 9.15. Homogeneous calcification. Dense and uniform calcification of a small right upper lobe nodule (*arrow*) is typical of a benign lesion, usually a tuberculoma.

FIG. 9.16. Dense central or "bull's-eye" calcification in a hamartoma. A round lung nodule (*arrows*) adjacent to the descending aorta shows dense central calcification. This is typical of histoplasmoma or hamartoma.

FIG. 9.18. Multiple confluent nodular foci of calcification ("popcorn" calcification; *arrow*) in a hamartoma. This appearance is typical of hamartoma and corresponds to the calcification of cartilage nodules.

The first three of these patterns are most typical of granulomas; the last is more typical of hamartoma. Calcified lesions thought to be benign should be followed up radiographically in most cases unless the calcification is diffuse.

Stippled calcification or eccentric foci of calcification (Figs. 9-19 and 9-20) may be seen in benign SPNs but are visible in as many as 10% to 15% of cancers; these patterns must be considered indeterminate (see Fig. 9-19).

Calcium in a tumor may reflect dystrophic calcification (occurring in areas of tumor necrosis), engulfing of a preexisting granuloma, or calcification of the tumor itself (as in mucinous adenocarcinoma, carcinoid tumor, or osteogenic sarcoma). A "benign" pattern of calcification occasionally is seen in patients with neoplasm. Carcinoid tumor and mucinous adenocarcinoma can show dense central calcification. Metastases from osteogenic sarcoma or chondrosarcoma can show homogenous calcification, but a history of the primary tumor allows a correct diagnosis.

Because of the high likelihood of cancer in patients with spiculated nodules or nodules exceeding 2 cm in diameter, it is inadvisable to call such a nodule benign on the basis of visible calcification, unless the calcification is diffuse and dense. A small central calcification is insufficient for determining whether such a nodule is benign.

Usually, a visible inspection of HRCT scans is sufficient for diagnosing calcification. However, the measurement of

FIG. 9.17. Concentric or "target" calcification (*arrow*). One or more rings of calcium may be seen. This pattern is typical of a histoplasmoma.

SMALL FLECKS   ECCENTRIC

FIG. 9.19. Indeterminate patterns of calcification. These may be seen in benign or malignant lesions.

FIG. 9.20. Eccentric calcification in an adenocarcinoma. A lobulated mass shows a small focus of eccentric calcification (*arrow*).

CT numbers can allow the detection of calcification, which is not clearly seen on the scans. This technique is termed *CT nodule densitometry*. Pixels denser than 100 HU indicate the presence of calcification.

High attenuation of a nodule or mass sometimes is seen using CT in patients who do not have calcification. This may be seen in patients with amiodarone toxicity resulting in focal organizing pneumonia: the drug contains iodine, which appears dense. Patients with conglomerate masses from talcosis may show high attenuation due to the talc.

Fat

The presence of fat in an SPN may be diagnosed accurately only on HRCT. On HRCT, fat can be accurately diagnosed if low CT numbers are seen (−40 to −120 HU). This most likely indicates the presence of hamartoma (see Figs. 3-49 and 3-51 in Chapter 3), lipoma, or lipoid pneumonia (see Figs. 20-1 and 20-2 in Chapter 20). On occasion, histoplasmoma may show fat deposition with growth (Table 9-10). Nearly 65%

TABLE 9.10 Causes of SPNs Containing Fat

Hamartoma
Lipoma
Liposarcoma (primary or metastatic)
Lipoid pneumonia
Histoplasmoma
Teratoma

of hamartomas show fat on HRCT, sometimes in association with dense popcorn calcification or flecks of calcium. The presence of fat within a lung nodule is sufficient for calling it benign, although follow-up is appropriate.

Low (Water or Fluid) Attenuation

Benign cystic lesions, such as pulmonary bronchogenic cyst, sequestration, congenital cystic adenomatoid malformation (CCAM), or a fluid-filled cyst or bulla (Table 9-11), occasionally may be diagnosed on CT by their low attenuation (0 to 20 HU) and very thin or invisible walls (see Fig. 1-6 in Chapter 1). Mucoid impaction also may appear to be of low attenuation. On the other hand, bronchogenic cysts or other cystic lesions may have a higher attenuation because of their protein content. A hematoma may have the attenuation of blood (50 HU) or may have low attenuation, depending on its age.

A necrotic neoplasm, conglomerate mass, or lung abscess or infarction may have a low attenuation center on CT, but these lesions have a thick and perceptible wall.

Contrast Enhancement

Cancers have a greater tendency to opacify following contrast infusion than do some types of benign nodules. Specific contrast enhancement techniques have been suggested to help diagnose malignancy. When using these techniques, sequential thin-collimation scans must be obtained through the center of a lung nodule for several minutes following contrast injection. Most SPNs show peak enhancement at either 3 or 4 minutes.

One currently recommended protocol uses scans at 1 minute intervals for 4 minutes following the start of the injection of 420 mg iodine/kg (usually 75 to 125 mL) at a rate of 2 mL/s. A region of interest encompassing about 60% of the nodule diameter is used to measure enhancement.

Using this protocol, carcinomas enhance by 14 to 165 HU (median, 38 HU; Fig. 9-21) and benign lesions exhibit a change in CT number of −20 to 96 HU (median, 10 HU). Using an enhancement of 15 HU or more to suggest

TABLE 9.11 Causes of Fluid Density SPNs

Bronchogenic cyst
Carcinoma (necrotic or infected)
Congenital cystic adenomatoid malformation
Conglomerate mass (necrotic)
Fluid-filled or infected cyst, cavity, or bulla
Hematoma
Lung abscess (bacterial and fungal)
Lymphoma (necrotic)
Metastatic neoplasm (necrotic)
Mucoid impaction
Sequestration

A   B

FIG. 9.21. Enhancement of a carcinoma. **A:** A lobulated right upper lobe nodule shown on HRCT represents a carcinoma. **B:** After contrast enhancement, the region of interest in the center of the nodule (*arrow*) showed an increase in attenuation of 40 HU (change from 8 to 48 HU). This is typical of malignant lesions.

malignancy, this test has a sensitivity of 98%, specificity of 58%, and accuracy of 77%. Specific benign lesions that show significant enhancement include active granulomas, inflammatory lesions, focal pneumonias, and some benign tumors such as hamartoma (Fig. 9-22; Table 9-12). Round atelectasis tends to enhance densely, as does any area of atelectasis.

It would seem most appropriate to use this technique when a nodule does not show typical findings of malignancy (e.g., spiculation, nodularity, cavitation, or growth) or typical features of a specific benign lesion. In such patients, this technique may help select which patients require surgery (i.e., if enhancement is present) or which can just be followed up carefully (i.e., if enhancement is absent).

FIG. 9.22. Enhancement of a hamartoma. HRCT through a left lung nodule during contrast enhancement showed an increase in attenuation of 22 HU (increase in attenuation from 20 to 42 HU) following contrast enhancement for the region of interest shown.

Contrast Opacification

Some solitary (or multiple) lesions opacify following contrast injection, thus representing vascular structures (Table 9-13). These have a limited differential diagnosis and specific morphology, described in the following sections.

Growth and Doubling Time

Carcinomas grow (Fig. 9-23). The growth rate of an SPN has been used to determine its likelihood of being malignant. *Doubling time*, the time required for a lesion to double in volume, is used to measure the growth rate. For easy reference, a 26% increase in nodule diameter is one doubling, and a doubling of diameter means that three volume doublings have occurred. However, not all carcinomas grow in a concentric fashion, and estimating their volume may be difficult (see Fig. 9-23).

The range of doubling times associated with carcinoma has been reported to be 1 week to 16 months, although reported values vary. Doubling times ranging from 1 month to 200 days encompass most cancers.

TABLE 9.12 Causes of an SPN With Contrast Enhancement

Carcinoma
Carcinoid tumor
Granuloma (active)
Hamartoma or other benign tumor
Hemangioma
Focal pneumonia
Round atelectasis
Vascular metastases

TABLE 9.13 SPNs Associated With Contrast Opacification

Arteriovenous malformation
Pulmonary vein varix
Pulmonary artery aneurysm

Average doubling times for different cell types of lung cancer have been estimated and vary with cell type. The average doubling time is estimated as 30 days for small cell carcinoma, 100 days for squamous cell and large cell carcinomas, and 180 days for adenocarcinoma. The doubling time of the slowest growing BACs may be more than 1,500 days.

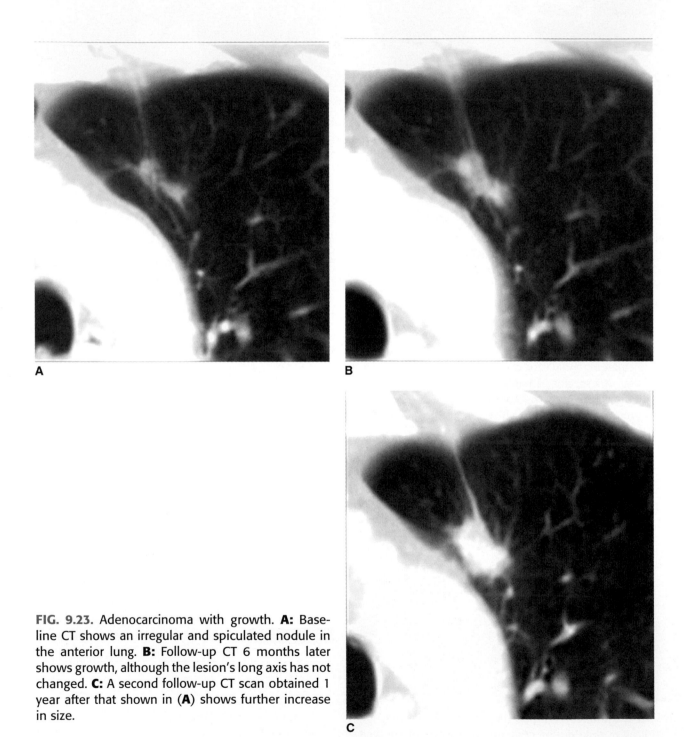

FIG. 9.23. Adenocarcinoma with growth. **A:** Baseline CT shows an irregular and spiculated nodule in the anterior lung. **B:** Follow-up CT 6 months later shows growth, although the lesion's long axis has not changed. **C:** A second follow-up CT scan obtained 1 year after that shown in (**A**) shows further increase in size.

Nearly all carcinomas will show some growth over a follow-up period of 2 years.

It has been suggested that a typical lung cancer has doubled approximately 30 times by the time it reaches a diameter of 1 cm and becomes visible radiographically. Metastasis occurring before the primary tumor is recognized radiographically probably accounts for the poor prognosis of many lung cancer patients.

A pulmonary nodule that doubles in volume in less than 1 month or more than 200 days is likely benign. Slower-growing lesions often are benign tumors or granulomas. More rapidly growing lesions usually are inflammatory.

However, the overlapping growth rates of benign and malignant lesions make it difficult to use doubling time as an absolute indicator that a nodule is benign. Nonetheless, it is generally agreed that an SPN that does not grow over a 2-year period likely is benign and does not require resection. It is important to note, however, that exceptions to this rule have been reported. If only 2 years of stability can be demonstrated, further follow-up to ensure stability is a good idea. This is particularly true for nodules of ground-glass opacity, which are more likely to represent BAC, and may have a very slow growth rate.

If no old examinations are available, or if prior examinations are not old enough to demonstrate lack of growth for 2 or more years, the diagnostic approach may be based on the patient's age and the plain radiographic appearance of a lesion. If the patient is younger than 30 years of age and the pulmonary nodule appears benign (e.g., it is small, round, and sharply defined), follow-up should be sufficient; lung cancers are rare in patients under the age of 30. However, if the patient is older than 30, has a history of an extrathoracic tumor (which raises the possibility of a solitary metastasis), or

if the lesion does not appear benign (i.e., it is large, irregular, ill defined, or spiculated), further diagnostic procedures must be performed. In most cases, CT would be appropriate.

PET and SPECT Imaging

Positron emission tomography (PET) obtained following an injection of 2-(fluorine-18)-fluoro-2-deoxy-D-glucose (FDG) may be used to characterize pulmonary nodules. FDG is a D-glucose analog labeled with a positron emitter (^{18}F) that is transported through the cell membrane and phosphorylated using normal glycolytic pathways. Increased uptake and accumulation of FDG have been shown to occur in tumor cells, although the effect is nonspecific and may be seen with inflammation.

The degree of FDG accumulation is measured using the standardized uptake value (SUV); the SUV of lung cancers usually is more than 2.5. FDG-PET has a sensitivity of about 95% in detecting malignant SPNs 1 cm or more in diameter, with a specificity of about 80% (Fig. 9-24). False-positive studies occur with inflammatory lesions. False-negative scans may occur with carcinoid tumors, BACs, and lesions smaller than 1 cm.

Radionuclide single-photon emission computed tomography (SPECT) employing depreotide (a somatostatin analog), thallium, or FDG also may be used to diagnose malignancy in a large lung nodule but is less sensitive than PET for nodules smaller than 2 cm.

Biopsy

Methods for biopsy of an SPN include fiberoptic bronchoscopy (FOB), transthoracic needle biopsy (TNB), and surgery, including video-assisted thoracoscopic surgery (VATS).

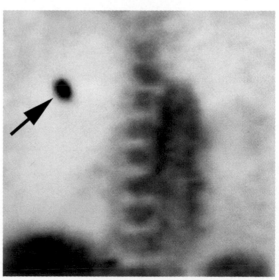

A
B

FIG. 9.24. FDG-PET in a patient with adenocarcinoma. **A:** HRCT shows a small right upper lobe nodule (*arrow*). **B:** PET (coronal plane) shows the nodule to have a very high activity (*arrow*). The size of the nodule on PET exceeds its real size. PET is poor at showing the specific location of abnormalities.

Fiberoptic Bronchoscopy

FOB with transbronchial biopsy and bronchial washing has a limited role in evaluating an SPN. Although transbronchial biopsy is accurate for assessing endobronchial lesions, the yield of FOB for peripheral nodules is less than 60% and is only 25% to 30% for an SPN smaller than 2 cm. The sensitivity of FOB is best when a bronchus leads directly to or is seen within the SPN (the "positive bronchus" sign; Fig. 9-25).

Transthoracic Needle Biopsy

TNB is often used for assessing an SPN. The sensitivity of TNB in diagnosing cancer is over 90%. Unfortunately, the accuracy of TNB for diagnosing benign disease other than active infections is limited. Malignancy cannot be ruled out if a biopsy is "negative" but no specific benign diagnosis is made; 30% of such cases later prove to represent cancer. Biopsy of nodules smaller than 1 cm in diameter is associated with an increased false-negative rate. Complications include pneumothorax, hemorrhage, and air embolism.

Video-assisted Thoracic Surgery

VATS also is used to assess indeterminate pulmonary nodules. Wedge resections and, less commonly, lobar resections may be performed using either an endoscopic stapler or a laser. CT nodule localization before surgery may be accomplished using methylene blue or a hooked wire.

A Strategy for Nodule Evaluation

If a nodule is definitely benign, based on lack of growth on sequential examinations or CT findings (i.e., it has specific morphologic characteristics of a benign lesion, contains fat, or benign calcification), further evaluation should be limited to plain film or perhaps CT follow-up.

For an indeterminate nodule (i.e., one that is not definitely benign), CT is often used for follow-up to determine if the nodule is stable in size or growing. The history and size of the nodule may be used to determine the appropriate interval for CT follow-up. The current recommendations of the Fleischner Society and the American College of Chest Physicians for CT follow-up of nodules 8 mm or smaller in size are similar and summarized in Table 9-14.

The management of an SPN larger than 8 mm is often based on an assessment of risk factors and the patient's likelihood of having lung cancer. The likelihood of lung cancer may be determined using published algorithms (see Schultz et al. in Selected Reading for an example), which consider various aspects of the patient's history and the size and appearance of the nodule. For patients with a low likelihood of lung cancer based on the absence of risk factors, age, small nodule size or appearance, and other factors, CT follow-up at 3, 6, 12, and 24 months is often appropriate. In patients with an intermediate probability of lung cancer, additional testing (i.e., PET, contrast-enhanced CT, needle

FIG. 9.25. The positive bronchus sign. A small right upper lobe nodule (*large arrow*) with a bronchus (*small arrow*) leading to it. This sign predicts a higher likelihood of a diagnosis being made at bronchoscopy.

TABLE 9.14 Fleischner Society and American College of Chest Physician Recommendations for CT Follow-up of Nodules 8 mm or Smaller in Size

Nodule Size[a]	Low-risk Patient	High-risk Patient
≤4 mm	No follow-up needed (f/u is optional)	f/u at 12 months; if unchanged, no further f/u[b]
>4–6 mm	f/u at 12 months; if unchanged, no further f/u	f/u CT at 6–12 months, then at 18–24 months if no change[b]
>6–8 mm	f/u CT at 6–12 months, then at 18–24 months if no change	f/u CT at 3–6 months, then at 9–12 and 24 months if no change[b]

[a]Average of length and width.
[b]Ground-glass or partly ground-glass nodules may require longer follow-up to exclude slowly growing BAC.
Low-risk patient, minimal or absent history of smoking or other known risk factors.
High-risk patient, history of smoking or other known risk factors.
(Modified from **MacMahon H, Austin JH, Gamsu G, et al.** Guidelines for management of small pulmonary nodules detected on CT scans: a statement from the Fleischner Society. Radiology 2005; 237:395–400, and **Gould MK, Fletcher J, Iannettoni MD, et al.** Evaluation of patients with pulmonary nodules: when is it lung cancer? ACCP evidence-based clinical practice guidelines [2nd ed]. Chest 2007; 132:108S–130S.)

biopsy, bronchoscopy) is appropriate. In patients with a high probability of cancer, VATS or resection is most appropriate.

For example, if an SPN larger than 8 mm has benign characteristics on CT (e.g., it is smooth, round, and sharply defined) but is not definitely benign and risk factors for cancer (e.g., history of malignancy, smoking history) are absent, follow-up using CT would be appropriate. However, depending on the clinician's or patient's wishes, needle biopsy or PET may be performed. If the patient is a smoker, has a history of malignancy, or the nodule has malignant characteristics on CT (e.g., it is uncalcified, irregular in shape or spiculated, or contains air bronchograms), a surgeon should generally be consulted. The surgeon may request a needle biopsy or PET scanning for further evaluation, or VATS or resection may be performed.

Occasionally, a patient with an acute process, such as pulmonary embolism, focal pneumonia, or other inflammatory process, can present with an SPN on chest radiographs or CT. Short-term follow-up may be indicated, particularly in patients with acute symptoms. A decrease in the size of a nodule suggests it is benign, although lung cancers sometimes show a transient decrease in size because of necrosis. A single follow-up study showing a decrease in the size of a lung nodule should not be considered proof of a benign process. Further follow-up showing continued resolution or stability is a good idea.

MULTIPLE NODULES AND MASSES

This section reviews the differential diagnosis of multiple large nodules (i.e., 1 cm or larger) and masses (Table 9-15). A nodular pattern of diffuse lung disease (i.e., innumerable nodules 1 cm or less in diameter) is discussed in Chapter 10. Obviously, there is some overlap in differential diagnosis.

Metastases should be considered most likely when multiple nodules or masses are visible (see Chapter 4). The initial evaluation of these abnormalities usually is based on history, clinical studies, and assessment of radiographic findings. Bronchoscopy or percutaneous biopsy may be needed for eventual diagnosis. An organized radiographic approach to the evaluation of multiple nodules and masses is more difficult to devise than for the SPN, but it is based on many of the same principles.

Size

Benign and malignant lesions may be either small or large. A clear-cut relation of size to malignancy does not exist as it does with SPN. There is a tendency for multiple nodular metastases to vary in size (see Fig. 4-8 in Chapter 4), whereas benign processes result in nodules of similar size.

Number

Multinodular metastases may be few in number or innumerable, but a large number of nodules suggest this diagnosis (see Figs. 4-8 to 4-11 in Chapter 4). Most infectious and inflammatory diseases result in less than a dozen nodules.

TABLE 9.15 Multiple Pulmonary Nodules or Masses

Congenital lesions and normal variants
Arteriovenous fistulas
Intrapulmonary lymph nodes

Malignant neoplasm
Bronchioloalveolar carcinoma
Carcinoma
Lymphoma
Lymphoproliferative disease
Metastatic neoplasm

Benign neoplasms and neoplasm-like conditions
Endometriomas
Lymphoproliferative disease
Multiple chondromas (Carney's triad)
Papillomas (papillomatosis)

Infection and parasites
Aspergillosis, angioinvasive
Bronchopneumonia
Echinococcus
Granulomatous infection or granulomas
  Tuberculosis
  Nontuberculous mycobacteria (e.g., *Mycobacterium avium-intracellulare* complex)
  Coccidioidomycosis
  Histoplasmosis
  Cryptococcus
Lung abscesses
Mycetomas (aspergillomas)
Paragonimiasis
Septic embolism

Inflammatory (noninfectious)
Churg-Strauss' syndrome
Focal organizing pneumonia
Rheumatoid nodules
Sarcoidosis
Wegener's granulomatosis

Airways and inhalational disease
Mucoid impaction (mucous plug)
  Asthma
  Allergic bronchopulmonary aspergillosis
  Bronchiectasis
  Cystic fibrosis
Conglomerate masses or progressive massive fibrosis (e.g., silicosis)
Lipoid pneumonia

Vascular lesions
Arteriovenous fistulas
Hematomas
Infarctions
Pulmonary artery aneurysms
Septic embolism

Idiopathic and miscellaneous
Amyloidosis
Fluid-filled bullae
Round atelectasis

Location

Metastases, infarction, and septic emboli have a predilection for the lung periphery and the lung bases. Abscesses related to aspiration often are posterior or basal in distribution.

Edge Appearance

Metastases usually are sharply marginated (see Figs. 4-8 to 4-11 in Chapter 4), as are nodules in amyloidosis, rheumatoid nodules, AVMs, hematomas, and Caplan's syndrome. Infectious lesions, diffuse BAC (see Figs. 3-8, 3-9, and 3-22 in Chapter 3), lymphoma (see Figs. 5-10 to 5-12 in Chapter 5), conglomerate masses and progressive massive fibrosis, and Wegener's granulomatosis are often ill defined.

An increase in sharpness of the edge of a lesion with time suggests the resolution of a benign inflammatory process. For example, septic emboli, lung abscesses, infections, and Wegener's granulomatosis result in masses that are ill defined early in their course and become sharply defined as they heal.

The halo sign may be seen in patients with multiple nodules; its differential diagnosis is described in Table 9-4.

Cavitation

As with SPNs, thick-walled cavities are consistent with malignancy, but thick walls may be seen with inflammatory, nonmalignant lesions as well. Very thin-walled cavities usually are benign, although metastatic tumors, particularly squamous cell carcinoma of the head and neck or sarcomas and tracheobronchial papillomatosis, may be associated with thin-walled lesions. As with SPNs, an air-fluid level tends to predict benign disease. The differential diagnosis of multiple cystic or cavitary lesions is reviewed in Table 9-6.

Growth

Rapid growth with an increase in size over a period of a few days suggests infection (e.g., bacterial infection or fungus or TB in an immunosuppressed patient). Progression over a period of a few weeks is typical of indolent infections (e.g., TB or fungus in an immunocompetent patient), noninfectious inflammatory disease, or rapidly progressing malignancy (Fig. 9-26). Nodules that appear stable over a period of weeks or show slow growth during a few months are likely to be either malignant or due to indolent inflammatory conditions (e.g., rheumatoid nodules). Masses that show little change over a period of months are typical of amyloidosis, AVMs, benign tumors, and conglomerate masses. Some metastatic tumors (e.g., thyroid carcinoma or benign metastasizing leiomyoma) may show very slow growth.

Resolution of lesions with or without treatment suggests benign disease. Slow resolution is typical of hematoma and infarction. Rapid resolution is typical of treated infections.

DIFFERENTIAL DIAGNOSIS OF LUNG NODULES, MASSES, AND CAVITIES

A large number of diseases and abnormalities associated with solitary or multiple nodules, masses, or cysts are reviewed in the following sections in alphabetical order. Many of these are discussed in more detail elsewhere in this book.

Amyloidosis

Patients with localized nodular amyloidosis usually are asymptomatic. Nodular amyloidosis may manifest as single or multiple lung nodules or masses, usually well-defined and round (see Fig. 21-5 in Chapter 21). Bilateral lung nodules

A   **B**

FIG. 9.26. Metastases from a spindle cell sarcoma with rapid growth. **A:** CT scan shows multiple small nodules (*arrows*). **B:** A follow-up scan 6 weeks later shows marked increase in size. Such rapid growth suggests an infectious or inflammatory process but may be seen with very rapidly growing neoplasms.

are most typical, and they tend to be peripheral or subpleural in location. Nodules range from 0.5 to 5 cm in diameter in most cases but may be as large as 10 cm. Calcification is visible radiographically in 30% to 50% of cases and may be stippled or dense. Cavitation may be seen in approximately 5%. Nodules may grow slowly or remain stable over a number of years. Needle biopsy may be diagnostic.

Arteriovenous Malformation

Congenital arteriovenous malformation, also known as arteriovenous fistula, is associated with Osler-Weber-Rendu syndrome in 35% to 67% of cases. *Simple AVM* represents a single, dilated vascular sac connecting one artery and one vein (see Figs. 1-10 to 1-15 in Chapter 1). It is the most common type and accounts for almost all cases of AVM. *Complex AVM* has multiple feeding arteries or draining veins. Radiographically, a simple fistula appears as a peripheral, well-defined, round, oval, lobulated, or serpentine opacity. Large vessels (feeders) extending centrally toward the hilum are easily seen on CT. AVMs typically are subpleural in location, and more than two thirds are found in the lower lobes. Fistulas are multiple in 35% of patients and bilateral in 10%. Multiple AVMs are most common in patients with Osler-Weber-Rendu syndrome. Enlargement of fistulas over a period of months or years is common, and a rapid increase in size can occur. Opacification occurs following contrast enhancement.

Aspergillosis

Angioinvasive Aspergillosis

Angioinvasive aspergillosis is characterized by the involvement of normal lung tissue by aspergillus organisms, usually resulting in significant tissue damage and necrosis. It almost always occurs in immunosuppressed patients and is particularly common in association with (1) neutropenia in patients with acute leukemia, (2) treatment using corticosteroids or other immunosuppressive agents, (3) organ transplantation, and (4) malignancy. Pathologic examination shows infiltration of lung tissue by fungus, with invasion of small arteries, vascular occlusion, and, often, infarction of the involved lung.

Early in the course of disease, ill-defined nodules up to several centimeters in diameter or focal areas of consolidation typically are seen on chest radiographs. At this stage, CT typically shows the halo sign, in which a halo of ground-glass opacity surrounds a central nodule (see Figs. 9-7 and 9-27). The halo and central nodule reflect, respectively, a rim of hemorrhage surrounding a central fungal nodule or infarct. In an immunosuppressed patient, the CT appearance of early invasive aspergillosis with a visible halo sign is sufficiently characteristic to justify a presumptive diagnosis and treatment. However, as described above, the halo sign can be associated with a variety of infectious and noninfectious processes.

If patients with angioinvasive aspergillosis survive their acute infection, nodules often cavitate, showing the air-crescent sign (see Fig. 9-27). The presence of an air crescent

FIG. 9.27. Angioinvasive aspergillosis with halo sign and air-crescent sign. CT scans at three adjacent levels in a patient with leukemia show an air-crescent sign (*large arrow*) outlining a "lung ball" within a cavity. Anterior to it is an ill-defined nodule with a halo sign (*small arrows*).

in angioinvasive aspergillosis reflects lung necrosis with the presence of a sequestrum or ball of devitalized and necrotic lung occupying part of the cavity. Although this appearance mimics that of a mycetoma, the two conditions are unrelated.

Cavitation, when present, generally occurs about 2 weeks after the appearance of nodular opacities and is associated with a white blood cell count of more than 1,000. Thus, the presence of cavitation is generally considered to be a good prognostic sign.

Semi-invasive (Chronic Necrotizing) Aspergillosis

Semi-invasive (chronic necrotizing) aspergillosis typically is associated with slowly progressive upper lobe abnormalities. Most patients have an underlying chronic lung disease such as TB, COPD, fibrosis, or pneumoconiosis. Patients may be mildly immunocompromised (e.g., chronic disease, advanced age, diabetes, poor nutrition, alcoholism, low-dose corticosteroid treatment) but lack the severe immune deficiencies typical of patients with invasive aspergillosis. Pathology reveals a combination of granulomatous inflammation, necrosis, and fibrosis similar to that seen in TB. Symptoms are nonspecific, consisting of cough, sputum production, weight loss, fever, and hemoptysis.

Radiographs and CT typically show upper lobe consolidation, with progressive cavitation over a period of weeks to months, indistinguishable from TB. It is common to see irregular thickening of the wall of a cavity or frond-like intracavity opacities representing growing fungus. Frank aspergillomas may develop in patients with semi-invasive aspergillosis. These may have a typical (i.e., air-crescent sign) or atypical appearance. With progressive disease, pleural and chest wall involvement may be present. Aspergillus infection is discussed in detail in Chapter 12.

Bronchiectasis

Bronchiectasis may result in the presence of multiple cystic lung lesions (i.e., cystic bronchiectasis). These often have thin but easily recognizable walls and may be focal or diffuse in distribution. Air-fluid levels are common, representing secretions and pus, and help to distinguish cystic bronchiectasis from cystic lung diseases such as lymphangiomyomatosis, histiocytosis, and lymphoid interstitial pneumonia. Because the cystic areas communicate with each other (via the bronchial tree), the amount of fluid in each "cyst" is similar or more fluid is seen in cysts located at the lung bases (Fig. 9-28).

Bronchogenic Cyst

Pulmonary bronchogenic cysts are most common in the medial lung and the lower lobes. Uninfected cysts are sharply circumscribed and round or oval in shape; their wall is invisible on CT or appears very thin. Fluid-filled bronchogenic cysts may appear low in attenuation on CT (0 to 20 HU; see Fig. 1-6 in Chapter 1) or may have high CT numbers (40 to 80 HU). Rarely, the cyst wall may calcify or the cyst may contain milk of calcium and appear dense. Infection eventually occurs in 75% of cases. In the presence of acute infection, a rapid increase in size of the cyst may be seen. In addition, the outer cyst wall may become less well-defined because of surrounding lung inflammation (Fig. 9-29A). A previously infected cyst may contain air, showing a thin and well-defined wall, and may contain an air-fluid level (see Fig. 9-29B and Fig. 1-7 in Chapter 1).

Bronchioloalveolar Carcinoma

BAC most often presents as a solitary nodule, often containing air bronchograms, associated with the halo sign, or appearing to be entirely ground-glass opacity. However, 40% of patients show radiographic findings of diffuse lung involvement (see Figs. 3-8, 3-9, and 3-22 in Chapter 3). Thirty

percent of these demonstrate multiple ill-defined nodules, which may be centrilobular in distribution on HRCT. The nodules are usually 5 mm to 1 cm in diameter and may be patchy in distribution or diffuse. Most (60%) of the remaining patients with diffuse BAC show patchy, lobar, or diffuse consolidation, with air bronchograms. Nodules and consolidation may be seen in combination.

Bullae

By definition, a bulla is a sharply demarcated area of emphysema, measuring 1 cm or more in diameter and possessing a wall less than 1 mm thick. Bullae usually are a manifestation of paraseptal emphysema but also may be seen in patients with centrilobular emphysema. Bullae usually are subpleural in location, largest at the lung apices, and very thin walled (Fig. 9-30A); these findings often allow their accurate diagnosis on chest radiographs or CT. On HRCT, other areas of emphysema usually are visible.

A bulla may contain fluid, showing an air-fluid level or appearing as a focal mass. This may result from infection, hemorrhage, tumor arising in a bulla, or bland fluid accumulation (see Fig. 9-30B and C). The identification of other bullae may be helpful in diagnosis. CT may show the fluid nature of the opacity or associated wall thickening in patients with tumor.

Carcinoma

Approximately one third of lung cancers present radiographically as an SPN or lung mass. The most common cell types presenting as a nodule or mass are adenocarcinoma

A

B

FIG. 9.28. Cystic bronchiectasis. A: Multiple thin-walled cysts represent cystic bronchiectasis. **B:** Detail view of the right lower lobe. Air-fluid levels are visible, with the largest amount of fluid being in cysts at the lung bases. This implies communication between the cysts and is diagnostic of bronchiectasis.

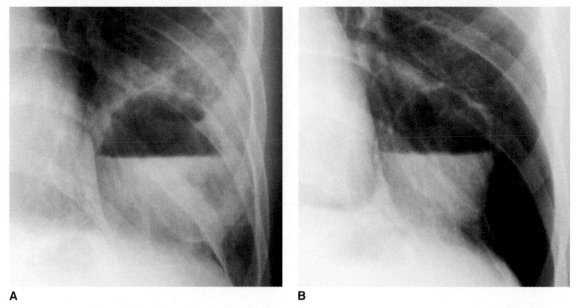

A   B

FIG. 9.29. Bronchogenic cyst. **A:** When it is acutely infected, the air- and fluid-filled cyst is very ill defined, resembling a lung abscess. **B:** After treatment, a thin-walled cystic lesion is visible in the left lung. This was found to represent a bronchogenic cyst. The presence of an air-fluid level indicates prior infection.

A   B

C

FIG. 9.30. Bullae. **A:** Bullous emphysema with large subpleural bullae. These appear very thin walled. Bronchiectasis also is visible, resulting in thicker-walled cystic structures in the central lung. **B:** Bullous emphysema with infection. Multiple thin-walled bullae with air-fluid levels are visible in the right lung. **C:** Carcinoma arising in a bulla. A patient with bullous emphysema shows a fluid-filled bulla (*white arrow*) in the left upper lobe. Masses (*black arrows*) within the bulla represent carcinoma.

(40%), squamous cell carcinoma (20%), large cell carcinoma (15%), and BAC (10%). Nearly two thirds of lung cancers presenting as a lung nodule occur in the upper lobes. Because they are not usually associated with symptoms, they often are relatively large when first detected; nearly 60% are larger than 2 cm, and 25% are larger than 3 cm. The appearances of lung carcinoma are described earlier in this chapter and in Chapter 3.

Multiple lung nodules may occur in patients with lung cancer in the presence of multiple synchronous primary tumors, satellite nodules associated with the primary tumor due to local spread, or hematogenous metastases to lung from the primary lung cancer or may occur in patients with diffuse BAC (see Figs. 3-8, 3-9, and 3-22 in Chapter 3). In patients with metastatic lung carcinoma, the primary lesion usually is visible as a dominant mass (Fig. 9-31).

Carcinoid Tumor

Carcinoid tumors account for 1% to 2% of tracheobronchial neoplasms. Approximately 20% of carcinoid tumors present as a peripheral nodule or mass. They often are well-defined, round or oval, and slightly lobulated in contour (see Fig. 3-44 in Chapter 3). Calcification is uncommonly seen on radiographs but is visible on CT in nearly 40%. Approximately 10% to 25% of carcinoid tumors can be classified as *atypical carcinoid tumor* because of histologic features suggesting a more aggressive behavior. Atypical carcinoid tumors tend to present as a lung nodule or mass somewhat larger than seen with carcinoid tumor. Cavitation is rare. Dense enhancement may be seen following contrast infusion.

Churg-Strauss Syndrome

Churg-Strauss' syndrome is characterized by a combination of necrotizing vasculitis, extravascular granulomas, and tissue infiltration by eosinophils. Patients with this syndrome usually are middle-aged (average onset, 40 to 50 years) and often have a history of allergic diseases including asthma, nasal polyps, or sinusitis. One or more ill-defined pulmonary nodules, up to 3.5 cm, are seen in 20% of cases. Cavitation is uncommon, a finding that is helpful in distinguishing Churg-Strauss syndrome from Wegener's granulomatosis, which may have a similar presentation. Other common radiographic abnormalities, which may be seen in combination, consist of transient multifocal areas of consolidation indistinguishable from simple pulmonary eosinophilia or chronic eosinophilic pneumonia. Pulmonary hemorrhage may be associated. Churg-Strauss syndrome is described in detail in Chapter 16.

Congenital Cystic Adenomatoid Malformation

CCAM consists of a multicystic, intralobar mass of disorganized lung tissue. About 70% of cases present during the first week of life, but 10% are diagnosed after the 1st year. Lower lobes are involved most often, but any lobe can be affected. CCAM often is classified into three types that have different histologies, gross pathologic findings, and radiographic appearances.

Type I CCAM (55% of cases) contains one or more cysts, which are larger than 2 cm in diameter (see Fig. 1-8 in Chapter 1). Type I CCAM usually presents as a large, air-filled, multicystic lesion, sometimes with air-fluid levels, which may occupy the entire hemithorax.

FIG. 9.31. Lung cancer with multiple nodules representing metastases. **A:** A patient with right upper lobe collapse due to right hilar carcinoma shows multiple small nodules (*arrows*) representing metastases. **B:** CT in a patient with left-sided carcinoma (*C*) who shows diffuse nodular metastases (*arrows*).

Type II CCAM (40% of cases) contains multiple cysts less than 2 cm in diameter. It presents as an air-filled multicystic mass or a solid mass or area of consolidation (see Fig. 1-9 in Chapter 1).

Type III CCAM (5% of cases) contains microscopic (less than 3 to 5 mm) cysts and presents radiographically as a solid mass.

Types I and II CCAM may become air filled over a period of days to weeks after birth. They often are associated with progressive air trapping and mediastinal shift to the opposite side. In adults, CCAM usually presents as an air-filled or air- and fluid-filled cystic or multicystic mass.

Conglomerate Masses

Large conglomerate masses may develop in patients with sarcoidosis (see Figs. 15-9 and 15-12 in Chapter 15), long-standing silicosis or coal worker's pneumoconiosis (see Figs. 18-10 and 18-11 in Chapter 18), and talcosis (see Fig. 18-13 in Chapter 18), and in association with some granulomatous infections. Their appearances are similar. In silicosis, conglomerate masses reflect the presence of progressive massive fibrosis.

These masses represent a conglomeration of small interstitial nodules in combination with a variable degree of fibrosis. A background pattern of multiple small lung nodules often is visible (*satellite nodules*). Conglomerate masses are typically, but not always, seen in the upper lobes or mid-lung, are usually oval or lenticular in shape, are distinct from the hila, and are separated from peripheral pleural surface (Fig. 9-32). Nearly all have irregular borders. They often are bilateral and symmetrical.

Distortion of lung architecture usually is evident due to fibrosis and volume loss. Traction bronchiectasis with

FIG. 9.32. Conglomerate masses (progressive massive fibrosis) in silicosis. Conglomerate masses typically—but not always—are seen in the upper lobes or mid-lung and usually are oval or lenticular in shape. They often are bilateral and symmetrical.

air bronchograms may be seen within the masses, and surrounding bullae may be present. Calcification in association with conglomerate masses is common. Central necrosis or cavitation may be present and may indicate superinfection by TB or bacteria. Cavities usually are thick walled. Talcosis, secondary to intravenous injection of talc, is seen almost exclusively in drug users who inject medications intended for oral use; the masses may appear high in attenuation on CT because of the talc they contain.

Cysts and Cystic Lung Disease

Cyst is a nonspecific term describing the presence of a thin-walled (usually less than 3 mm), well-defined and circumscribed, air- or fluid-containing lesion, 1 cm or more in diameter, having an epithelial or fibrous wall. The term usually is used to describe the presence of a thin-walled lesion when a more specific diagnosis cannot be made. Cysts may be congenital (e.g., bronchogenic cyst) or acquired (e.g., honeycombing, bullae, pneumatocele). It is not uncommon to see one or more (i.e., up to a few) lung cysts in an asymptomatic patient without known disease. These are usually undiagnosed and are rarely of significance.

Multiple lung cysts as a manifestation of diffuse lung disease are seen in patients with Langerhans' histiocytosis, lymphangiomyomatosis, sarcoidosis, and lymphoid interstitial pneumonia (see Chapter 25).

Lung cysts may contain fluid as a result of accumulated secretions or in the presence of infection, hemorrhage, or tumor. Thickening of the wall of a cyst suggests infection or tumor. Fluid filling cysts is uncommon in patients with cystic lung diseases such as lymphangiomyomatosis, histiocytosis, and lymphoid interstitial pneumonia.

Dirofilaria immitis

Dirofilaria immitis is the dog heartworm. Humans may become infected by a mosquito bite. Larvae travel to right-sided cardiac chambers, but cannot live in humans, and eventually embolize to the pulmonary vascular bed, where they result in an infarct and granulomatous response. A small lung nodule may result, usually less than 2 cm in diameter, rounded, sharply marginated, and subpleural in location (Fig. 9-33). Calcification may be visible on CT. Eosinophilia usually is absent. It is most common in eastern and southern states.

Echinococcosis

Echinococcus granulosus and *Echinococcus multilocularis* are intestinal tapeworms of canine carnivores such as the dog and wolf. Ova are dispersed in feces and ingested by an intermediate host. Larvae develop in the intestine of the intermediate host and migrate via the circulation to organs such as the liver and lungs, where they develop and encyst. When the larva is consumed by the carnivore (at the same time the intermediate host is consumed), the adult tapeworm develops in the carnivore.

A B

FIG. 9.33. Lung nodule secondary to *Dirofilaria immitis* infection. **A:** A sharply marginated, rounded nodule (*arrows*) is visible in the peripheral right lung. **B:** The histologic specimen following resection shows an intravascular worm (*arrows*) within the nodule.

The development of parasites in the intermediate host results in one or more hydatid cysts, usually in the liver or lungs, an occurrence termed *hydatid disease*. Hydatid disease occurs in two forms. In the *pastoral* form, a dog is the primary host and sheep are the intermediate host; it occurs in sheep-raising countries and is most common in the Mediterranean regions of Europe and North Africa, in South America, and in Australia. In the *sylvatic* or *sylvian* form, the wolf is the primary host, and wild animals such as deer, moose, or caribou are intermediate hosts; it is endemic in Arctic regions such as Alaska or Siberia. Humans may serve as an intermediate host of either form.

Pulmonary lesions have three components, knowledge of which is important in understanding the radiographic appearance of pulmonary hydatid cysts. The outermost part is termed the *pericyst*. It consists of compressed lung tissue and fibrosis adjacent to the parasite. The parasite itself is composed of two layers, an outer layer or *ectocyst* and an inner layer or *endocyst*, from which daughter cysts bud.

Uncomplicated pulmonary hydatid cysts are fluid filled, rounded, and may be quite large (over 10 cm; Fig. 9-34). Pulmonary cysts are solitary in more than half of cases. They occur most commonly in the lower lobes. Rapid growth may be seen. CT may show a wall ranging up to 1 cm in thickness, largely depending on the thickness of the pericyst. Cyst contents are of fluid attenuation on CT, but septations may be visible, representing the walls of daughter cysts. Although common in the liver, calcification of the walls of cysts is rare in the lung. Liver cysts may or may not be present in a patient with lung cysts.

Rupture of the pericyst leads to dissection of air between the pericyst and the ectocyst, resulting in an air-crescent sign. Rupture of the exocyst, with the expulsion of some fluid contents, produces an air-fluid level and allows the endocyst to

collapse. The presence of the endocyst floating on the fluid may be visible as the "water lily" or *camalote* sign. Rupture of the cyst into the pleural space may result in effusion or seeding of the pleural space with cysts. Rupture of the cyst into a bronchus may be associated with an allergic reaction or infection. Mediastinal cysts may be seen. Diagnosis usually is based on serologic tests. Biopsy should be avoided because of the risk of rupture. Echinococcosis is discussed in detail in Chapter 12.

Endometrioma

Nodules of the endometrium may rarely involve the lung parenchyma. They typically occur in women who have previously given birth or have had uterine surgery and probably

FIG. 9.34. Pulmonary hydatid cyst (*arrows*) resulting from the sylvatic form of disease. A fisherman from Alaska shows a focal rounded opacity.

reflect embolism and implantation of endometrial tissue. Pelvic endometriosis need not be present. Pulmonary endometrioma may result in catamenial hemoptysis or pulmonary hemorrhage, symptoms that strongly suggest the diagnosis. Pneumothorax may result if the implants involve the pleural surface. Pulmonary endometrioma usually is solitary, appearing in most cases as a well-defined, rounded nodule up to a few centimeters in diameter. Cavitation may occur, with the cavity often appearing thin walled. Treatment is hormonal or by excision.

Focal Organizing Pneumonia

Organizing pneumonia (OP), also known as bronchiolitis obliterans organizing pneumonia (BOOP), is characterized pathologically by the presence of granulation tissue polyps within bronchioles and alveolar ducts and patchy areas of inflammation in the surrounding lung (organizing pneumonia). Many cases are idiopathic, but OP also may be seen in patients with pulmonary infection, drug reactions, collagen-vascular diseases, Wegener's granulomatosis, and after inhalation of toxic fumes.

Most often, OP presents with patchy, unilateral or bilateral areas of air-space consolidation, which may be peripheral or peribronchial. Small or large nodules are seen in up to 50%, with or without associated consolidation (see Figs. 13-18 and 13-19 in Chapter 13 and Fig. 17-3 in Chapter 17). Large nodules or masses usually are multiple and may appear very irregular in shape, mimicking carcinoma. A finding termed the *atoll sign* or *reversed-halo sign*, in which ring-shaped or crescentic opacities are seen, often with ground-glass opacity in the center of the ring (resembling a coral atoll or the opposite of the halo sign), may be seen with OP. This finding strongly suggests the diagnosis. High-attenuation nodules or masses may be seen in patients with OP related to amiodarone toxicity due to its iodine content. Cavitation and calcification do not occur.

Focal (Round) Pneumonia

Pneumonias may be focal, mimicking the appearance of carcinoma. This configuration has been termed "round pneumonia." Findings suggestive of focal pneumonia include satellite nodules (Fig. 9-35A), tree-in-bud, centrilobular nodules, or a lobular or multilobular pattern, but these

A

C

B

FIG. 9.35. Focal (round) pneumonia. **A:** An irregular nodule is visible in the right lung, associated with satellite nodules in a patient with bacterial infection. This appearance may be seen in patients with infection from a variety of organisms. **B:** Cryptococcal pneumonia with multiple focal areas of consolidation. **C:** *Pneumocystis jiroveci* (*P. carinii*) infection in a patient with AIDS. Patchy ground-glass opacity is visible bilaterally, typical of this infection. A focal mass with a halo sign within the right lung (*arrow*) also represented *Pneumocystis* infection.

do not need to be seen to establish the diagnosis. Focal infections are common with bacterial bronchopneumonia (see Fig. 9-34A), TB, nontuberculous mycobacteria, and fungal infection (see Fig. 9-34B) and occasionally are seen with viral infection or infection with *Pneumocystis jiroveci* (formerly *P. carinii*; see Fig. 9-34C). Focal opacities associated with infection may be solitary or multiple. The halo sign is common with angioinvasive aspergillosis (see Figs. 9-7 and 9-27) but may be seen with focal infection of various causes (see Fig. 9-34C).

Granuloma

Granulomas usually result from TB, nontuberculous mycobacteria, and fungal infections, most commonly coccidioidomycosis and histoplasmosis. They usually are well-defined and rounded (see Fig. 9-3). Granulomas associated with surrounding lung fibrosis (common in TB) may appear very irregular and spiculated in contour, mimicking carcinoma. Granulomas also may be associated with irregular cavitation. Calcification is common but may have a variety of appearances—dense and homogeneous, central, lamellar, eccentric, or stippled.

Granulomas usually are smaller than 2 cm in diameter and often are solitary or few in number. Numerous small granulomas, a few millimeters in diameter, also may be seen.

Hamartoma

Hamartoma is the most common mesenchymal lung tumor and accounts for more than 75% of benign lung tumors. More than 85% appear radiographically as an SPN. Peripheral hamartomas usually are 1 to 4 cm in diameter, well-defined, sharply circumscribed, and often lobulated (see Fig. 9-4 and Figs. 3-50 to 3-52 in Chapter 3). Calcification is visible on

plain radiographs in approximately 30% of hamartomas and is seen more commonly on CT. The calcification of hamartomas can be stippled or conglomerate, referred to as "popcorn" calcification. Nearly 65% of hamartomas may be diagnosed using HRCT because of visible fat (−40 to −120 HU), either focal or diffuse or a combination of fat and calcification. Cavitation is rare.

Other benign tumors may arise from mesenchymal tissues. They are usually solitary, well-defined, and rounded in shape. Benign tumors usually are solitary. Multiple chondromas may be associated with *Carney's triad* (i.e., multiple pulmonary chondromas, gastric epithelioid leiomyosarcoma, and extra-adrenal paraganglioma).

Hematoma and Laceration

Hematomas are often the result of trauma (blunt or penetrating), representing focal lung contusion or pulmonary laceration containing blood. *Contusion* represents focal bleeding without disruption of lung architecture. *Traumatic laceration* is associated with tearing of lung; a laceration contains blood or air (or both), with air-fluid levels sometimes visible (Figs. 9-36 and 9-37). These lesions usually are thin walled. They may be solitary or multiple. High-attenuation clot may be detectable using CT. Focal hematoma also may result from other causes of bleeding.

Infarction

Focal consolidation distal to a pulmonary embolus may be due to ischemia with focal pulmonary hemorrhage or frank infarction. Because the lung is supplied by both pulmonary and bronchial arteries, pulmonary infarction occurs in the minority (10% to 15%) of patients with pulmonary embolism

A

B

FIG. 9.36. Pulmonary laceration with hematoma in a hockey player with hemoptysis after a "bad body check." **A:** A focal lung opacity (*arrow*) represents a focal hematoma. Some surrounding ground-glass opacity is due to hemorrhage. **B:** At a different level, an air-fluid level (*arrow*) is visible within a focal cystic lesion.

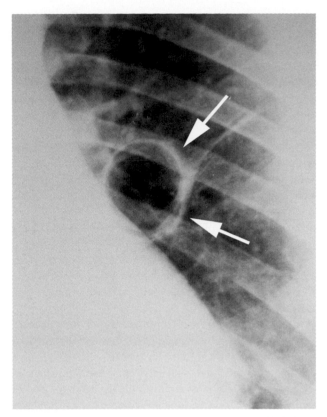

FIG. 9.37. Pulmonary laceration. A cystic air-filled lesion in the left lung (*arrows*) represents a laceration from a stab wound.

FIG. 9.38. Pulmonary infarction in a patient with pulmonary embolism. CT shows a pulmonary embolus in the right interlobar pulmonary artery (*large arrow*). A wedge-shaped opacity (*small arrows*) is visible in the peripheral lung, contacting the pleural surface, and associated with surrounding ground-glass opacity (halo sign). A vessel is noted at the apex of the opacity. A pleural effusion is associated.

and often is associated with underlying cardiovascular disease, the presence of peripheral emboli, or multiple emboli.

Hemorrhage or infarction in the peripheral lung may result in a wedge-shaped or rounded, pleural-based opacity, the classic *Hampton hump*. Subpleural opacities are seen more often in the lower lobes, where most emboli occur. On plain films, these opacities usually are unassociated with air bronchograms; the absence of air bronchograms is likely due to blood filling the bronchi. Pulmonary opacities due to hemorrhage usually resolve within a week, but pulmonary infarctions may require months to heal. They typically resolve by maintaining the same shape while decreasing in size, an occurrence called the "melting sign" because of its resemblance to a melting ice cube. Infarctions often leave linear scars.

On CT (Fig. 9-38), a pulmonary infarction may be characterized by the following features:

1. A wedge-shaped opacity (sometimes with a truncated apex)
2. Contact with the pleural surface
3. Convex borders
4. A linear opacity directed from the apex of the density toward the hilum (i.e., its feeding vessel)
5. Scattered areas of low attenuation (necrosis) within the lesion
6. A halo sign due to adjacent hemorrhage

Some or all of these findings are seen on CT in about half of patients with pulmonary embolism.

Following the administration of a bolus of intravenous contrast medium, the perimeter of an infarct characteristically enhances, possibly because of collateral blood flow from adjacent bronchial arteries, while the center of the lesion remains lucent. Cavitation of an infarction suggests septic embolism or infection of a bland infarct.

Intrapulmonary Lymph Nodes

Intrapulmonary lymph nodes may be visible as a small peripheral lung nodule, usually well-defined, smooth, and rounded in contour. They may be located immediately beneath the visceral pleural surface or within 2 cm of the pleura and are most common at the lung bases. They usually measure a few millimeters in diameter but may be as large as 1 cm. They are almost always solitary.

Lipoid Pneumonia

Lipoid pneumonia (lung consolidation containing lipid) may be endogenous or exogenous.

Endogenous lipoid pneumonia may occur due to bronchial obstruction with accumulation of lipid-rich cellular debris distal to the obstructing lesion.

Exogenous lipoid pneumonia results from the chronic aspiration of animal-, vegetable-, or petroleum-based oils or fats. Consolidation, ill-defined masses, or (sometimes) findings of fibrosis are seen on chest radiographs. A posterior or lower lobe distribution is typical. Opacities may be bilateral or unilateral. If a large amount of lipid has been aspirated, CT can show rounded or irregular areas of low-attenuation consolidation (−35 to −75 HU); this appearance is most common in patients with chronic mineral oil aspiration (see Figs. 20-1 and 20-2 in Chapter 20). Because inflammation or fibrosis may accompany the presence of the lipid material, the CT attenuation of the consolidation need not be low, but in many cases, small areas of low-attenuation oil are visible within larger masses. In some patients, necrosis and cavitation may be present.

Lung Abscess

Lung abscess represents an infected, necrotic, pus-filled cavity. If communication with a bronchus occurs, partial drainage of the abscess contents may occur. With a chronic abscess, the wall of the cavity may be surrounded by granulation tissue or fibrosis.

Lung abscess may result from pyogenic bacteria, mycobacteria, fungal organisms, parasites, and, rarely, viral infections.

Many cases are caused by anaerobic organisms in association with poor oral hygiene and periodontal disease, conditions predisposing to aspiration, and old age. Lung abscess may also be associated with infection by *Klebsiella pneumoniae*, *Staphylococcus aureus*, *Pseudomonas aeruginosa*, *Nocardia* spp., *Actinomyces* spp., and TB. They may occur as complications of infarction, cavitary neoplasm, and cavitary conglomerate mass.

In patients with an anaerobic abscess, symptoms include low-grade fever, cough, and sputum production, often of several weeks' duration. In patients with other causes of bacterial abscess, symptoms usually are acute and resemble those of pneumonia.

On plain radiographs, acute lung abscesses usually appear as irregular masses. The outer aspect of an abscess may be very ill defined because of surrounding inflammation and lung consolidation. An air-fluid level may be seen if communication with a bronchus and partial drainage have occurred.

On CT, when contrast medium is infused, lung abscesses typically show a densely enhancing wall that is variable in thickness and irregular in contour (Fig. 9-39A). The internal wall of the abscess cavity often is shaggy (Fig. 9-40). The outer wall may be sharply marginated and smooth, irregular, or obscured by surrounding consolidation. The contents of a lung abscess appear low in attenuation (i.e., fluid attenuation) compared to the density of the enhancing wall or surrounding consolidated lung. An air-fluid level may be seen (see Fig. 9-10). Bronchi

A

B

FIG. 9.39. Lung abscess. **A:** Acutely, an irregular, fluid-filled abscess is visible in the left lung on contrast-enhanced CT. Its wall enhances. A small amount of air (*arrow*) is visible within the fluid-filled cavity. **B:** After healing, a thin-walled cystic lesion is visible in the left lower lobe.

FIG. 9.40. Lung abscess. Both the internal and the external walls of the cavitary lesion appear irregular or shaggy. An air bronchogram is seen within the abscess.

may be seen entering the abscess, an appearance that helps to distinguish lung abscess from empyema.

With healing, the wall of an abscess becomes thinner and more sharply defined (see Fig. 9-39B). The abscess tends to decrease in size, and the amount of fluid in the abscess decreases. Complete resolution or focal scarring is typical.

In patients with clinical symptoms of infection, the diagnosis of lung abscess usually is not difficult. However, the appearance of a peripheral abscess may overlap that of an empyema. This distinction is important to make because an empyema is often treated by tube drainage, whereas an abscess is not. Several findings usually assist in distinguishing these two entities.

Lung abscesses typically are round or oval in shape and form acute angles where they touch the pleural surface. Abscesses tend to have an irregularly thick wall in their acute stage. Because an abscess represents necrotic lung, pulmonary vessels or bronchi may be seen entering an abscess wall or may be seen within its center.

Empyemas typically are oval, lenticular, or crescentic in shape and usually show obtuse angles at the pleural surface. The walls of an empyema cavity tend to be smooth and uniform in thickness, although the wall may be partially obscured by adjacent atelectasis. Pulmonary vessels and bronchi are displaced by an empyema.

Lymphoma

Lymphoma may be associated with single or multiple lung nodules, masses, or focal masslike areas of consolidation. Cavitation may occur. The presence of associated lymph node enlargement is variable. Lymphomas are discussed in detail in Chapter 5.

Hodgkin's Disease

Hodgkin's disease (HD) involves lung in 10% of patients at the time of presentation. It is uncommon in untreated patients in the absence of radiographically visible mediastinal or ipsilateral hilar adenopathy. However, lung recurrence can be seen without node enlargement in patients with prior mediastinal and hilar radiation. Discrete, single or multiple, well-defined or ill-defined, large or small nodules or masslike lesions, or localized areas of air-space consolidation associated with air bronchograms, may all be seen (see Figs. 5-10 to 5-12 in Chapter 5). These can cavitate, with either thick or thin walls. Peripheral, subpleural masses are common.

Non-Hodgkin's Lymphoma

Non-Hodgkin's lymphoma (NHL) usually is a disseminated disease, and the lung is involved in 10% to 15% of cases. Lung involvement may appear as discrete nodules or masses, air-space consolidation, or infiltration contiguous with enlarged lymph nodes (see Figs. 5-21 and 5-29 in Chapter 5). Specific types of NHL include primary pulmonary lymphoma, AIDS-related lymphoma, mycosis fungoides, and plasmacytoma.

Primary pulmonary lymphoma is considered to be present if there is no evidence of extrathoracic disease for at least 3 months after the initial diagnosis of lung lymphoma. Primary pulmonary lymphoma may be classified as a low-grade B-cell lymphoma, usually derived from bronchus or mucosa-associated lymphoid tissue (malt lymphoma or MALToma), or high-grade lymphoma. Both may present as a solitary nodule or mass, multiple nodules or masses, or multifocal areas of consolidation, with or without associated lymph node enlargement.

AIDS-related lymphoma originates primarily in extranodal locations and commonly involves multiple sites, including the lung. Multiple pulmonary nodules and masses, ranging in size from 1 to 5 cm, are seen most commonly on radiographs or CT. The nodules usually are well-defined. Cavitation may be present but is not common.

Mycosis fungoides is a T-cell lymphoma that primarily affects the skin. Radiographic findings in patients with disseminated disease are similar to those of other lymphomas and include lung nodules, areas of lung consolidation, and hilar or mediastinal lymph node enlargement.

Plasmacytoma usually originates in bone; much less common is extramedullary plasmacytoma. Pulmonary nodules or mass lesions may be seen.

Lymphoproliferative Disease

In addition to HD and NHLs, pulmonary lymphoproliferative diseases represent a spectrum of focal and diffuse lung abnormalities associated with either a benign or a malignant course. As with the lymphomas, these may be associated with single or multiple lung nodules, masses, or focal masslike areas of consolidation, and cavitation may occur.

Focal lymphoid hyperplasia is an uncommon benign condition characterized histologically by localized proliferation of benign mononuclear cells including polyclonal lymphocytes, plasma cells, and histiocytes. Its most common radiologic manifestation is that of a solitary nodule or a focal area of consolidation, often containing air bronchograms (see Fig. 5-31 in Chapter 5). There is no associated lymphadenopathy.

Lymphomatoid granulomatosis encompasses a group of angiocentric, angiodestructive abnormalities characterized by a lymphoid infiltrate and a variable degree of cellular atypia. Progression to lymphoma may occur. The lung is the primary site of disease. Radiographic and CT findings consist of bilateral, poorly defined nodular lesions, ranging from 0.5 to 8 cm in diameter, with a basal predominance. Lesions may progress rapidly and cavitate, mimicking Wegener's granulomatosis.

Posttransplantation lymphoproliferative disorder (PTLD). Several histologic patterns of disease, ranging from a benign proliferation of lymphocytes to overtly malignant lymphoma, can occur after bone marrow or solid organ transplantation. These are known collectively as PTLD. PTLD can manifest as localized or disseminated disease and has a predilection for extranodal involvement. Lung involvement may occur as part of multiorgan disease or in isolation. In 85% of cases, radiographs and CT show single or multiple pulmonary nodules, which may be small or large (0.3 to 5 cm), well-defined or ill defined (see Fig. 5-33 in Chapter 5). Other findings include patchy or focal consolidation. Hilar or mediastinal lymphadenopathy is common.

Metastatic Neoplasm

Lung nodules are the most common thoracic manifestation of metastatic tumors, usually due to hematogenous spread (see Chapter 4).

Nodules of metastatic tumor tend to be sharply marginated. Poorly marginated nodules may be seen in the presence of surrounding hemorrhage, local invasion of adjacent lung, or lepidic growth. They tend to predominate in the lung bases because of relatively greater blood flow. Individual metastases may arise from the tips of small arteries, suggesting their hematogenous origin (i.e., the feeding vessel sign). Nodules may be of any size.

Cavitation of metastases is not as common as with primary lung carcinoma, but it does occur in 5% of cases. The likelihood of cavitation varies with histology. Cavitation is most common with squamous cell tumors, but it also may be seen in adenocarcinomas and in some sarcomas.

Calcification of metastases occurs most commonly with osteogenic sarcoma, chondrosarcoma, synovial sarcoma, thyroid carcinoma, and mucinous adenocarcinoma.

A subpleural predominance of nodules is common unless the nodules are very numerous. On HRCT, numerous nodules tend to involve the lung in a diffuse fashion without regard for specific anatomic structures, a distribution termed "random."

Multiple nodules are most common, and often the nodules vary in size. Benign nodular disease most often results in nodules of similar size. The size and number of nodules vary

greatly. Nodules may be small and very numerous (i.e., miliary); this appearance often is seen with very vascular tumors. Fewer, larger metastases also may be seen; when these are well-defined, they are referred to as *cannonball metastases.*

Most patients (80% to 90%) with multiple metastases have a history of neoplasm. In some patients, however, a history of a primary tumor is lacking at the time of diagnosis; in others, the primary tumor may never be found.

A metastatic tumor occasionally presents as a solitary nodule. About 5% to 10% of solitary nodules represent a solitary metastasis. Solitary metastases are most common with carcinoma of the colon, sarcomas, melanoma, and carcinomas of the kidney and testicle. Solitary metastases more often have a smooth margin than do the lesions of primary lung carcinoma.

Solitary metastases are least common in patients with carcinomas of the head and neck, bladder, breast, cervix, bile ducts, esophagus, ovary, prostate, and stomach; in patients with these tumors, a solitary nodule more likely represents a primary lung carcinoma.

Multiple pulmonary "leiomyomas" associated with smooth muscle tumors of the uterus in women (*benign metastasizing leiomyoma*) represent pulmonary metastases from a low-grade uterine leiomyosarcoma. Single or multiple lung masses usually are seen. They may be quite large, may calcify, and grow very slowly over a period of years.

Mucoid Impaction (Mucous Plug)

Mucous plugs mimicking the appearance of a lung nodule or nodules may be seen in a variety of conditions, including bronchial atresia (see Figs. 1-4 and 1-5 in Chapter 1), bronchial obstruction by a stricture or tumor, asthma, allergic bronchopulmonary aspergillosis, cystic fibrosis, and other causes of bronchiectasis (Fig. 9-41). In many cases, the characteristic branching appearance of the mucoid impaction allows it to be distinguished from other causes of a lung nodule. Air trapping or atelectasis may be associated. Mucous plugs often appear low in attenuation on CT, being less dense than the bronchial wall. High-attenuation mucous plugs may be seen on CT in patients with allergic bronchopulmonary aspergillosis due to calcification associated with the presence of aspergillus. Resolution of the mucous plug, revealing a dilated bronchus, may mimic cavitation of a solid lesion.

Mycetoma (Aspergilloma)

In patients with a preexisting cyst or cavity, a mycetoma or fungus ball can form as a result of saprophytic infection, usually by aspergillus; other fungi occasionally are involved. Patients may be asymptomatic. However, hemoptysis and hemorrhage are common presenting complaints because of inflammation in the wall of the cyst.

Chest radiographs often show a cyst or cavity containing a mass within its dependent portion (Fig. 9-42). Cysts are

FIG. 9.41. Mucoid impaction in bronchial atresia. A large oval mass in the right upper lobe represents a mucous plug distal to the atretic bronchial segment. Air in the dilated bronchial lumen (*arrows*) outlines the bronchial wall and mucous plug, resulting in an air-crescent sign.

commonly found in upper lobe and often result from prior TB or sarcoidosis (see Figs. 15-17 and 15-18 in Chapter 15). However, early in the development of the mycetoma, thickening of the wall of the preexisting cyst or adjacent pleural thickening may be the only recognizable finding and should

suggest the diagnosis. Gravitational shift of the intracavity mass may be seen with change in the patient's position. A rim of air outlining the top of the mycetoma and the inner wall of the cavity is characteristic and is termed the "air-crescent" sign (see Table 9-7).

On CT, a round or oval mass (the fungus ball) can be seen within the cavity, usually in a dependent location. An air-crescent sign may be seen. The wall of the associated cyst or cavity usually is thick. In patients with a developing mycetoma, the fungus ball can contain multiple bubbles of air.

Papillomatosis

In 2% to 5% of patients with a history of laryngeal papillomas, distal spread occurs, with involvement of the tracheobronchial tree, a condition referred to as *tracheobronchial papillomatosis*. The extension of papillomas to the bronchi, bronchioles, and lung parenchyma is rare but may occur. Papillomas may be visible radiographically as nodular mass lesions within the lung, usually multiple, which often cavitate. Eventually, cavitary lesions may progress to large, thick- or thin-walled cysts. Nodules representing papillomas may be seen within cysts (Fig. 9-43; see also Figs. 3-55 and 3-56 in Chapter 3). Squamous cell carcinoma may develop.

Paragonimiasis

Paragonimiasis results from infection by the lung fluke *Paragonimus westermani*. It is common in Southeast Asia and thus may be seen in recent immigrants to the United States. It is acquired by eating freshwater crustaceans. Flukes migrate through the bowel wall, peritoneum, diaphragm,

A   B

FIG. 9.42. Mycetoma (aspergilloma) seen on chest radiograph. **A:** Cystic lung disease in the left upper lobe is associated with an intracavity mass (*arrow*). **B:** On the prone image, the mass moves anteriorly (*arrow*).

FIG. 9.44. Paragonimiasis in a world traveler with hemoptysis. Radiograph coned to the right lung base shows multiple small nodules. Some cystic or cavitary lesions also are visible.

FIG. 9.43. Papillomatosis with multiple nodules. Detail view of the right lower lobe. Multiple well-defined nodules are visible, one of which is cavitary (*arrow*).

and pleura to reach the lungs, where they develop. They may result in the presence of ill-defined nodules or linear opacities, often multiple, with predominance at the lung bases (Fig. 9-44). Cysts or cavities may also be seen; irregular wall thickening may reflect the presence of the adult worm within a lung cyst.

Pneumatocele

Pneumatoceles are thin-walled, air-filled cysts that typically occur in association with infection. They may increase in size due to air trapping. Pneumatoceles are commonly seen in patients with *P. jiroveci* (*P. carinii*) pneumonia in association with AIDS, *S. aureus* pneumonia, and other bacterial infections. In distinction to lung abscess or pulmonary gangrene, the wall of an air-filled pneumatocele tends to be thin and of uniform thickness (Fig. 9-45).

Pulmonary Artery Aneurysm

Pulmonary artery aneurysms are rare. When they occur in relation to lobar, segmental, or smaller arteries, they may present as a lung nodule (Fig. 9-46). CT with contrast infusion is diagnostic, resulting in dense opacification. Pulmonary artery aneurysms may be (1) mycotic (see Fig. 9-46); (2) the result of catheter-related complications; or (3) associated with pulmonary hypertension (see Fig. 6-29 in Chapter 6) or diseases

such as Takayasu's arteritis, Williams' syndrome, Behçet's syndrome (Fig. 19-8 in Chapter 19), and prenatal varicella.

Rasmussen aneurysm is a mycotic aneurysm occurring in relation to an infectious cavity and is most typical of TB.

Pulmonary Vein Varix

Pulmonary vein varix represents a segmental dilatation of a pulmonary vein at or near its junction with the left atrium. Although varix may result from a congenital defect of the vein wall, many varices are associated with elevated pulmonary venous pressure and mitral valve disease. They are radiographically visible as round or oval densities in the medial third of either lung, typically adjacent to the left atrial shadow (Fig. 9-47). On the lateral view, they are noted in the typical location of pulmonary veins. They rarely cause symptoms

FIG. 9.45. Pneumatoceles in *Pneumocystis jiroveci* (*P. carinii*) pneumonia. High-resolution CT in a patient with AIDS shows ground-glass opacity consistent with *P. jiroveci* pneumonia. Thin-walled pneumatoceles are visible bilaterally.

FIG. 9.46. Pulmonary artery aneurysm following septic embolism. A small, densely opacified aneurysm (*arrow*) is visible at the left lung apex.

but can enlarge in response to increasing left atrial pressure and may rupture with hemorrhage. CT is diagnostic.

Pulmonary Gangrene

Rarely, patients with a lung infection develop an abscess containing a sequestrum of necrotic lung, identical to what is seen in patients with angioinvasive aspergillosis. This is termed *pulmonary gangrene*. Lung necrosis may be the result of direct action by bacterial toxins or ischemia resulting from thrombosis of small pulmonary arteries. It may occur in patients infected with *Klebsiella*, *Streptococcus pneumonia*, *Haemophilus influenzae*, *S. aureus*, or anaerobic bacteria. The presence of a mass in a cavity or an air-crescent sign is typical on radiographs or CT (Fig. 9-48).

Rheumatoid Nodules and Caplan's Syndrome

Rheumatoid (necrobiotic) nodules are an uncommon manifestation of rheumatoid arthritis. They often are asymptomatic but tend to appear and disappear in conjunction with subcutaneous nodules. They range in size from a few millimeters to 5 cm or more and may be solitary or multiple and numerous (Fig. 9-49). Rheumatoid nodules predominate in the lung periphery and typically are well-defined. They may cavitate, having thick walls that become thin with healing. Pleural effusion may be associated and cavitary nodules in the periphery may lead to pneumothorax.

Caplan's syndrome is a rare manifestation of rheumatoid arthritis that occurs in coal miners or patients with silicosis. It is characterized by single or multiple lung nodules ranging from a few millimeters to 5 cm in diameter, similar to those seen with rheumatoid nodules. Nodules may have an upper lobe predominance, resembling the appearance of silicosis, but nodules in Caplan's syndrome appear rapidly and in "crops," in contrast to the slow progression of pneumoconiosis.

Round Atelectasis

Round atelectasis represents focal rounded lung collapse, usually associated with pleural thickening or effusion. It typically appears as a focal mass lesion and is described in detail in Chapter 2.

Round atelectasis often shows characteristic findings on chest radiographs or CT. It usually is (1) round or oval in shape; (2) peripheral in location and abutting the pleural surface; (3) associated with curving of pulmonary vessels or bronchi into the edge of the lesion (the "comet-tail" sign);

A

B

FIG. 9.47. Pulmonary vein varix in mitral stenosis. **A:** On the PA radiograph, a well-defined oval opacity (*arrows*) overlies the shadow of the left atrium. **B:** On the lateral view, the opacity is localized to the junction of the pulmonary veins with the left atrium (*arrows*).

A   B

FIG. 9.48. Pulmonary gangrene in *Staphylococcus aureus* infection. **A:** Chest radiograph shows a thin-walled cavity (*arrows*) in the left upper lobe. The cavity contains an ill-defined opacity, representing a sequestrum of necrotic lung. **B:** HRCT shows the thin-walled cavity, a sequestrum of necrotic lung, and an air-crescent sign. This appearance is very similar to that seen with angioinvasive aspergillosis.

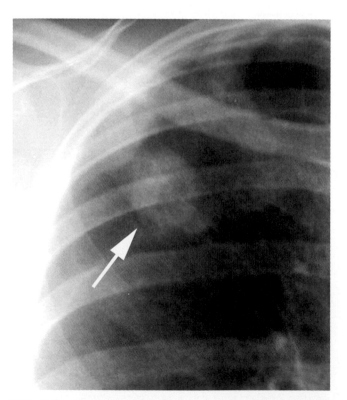

FIG. 9.49. Rheumatoid nodule. A well-defined nodule (*arrow*) is visible in the peripheral right upper lobe. A central lucency represents cavitation. Focal pleural thickening is visible adjacent to the nodule.

and (4) associated with an ipsilateral pleural abnormality, either effusion or pleural thickening, with the lesion contacting the abnormal pleural surface. If these criteria for rounded atelectasis are met, a confident diagnosis usually can be made, and radiographic follow-up should be sufficient. Rounded atelectasis is most common in the posterior lower lobes and, sometimes, is bilateral or symmetrical (see Figs. 2-42 to 2-46 in Chapter 2).

Sarcoidosis

Large masses or areas of consolidation, measuring 4 cm in diameter or larger, are seen in 15% to 25% of patients with active sarcoidosis (see Figs. 15-9 and 15-10 in Chapter 15). Because they may contain air bronchograms, they sometimes are termed *alveolar sarcoid*. These masses are due to the confluence of large numbers of small interstitial granulomas. They may be parahilar or peripheral in location, and they rarely cavitate. On CT, small nodules (*satellite nodules*) often are visible at the periphery of these masses. This occurrence is also termed the *galaxy sign*.

Pulmonary masses also may be seen in patients with end-stage sarcoidosis (see Fig. 15-12 in Chapter 15). Progressive fibrosis may lead to abnormal central conglomeration of parahilar bronchi and vessels, associated with masses of fibrous tissue, typically most marked in the upper lobes. This finding often is associated with bronchial dilation, a finding referred to as *traction bronchiectasis*. It is similar in appearance to that of progressive massive fibrosis in silicosis.

Septic Embolism With Infarction

Septic pulmonary emboli, with or without infarction, generally result in multiple parenchymal abnormalities; rarely does septic embolism present as a solitary lesion. The correct radiographic diagnosis usually is suggested by the finding of relatively well-defined, bilateral peripheral nodules with or without cavitation, especially in the setting of known intravenous drug abuse, or some other known source of sepsis.

In patients with septic embolism, peripheral nodules in varying stages of cavitation often are present, presumably due to intermittent seeding of the lungs by infected material (Fig. 9-50). The feeding vessel sign is visible in 65% of cases (see Fig. 9-50C). CT is helpful in showing the peripheral and subpleural location of the nodules (see Fig. 9-50B and C).

Sequestration

Sequestration represents an area of disorganized pulmonary parenchyma without normal pulmonary arterial or bronchial communications. Sequestration usually receives its blood supply from branches of the thoracic or abdominal aorta. There are two forms of sequestration, intralobar and extralobar.

Intralobar sequestration is more common. Two thirds of intralobar sequestrations are found adjacent to the diaphragm in relation to the posterior basal segment of the left lower lobe. Intralobar sequestration usually presents in adults or older children. Uncomplicated intralobar sequestration can have a variety of appearances. It may appear as (1) a homogeneous and well-defined mass lesion, (2) a cystic or multicystic air- and fluid-filled lesion, (3) a hyperlucent and hypovascular region of lung, or (4) a combination of these. Bilateral intralobar sequestrations may occur (see Figs. 1-26 to 1-29 in Chapter 1).

Extralobar sequestration represents an anomaly in which the sequestered tissue is enclosed within its only pleural envelope; it is less common than intralobar sequestration and

FIG. 9.50. Septic embolism in a patient with intravenous drug abuse and endocarditis. **A:** Chest radiograph shows lung nodules, which appear cavitary (*arrows*). **B:** CT shows the peripheral nature of the nodules (*arrows*), relatively well-defined margins, and a variable degree of cavitation. **C:** Several examples of the feeding vessel sign are visible (*arrow*). The nodules are peripheral in location.

often is diagnosed in neonates. Approximately 90% of cases are visible at the left lung base, contiguous with the left hemidiaphragm (see Figs. 1-30 and 1-31 in Chapter 1). Extralobar sequestration appears as a sharply marginated mass lesion, which does not contain air (unlike intralobar sequestration). It usually is homogeneous in appearance but may contain cystic areas. Its supplying artery may be seen on CT.

Wegener's Granulomatosis

Wegener's granulomatosis is a multisystem disease of unknown cause associated with the involvement of the upper respiratory tract (nasal, oral, or sinus inflammation), lower respiratory tract (airway or lung), and kidney (see Chapter 19). The presence of antineutrophilic cytoplasmic antibody (C-ANCA) is characteristic and is seen in 90% of cases.

Patients usually are between the ages of 30 and 60. At presentation, chest radiographic abnormalities are visible in 75% of patients with Wegener's granulomatosis. The most common radiographic abnormality is multiple lung nodules or masses; these are visible in more than half of patients at presentation. Typically, fewer than a dozen nodules are visible, but they may be more numerous. In most cases, the nodules are bilateral and widely distributed without predominance

in any lung region. A solitary nodule or mass may be seen, but this appearance is less common.

Masses usually range from 2 to 4 cm but may be up to 10 cm in diameter (Fig. 9-51; see also Figs. 19-9 and 19-10 in Chapter 19). Masses are round or oval in shape and may be well- or poorly defined. Cavitation occurs in approximately 50% of cases. Cavities usually are thick walled with an irregular inner margin. Air-fluid levels may be present. Calcification of the masses does not occur.

With the progression of disease, nodules and masses tend to increase in size and number. With treatment, nodules usually resolve over a period of months. Typically, cavitary nodules and masses become thin walled and decrease in size with treatment. Complete resolution may occur.

SELECTED READING

Au V, Leung AN. Radiologic manifestations of lymphoma in the thorax. AJR Am J Roentgenol 1997; 168:93–98.

Balakrishnan J, Meziane MA, Siegelman SS, Fishman EK. Pulmonary infarction: CT appearance with pathologic correlation. J Comput Assist Tomogr 1989; 13:941–945.

Bankoff MS, McEniff NJ, Bhadelia RA, et al. Prevalence of pathologically proven intrapulmonary lymph nodes and their appearance on CT. AJR Am J Roentgenol 1996; 167:629–630.

Bernard A, Azorin J, Bellenot F, et al. Resection of pulmonary nodules using video-assisted thoracic surgery. Ann Thorac Surg 1996; 61:202–204.

Calhoun P, Feldman PS, Armstrong P, et al. The clinical outcome of needle aspirations of the lung when cancer is not diagnosed. Ann Thorac Surg 1986; 41:592–596.

Davis SD. CT evaluation for pulmonary metastases in patients with extrathoracic malignancy. Radiology 1991; 180:1–12.

Dewan NA, Shehan CJ, Reeb SD, et al. Likelihood of malignancy in a solitary pulmonary nodule: comparison of Bayesian analysis and results of FDG-PET scan. Chest 1997; 112:416–422.

Gaeta M, Pandolfo I, Volta S, et al. Bronchus sign on CT in peripheral carcinoma of the lung: value in predicting results of transbronchial biopsy. AJR Am J Roentgenol 1991; 157:1181–1185.

Gould MK, Fletcher J, Iannettoni MD, et al.; American College of Chest Physicians. Evaluation of patients with pulmonary nodules: when is it lung cancer?: ACCP evidence-based clinical practice guidelines (2nd ed.). Chest 2007; 132:108S–130S.

Gupta NC, Maloof J, Gunel E. Probability of malignancy in solitary pulmonary nodules using fluorine-18-FDG and PET. J Nucl Med 1996; 37:943–948.

Gurney JW. Determining the likelihood of malignancy in solitary pulmonary nodules with Bayesian analysis. Part 1: theory. Radiology 1993; 186:405–413.

Gurney JW, Lyddon DM, McKay JA. Determining the likelihood of malignancy in solitary pulmonary nodules with Bayesian analysis. Part II: application. Radiology 1993; 186:415–422.

Hasegawa M, Sone S, Takashima S, et al. Growth rate of small lung cancers detected on mass CT screening. Br J Radiol 2000; 73:1252–1259.

Hirakata K, Nakata H, Haratake J. Appearance of pulmonary metastases on high-resolution CT scans: comparison with histopathologic findings from autopsy specimens. AJR Am J Roentgenol 1993; 161:37–43.

Huang RM, Naidich DP, Lubat E, et al. Septic pulmonary emboli: CT-radiographic correlation. AJR Am J Roentgenol 1989; 153:41–45.

Jang HJ, Lee KS, Kwon OJ, et al. Bronchioloalveolar carcinoma: focal area of ground-glass attenuation at thin-section CT as an early sign. Radiology 1996; 199:485–488.

Kuhlman JE, Fishman EK, Siegelman SS. Invasive pulmonary aspergillosis in acute leukemia: characteristic findings on CT, the CT halo sign, and the role of CT in early diagnosis. Radiology 1985; 157:611–614.

Kui M, Templeton PA, White CS, et al. Evaluation of the air bronchogram sign on CT in solitary pulmonary lesions. J Comput Assist Tomogr 1996; 20:983–986.

FIG. 9.51. Wegener's granulomatosis with multiple nodules. Multiple, poorly marginated nodules are visible in the right lung. Some appear cavitary. Free intraperitoneal air is the result of peritoneal dialysis for associated renal failure.

Kushihashi T, Munechika H, Ri K, et al. Bronchoalveolar adenoma of the lung: CT-pathologic correlation. Radiology 1994; 193:789–793.

Li HQ, Boiselle PM, Shepard JAO, et al. Diagnostic accuracy and safety of CT-guided percutaneous needle aspiration biopsy of the lung: comparison of small and large pulmonary nodules. AJR Am J Roentgenol 1996; 167:105–109.

Libby DM, Henschke CI, Yankelevitz DF. The solitary pulmonary nodule: update 1995. Am J Med 1995; 99:491–496.

MacMahon H, Austin JH, Gamsu G, et al.; Fleischner Society. Guidelines for management of small pulmonary nodules detected on CT scans: a statement from the Fleischner Society. Radiology 2005; 237:395–400.

Mahoney MC, Shipley RT, Cocoran HL, Dickson BA. CT demonstration of calcification in carcinoma of the lung. AJR Am J Roentgenol 1990; 154:255–258.

Munden RF, Pugatch RD, Liptay MJ, et al. Small pulmonary lesions detected at CT: clinical importance. Radiology 1997; 202:105–110.

Nathan MH, Collins VP, Adams RA. Differentiation of benign and malignant pulmonary nodules by growth rate. Radiology 1962; 79:221–231.

Patz EF, Lowe VJ, Hoffman JM. Focal pulmonary abnormalities: evaluation with F-18 fluorodeoxyglucose PET scanning. Radiology 1993; 188: 487–490.

Primack SL, Hartman TE, Lee KS, Müller NL. Pulmonary nodules and the CT halo sign. Radiology 1994; 190:513–515.

Quint LE, Park CH, Iannettoni MD. Solitary pulmonary nodules in patients with extrapulmonary neoplasms. Radiology 2000; 217:257–261.

Remy J, Remy-Jardin M, Giraud F, Wattinne L. Angioarchitecture of pulmonary arteriovenous malformations: clinical utility of three-dimensional helical CT. Radiology 1994; 191:657–664.

Schultz EM, Sanders GD, Trotter PR, et al. Validation of two models to estimate the probability of malignancy in patients with solitary pulmonary nodules. Thorax 2008; 63:335–341.

Siegelman SS, Khouri NF, Leo FP, et al. Solitary pulmonary nodules: CT assessment. Radiology 1986; 160:307–312.

Siegelman SS, Khouri NF, Scott WW, et al. Pulmonary hamartoma: CT findings. Radiology 1986; 160:313–317.

Theros EG. Varying manifestations of peripheral pulmonary neoplasms: a radiologic-pathologic correlative study. AJR Am J Roentgenol 1977; 128:893–914.

Webb WR. Radiologic evaluation of the solitary pulmonary nodule. AJR Am J Roentgenol 1990; 154:701–708.

Webb WR. The pleural tail sign. Radiology 1978; 127:309–313.

Weisbrod GL, Towers MJ, Chamberlain DW, et al. Thin-walled cystic lesions in bronchioalveolar carcinoma. Radiology 1992; 185: 401–405.

Zwiebel BR, Austin JHM, Grines MM. Bronchial carcinoid tumors: assessment with CT of location and intratumoral calcification in 31 patients. Radiology 1991; 179:483–486.

Zwirewich CV, Vedal S, Miller RR, Müller NL. Solitary pulmonary nodule: high-resolution CT and radiologic-pathologic correlation. Radiology 1991; 179:469–476.

Plain Film and High-resolution Computed Tomographic Assessment of Diffuse Infiltrative Lung Disease

W. RICHARD WEBB

Diffuse infiltrative lung diseases (DILDs) may be acute or chronic, involving the interstitium, alveolar spaces, or both. Specific DILDs are discussed in other chapters in this book. This chapter reviews the radiographic and high-resolution computed tomography (HRCT) diagnosis of DILDs, including important findings and the differential diagnosis of various patterns of disease. Airways disease and emphysema, although diffuse lung diseases, are not considered DILDs and are discussed in Chapters 23 and 24.

PLAIN RADIOGRAPHIC ASSESSMENT OF DIFFUSE INFILTRATIVE LUNG DISEASE

On plain radiographs, infiltrative diseases usually are classified according to the pattern of abnormality they produce. There are six basic patterns:

1. Air-space or alveolar consolidation
2. Linear or septal
3. Reticular
4. Nodular
5. Reticulonodular
6. Ground-glass opacity

Air-space or Alveolar Consolidation

The terms *air-space consolidation* and *alveolar consolidation* refer to diseases associated with pathologic filling of alveoli (i.e., replacement of alveolar air) as the predominant abnormality. As discussed in detail in Chapter 2, radiographic abnormalities indicating the presence of air-space or alveolar disease include (1) confluent or homogeneous opacities obscuring vessels, (2) air bronchograms, (3) ill-defined or fluffy opacities, (4) air alveolograms, (5) "acinar" or air-space nodules, (6) preserved lung volume, and (7) a tendency for opacities to extend to pleural surfaces.

The differential diagnosis of diffuse air-space consolidation is reviewed in detail in Chapter 2 and Table 2-1. Alveolar filling may be caused by

1. Water (e.g., pulmonary edema)
2. Blood (e.g., pulmonary hemorrhage)
3. Pus (e.g., pneumonia)
4. Cells (e.g., bronchioloalveolar carcinoma, lymphoma, eosinophilic pneumonia, organizing pneumonia (also known as bronchiolitis obliterans or BOOP), hypersensitivity pneumonitis, interstitial pneumonia)
5. Other substances (e.g., lipoprotein in alveolar proteinosis, lipid in lipoid pneumonia)

Linear or Septal Pattern

A linear pattern is defined by the presence of Kerley's A or B lines. Kerley's A and B lines result from thickening of interlobular septa; this pattern also may be referred to as *septal* (Table 10-1).

Kerley B lines are most common (Fig. 10-1). They are horizontal lines, 1 to 2 cm in length. They are seen in contact with the pleural surface and are best seen laterally at the costophrenic angles. The characteristic appearance of Kerley B lines results from the consistent size and regular organization of pulmonary lobules at the lung bases.

TABLE 10.1 Linear or Septal Pattern: Differential Diagnosis

Pulmonary edema (hydrostatic most common), typically symmetric
Lymphangitic spread of neoplasm, often asymmetric
Chronic or recurrent pulmonary hemorrhage and hemosiderosis
Pulmonary fibrosis (sarcoidosis most common)

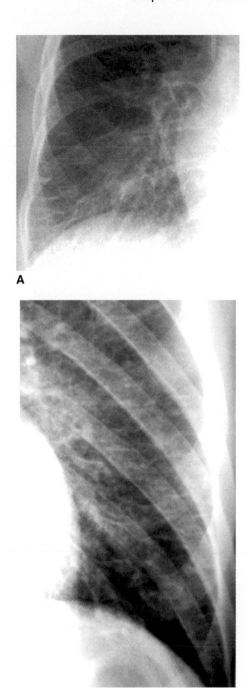

A

B

FIG. 10.1. Kerley B lines. Coned-down views of the right (**A**) and left (**B**) lateral costophrenic angles in two different patients with cardiogenic interstitial pulmonary edema. Thin horizontal lines in the lung periphery represent Kerley B lines. These represent thickened interlobular septa.

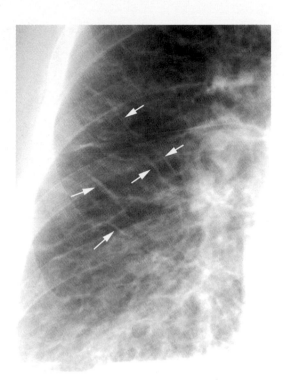

FIG. 10.2. Kerley A lines. A patient with pulmonary edema associated with fluid overload shows multiple Kerley A lines. Thin oblique lines in the parahilar lung (*arrows*) represent A lines. Thickening of the minor fissure also is seen.

Kerley C lines are seen at the lung bases and represent interlobular septa en face rather than in profile. They result in a nonspecific, reticular pattern and are unimportant in diagnosis, because B lines invariably are visible as well.

Peribronchial cuffing results from thickening of the peribronchovascular interstitium and also contributes to a linear pattern. This abnormality is seen as thickening of end-on bronchi or as lines radiating outward from the hila. To some extent, peribronchial cuffing contributes to the appearance of Kerley A lines on chest radiographs.

Well-defined and easily recognized Kerley's lines are indicative of interstitial lung disease and have a limited differential diagnosis. They are typical of interstitial pulmonary edema and lymphangitic spread of carcinoma. Edema usually is symmetrical. Lymphangitic spread often is asymmetrical; asymmetrical Kerley's lines strongly suggest lymphangitic spread of carcinoma.

Although consolidation may be seen with any type of pulmonary edema (e.g., hydrostatic, increased permeability with or without diffuse alveolar damage, or mixed), a septal pattern more often represents hydrostatic edema or increased permeability edema occurring in the absence of diffuse alveolar damage (see Chapter 11).

A septal pattern also can result from chronic or recurrent pulmonary hemorrhage and hemosiderosis.

Pulmonary fibrosis sometimes can result in well-defined Kerley's lines, but a reticular pattern is more typical. Kerley's

Kerley A lines are seen less often. They are oblique in orientation, several centimeters in length, and are located within the central or parahilar lung. Kerley A lines (Fig. 10-2) also represent thickened septa, but their appearance is different from that of B lines because of the different arrangement of pulmonary lobules in the parahilar lungs.

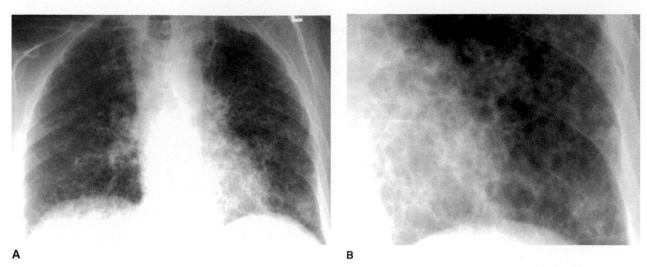

A   **B**

FIG. 10.3. Reticular pattern in rheumatoid lung disease. **A:** Chest radiograph shows decreased lung volumes and irregular reticular opacities at the lung bases. Kerley B lines are inconspicuous. The lines appear to outline spaces 1 cm or less in diameter, representing a medium reticular pattern. **B:** Coned-down view of the left lower lobe in the same patient shows the irregular reticular pattern.

lines in patients with fibrosis are seen most commonly in patients with sarcoidosis.

Reticular Pattern

"Reticular" means "netlike," which is an excellent description of the appearance of this pattern. A reticular pattern is characterized by multiple intersecting lines, often irregular in appearance, outlining round or irregular spaces (Fig. 10-3). Although a few Kerley lines may be visible, they do not predominate (if they did, the pattern would be linear). A reticular pattern indicates the presence of interstitial lung disease (Table 10-2).

The reticular pattern has been subdivided into three subpatterns, based on the size of the "spaces" surrounded by lines: a fine pattern (spaces smaller than 3 mm; Fig. 10-4), a medium pattern (spaces 3 to 10 mm; Fig. 10-5), and coarse pattern (spaces larger than 10 mm; Fig. 10-6). It should be kept in mind, however, that the size of the spaces visible on chest radiograph do not necessarily reflect the presence or size of the spaces present pathologically. Superimposition of the reticular opacities often confuses the picture; in the presence of extensive reticulation, the outlined spaces usually appear smaller than they really are (see Fig. 10-4). Medium or coarse patterns are the most common and the most easily seen on chest radiographs.

A medium pattern is typical of patients with pulmonary fibrosis and "honeycombing"; the reticulation often appears to have a peripheral, posterior, and lower lobe predominance (see Figs. 10-3 and 10-5). The abnormality often is best seen on the lateral view, just above the diaphragm, in the posterior costophrenic angles. Because of lung fibrosis, lung volumes usually appear reduced.

Honeycombing with a medium reticular pattern usually indicates the presence of *usual interstitial pneumonia* (UIP).

UIP can be seen in a variety of conditions; however, over 90% of cases of honeycombing result from a small group of diseases, including idiopathic pulmonary fibrosis (IPF), collagen-vascular disease, drug-related fibrosis, asbestosis, end-stage hypersensitivity pneumonitis, or end-stage sarcoidosis. *Nonspecific interstitial pneumonia* (NSIP) less commonly results in honeycombing; it often is associated with collagen-vascular disease. Honeycombing also may result from radiation lung fibrosis, as an end-stage of acute respiratory distress syndrome, and other entities. Lung volumes are characteristically reduced in the presence of honeycombing.

Some cystic lung diseases (e.g., Langerhans' cell histiocytosis, lymphangiomyomatosis [LAM]) result in a reticular pattern because of superimposition of the walls of cysts

TABLE 10.2 Reticular Pattern: Differential Diagnosis

Usual interstitial pneumonia
    Idiopathic pulmonary fibrosis
    Collagen-vascular disease
    Drug-related fibrosis
    Asbestosis
    End-stage hypersensitivity pneumonitis
    End-stage sarcoidosis
Nonspecific interstitial pneumonia
Radiation
End-stage adult respiratory distress syndrome
Cystic lung disease
    Langerhans' cell histiocytosis
    Lymphangiomyomatosis
    Tuberous sclerosis
    Sjögren's syndrome with LIP
    Lymphoid interstitial pneumonia (LIP)
    Cystic bronchiectasis
    Pneumonia with pneumatoceles (e.g., pneumocystis)
    Papillomatosis

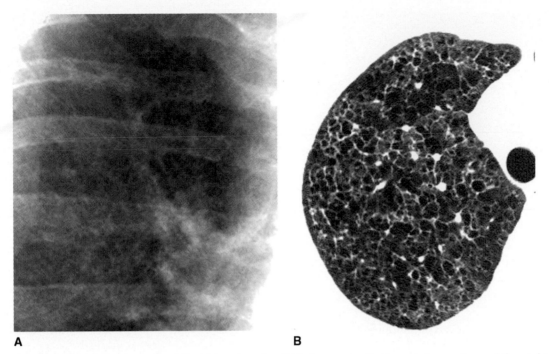

FIG. 10.4. Fine reticular pattern in Langerhans' cell histiocytosis. **A:** Coned-down view of the right upper lobe shows fine reticular opacities with poor definition of pulmonary arteries. **B:** HRCT shows cystic disease. Superimposition of the cyst walls results in the fine reticular pattern that is visible on chest radiographs.

FIG. 10.5. Medium reticular pattern in rheumatoid lung disease. **A:** Chest radiograph shows irregular reticular opacities, best classified as a medium pattern. **B:** HRCT shows reticular opacities associated with honeycombing in the anterior lung.

FIG. 10.6. Coarse reticular pattern in cystic lung disease. Coned-down view of the right apex shows reticular opacities outlining spaces exceeding 1 cm.

ranging in size from several millimeters to several centimeters in diameter (see Fig. 10-6). Depending on the size of the cysts, the pattern may be fine, medium, or coarse. This appearance can mimic honeycombing, but significant lung fibrosis is absent, and lung volumes are not reduced. In many such patients, lung volumes appear increased. An upper lobe predominance may be seen rather than predominance at the lung bases, depending on the responsible disease.

A fine reticular pattern may indicate fine lung fibrosis or lung infiltration by a variety of processes (see Fig. 10-4). This pattern is less common, more difficult to see, and less specific.

Nodular Pattern

Innumerable small nodules, ranging from a few millimeters to 1 cm in diameter, may indicate interstitial or air-space disease. The differential diagnosis of multiple larger nodules and masses is reviewed in Chapter 9.

Interstitial nodules usually are sharply marginated, despite being very small (Figs. 10-7 and 10-8). Air-space disease also may result in nodules (air-space or acinar nodules), typically 5 to 10 mm in diameter and poorly marginated. The term *miliary pattern* describes the presence of diffuse or widespread, well-defined nodules, 2 mm or less in diameter (see Figs. 10-7 and 10-8). Miliary nodules usually are interstitial.

Nearly all patients with nodules that are 5 mm or less in size, either well defined or ill defined, have a predominant interstitial abnormality; many will have metastases (Fig. 10-9) or a granulomatous disease (see Figs. 10-7 and 10-8; Table 10-3). Granulomatous diseases that may produce this appearance include infections (e.g., miliary

A   B   C

FIG. 10.7. Miliary nodules in hematogenous spread of coccidioidomycosis. Coned-down views from PA (**A**) and lateral (**B**) radiographs show innumerable nodules a few millimeters in diameter. **C:** HRCT shows innumerable, very small lung nodules.

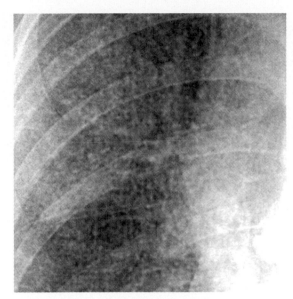

FIG. 10.8. Miliary tuberculosis. Coned-down view of the right upper lobe shows innumerable, discrete, very small nodules.

tuberculosis and fungus), noninfectious granulomatous diseases (e.g., sarcoid, histiocytosis, hypersensitivity pneumonitis), and some pneumoconioses (primarily silicosis and coal worker's pneumoconiosis [CWP]). Metastases tend to have a basal predominance because of greater blood flow to the bases (see Fig. 10-9); the granulomatous diseases and pneumoconioses, for a variety of reasons, often have an upper lobe predominance.

Nodules measuring 5 to 10 mm in diameter may be seen in these same diseases but are more typical of infection, particularly endobronchial spread of infection or bronchopneumonia. Common causes include tuberculosis (Fig. 10-10) and other mycobacterial, bacterial, viral infections such as cytomegalovirus or varicella, and *Pneumocystis* infection in patients with AIDS. Other causes of air-space consolidation also may result in ill-defined nodules. Diffuse bronchioloalveolar carcinoma often results in this appearance.

Reticulonodular Pattern

The term *reticulonodular*, indicating a perceived combination of lines and dots, is used commonly by radiologists but is of limited value in diagnosis. Reticulonodular opacities observed on plain radiographs often are artifactual, resulting from the superimposition of mostly lines or mostly nodules. Thus, it is generally a good idea, if a reticulonodular pattern is detected on plain radiographs, to decide whether a reticular or nodular pattern predominates and use that finding for differential diagnosis. Cases actually characterized histologically by a combination of reticular and nodular opacities are relatively uncommon but include sarcoidosis, lymphangitic spread of tumor, and diffuse amyloidosis.

Ground-glass Opacity

Ground-glass opacity represents an increase in lung density without the presence of frank consolidation (Fig. 10-11A). A slight fuzziness of pulmonary vessels usually is visible,

FIG. 10.9. Small nodules in metastatic melanoma. **A:** Numerous small nodules are visible, with a basal predominance. **B:** Detailed view of the right lower lobe shows small nodules.

TABLE 10.3 **Nodular Pattern: Differential Diagnosis**

Metastases: diffuse or basal, well-defined
Diffuse bronchioloalveolar carcinoma (diffuse or patchy, ill defined)
Miliary tuberculosis (diffuse, well-defined, may be upper lobe)
Miliary fungus (diffuse, well-defined)
Sarcoidosis (upper lobe, may be asymmetric, adenopathy)
Silicosis and CWP (posterior, upper lobe predominance, symmetric, adenopathy with eggshell calcification)
Histiocytosis (upper lobe predominance, cysts)
Hypersensitivity pneumonitis (ill defined)
Endobronchial infection (diffuse or patchy, ill defined)

FIG. 10.10. Endobronchial spread of tuberculosis. Ill-defined nodules ranging from 5 to 10 mm in diameter are visible.

but this abnormality can be quite subtle and difficult to diagnose with certainty. It is a nonspecific pattern (see the following section on HRCT) and can be seen in the presence of either air-space disease or interstitial disease. Because it is nonspecific, its differential diagnosis is very long. It may be seen with edema, hemorrhage, infections, and a wide variety of different DILDs. When visible on a chest film, it is best evaluated by assessment of the history and clinical presentation in patients with acute symptoms or by further imaging (e.g., HRCT) in patients with chronic symptoms (see Fig. 10-11B).

HRCT ASSESSMENT OF DIFFUSE INFILTRATIVE LUNG DISEASES

HRCT techniques optimize the radiographic demonstration of lung architecture and are invaluable in the assessment of patients with suspected DILD. The use of thin collimation

A

B

FIG. 10.11. Ground-glass opacity in exogenous lipoid pneumonia. **A:** Chest radiograph shows a subtle increase in lung opacity in the right parahilar region. Pulmonary vessels are poorly defined. **B:** HRCT coned down to the right lung shows patchy ground-glass opacity.

(1.5 mm or less) and a high-resolution algorithm for image reconstruction is essential.

HRCT may be obtained with volumetric imaging or with isolated spaced scans. Spaced axial images are usually sufficient for diagnosis of a diffuse lung disease and result in a significant reduction in radiation dose. Scanning at 1-cm intervals in the supine position is commonly employed.

Obtaining prone scans also is advisable. Some dependent (posterior) lung collapse often is seen on supine scans (Fig. 10-12A). Prone scans are valuable in distinguishing true posterior lung disease from dependent collapse; posterior lung collapse clears in the prone position (Fig. 10-12B). If spaced axial imaging is employed, scanning at 2-cm intervals in both the supine and the prone positions would be an appropriate protocol. In patients having volumetric HRCT, prone scans may be obtained volumetrically or at spaced intervals. Patients with normal or minimal chest film abnormalities benefit the most from prone scans.

Postexpiratory scans at selected levels can demonstrate air trapping and may be valuable in diagnosing airway disease in patients with normal inspiratory scans. Appropriate lung windows for viewing HRCT are mean −700 and width 1,000 HU or −600/1,500 HU.

NORMAL ANATOMY: THE SECONDARY PULMONARY LOBULE AND ACINUS

A *secondary pulmonary lobule* (also simply known as a *pulmonary lobule*) ranges from 1 to 2.5 cm in size and is marginated by connective tissue interlobular septa, which contain pulmonary veins and lymphatics (Figs. 10-13 and 10-14). Within the peripheral lung, interlobular septa are at the lower limit of HRCT resolution. On clinical HRCT in normal patients, a few interlobular septa often can be seen, but they tend to be inconspicuous.

The central portion of the secondary lobule, referred to as the *centrilobular region*, contains the pulmonary artery and bronchiolar branches that supply the lobule. The pulmonary artery supplying a secondary lobule measures somewhat less than 1 mm in diameter and can be seen in normal lungs as a dot or branching structure 5 to 10 mm from the pleural surface; the centrilobular bronchiole normally is invisible.

An *acinus* is the largest unit of lung structure in which all airways participate in gas exchange. Anatomically, it is located distal to a terminal bronchiole and is supplied by a first-order respiratory bronchiole (see Fig. 10-13). Acini average 7 to 8 mm in diameter. A pulmonary lobule usually consists of a dozen or fewer acini, although large lobules may contain twice that number. Acini are not visible on HRCT.

HRCT FINDINGS IN DIFFUSE INFILTRATIVE LUNG DISEASES

Chest films are normal in 10% to 15% of patients with interstitial lung disease. HRCT is more sensitive, specific, and accurate. HRCT characterizes morphologic abnormalities much more precisely and allows a more accurate diagnosis than do chest radiographs.

An approach to the HRCT diagnosis of DILD is fundamentally based on the recognition of specific abnormalities in lung anatomy, together with an assessment of their distribution. Generally speaking, HRCT findings of lung disease can be considered in four groups or categories, which reflect the types of histologic abnormalities present. These abnormalities include reticular opacities, nodular opacities, increased lung opacity, and decreased lung opacity or cystic lesions.

A

B

FIG. 10.12. Normal dependent lung collapse and the use of prone scans. **A:** Supine HRCT in a normal subject shows increased opacity in the posterior (dependent) lung. This appearance cannot be distinguished from lung disease. **B:** Prone scan shows that the posterior lung is normal.

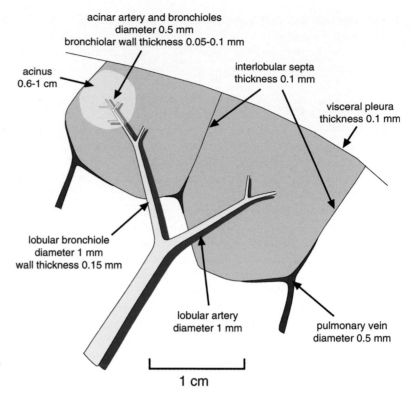

FIG. 10.13. Normal anatomy of the pulmonary lobule. Two lobules are shown.

Within each of these four categories, a relatively short list of findings may be recognized. Although some findings (e.g., "tree-in-bud" pattern, emphysema, mosaic perfusion, and air trapping) are features of airways and obstructive lung diseases rather than DILDs, they are discussed briefly in this chapter in order to describe an overall approach to HRCT.

Reticular Opacities

Thickening of the interstitial fiber network of the lung by fluid or fibrous tissue, or because of cellular infiltration, results in an increase in reticular lung opacities.

FIG. 10.14. Normal HRCT. **A:** The lung appears homogeneous in attenuation, with the posterior lung appearing slightly denser than the anterior lung. Fissures are smooth and uniform in thickness. Vessels are smooth in contour and sharply marginated. The most peripheral vessels visible are 5 to 10 mm from the pleural surface and represent centrilobular arteries or, sometimes, veins in interlobular septa. Centrilobular bronchioles and interlobular septa are not visible. **B:** Coneddown HRCT of the left lower lobe. Two pulmonary lobules are outlined by pulmonary veins within interlobular septa (*black arrows*). Centrilobular arteries are visible as dots (*white arrows*).

Interlobular Septal Thickening

Thickened interlobular septa can be recognized because they outline the margins of pulmonary lobules, which have a characteristic size and shape. In the peripheral lung, thickened septa measure 1 to 2 cm in length and often are seen extending to the pleural surface; in the central lung, the thickened septa can outline lobules that are 1 to 2.5 cm in diameter and appear polygonal in shape (Figs. 10-15 and 10-16). Visible lobules commonly contain a central dotlike or branching centrilobular artery.

Associated findings, regardless of the cause of septal thickening, often include peribronchial interstitial thickening recognized as peribronchial cuffing, thickening of fissures, and abnormal prominence of the centrilobular arteries (see Fig. 10-16).

Septal thickening can be smooth, nodular, or irregular in contour in different pathologic processes. *Smooth septal thickening* is most typical of pulmonary edema (see Fig. 10-15), lymphangitic spread of tumor (see Fig. 10-16), or, rarely, amyloidosis (Table 10-4). *Nodular septal thickening* reflects a perilymphatic distribution of nodules and is typical of sarcoidosis and lymphangitic spread of tumor. Septal thickening is not common in patients with interstitial fibrosis, except for those with sarcoidosis; when visible, septal thickening due to fibrosis often is irregular in appearance and associated with distortion of lung architecture.

Honeycombing

Honeycombing reflects extensive lung fibrosis with alveolar destruction and results in a characteristic reticular

FIG. 10.16. Interlobular septal thickening in lymphangitic spread of lung cancer. Smooth thickening of septa is visible within the right lung. The left lung appears normal. Peribronchial interstitial thickening recognized as peribronchial cuffing on the right. The right bronchi appear thicker walled than those on the left. A right pleural effusion also is present.

appearance. On HRCT, honeycombing results in thick-walled, air-filled cysts, usually measuring from 3 mm to 1 cm in diameter (although they may be larger or smaller), immediately beneath the pleural surface. When extensive honeycombing is present, the cysts occur in several layers and characteristically share walls (Fig. 10-17). With early or minimal honeycombing, scattered cysts are visible beneath the pleural surface, rather than layers of clusters of cysts (Fig. 10-17C and D).

When honeycombing is present, normal lung architecture is distorted, and secondary lobules are difficult or impossible to recognize. Associated findings of fibrosis, including reticular opacities, traction bronchiectasis, and traction bronchiolectasis, are usually present.

The presence of honeycombing usually predicts the presence of UIP. The differential diagnosis of honeycombing is that of UIP and includes IPF, which accounts for 60% to 70% of cases of honeycombing; collagen-vascular diseases (most often rheumatoid arthritis and scleroderma); fibrotic drug reactions; asbestosis, chronic or end-stage hypersensitivity pneumonitis; and, occasionally, sarcoidosis (Table 10-5). This appearance also may be seen with fibrotic NSIP. It usually is easy to distinguish honeycombing from cystic disease on HRCT (as opposed to plain radiographs), and diseases such as histiocytosis and LAM usually are not considered in the differential diagnosis.

FIG. 10.15. Interlobular septal thickening in interstitial pulmonary edema. Smooth thickening of numerous septa is visible in the right lung. The thickened septa outline lobules of characteristic size and shape. Centrilobular arteries (*arrows*) are visible within many of the lobules.

TABLE 10.4 Smooth Interlobular Septal Thickening: Differential Diagnosis

Lymphangitic spread of tumor (asymmetrical or symmetrical)
Pulmonary edema (symmetrical)
Amyloidosis (rare)

FIG. 10.17. Honeycombing. A: Patchy areas of subpleural honeycombing (*arrows*) are visible in a patient with rheumatoid arthritis and lung fibrosis. The cysts share walls and occur in multiple layers in the subpleural lung. **B:** Honeycombing in a patient with scleroderma. Cysts tend to be clustered. Several cysts are larger than 1 cm. **C:** Honeycombing in a patient with idiopathic pulmonary fibrosis. In the posterior lung, cysts are seen in a single layer. **D:** Early honeycombing in a patient with lupus. Focal fibrosis is visible posteriorly on a prone scan. Scattered subpleural honeycomb cysts are visible (*arrows*).

TABLE 10.5 Honeycombing: Differential Diagnosis

Usual interstitial pneumonia
   Idiopathic pulmonary fibrosis
   Collagen-vascular disease (often rheumatoid arthritis or
     scleroderma)
   Drug-related fibrosis
   Asbestosis
   End-stage hypersensitivity pneumonitis
   End-stage sarcoidosis
Nonspecific interstitial pneumonia
Radiation
End-stage acute respiratory distress syndrome

A

The identification of honeycombing on HRCT is of great clinical importance for the following reasons:

1. It indicates end-stage disease in most patients, although progression can be seen in some patients with honeycombing.
2. It indicates that a lung biopsy probably will not prove diagnostic (other than showing UIP). Lung biopsy is not often performed in patients with obvious honeycombing.
3. In a patient without an associated disease (e.g., collagen-vascular disease) or exposure (e.g., asbestos, drugs, organic antigens), IPF is likely the diagnosis.
4. It points to a poor prognosis in patients with IPF (5-year survival rate in patients with IPF is 20%).

Nonspecific Reticular Patterns

Reticular patterns other than interlobular septal thickening and honeycombing are somewhat nonspecific and may indicate lung fibrosis or lung infiltration without fibrosis. The reticular opacities may be very fine and difficult to see or may be coarse and irregular. They often reflect the presence of intralobular interstitial thickening, or thickening of the lung interstitium at a sublobular level (Fig. 10-18).

A reticular pattern not associated with traction bronchiectasis may represent mild fibrosis (see Fig. 10-18A) or may be seen in association with ground-glass opacity, nodules, or other findings in patients with infiltrative or inflammatory lung disease (see Fig. 10-18B). When this is the case, it is most appropriate to ignore the reticulation and base the differential diagnosis on the other findings present. When reticular opacities are visible, the presence of "traction bronchiectasis" is important in determining that fibrosis is present.

Traction Bronchiectasis

The term *traction bronchiectasis* refers to bronchial dilatation occurring as a result of lung fibrosis. It typically is associated with a reticular pattern, lung distortion, or honeycombing. Bronchi tend to be quite irregular or corkscrewed in appearance (Fig. 10-19). In comparison to garden variety bronchiectasis associated with infection, mucous plugging

B

FIG. 10.18. Fine reticular opacities (intralobular interstitial thickening). **A:** Prone HRCT in a patient with scleroderma shows fine reticular opacities in the posterior left lung (*arrows*). This represents mild lung fibrosis. **B:** HRCT in a patient with alveolar proteinosis shows a fine reticular pattern in the right lung associated with ground-glass opacity. Some septal thickening is also visible. This appearance represents interstitial infiltration rather than fibrosis.

or fluid within the bronchi is absent. The appearance of traction bronchiectasis in the peripheral lung may overlap with that of honeycombing.

Dilatation of small peripheral bronchioles also may be seen in the presence of lung fibrosis and is termed *traction bronchiolectasis*. Normally, bronchi are not visible in the peripheral 1 to 2 cm of lung; if they are visible, bronchiolectasis is present. If this finding is seen in combination with a reticular pattern, fibrosis is the likely cause.

Traction bronchiectasis and traction bronchiolectasis are very helpful in suggesting the presence of fibrosis when honeycombing is absent (Fig. 10-19B and C). Although the differential diagnosis of traction bronchiectasis without honeycombing includes UIP, other diseases are more likely when this pattern of fibrosis is present, including sarcoidosis, hypersensitivity pneumonitis, and NSIP (Table 10-6). Because of this possibility and the greater likelihood that treatment may be effective when this pattern is present, lung biopsy may be performed.

FIG. 10.19. Reticular opacities with traction bronchiectasis. **A:** Prone HRCT in a patient with lung fibrosis shows an extensive reticular pattern associated with multiple irregularly dilated (cork-screwed) bronchi (*large arrows*). This is termed *traction bronchiectasis*. A few scattered subpleural honeycomb cysts also are visible in the posterior subpleural lung (*small arrows*). **B:** A patient with NSIP shows reticular opacities with irregular dilatation of multiple bronchi. This finding indicates the presence of lung fibrosis. There is no evidence of honeycombing. **C:** Prone HRCT in a patient with mixed connective tissue disease shows a fine reticular pattern. This appearance is nonspecific, but the presence of multiple dilated bronchi (*arrows*) indicates that lung fibrosis is present. There is no evidence of honeycombing. This appearance probably is due to nonspecific interstitial pneumonia. **D:** Lung slice in a patient with idiopathic pulmonary fibrosis, traction bronchiectasis (*arrows*), and honeycombing in the subpleural lung.

TABLE 10.6 Traction Bronchiectasis without Honeycombing: Differential Diagnosis

Nonspecific interstitial pneumonia
Usual interstitial pneumonia and its causes (see above)
Sarcoidosis
Hypersensitivity pneumonitis
Radiation
End-stage acute respiratory distress syndrome

Nodules

Nodules as small as 1 to 2 mm in diameter can be detected on HRCT in patients with DILD. Nodules can be classified by (1) their appearance as well defined (and thus most likely interstitial) or ill defined (and most likely "air-space"), (2) their overall distribution, or (3) their specific anatomic distribution relative to lung structures. Although taking account of each of these features is important, recognition of the specific anatomic distribution of nodules is fundamental to their accurate diagnosis.

Nodules can be classified as perilymphatic, random, or centrilobular in distribution on HRCT.

Perilymphatic Nodules

Perilymphatic nodules occur in relation to lung lymphatics. They usually are well defined. They involve specific lung regions: (1) the subpleural interstitium at the pleural surfaces and fissures, (2) the peribronchovascular interstitium in the parahilar lung, (3) the interlobular septa, and (4) the peribronchovascular interstitium in a centrilobular location (Fig. 10-20).

In clinical practice, perilymphatic nodules usually are the result of sarcoidosis (see Chapter 15), which tends to have a peribronchovascular and subpleural predominance of nodules (Fig. 10-21), or lymphangitic spread of tumor (see Chapter 4), which typically predominates in relation to interlobular septa and the peribronchovascular interstitium (Fig. 10-22; Table 10-7). Sarcoidosis usually shows more extensive abnormalities in the upper lobes and may be symmetrical or asymmetrical. Lymphangitic spread of carcinoma usually is most severe at the lung bases and often is asymmetrical.

Silicosis and CWP also may result in this pattern, predominating in the subpleural and centrilobular peribronchovascular regions (see Chapter 18). However, silicosis and CWP are best recognized by a symmetrical, posterior, upper lobe predominance of nodules. Also, an exposure history usually is available. Rarely, amyloidosis (see Chapter 21) or lymphoid interstitial pneumonitis (LIP; see Chapter 13) results in this pattern.

Random Nodules

Random nodules are randomly distributed relative to structures of the secondary lobule and lung and appear diffuse and uniform in distribution (Figs. 10-23 and 10-7C). Subpleural nodules often are seen. Nodules usually are well defined.

The random nodule pattern is most typical of miliary tuberculosis (Fig. 10-24) or fungal infection (see Fig. 10-7C) and hematogenous metastases (Fig. 10-25), but sarcoidosis, when diffuse, also can show this pattern (Table 10-8).

FIG. 10.20. Locations of "perilymphatic" nodules. **A:** Nodules are visible in the subpleural regions and adjacent to fissures, the parahilar region adjacent to vessels and bronchi, the interlobular septa, and the peribronchovascular interstitium in a centrilobular location. **B:** Simulated perilymphatic nodules. Nodules are visible in the subpleural regions (*black arrow*), peribronchovascular regions (*large white arrow*), and in relation to interlobular septae (*small white arrow*).

A   B

FIG. 10.21. A, B: Perilymphatic nodules on HRCT in two patients with sarcoidosis. Nodules involve the subpleural interstitium (*large arrows*) in the lung periphery and adjacent to the fissure. Parahilar peribronchovascular nodules (*small arrows*) also are visible. Septal nodules and centrilobular nodules are visible but are less numerous.

Centrilobular Nodules

Centrilobular nodules often reflect bronchiolar or peribronchiolar abnormalities in a centrilobular location, although abnormalities occurring in relation to small vessels also may result in this finding. Most peripheral nodules often are centered 5 to 10 mm from the pleural surface and do not touch the pleura unless they are large (unlike the other two patterns) (Fig. 10-26). Because lobules are all of similar size, centrilobular nodules tend to be evenly spaced. Nodules may be well- or ill defined, or a centrilobular rosette of small nodules may be seen (Fig. 10-27). Nodules may involve the lung diffusely or be patchy.

Centrilobular nodules can be seen in endobronchial spread of tuberculosis or other causes of bronchopneumonia (see Fig. 10-27A), endobronchial spread of tumor (e.g., bronchioloalveolar carcinoma [BAC]; see Fig. 3-8 in Chapter 3), hypersensitivity pneumonitis (see Fig. 10-27B and C); organizing pneumonia (BOOP), silicosis and CWP, histiocytosis, or vascular diseases such as vasculitis and pulmonary edema (Table 10-9).

When centrilobular nodules are the predominant finding, diseases involving the small airways are most likely. Consider infection, hypersensitivity pneumonitis (which may be diagnosed by history), and remember BAC.

Centrilobular Tree-in-bud Pattern

When a centrilobular distribution of nodules is present, the "tree-in-bud" pattern should be sought (see Fig. 10-26A). This finding nearly always represents the presence of dilated and fluid-filled (with mucus or pus) centrilobular bronchioles (Fig. 10-28). Nodular branching opacities are visible in the lung periphery, and these are considerably larger than normal branching vessels. Trees-in-bud, which are centrilobular, tend to be centered 5 to 10 mm from the pleural surface when they

FIG. 10.22. Lymphangitic spread of breast carcinoma. Multiple nodules (*arrows*) are visible in relation to interlobular septa.

TABLE 10.7	Perilymphatic Nodules: Differential Diagnosis

Sarcoidosis
Lymphangitic spread of tumor
Silicosis and coal-worker's pneumoconiosis
Amyloidosis (rare)
Lymphoid interstitial pneumonitis (rare)

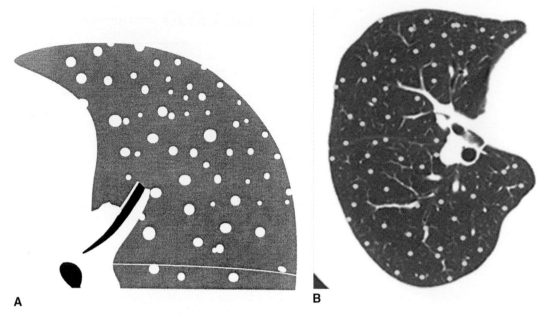

A   **B**

FIG. 10.23. Random nodules. A: Nodules may involve the pleural surfaces, peribronchovascular interstitium, and interlobular septa but do not show a predominance in relation to these structures as is present with a perilymphatic pattern. The overall distribution appears diffuse and uniform. **B:** Simulated random nodules. Compare with Figure 10-20B.

are seen in the peripheral lung. Centrilobular nodules or clusters of nodules (rosettes) also may be seen.

The presence of the tree-in-bud pattern is of great value in differential diagnosis. Because this finding represents dilatation and impaction of small centrilobular bronchioles, it confirms the presence of airway disease. Furthermore, the tree-in-bud appearance almost always indicates the presence of infection (e.g., tuberculosis, *Mycobacterium avium* com-

plex, bacteria, fungus) or infected airway disease (e.g., bronchiectasis, cystic fibrosis; Fig. 10-28). On occasion, it may be due to aspiration, asthma with mucous plugging, allergic bronchopulmonary aspergillosis, or endobronchial spread of tumor (Table 10-10).

This finding means the diagnosis should be made by examination or culture of sputum. If not, bronchoalveolar lavage is likely to be diagnostic.

A   **B**

FIG. 10.24. Random nodules in two patients with miliary tuberculosis. A: The nodules are small, sharply defined, and diffuse and uniform in distribution. **B:** Nodules involve the pleural surfaces and are diffuse.

FIG. 10.25. Random nodules of metastatic lung carcinoma. The primary carcinoma is visible in the left upper lobe. The nodules are diffuse and uniform in distribution.

Distribution of Nodules: A Diagnostic Algorithm

On HRCT, it is possible to distinguish these three specific distributions of nodules—perilymphatic, random, or

TABLE 10.8	Random Nodules: Differential Diagnosis

Miliary infections
Hematogenous metastases
Sarcoidosis

centrilobular nodules (and tree-in-bud)—by using a simple algorithm (Fig. 10-29).

The first step is to look for subpleural nodules and nodules seen in relation to the fissures. If they are absent, the nodules are centrilobular. Once it has been confirmed that the nodules are centrilobular, the presence of tree-in-bud should be sought.

If pleural or fissural nodules are present, then the pattern is either perilymphatic or random. These two patterns are then distinguished by looking at the distribution of other nodules. If they are patchy in distribution, particularly if a distinct peribronchovascular or septal distribution is present, then the nodules are perilymphatic; if the nodules are diffuse and uniform, the pattern is random. Using this approach, 94% of cases can be accurately classified.

Increased Lung Opacity

Increased lung opacity may be classified as consolidation or ground-glass opacity.

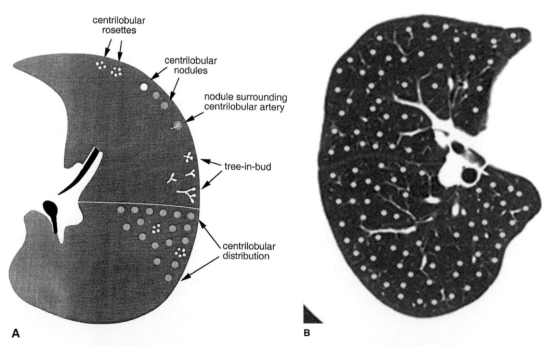

A　　　　　　　　　　　**B**

FIG. 10.26. Centrilobular nodules. **A:** Nodules spare the pleural surfaces unless they are large and tend to be centered 5 to 10 mm from the pleural surface or fissures. Because lobules are of similar size, nodules appear evenly spaced. Nodules may be well- or ill defined or may appear as a rosette of smaller nodules. The finding of the tree-in-bud pattern, which almost always represents dilatation and impaction of bronchioles, also is centrilobular in location. **B:** Simulated centrilobular nodules. Compare with Figure 10-20B.

A

B

C

FIG. 10.27. Centrilobular nodules. A: Bacterial bronchopneumonia with patchy centrilobular nodules in the lower lobe. The most peripheral nodules are centered 5 to 10 mm from the pleural surface and spare the pleura. Small rosettes also are visible. **B:** Centrilobular nodules in hypersensitivity pneumonitis. Note that the nodules spare the fissure (*arrow*) and pleural surface. The nodules are diffuse and appear evenly spaced. **C:** Hypersensitivity pneumonitis with centrilobular nodules of ground-glass opacity.

TABLE 10.9 **Centrilobular Nodules: Differential Diagnosis**

Bronchopneumonia or infectious bronchiolitis of any cause
Endobronchial spread of infection (bacteria, virus, tuberculosis, mycobacteria, fungus)
Endobronchial spread of tumor (bronchioloalveolar carcinoma)
Hypersensitivity pneumonitis
Respiratory bronchiolitis in a smoker
Follicular bronchiolitis
Organizing pneumonia (BOOP)
Silicosis and coal-worker's pneumoconiosis
Histiocytosis
Aspiration
Pulmonary edema or hemorrhage
Vasculitis

Air-space Consolidation

Air-space consolidation is said to be present when alveolar air is replaced by fluid, cells, or other substances. On HRCT, consolidation results in an increase in lung opacity associated with obscuration of underlying vessels. Air bronchograms may be present.

If another pattern also is present (e.g., small nodules), the consolidation probably represents confluent disease and should be ignored for the purposes of differential diagnosis.

The differential diagnosis of consolidation is based primarily on the duration of symptoms. In patients with acute symptoms, pneumonia, pulmonary edema, pulmonary hemorrhage, and acute lung injury (resulting in the acute respiratory distress syndrome) are most likely (see Table 10-10).

FIG. 10.28. Tree-in-bud. **A:** Tree-in-bud (*arrows*) in the right lower lobe in a patient with cystic fibrosis. A branching opacity in the peripheral lung (i.e., the tree) represents a dilated centrilobular bronchiole impacted with mucus and pus. Small, rounded opacities at the tips of the branches (i.e., the buds) represent peribronchiolar inflammation. Bronchial wall thickening and mosaic perfusion also are visible. **B:** Several examples of tree-in-bud (*arrows*) in another patient with airway infection. These appear larger than normal branching vessels in the peripheral lung, visible posteriorly. **C:** Tree-in-bud in a patient with *Pseudomonas bronchopneumonia*. **D:** Centrilobular nodules and tree-in-bud in a patient with *Haemophilus influenzae* bronchopneumonia.

TABLE 10.10 Tree-in-bud: Differential Diagnosis

Endobronchial spread of infection (bacteria, tuberculosis, mycobacteria, fungus)
Airways diseases with infection (e.g., cystic fibrosis, bronchiectasis)
Mucous plugging (asthma, allergic bronchopulmonary aspergillosis)
Aspiration
Bronchioloalveolar carcinoma (rare)

Among patients with chronic symptoms, the most common causes of this finding include chronic eosinophilic pneumonia (Fig. 10-30A), organizing pneumonia (BOOP; Fig. 10-30B), and interstitial pneumonia such as NSIP (Table 10-11). BAC also may result in this pattern.

Ground-glass Opacity

Ground-glass opacity is a nonspecific term referring to a hazy increase in lung opacity that is not associated with

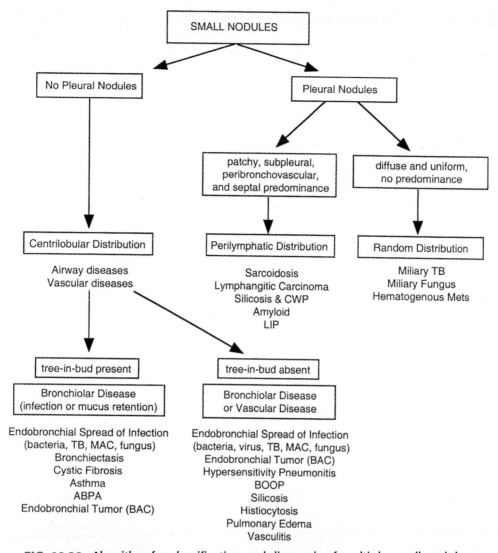

FIG. 10.29. Algorithm for classification and diagnosis of multiple small nodules.

A   B

FIG. 10.30. Consolidation. A: Homogeneous areas of consolidation are visible in the peripheral lung. This represents chronic eosinophilic pneumonia. **B:** Patchy areas of consolidation with air bronchogram in a patient with organizing pneumonia (BOOP).

TABLE 10.11 Air-space Consolidation: Differential Diagnosis

Acute symptoms
    Pneumonia
    Pulmonary edema
    Pulmonary hemorrhage
    Acute respiratory distress syndrome

Chronic symptoms
    Chronic eosinophilic pneumonia or other eosinophilic
      disease
    Organizing pneumonia (BOOP)
    Interstitial pneumonias
    Lipoid pneumonia
    Bronchioloalveolar carcinoma

obscuration of underlying vessels (see Figs. 10-11B, 10-18B, and 10-31), although they may appear fuzzy. This finding can reflect the presence of a number of diseases and can be seen in patients with either minimal interstitial thickening or minimal air-space disease. Although ground-glass opacity is a nonspecific finding, its presence is very significant. As with consolidation, the differential diagnosis is based primarily on the duration of symptoms.

In patients with acute symptoms, the presence of ground-glass opacity reflects active disease such as pulmonary edema (Fig. 10-31A) or hemorrhage, pneumonia (e.g., *Pneumocystis* or viral pneumonias (Fig. 10-31B and C), diffuse alveolar damage, acute interstitial pneumonia, and hypersensitivity pneumonitis (Table 10-12).

A

C

B

FIG. 10.31. Ground-glass opacity. **A:** A peripheral increase in lung attenuation represents ground-glass opacity. Vessels remain visible in the dense lung regions. This patient had acute dyspnea due to pulmonary edema. **B:** Patchy ground-glass opacity is visible in the upper lobes. This immunosuppressed patient had symptoms of acute fever and cough. Bronchoscopy revealed cytomegalovirus pneumonia. **C:** Parahilar ground-glass opacity in a patient with acute dyspnea related to *Pneumocystis* pneumonia. **D:** Patchy ground-glass opacity in a patient with progressive dyspnea over a period of months due to hypersensitivity pneumonitis.

D

TABLE 10.12 Ground-glass Opacity: Differential Diagnosis

Acute symptoms
Pulmonary edema
Hemorrhage
Pneumonia (e.g., *Pneumocystis jiroveci* [*P. carinii*] or viral pneumonias)
Diffuse alveolar damage
Acute interstitial pneumonia
Hypersensitivity pneumonitis (acute)

Chronic symptoms
Nonspecific interstitial pneumonia
Desquamative interstitial pneumonitis
Hypersensitivity pneumonitis (subacute or chronic)
Alveolar proteinosis
Sarcoidosis
Lipoid pneumonia
Bronchioloalveolar carcinoma

In patients with subacute or chronic symptoms, ground-glass opacity usually (60% to 80% of cases) indicates an acute, active, and potentially treatable process, such as NSIP, desquamative interstitial pneumonitis, hypersensitivity pneumonitis (Fig. 10-31D), alveolar proteinosis (see Figs. 10-18B and 10-32), sarcoidosis, lipoid pneumonia (see Fig. 10-11B), and BAC. Because of its association with active lung disease, the clinical diagnosis should be pursued. The presence of this finding often leads to lung biopsy, depending on the clinical status of the patient.

The combination of ground-glass opacity and interlobular septal thickening is termed *crazy paving* (see Fig. 10-32). This appearance is nonspecific and may be seen with a variety of acute lung diseases such as *Pneumocystis* or viral pneumonia, edema, hemorrhage, and acute lung injury. Among patients with chronic lung disease, it often is the result of alveolar proteinosis, although it may be seen in any chronic infiltrative lung disease characterized by ground-glass opacity.

When ground-glass opacity is associated with reticulation and findings of fibrosis such as traction bronchiectasis (Fig. 10-33) and particularly when they are seen in the same lung regions, the ground-glass opacity is likely to be due to fibrosis rather than active disease. In this situation, it is necessary to hedge in the interpretation; in most cases, the differential diagnosis is the same as for traction bronchiectasis (Table 10-6). Biopsy may be warranted and can be directed to areas showing the least evidence of fibrosis.

Decreased Lung Opacity and Cystic Lesions

Geographic areas of decreased lung attenuation may represent emphysema, mosaic perfusion, or air trapping (on expiratory scans). Circumscribed areas of decreased lung attenuation may represent emphysema or lung cysts.

Emphysema

Emphysema results in areas of very low attenuation, usually less than −950 HU. The appearance of emphysema is characteristic and depends on the type of emphysema present (Fig. 10-34). Typical appearances are as follows:

Centrilobular emphysema: focal areas of lucency without visible walls, usually with an upper lobe predominance (see Fig. 24-6 in Chapter 24)

Panlobular emphysema: large areas of low attenuation, usually diffuse and associated with decreased vessel size (see Fig. 24-9 in Chapter 24)

Paraseptal emphysema: subpleural lucencies marginated by interlobular septa, or subpleural bullae, usually with an upper lobe predominance (see Fig. 24-11 in Chapter 24).

Lung Cysts

Lung cyst is a nonspecific term, used to describe a thin-walled (usually less than 3 mm), well-defined and circumscribed, air-containing lesion, 1 cm or more in diameter.

FIG. 10.32. Ground-glass opacity with "crazy paving." Patchy ground-glass opacity is associated with interlobular septal thickening in the abnormal regions. This represents alveolar proteinosis.

FIG. 10.33. Ground-glass opacity associated with traction bronchiectasis. Fibrosis in the posterior lung bases is associated with ground-glass opacity and reticulation. The presence of traction bronchiectasis (*arrows*) indicates that the ground-glass opacity is likely due to fibrosis.

FIG. 10.34. Appearances of emphysema. **A:** Centrilobular emphysema. Focal areas of lucency without visible walls are visible in the left upper lobe. **B:** Panlobular emphysema in a patient with a left lung transplant. The right lung is hyperlucent, and vessels are reduced in size and number. **C:** Paraseptal emphysema. Subpleural lucencies marginated by interlobular septae and subpleural bullae are visible.

Cysts may be seen in cystic lung disease or may represent bullae in association with emphysema, honeycombing in patients with fibrosis, pneumatoceles in association with pneumonia, or cystic bronchiectasis (see Table 10-12). Bullae, honeycombing, pneumatoceles, and cystic bronchiectasis usually can be distinguished from cystic lung disease by associated findings. Scattered lung cysts may be seen in some patients with hypersensitivity pneumonitis.

Cystic lung diseases (i.e., lung disease characterized by numerous cysts) are rare. LAM and Langerhans' cell histiocytosis often are associated with multiple lung cysts as a primary manifestation. The cysts have a thin but easily

FIG. 10.35. Lung cysts. **A:** HRCT in a young woman with lymphangiomyomatosis (LAM). Multiple lung cysts are visible, having thin but easily discernible walls. In this disease, the cysts usually are interspersed within areas of normal-appearing lung and appear rounded. **B:** Lung cysts in histiocytosis. The cysts are more irregular in shape than those in patients with LAM and have an upper lobe predominance. In this patient, the cysts appear thick walled.

TABLE 10.13 Lung Cysts: Differential Diagnosis

Common causes of cysts
  Bullae
  Honeycombing
  Pneumatoceles in association with pneumonia
  Cystic bronchiectasis
  Cysts in hypersensitivity pneumonitis
Cystic lung disease (uncommon)
  Lymphangiomyomatosis
  Langerhans' cell histiocytosis
  Tuberous sclerosis
  Sjögren's syndrome
  Lymphoid interstitial pneumonia
  Papillomatosis

discernible wall, ranging up to a few millimeters in thickness (Fig. 10-35). In these diseases, the cysts usually are interspersed with areas of normal-appearing lung. LAM occurs only in women, usually of childbearing age, and typically the cysts are uniformly distributed, round, and similar in size and shape (see Fig. 10-35A). A small percentage of patients with tuberous sclerosis have LAM. In patients with histiocytosis, the cysts can be irregularly or bizarrely shaped (see Fig. 10-35B), have an upper lobe predominance, and tend to spare the costophrenic angles. Multiple cysts also may be seen in LIP, particularly in patients with Sjögren's syndrome and other collagen-vascular diseases (Table 10-13).

Mosaic Perfusion

Patchy areas of decreased lung attenuation sometimes can be recognized on HRCT in patients with abnormal lung perfusion and reduced regional pulmonary blood volume (Fig. 10-36). The term *mosaic perfusion* is used to describe this appearance. Mosaic perfusion most often results from airway disease such as cystic fibrosis or bronchiolitis obliterans; in this setting, abnormal regional lung ventilation leads to vasoconstriction and decreased perfusion. Mosaic perfusion also can be seen with vascular obstruction (e.g., chronic pulmonary embolism; Table 10-14).

A

C

B

FIG. 10.36. Mosaic perfusion due to bronchiolitis obliterans. **A:** HRCT shows decreased lung attenuation in the lower lobes and left upper lobe (*small arrows*). Note that vessels appear smaller in these regions than in the relatively dense right upper lobe (*large arrow*). This is typical of mosaic perfusion. Abnormal bronchi are also seen in the lucent lung regions, suggesting an airway disease as the cause. **B:** Minimum-intensity projection from a stack of HRCT images at the same level shows the density differences between lung regions resulting from differences in lung perfusion. **C:** Maximum intensity projection at the same level shows the difference in vascular size between lucent and dense lung regions.

TABLE 10.14	**Mosaic Perfusion: Differential Diagnosis**

Airway diseases

    Large airway diseases (e.g., cystic fibrosis, bronchiectasis)

    Small airway diseases (e.g., asthma, hypersensitivity pneumonitis, bronchiolitis obliterans, small airway infection, or mucous plugging)

Vascular diseases

    Chronic pulmonary embolism

    Other causes of vascular obstruction

The key to diagnosing mosaic perfusion as the cause of inhomogeneous lung attenuation on HRCT is recognizing the presence of reduced vessel size in relatively lucent lung regions (see Figs. 10-36A and 10-38A). If abnormal bronchi are visible in lucent lung regions (see Fig. 10-36A), and bronchi appear normal in relatively dense regions, airway disease very likely is the cause.

Air Trapping on Expiratory Computed Tomography

In patients with mosaic perfusion resulting from airway disease, air trapping often is visible on expiratory scans in lucent lung regions. Although mosaic perfusion and air trapping look the same, and often are related, they are distinct findings. Mosaic perfusion is an inspiratory scan finding, and air trapping is an expiratory scan finding. Also, in some patients with airway disease, air trapping may be visible on expiratory scans even though inspiratory scans are normal.

A variety of techniques can be used to obtain expiratory scans. Postexpiratory scans may be obtained following exhalation (i.e., the patient breathes out and suspends respiration). Dynamic expiratory scans are more sensitive. These are obtained with a spiral scanner by continuing to rotate the gantry as the patient exhales, obtaining a series of five or six scans at a single level. This may be done with reduced milliamperage settings so that the entire dynamic series equals the radiation dose of a single HRCT slice.

Normally, lung increases homogeneously in attenuation on expiratory scans (usually by more than 100 HU), although dependent lung increases more than nondependent lung (Fig. 10-37). In the presence of air trapping, the lung remains lucent on expiration, with little increase in measured attenuation, and shows little change in volume (see Fig. 10-38). Patchy air trapping is characteristic of small airway diseases. Larger areas of air trapping (e.g., an entire lobe) suggest a large airway abnormality. Air trapping on HRCT is associated principally with bronchiolitis; its appearance is discussed in detail in Chapter 23.

A

B

FIG. 10.37. Normal expiratory HRCT. **A:** Inspiratory scan shows the lung to be homogeneous in attenuation. **B:** Following expiration, the lung increases in attenuation. Posterior, dependent lung usually increases in density more than nondependent lung. Mild air trapping posterior to the major fissures in the superior segments of the lower lobes (*arrows*) is common in healthy individuals.

A   **B**

FIG. 10.38. Mosaic perfusion and air trapping in a patient with bronchiolitis obliterans secondary to lung transplant rejection. **A:** Inspiratory scan shows inhomogeneous lung attenuation due to mosaic perfusion. Several lung regions (*arrows*) appear relatively dense and contain larger vessels. Other lung regions appear relatively lucent and contain small vessels. **B:** Expiratory scan shows a normal increase in attenuation of the dense regions shown in (**A**). The relatively lucent regions in (**A**) show little change in attenuation on the expiratory scan due to air trapping.

SELECTED READING

Aquino SL, Gamsu G, Webb WR, Kee SL. Tree-in-bud pattern: frequency and significance on thin section CT. J Comput Assist Tomogr 1996; 20:594–599.

Arakawa H, Webb WR. Expiratory high-resolution CT scan. Radiol Clin North Am 1998; 36:189–209.

Austin JH, Müller NL, Friedman PJ, et al. Glossary of terms for CT of the lungs: recommendations of the Nomenclature Committee of the Fleischner Society. Radiology 1996; 200:327–331.

Colby TV, Swensen SJ. Anatomic distribution and histopathologic patterns in diffuse lung disease: correlation with HRCT. J Thorac Imaging 1996; 11:1–26.

Felson B. A new look at pattern recognition of diffuse pulmonary disease. AJR Am J Roentgenol 1979; 133:183–189.

Godwin JD, Müller NL, Takasugi JE. Pulmonary alveolar proteinosis: CT findings. Radiology 1988; 169:609–613.

Gruden JF, Webb WR, Naidich DP, McGuinness G. Multinodular disease: anatomic localization at thin-section CT—multireader evaluation of a simple algorithm. Radiology 1999; 210:711–720.

Gruden JF, Webb WR, Warnock M. Centrilobular opacities in the lung on high-resolution CT: diagnostic considerations and pathologic correlation. AJR Am J Roentgenol 1994; 162:569–574.

Johkoh T, Müller NL, Cartier Y, et al. Idiopathic interstitial pneumonias: diagnostic accuracy of thin-section CT in 129 patients. Radiology 1999; 211:555–560.

Lee KS, Kim TS, Han J, et al. Diffuse micronodular lung disease: HRCT and pathologic findings. J Comput Assist Tomogr 1999; 23:99–106.

Leung AN, Miller RR, Müller NL. Parenchymal opacification in chronic infiltrative lung diseases: CT-pathologic correlation. Radiology 1993; 188:209–214.

Mayo JR. High resolution computed tomography: technical aspects. Radiol Clin North Am 1991; 29:1043–1049.

Müller NL, Miller RR. Diseases of the bronchioles: CT and histopathologic findings. Radiology 1995; 196:3–12.

Müller NL, Miller RR. Computed tomography of chronic diffuse infiltrative lung disease: part 1. Am Rev Respir Dis 1990; 142:1206–1215.

Müller NL, Miller RR. Computed tomography of chronic diffuse infiltrative lung disease: part 2. Am Rev Respir Dis 1990; 142:1440–1448.

Primack SL, Hartman TE, Hansell DM, Müller NL. End-stage lung disease: CT findings in 61 patients. Radiology 1993; 189:681–686.

Webb WR. High resolution lung computed tomography: normal anatomic and pathologic findings. Radiol Clin North Am 1991; 29:1051–1063.

Webb WR. Thin-section CT of the secondary pulmonary lobule: anatomy and the image—The 2004 Fleischner lecture. Radiology 2006; 239:322–338.

Pulmonary Edema, the Acute Respiratory Distress Syndrome, and Radiology in the Intensive Care Unit

W. RICHARD WEBB

C hest radiographs are obtained daily in critically ill patients in the intensive care unit. Radiographs are used to detect significant changes in cardiopulmonary status; to search for pleural abnormalities; to evaluate the position of the numerous tubes, lines, and catheters used in monitoring and treatment; and to detect complications arising from the use of monitoring and support devices.

Radiographs obtained routinely or following placement of a tube or catheter show significant abnormalities not suspected clinically in 35% to 65% of patients in the ICU, and these findings often result in an intervention or change in treatment. The American College of Radiology (www.acr.org) recommends daily portable radiographs in patients requiring mechanical ventilation and in those with acute cardiac or pulmonary disease. Radiographs are also recommended following placement of support and monitoring devices such as endotracheal tubes, tracheostomy tubes, central venous catheters, nasogastric tubes, chest tubes, pacemakers, and intraaortic balloon pump.

RADIOGRAPHIC TECHNIQUE

Adequate radiographs are difficult to obtain in the ICU. Portable chest radiographs usually are done using relatively low kilovoltage, long exposure times, no grids, and short source (tube)-to-detector (film or digital medium) distance. These result in high-contrast films, often with portions of the mediastinum or pulmonary parenchyma poorly seen (*note*: digital techniques help solve this problem), motion-related blur, and increased scatter radiation. The American College of Radiology has recommended technical standards for the performance of bedside portable radiographs (Table 11-1).

Even if the technique is optimized, it often is not possible to obtain optimal radiographs because of the patient's inability to cooperate. Patients in the ICU often are too ill

to be positioned perfectly for radiographic examinations. Portable radiographs are performed in the anteroposterior (AP) projection, usually supine or semierect rather than upright. Position must be taken into account in interpreting radiographs for the presence of cardiomegaly, pulmonary vascular congestion, and pleural effusion. Furthermore, variation in patient position from day to day also must be considered.

PULMONARY DISEASE IN THE CRITICALLY ILL PATIENT

Common pulmonary complications that occur in critically ill patients include pulmonary edema (hydrostatic; increased capillary permeability), acute lung injury (ALI) and the

TABLE 11.1 American College of Radiology Technical Standards for Bedside Portable Radiographs

1. 72-in. source to image distance and upright position when possible (although this is uncommonly possible in ICU patients), or
2. 40-in. or more source to image distance for supine or semierect radiographs in uncooperative patients
3. kVp of 70–100 should be used in radiographs obtained without a grid
4. kVp of more than 100 may be used for radiographs obtained with a grid
5. Exposure times as short as possible
6. Technical parameters such as mAs, kVp, distance, and patient position should be recorded (to allow consistency in performance)
7. The radiographic beam should be collimated to limit radiation exposure

(Adapted from www.acr.org.)

acute respiratory distress syndrome (ARDS), atelectasis, pneumonia, aspiration, pulmonary embolism, and pulmonary hemorrhage. To some extent, the radiographic distribution of pulmonary disease, the time course of radiographic abnormalities, and associated radiographic findings may help in reaching a useful differential diagnosis. However, the radiographic findings in a patient in the ICU with acute pulmonary disease may be nonspecific, and knowledge of the clinical history or physical findings often is essential in suggesting the appropriate diagnosis.

PULMONARY EDEMA AND THE ACUTE RESPIRATORY DISTRESS SYNDROME

Pulmonary edema often is classified as either hydrostatic (cardiogenic) or due to increased capillary permeability (noncardiogenic). It should be recognized, however, that it is not always possible—or entirely appropriate—to make a simple distinction between hydrostatic edema and permeability edema. A classification as (1) hydrostatic edema, (2) increased permeability edema associated with diffuse alveolar damage (DAD), (3) increased permeability edema without associated DAD, and (4) mixed edema agrees better with pathology, physiology, and radiology. Although these types of edema cannot always be distinguished on the basis of plain film or CT findings, their appearances do tend to differ.

HYDROSTATIC PULMONARY EDEMA

Hydrostatic pulmonary edema results from alterations in the normal relation between intra- and extravascular hydrostatic and oncotic pressures. In most cases, an increased intravascular pressure due to pulmonary venous hypertension is the predominant cause, resulting in loss of fluid into the interstitium. This may result from left heart failure, left atrial or pulmonary venous obstruction, volume overload in renal failure, or overhydration. Low intravascular oncotic pressure resulting from hypoalbuminemia, liver failure, or renal failure also can result in an increased interstitial transudation of fluid.

Radiographic abnormalities associated with hydrostatic or cardiogenic pulmonary edema may be difficult to evaluate on portable radiographs. Heart size is difficult to determine accurately on portable AP radiographs, particularly when lung volume is reduced. Pulmonary vascular congestion also may be difficult to identify with certainty because of patient position. Upper lobe vessels appear larger than normal when patients are supine or semierect. Similarly, dilatation of the azygos vein, useful as a sign of increased right atrial pressure, occurs normally in the supine position. The apparent width of the mediastinum (vascular

pedicle) is increased by supine position, AP projection, and decreased inspiratory level. Associated pleural effusion is common, but may be difficult to see on supine radiographs.

In patients with hydrostatic pulmonary edema, plain radiographs and high-resolution CT (HRCT) may show findings of interstitial or air-space edema or both.

Interstitial Edema

Interstitial edema is manifested on chest radiographs by (1) Kerley's A or B lines, (2) thickening of the fissures, (3) "peribronchial cuffing," and (4) poor definition of pulmonary vessels or "perihilar haze." On CT, these findings correspond to the presence of (1) smooth interlobular septal thickening, (2) subpleural edema, (3) thickening of the peribronchovascular interstitium, and (4) ground-glass opacity.

Kerley's Lines (Thickening of Interlobular Septa)

Kerley's B lines visible on chest radiographs result from thickening of interlobular septa (Fig. 11-1; see also Fig. 10-1 in Chapter 10). They are horizontal, 1 to 2 cm in length, touch the pleural surface, and are best seen laterally in the costophrenic angles. Their characteristic appearance results from the regular organization of pulmonary lobules at the lung bases.

Kerley's A lines (see Fig. 11-1; see also Fig. 10-2 in Chapter 10) are less commonly seen. They are oblique, several centimeters in length, and are seen within the central or perihilar lung. They also represent thickened septa, but their appearance is different from that of B lines because of the different organization of lobules in this location.

In patients with Kerley's lines visible on radiographs, HRCT shows smooth interlobular septal thickening (Fig. 11-2; see also Fig. 10-15 in Chapter 10).

Thickening of the Fissures (Subpleural Edema)

The subpleural interstitial space is contiguous with peripheral interlobular septa. If interlobular septal thickening and Kerley's lines are present, subpleural interstitial thickening is often visible as well. It is recognized as thickening of the fissures on both chest radiographs and CT (see Figs. 11-1B and 11-2). This finding also may be due to pleural effusion thickening the fissure.

Peribronchial Cuffing (Thickening of the Peribronchovascular Interstitium)

Thickening of the peribronchovascular interstitium often occurs in patients with interstitial edema, resulting in apparent bronchial wall thickening on chest radiographs, or *peribronchial cuffing* (see Fig. 11-2). Peribronchial cuffing is

A

B

C

FIG. 11.1. Acute hydrostatic pulmonary edema with Kerley's lines in a patient with aortic stenosis and fluid overload. **A:** Baseline chest radiograph is normal. **B:** One hour later, after rapid infusion of fluid, Kerley's A and B lines are visible, with a perihilar predominance. Thickening of the right minor fissure also is visible (*arrow*) as a result of subpleural edema. The patient was acutely short of breath. **C:** Detail view of the left lower lobe shows interlobular septal thickening.

easiest to recognize in the perihilar regions where bronchi are seen end-on; sometimes lines radiating outward from the hila reflect the thickened peribronchial interstitium. On CT, thickening of the peribronchovascular interstitium resembles bronchial wall thickening; pulmonary arteries adjacent to the bronchi appear increased in diameter because the thickened interstitium surrounds them as well.

Poor Definition of Perihilar Vessels and Perihilar Haze (Ground-glass Opacity)

On chest radiographs, edema fluid surrounding pulmonary vessels blurs their margins, making them difficult to see or poorly defined on chest radiographs. This finding is easiest

to recognize when comparison films are available. Poor definition of lower lobe vessels usually is the first abnormality noted in pulmonary edema and may be seen when Kerley's lines are unrecognizable.

Poor definition of hilar or perihilar vessels is a common finding in patients with mild pulmonary edema (Fig. 11-3). On radiographs, this finding, sometimes referred to as *perihilar haze*, is often useful in diagnosing pulmonary edema in bedridden patients with lower lobe atelectasis or pneumonia in whom the lower lobe vessels cannot be assessed. This appearance may progress to a frank "batwing" pattern of pulmonary edema.

An overall increase in lung water or interstitial thickening often is recognizable as a poorly defined, generalized increase

A   B

FIG. 11.2. Interlobular septal thickening on HRCT in acute hydrostatic pulmonary edema in two different patients. **A:** There is extensive thickening of interlobular septa. Subpleural edema results in thickening of the fissures (*large arrow*). Apparent parahilar bronchial wall thickening ("peribronchial cuffing") results from edema fluid thickening the peribronchovascular interstitium (*small arrows*). Bilateral pleural effusions also are present. **B:** Interlobular septal thickening and thickening of the left major fissure are visible. Peribronchial cuffing (*arrows*) is well seen in this case. Patchy areas of increased lung attenuation represent ground-glass opacity, which may be seen with or without septal thickening in patients with interstitial edema.

in lung density, or ground-glass opacity. It may be difficult to recognize on chest radiographs in the absence of comparison films, but is easily seen on HRCT (Fig. 11-4). In patients with perihilar haze visible on chest radiographs, ground-glass opacity often is seen on HRCT.

On HRCT, ground-glass opacity due to edema may be perihilar and perivascular (see Fig. 11-4B), peripheral and subpleural (see Fig. 10-31A in Chapter 10), patchy (Fig. 11-5) and lobular, or centrilobular in distribution. It may be seen in isolation or in combination with septal thickening (see Fig. 11-2B).

A   B

FIG. 11.3. Poor definition of perihilar and lower lobe vessels ("perihilar haze") in two patients with hydrostatic edema. **A:** Chest radiograph in a patient with congestive heart failure and cardiomegaly shows poor definition of perihilar and lower lobe vessels as the first sign of pulmonary edema. **B:** In another patient with cardiomegaly and pulmonary edema, hazy opacity obscures perihilar and lower lobe vessels.

FIG. 11.8. Left-sided Swyer-James syndrome with predominant right-sided pulmonary edema. **A:** Baseline chest radiograph shows a hyperlucent and hypovascular left upper lobe. This appearance is typical of Swyer-James syndrome. **B:** Subsequently, congestive heart failure with cardiomegaly is associated with pulmonary edema. The edema spares the left upper lobe.

symptoms appear. However, it is important to recognize that hydrostatic edema may be visible on chest radiographs before the symptoms develop (clinical lag) or after pulmonary venous pressure has returned to normal (radiographic lag).

Because hydrostatic edema is relatively low in protein, it may show rapid clearing with improvement in patient status. Similarly, a gravitational shift in the distribution of edema fluid may occur within minutes to hours of a change in patient position. Air-space edema reacts more slowly than interstitial edema to changes in patient status.

Although a progression of edema from an interstitial to an air-space pattern may be seen with worsening, this is not always the case. Many patients show air-space edema as the initial finding. Similarly, in patients with air-space edema, the edema does not typically assume an interstitial appearance as it clears.

INCREASED PERMEABILITY EDEMA WITH DIFFUSE ALVEOLAR DAMAGE: ACUTE LUNG INJURY AND THE ACUTE RESPIRATORY DISTRESS SYNDROME

Permeability edema is a manifestation of capillary endothelial injury with resultant loss of fluid and protein into the lung interstitium. It results in a high-protein edema and, therefore, is slow to clear. It often is associated with respiratory epithelial injury, and *diffuse alveolar damage (DAD)*. This combination often results in the clinical entities known as *acute lung injury (ALI)* and the *acute respiratoy distress syndrome (ARDS)*.

ALI and ARDS are characterized by progressive dyspnea and hypoxemia over a period of hours to days. Their definitions differ only in the degree of hypoxemia. Specific criteria for the diagnosis of ALI and ARDS include the following:

1. Acute onset of respiratory failure
2. Diffuse bilateral infiltrates on chest radiographs
3. Absence of left atrial hypertension (pulmonary artery occlusive pressure* [PAOP] ≤ 18 mm Hg) or no clinical evidence of left atrial hypertension
4. Hypoxemia is defined as

PaO_2/FIO_2 300 mm Hg or less (ALI)
PaO_2/FIO_2 200 mm Hg or less (ARDS)
where FIO_2 is the fraction of inspired O_2

ALI and ARDS can be related to a variety of pathologic processes, including the following:

1. Infection (e.g., pneumonia and sepsis)
2. Inhalation or aspiration of toxic or irritating substances
3. Trauma with lung or extrathoracic injury
4. Hemodynamic abnormalities (e.g., shock, high altitude, anaphylaxis)
5. Hematologic disorders (e.g., disseminated intravascular coagulation, transfusion reaction)
6. Embolic disease (e.g., fat embolism, amniotic fluid embolism)
7. Drugs, either therapeutic or nontherapeutic
8. Metabolic disorders (e.g., pancreatitis, ketoacidosis)
9. Neurologic disease (e.g., head injury, stroke).

An idiopathic form of ALI or ARDS is termed acute interstitial pneumonia (AIP). AIP is discussed in Chapter 13.

Most simply, the mechanism of lung injury in ALI and ARDS may be considered to be *direct*, in which the lungs

TABLE 11.3 Direct and Indirect Causes of ALI and ARDS

Direct injury
Pneumonia (including virus, bacteria, mycoplasma, fungus, tuberculosis, *Pneumocystis jiroveci* [*P. carinii*] pneumonia, rickettsia)
Miliary tuberculosis or other disseminated infections
Inhalation (smoke, toxic gases, oxygen in high concentration)
Aspiration (gastric acid, ingested substances, drowning, chemicals, blood)
Thoracic trauma with contusion or crush injury
Thoracic radiation
Cardiopulmonary bypass
Fat embolism
Air embolism
Amniotic fluid embolism
Reexpansion or reperfusion edema
Sickle cell crisis
Acute interstitial pneumonia
Usual interstitial pneumonia with acute exacerbation

Indirect injury
Sepsis (particularly gram negative organisms)
Shock
Toxic shock syndrome
Disseminated intravascular coagulation
Extrathoracic trauma
Burns
Neurogenic edema
Drugs
Anaphylaxis
Transfusion reactions
Leukoagglutinin reactions
Diabetic ketoacidosis
Pancreatitis
Uremia
High altitude

themselves are injured (e.g., pneumonia, aspiration, and inhalational injury) or *indirect*, in which extrapulmonary abnormalities (e.g., sepsis, shock, pancreatitis) lead to lung injury (Table 11-3).

The Stages of ALI and the Acute Respiratory Distress Syndrome

ALI and ARDS are considered to occur in stages, within the time frame of hours, days, weeks, and months (Table 11-4), which have close pathologic and radiographic correlates.

Pathologic Abnormalities

Pathologic abnormalities in ARDS are similar regardless of its cause. The histologic abnormalities occurring in ARDS are usually referred to as *DAD*.

Hours. Within hours of the precipitating insult, endothelial cell edema, widening of intracellular junctions, congestion of capillaries, and limited interstitial pulmonary edema and hemorrhage are present. These manifestations represent the early *exudative (injury) stage* of ALI and ARDS.

Days. The period from a day to a week after the initial insult is characterized by progressive capillary endothelial injury, necrosis of alveolar lining cells (type I pneumocytes), proteinaceous interstitial and alveolar edema, and hemorrhage. Hyaline membranes form within the alveoli. This represents the late *exudative (injury) stage*.

Weeks. The *proliferative (reparative) stage* usually occurs from 1 week to 1 month following the onset of ARDS. It is characterized by proliferation of type II pneumocytes, which reline the denuded alveolar walls, organization of the alveolar exudates, fibroblast proliferation within the alveolar walls and interstitium, and deposition of collagen.

Months. In many patients, these abnormalities resolve, and little respiratory disability results. In patients with more severe lung injury, interstitial fibrosis develops. This is termed the *fibrotic stage*.

Radiographic Abnormalities

Hours. Radiographs typically are normal for the first 12 to 24 hours after the acute injury, despite the presence of dyspnea (Fig. 11-9A). This latent period is suggestive of ALI or ARDS (Table 11-4).

TABLE 11.4 The Stages of ALI and ARDS

Time Frame	Stage	Pathologic Findings	Radiologic Findings
Hours	Early exudative (injury)	Endothelial edema, early edema	Normal
Days	Late exudative (injury)	Progressive endothelial injury, necrosis of alveolar lining cells, progressive alveolar edema and hemorrhage	Patchy consolidation, often peripheral, progressive confluence, dependent atelectasis
Weeks	Proliferative (reparative)	Proliferation of alveolar lining cells, organization of alveolar exudates, fibroblast proliferation in alveolar walls	Slow resolution of consolidation, development of reticular opacities
Months	Fibrosis	Depending on the degree of injury, resolution or fibrosis	Persistence of reticular opacities and honeycombing, often anterior

FIG. 11.38. Pulmonary artery anatomy on the chest radiograph. A Swan-Ganz catheter tip should overlie the main or hilar arteries. The thoracic systemic veins are shown in blue as in Fig 11-32. The right atrium (*RA*) and location of the tricuspid valve are shown. PA = pulmonary artery; RPA = right pulmonary artery; R ILPA = right interlobar pulmonary artery; LPA = left pulmonar artery.

FIG. 11.39. Properly positioned Swan-Ganz catheter. The catheter tip (*arrow*) overlies the hilar shadow and is within the right interlobar pulmonary artery.

interlobar pulmonary artery is usually adequate for pressure measurements (Figs 11-38). Thus, the catheter tip should overlie the main or hilar arteries (Fig 11-39). If the catheter lies in a small (lobar or segmental) artery, it may remain wedged with the balloon uninflated, and thrombosis and pulmonary infarction or pulmonary artery aneurysm can result (Fig. 11-40). Care also must be taken that the balloon does not remain inflated between measurements; continued inflation also may result in infarction. Coiling of the catheter within the heart should be avoided. Coiling can result in knotting or sudden peripheral migration of the catheter with wedging.

Transvenous Pacemakers

Transvenous pacemaker and implanted defibrillator leads vary in number and location in different patients. A right ventricular is typically positioned with its tip in the apex of the right ventricle, pointing to the left, anteriorly, and inferiorly (Fig 1-41A). Placement of the tip into the coronary sinus usually results in a superior and posterior deviation of the pacemaker lead.

A

B

FIG. 11.40. Peripheral location of a Swan-Ganz catheter with infarction. **A:** A patient with cardiomegaly shows a peripherally located (segmental or subsegmental) Swan-Ganz catheter (*arrow*). The catheter should overlie the large hilar vessels. **B:** Following withdrawal of the catheter 1 day later, a focal opacity representing a lung infarction is visible in the right lung (*arrow*).

A   B

FIG. 11.41. Tranvenous pacemaker (implanted defibrillator) leads. **A** and **B:** Pacemaker leads are positioned with tips in right ventricular apex (*white arrows*) and right atrial appendage (*black arrows*). The dense bands along the pacemaker leads indicate this is an implanted defibrillator.

A second lead is often present, positioned in the right atrium, with its tip usually directed anteriorly into the atrial appendage (Fig 11-41B) or laterally against the right atrial wall. In some patients, a third lead is positioned in a coronary vein by means of the coronary sinus.

Rarely, pacemaker leads perforate the coronary sinus or myocardium, resulting in pericardial tamponade or diaphragmatic pacing (with hiccoughs). If this occurs, the lead tip may be seen very close to the edge of the heart shadow or may project beyond it.

Pacemaker failure may result from poor lead position, fracture of the pacemaker lead usually near the pacemaker (this often is difficult to see), or failure of the pacemaker itself. Some patients play with their pacemaker device (so-called "twiddler's syndrome"), which may result in coiling of the pacemaker wire around the pacemaker and retraction of the lead tip into the right atrium or vena cava.

Pleural Drainage Tubes

Pleural drainage tubes commonly are used to evacuate pneumothorax or pleural effusion. Ideally, tubes placed for pneumothorax should occupy the least dependent portion of the pleural space (anterosuperior in a bedridden patient). For the treatment of pleural fluid, tubes should be placed within the dependent portion of the pleural space (postero-inferior).

If a tube functions poorly, it may be occluded or kinked, it may be positioned in the chest wall or with its side hole (marked by a discontinuity in the radiopaque tube marker)

outside the thoracic cavity, or may be positioned in the major fissure with the two adjacent lobes occluding the tube. A tube located within the major fissure is most easily recognized by comparing its position on the frontal and lateral radiographs, and localizing this to the plane of the fissure.

Rarely, the lung may be perforated during tube placement with the tube tip lying within lung parenchyma. Obviously, such tubes function poorly and lead to pneumothorax. CT may be needed to confirm this location.

Nasogastric Tubes

Nasogastric tubes or feeding tubes occasionally may be placed in the tracheobronchial tree (Figs. 11-42). This placement may result in perforation of the visceral pleura and pneumothorax, bronchial obstruction and atelectasis, or delivery of a tube feeding into the lung, which may result in severe pneumonia. Coiling of a nasogastric tube in the hypopharynx can contribute to aspiration. If the tube is coiled in the esophagus, gastric distention and aspiration may result. Feeding tubes characteristically have a dense marker at their tip; nasogastric tubes placed for suction have a dense marker along their length.

Aortic Balloon Pump

A catheter-based, gas-filled intraaortic balloon pump may be used to improve peripheral blood flow in patients with left ventricular failure and low cardiac output. The long (nearly 30 cm), sausage-shaped balloon may be visible when inflated as

A   B

FIG. 11.42. Feeding tubes placed in the tracheobronchial tree. **A:** A feeding tube (*arrow*) is placed in the left lower lobe, and is oriented along the course of bronchi. **B:** In another patient, the tube follows the course of bronchi in the central lung, but curves in a manner inconsistent with an endobronchial location in the periphery (*arrow*). This suggests perforation of the visceral pleura, with the tube tip in the pleural space.

FIG. 11.43. Aortic balloon pump. The balloon tip (*white arrow*) is radiopaque, and is properly positioned slightly below the superior aspect of the aortic arch. In this patient, the balloon (*black arrows*) was inflated at the time the radiograph was performed, and is visible as a long lucency overlying the descending aorta.

a relative lucency within the descending aorta (Fig. 11-43). The catheter itself is difficult to see, although a small radiopaque line usually marks its tip. Ideally, the catheter tip is positioned just below the origin of the left subclavian artery, and therefore should overlie the aortic knob on the radiograph (see Fig. 11-43). If advanced too far, the catheter may occlude the left vertebral artery; if located too low, it is less effective, and its lower portion may partially obstruct the renal arteries.

SELECTED READING

Bartsch P. High altitude pulmonary edema. Respiration 1997; 64:435–443.

Bernard GR, Artigas A, Brigham KL, et al. The American-European Consensus Conference on ARDS. Definitions, mechanisms, relevant outcomes, and clinical trial coordination. Am J Respir Crit Care Med 1994; 149:818–824.

Desai SR, Wells AU, Rubens MB, et al. Acute respiratory distress syndrome: CT abnormalities at long-term follow-up. Radiology 1999; 210:29–35.

Gluecker T, Capasso P, Schnyder P, et al. Clinical and radiologic features of pulmonary edema. Radiographics 1999; 19:1507– 1531.

Goodman LR, Fumagalli R, Tagliabue P, et al. Adult respiratory distress syndrome due to pulmonary and extrapulmonary causes: CT, clinical, and functional correlations. Radiology 1999; 213:545–552.

Hommeyer SH, Godwin JD, Takasugi JE. Computed tomography of air-space disease. Radiol Clin North Am 1991; 29:1065–1084.

Ketai LH, Godwin JD. A new view of pulmonary edema and acute respiratory distress syndrome. J Thorac Imaging 1998; 13:147–171.

Müller-Leisse C, Klosterhalfen B, Hauptmann S, et al. Computed tomography and histologic results in the early stages of endotoxin-injured pig lungs as a model for adult respiratory distress syndrome. Invest Radiol 1993; 28:39–45.

Murata K, Herman PG, Khan A, et al. Intralobular distribution of oleic acid–induced pulmonary edema in the pig: evaluation by high-resolution CT. Invest Radiol 1989; 24:647–653.

Owens CM, Evans TW, Keogh BF, Hansell DM. Computed tomography in established adult respiratory distress syndrome. Correlation with lung injury score. Chest 1994; 106:1815–1821.

Schuster DP. What Is Acute Lung Injury? Chest 1995; 107:1721–1726.

Storto ML, Kee ST, Golden JA, Webb WR. Hydrostatic pulmonary edema: high-resolution CT findings. AJR Am J Roentgenol 1995; 165:817–820.

Pulmonary Infections

MICHAEL B. GOTWAY AND W. RICHARD WEBB

P ulmonary infections are among the most common causes of morbidity and mortality worldwide and contribute substantially to annual medical expenditures in the United States. The causes of pulmonary infection are numerous, and the clinical presentations of pulmonary infection are frequently nonspecific. Thoracic imaging plays a central role in the evaluation of patients suspected of pulmonary infection.

MECHANISMS

Microorganisms gain access to the respiratory system and cause infection in a variety of ways. The most common route of entry is inoculation via the tracheobronchial tree, usually by the inhalation of aerosolized respiratory droplets, less commonly by the aspiration of oropharyngeal secretions, and rarely by the direct extension of organisms into the respiratory system from adjacent sources, such as infected mediastinal or hilar lymph nodes. Pulmonary infections may also occur through inoculation via the pulmonary vasculature, usually in the presence of a definable extrapulmonary infectious source, such as endocarditis or thrombophlebitis. Finally, pulmonary infections may occur as a result of extension of an infectious process from an adjacent organ, such as transdiaphragmatic spread from a liver abscess or esophageal rupture with esophagopulmonary fistula formation.

Whether or not overt pulmonary infection takes place depends on a variety of factors, including the number of inoculating organisms, the integrity of the host's immune system, and the virulence of the infecting organisms. Many organisms exhibit characteristics that enhance the likelihood of pulmonary infection and promote tissue destruction.

PATTERNS

Pathologically, pulmonary infections may be divided into infections involving the central airways (tracheobronchitis), the small airways (bronchiolitis), and the pulmonary parenchyma (pneumonia).

Pneumonia may be subdivided into several categories: lobar pneumonia, bronchopneumonia, and interstitial pneumonia. Lung abscess is an additional pattern of pulmonary infection that may be seen with lobar pneumonia or bronchopneumonia.

Imaging manifestations often are sufficiently different to allow the recognition of these patterns of infection. Although it is usually not possible to suggest a specific microbiological diagnosis in individual cases, specific patterns tend to be associated with specific organisms.

Tracheobronchitis

Infection of the central airways may predominantly affect the trachea, the central bronchi, or both. Tracheobronchitis is often the result of viral infection.

Viral tracheobronchitis, also known as croup, is a common infection in children, particularly those under the age of 3 years. Narrowing of the subglottic trachea may be seen on chest radiographs.

In adults, viral tracheobronchitis is usually of little clinical consequence, and patients rarely undergo imaging. Occasionally, viral infections impair host immunity sufficiently to predispose to bacterial superinfection, in which case the radiographic pattern will primarily be that of a bacterial pneumonia.

Bacterial tracheitis is rare. It most often affects children, although adults may be affected as well. It often occurs after an upper respiratory viral infection. The most common etiologic agents are *Staphylococcus aureus* and *Haemophilus influenzae*; anaerobes and *Corynebacterium diphtheriae* are rare causes. Bacterial tracheitis produces inflammatory exudates that may lead to obstruction of the tracheal lumen.

Bacterial bronchial infections in adults are most common in patients with chronic obstructive pulmonary disease (COPD) or cystic fibrosis. Bacterial bronchitis is usually diagnosed clinically and treated conservatively. Imaging is not necessary in most cases, although airway wall thickening may be visible on chest radiographs. Often, chest radiographs are performed to exclude associated pneumonia. CT, particularly high-resolution CT (HRCT), may show airway wall thickening, and air trapping may be evident on postexpiratory imaging.

Airway inflammation and stenoses may result from tuberculosis. Smooth, tapered narrowing affecting the lobar bronchi and associated with bronchial wall thickening is most typical. The distal trachea may be involved, usually in concert with main stem bronchial involvement.

Acute tracheobronchitis may be seen with *Aspergillus fumigatus* infection. It is an uncommon form of invasive aspergillosis occurring in immunosuppressed patients. Chest radiography and CT are often normal in this form of disease. Focal airway wall thickening or plaques are seen on CT in some cases (Fig. 12-1).

Bronchiolitis

The term *bronchiolitis* refers to inflammation of small airways, particularly membranous and respiratory bronchioles.

Acute bronchiolitis consists of predominantly peribronchiolar neutrophilic and lymphocytic inflammation associated with necrosis of the respiratory epithelium. The organisms most commonly associated with acute bronchiolitis are viruses, especially respiratory syncytial virus (RSV) but also human metapneumovirus (hMPV), parainfluenza virus, adenovirus types 3, 7, and 21, and rhinoviruses. *Mycoplasma pneumoniae* and *Chlamydia* spp. may also cause acute bronchiolitis. Bacterial and fungal organisms involving the large airways may also result in infectious bronchiolitis.

Most clinically significant viral bronchiolar infections are encountered in small children. RSV is the most common offending agent and usually afflicts children between the ages of 2 months and 2 years. Infants below the age of 6 weeks may be relatively protected by maternal IgG. hMPV is a relatively recently recognized viral pathogen that is responsible for infant bronchiolitis in 5% to 15% of cases. Serologic studies suggest that infection with hMPV is nearly ubiquitous by the age of 5.

Chest radiographic findings of acute bronchiolitis may show a combination of peribronchiolar thickening, perihilar linear opacity, and peribronchiolar consolidation, often bilateral (Fig. 12-2A). Air trapping, manifested as areas of increased lucency, is also common in patients with acute bronchiolitis. Air trapping may be effectively demonstrated with postexpiratory imaging. In very young patients who are unable to cooperate with the instructions required for postexpiratory imaging, lateral decubitus imaging may be used to demonstrate air trapping.

A

B

FIG. 12.1. *Aspergillus* tracheobronchitis. Axial CT image in an immunosuppressed heart transplant recipient shows irregular, mildly high-attenuation plaques (*arrows*) along the posterior and left lateral tracheal wall, consistent with *Aspergillus* tracheobronchitis.

FIG. 12.2. Viral bronchiolitis in a 3-year-old boy. **A:** Frontal chest radiograph shows bilateral perihilar linear opacities (*arrows*) consistent with bronchial wall thickening and atelectasis. **B:** Axial CT image shows patchy atelectasis (*large arrow*) and lobular air trapping (*small arrows*).

A   B

FIG. 12.3. Swyer-James syndrome. **A:** Frontal chest radiograph shows a diminutive left hilum (*arrow*) and relatively decreased attenuation throughout the left upper lobe. Note the leftward shift of the trachea, indicating diminished left upper lobe volume. **B:** Axial CT image shows relatively decreased attenuation of the left upper lobe associated with irregular bronchial wall thickening and dilation (*arrow*).

CT and HRCT manifestations of acute bronchiolitis include patchy areas of atelectasis, frequently combined with bronchial wall thickening and mosaic perfusion (see Fig. 12-2B), the latter due to air trapping.

Acute bronchiolitis, particularly related to adenovirus infection acquired during early childhood, may result in the Swyer-James syndrome (constrictive bronchiolitis or bronchiolitis obliterans). Histopathology in the Swyer-James syndrome shows constrictive bronchiolitis, chronic bronchiolitis, bronchiectasis, and some destruction of the lung parenchyma.

The Swyer-James syndrome is usually encountered incidentally in a patient undergoing radiography for unrelated reasons. Patients occasionally complain of dyspnea on exertion. Many patients provide a history of childhood infection.

Inspiratory chest radiographs in patients with Swyer-James syndrome show increased lucency involving all or part of one lung. The inspiratory volume of the affected lung or lobe is usually normal or perhaps slightly diminished. The area of lucency shows attenuated peripheral vasculature. The hilum on the affected side is usually small (Fig. 12-3A). Postexpiratory imaging shows air trapping in the affected lung or lobe, with shift of the mediastinum away from the affected side. CT and HRCT easily demonstrate the findings of Swyer-James syndrome. CT shows increased lucency with diminished vascular size in the affected area in most patients (see Fig. 23-23 in Chapter 23). Bronchiectasis is often seen as well (see Fig. 12-3B). Air trapping, seen as failure of the expected increase in lung attenuation (and decrease in volume) following exhalation, or a paradoxical decrease in attenuation following exhalation, is always present.

Lobar Pneumonia

Lobar pneumonia is typically caused by organisms such as *Streptococcus pneumoniae* (*Pneumococcus*) and *Klebsiella pneumoniae*. This pattern is characterized by the initial development of peripheral opacity that rapidly evolves into confluent, homogeneous consolidation (Fig. 12-4

FIG. 12.4. Lobar pneumonia. Frontal chest radiograph shows homogeneous right middle lobe consolidation (*arrows*), representing pneumococcal pneumonia.

FIG. 12.5. Air-space pneumonia: air bronchograms. Frontal chest radiograph in a patient with pneumococcal pneumonia shows homogenous consolidation associated with tubular lucencies (*arrows*), representing air bronchograms.

FIG. 12.6. Air-space pneumonia: the bulging fissure sign. Frontal chest radiograph shows homogenous right upper lobe consolidation associated with inferior displacement of the major fissure. *K. pneumoniae* was recovered in both blood and sputum.

and Fig. 2-12 in Chapter 2), often conforming to anatomic boundaries such as the interlobar fissures. Lobar pneumonia uncommonly affects the entire lobe, and the term *air-space pneumonia* is often used instead. Air bronchograms are common with lobar or air-space pneumonia (Fig. 12-5). Usually, lobar or air-space pneumonia is nonsegmental, meaning that it easily crosses pulmonary segments (bronchopneumonia is usually segmental and patchy—see below). Lobar or air-space pneumonia may produce expansion of a lobe, the "bulging fissure" sign (Fig. 12-6 and Fig. 2-12 in Chapter 2); this sign has been associated with *K. pneumoniae* infection but probably is more commonly the result of pneumococcal pneumonia owing to the latter's greater prevalence. If the patient survives the infection, air-space pneumonia usually heals without sequelae.

Bronchopneumonia

Bronchopneumonia begins with infection of the airway mucosa and subsequently extends into the adjacent alveoli. The bronchopneumonia pattern consists of patchy areas of consolidation that may be initially limited to one or more pulmonary segments (Fig. 12-7), but it then progresses to multifocal, often bilateral, consolidation (see Fig. 2-4 in Chapter 2). Air-space nodules (also known as acinar nodules) are commonly encountered with the bronchopneumonia pattern. These nodules are ill defined and usually range from 5 to 10 mm in size; they represent infection of the terminal and respiratory bronchioles with peribronchiolar consolidation. Because of the prominent airway involvement with bronchopneumonia, some volume loss is common. The bronchopneumonia

pattern is often associated with virulent organisms such as *S. aureus* or Gram-negative organisms. Because these organisms are commonly aggressive, tissue destruction is common and complications such as abscess may occur. Healing of bronchopneumonia often results in scarring.

Interstitial Pneumonia

Infectious interstitial pneumonias are commonly caused by viruses, *M. pneumoniae*, and *Pneumocystis jiroveci* pneumonia. Pathologically, inflammation in interstitial pneumonia is primarily limited to the pulmonary interstitium, although not exclusively so. The typical chest radiographic appearance of interstitial pneumonia is bilateral, symmetric, linear or reticular opacities (Fig. 12-8). Interstitial pneumonias, particularly *P. jiroveci* pneumonia, may produce a fine granular or ground-glass pattern on chest radiography that subsequently evolves to consolidation if not treated. Ground-glass opacity or consolidation is usually associated with alveolar filling superimposed on the interstitial abnormality. Treated infectious interstitial pneumonias typically resolve without sequelae, if the patient survives.

Lung Abscess

A lung abscess represents a localized infection that undergoes tissue destruction and necrosis. When a communication with the tracheobronchial tree is present, cavitation and an air-fluid level may be evident (Fig. 12-9 and Figs. 9-10, 9-39, and 9-40 in Chapter 9). The inner wall of an abscess varies from smooth

A

B

C

FIG. 12.7. Bronchopneumonia. **A:** Frontal chest radiograph shows patchy right lower lobe consolidation, consistent with bronchopneumonia. **B:** Axial CT image shows numerous small nodules throughout the right lower lobe, some with a branching appearance (*arrow*) typical of tree-in-bud appearance. This represents endobronchial spread of infection. **C:** Gross specimen shows tree-in-bud opacities (*arrows*). (Image courtesy of Martha L. Warnock, MD, Professor Emerita, Department of Pathology, University of California, San Francisco.)

FIG. 12.8. Infectious interstitial pneumonia. Frontal chest radiograph shows diffuse, bilateral interstitial prominence. *P. jiroveci* was recovered with sputum induction.

FIG. 12.9. Pulmonary abscess. **A:** Frontal and (**B**) lateral chest radiography shows a focal lucency within the left lower lung associated with an air-fluid level (*arrows*), representing a pulmonary abscess. **C:** Axial CT image shows that the left lung abscess (*arrows*) is relatively thin walled anteriorly and contains an air-fluid level. The patient was septic and unresponsive to conservative therapy and underwent resection. **D:** Gross left lung specimen shows the cavity (*arrows*).

to shaggy and irregular, and maximum wall thickness usually ranges from 5 to 15 mm. Pulmonary abscesses are most commonly caused by mixed anaerobic infections, followed in frequency by *S. aureus* and *Pseudomonas aeruginosa*. Such infections are often the result of aspiration. Consequently, a lung abscess is often encountered in patients at risk for aspiration, such as patients with poor dental hygiene, impaired consciousness, esophageal motility disorders, and neurologic diseases. Multiple abscesses may result from septic embolism.

APPROACH TO IMAGING OF THE IMMUNOCOMPROMISED PATIENT

Imaging of immunocompromised patients, including those with HIV infection, organ transplantation, and patients with bone marrow transplantation or suppression, requires special consideration. An organized approach to the imaging evaluation of such patients is critical to ensure accurate and timely diagnosis.

It is critical to understand the pathogenesis of the various causes of immunosuppression for such patients and to recognize that the use of any prophylactic medications may alter the interpretation of imaging studies. For example, the pathogenesis of immunosuppression for patients with HIV infection is related to progressive depletion of T-cell immunity (specifically depletion of CD4 cells). Because opportunistic infections occur with greater frequency as the CD4 cell count falls, awareness of the CD4 cell count is critical for accurate interpretation of imaging studies. Furthermore, because the use of highly active antiretroviral therapy (HAART) has dramatically changed the course of HIV infection, every effort should be made to determine whether a patient is receiving HAART before providing a differential diagnosis for abnormal thoracic imaging findings.

For patients with bone marrow suppression from chemotherapy or bone marrow transplantation and for patients with organ transplantation, certain infectious and noninfectious complications are more likely to occur at different times following the institution of chemotherapy or transplantation. Awareness of these time courses is important for accurate diagnosis.

Imaging of immunosuppressed patients usually begins with chest radiography. While chest radiographic findings in immunosuppressed patients are often nonspecific, recognizing certain basic radiographic patterns is important. The discussion below details a basic imaging approach to the immunosuppressed patient.

Focal Air-space Opacities

Infected immunosuppressed patients with focal air-space opacities are most likely to have bacterial infection, particularly if such opacities are unilateral, if they show air bronchograms and/or pleural effusions, or if either a segmental or a lobar distribution is evident. This is true for patients with HIV infection, regardless of CD4 count, and is generally the case for patients with immunosuppression unrelated to HIV infection. With advancing severity of immunosuppression, infection with *Mycobacterium tuberculosis* (MTB) must be considered as a cause of focal air-space consolidation. Although uncommon in patients with HIV infection, *Nocardia asteroides* infection may present with focal, often mass-like, air-space opacity, particularly in organ transplant recipients (Fig. 12-10). This pattern may reflect lobar pneumonia or bronchopneumonia.

Multifocal Air-space Opacities

When bilateral opacities are present, the differential diagnosis must be expanded, and it becomes very important to integrate information regarding the degree of immunosuppression in the imaging assessment of such patients. Bilateral opacities may represent bacterial pneumonia, but for severely immunosuppressed patients (HIV infection with CD4 cell counts below 200 cells/μL and non–HIV immunosuppressed patients with neutropenic fever), opportunistic infections, such as *P. jiroveci* pneumonia (still often referred to as *Pneumocystis carinii* pneumonia or PCP), fungal infections (most commonly *Cryptococcus neoformans* and *A. fumigatus*), and, less commonly, viruses and infection with unusual bacterial organisms, such as mycobacteria and *N. asteroides*, must be considered. Fungal, mycobacteria, or *N. asteroides* infections are more likely if the radiographic abnormalities are nodular in appearance, whereas PCP or viral infections are more likely when opacities are interstitial appearing (see Fig. 12-8) or have a ground-glass appearance and are unaccompanied by either pleural effusion or lymphadenopathy.

Linear (Interstitial-appearing) Opacities

Linear, or interstitial-appearing, radiographic abnormalities in immunosuppressed patients may reflect atypical pneumonia, such as viral infections or PCP. These

FIG. 12.10. *Nocardia asteroides* infection in a heart transplant recipient. Axial CT image shows nodular right lung consolidation with central cavitation (*arrow*). *N. asteroides* was recovered following biopsy of this lesion.

infections usually occur in HIV-infected patients with CD4 cell counts below 200 cells/μL and in bone marrow transplant patients between 1 and 6 months after transplantation, although viral infections may occur in lung transplant recipients any time after lung transplantation. PCP is, however, very uncommon in patients receiving appropriate prophylactic therapy.

Cavitation

Cavitation within either focal or diffuse lung parenchymal opacities in immunosuppressed patients is usually caused by bacterial infection, including *N. asteroides* (see Fig. 12-10) and mycobacterial infections, and fungal infection. In patients with severe bone marrow suppression, such as chemotherapy patients or patients several weeks after bone marrow transplantation, bilateral, multifocal, nodular opacities that quickly undergo cavitation are very suggestive of invasive aspergillosis.

Cavitation of upper lobe parenchymal opacities may occur in relatively immunocompetent patients with mycobacterial infections. Cavitation in mycobacterial infections in HIV-infected patients with CD4 cell counts below 200 cells/μL is uncommon, however, and the presence of cavitation within focal or diffuse opacities in such patients favors either necrotizing pyogenic pneumonia or fungal infection.

Pleural Effusions

Pleural effusions are commonly present in immunosuppressed patients with pyogenic bacterial infections of any etiology. They may be present in patients with fungal infections, although they are extremely uncommon in patients with PCP.

FIG. 12.11. *Mycobacterium tuberculosis* infection in an AIDS patient with a low CD4 cell count. Frontal chest radiograph shows right paratracheal lymph node enlargement (*arrows*).

Lymphadenopathy

Lymphadenopathy is commonly encountered in immunosuppressed patients with pyogenic bacterial infections, although enlarged nodes are usually seen only with CT and not on chest radiographs. Visibly enlarged nodes on chest radiographs in HIV-infected patients with CD4 cell counts below 200 cells/µL should specifically suggest the diagnosis of MTB (Fig. 12-11). The development of lymphadenopathy in patients who have recently been started on HAART therapy has been associated with mycobacterial infection. It has been postulated that HAART allows the reconstituted immune system to react to latent pulmonary infection. It is therefore important to know whether an HIV-infected patient is taking HAART, and when HAART was started, if lymphadenopathy is encountered on chest radiographs in patients with AIDS.

SPECIFIC INFECTIONS

The epidemiology, pathogenesis, clinical presentation, and imaging findings of specific infections (Table 12-1) are reviewed in this section.

Bacteria

Gram-positive Cocci

Streptococcus pneumoniae

Streptococcus pneumoniae is overwhelmingly the most common cause of pneumonia associated with Gram-positive cocci (Table 12-2). Numerous antigenic types have been identified. Pneumococcus may colonize nearly 20% of the population, and this figure is higher in COPD patients.

The development of pneumococcal pneumonia has been associated with several risk factors, including advanced age, immunosuppression, chronic heart, lung, and renal diseases, sickle cell disease, cirrhosis, prior splenectomy, and hematologic malignancies. *S. pneumoniae* is the most commonly isolated pathogen in hospitals, and pneumococcal pneumonia is the most common cause of pneumonia requiring hospitalization or resulting in death. In recent years, the emergence of resistant strains of *S. pneumoniae* has caused great concern in the medical community.

Pulmonary infection with *S. pneumoniae* is typically preceded by colonization of the nasopharynx. Once the organism reaches the lower respiratory tract, infection is facilitated by several virulence factors, including the antiphagocytic properties of the organism's capsule as well as the organism's ability to elaborate various proteins that augment the infection.

Pneumococcal pneumonia classically presents with the abrupt onset of high fever, cough that may be productive of rusty brown sputum, shaking chills, and pleuritic chest pain. Manifestations of pneumococcal pneumonia in the elderly may be somewhat atypical and are occasionally overshadowed by other chronic illnesses. Physical examination may reveal crackles, dullness to percussion, decreased breath sounds, and bronchial breathing.

Complications of pneumococcal pneumonia include empyema, meningitis, disseminated intravascular coagulation, hepatocellular damage, renal damage, and acute respiratory distress syndrome (ARDS). Pneumococcal pneumonia may leave the patient vulnerable to superinfection by other bacterial organisms.

Imaging Findings. Pneumococcal pneumonia appears on the chest radiograph as classical air-space pneumonia: consolidation extending to pleural surfaces, often with air bronchograms (Fig. 12-12). Volume loss is minimal. Pneumococcal pneumonia may also present with patchy, multifocal consolidation consistent with bronchopneumonia or, rarely, as an interstitial-appearing process associated with some air-space consolidation. Occasionally, pneumococcal pneumonia appears as a focal nodule or mass (Fig. 12-13), often referred to as "round pneumonia." Cavitation and abscess formation are uncommon. Pleural disease, either pleural effusion or empyema, is found in 50% or fewer patients. Thoracic CT often shows lobar air-space consolidation, often with areas of ground-glass opacity surrounding the consolidation, lobular opacity, poorly defined centrilobular nodules measuring 3 to 10 mm, bronchial wall thickening, and smooth interlobular septal thickening. Localization of opacity in the middle and outer third of the lung is common. It has been suggested that small (less than 3 mm) centrilobular nodules are less commonly seen in bacterial pneumonias, such as pneumococcus, and may favor another infectious etiology, such as *M. pneumoniae* or viral pneumonia.

With appropriate treatment, pneumococcal pneumonia may completely resolve within 14 days, although complete resolution may take longer in elderly or very ill patients.

TABLE 12.1   **Classification of Important Pulmonary Infections by Organism**

Bacteria
Gram-positive cocci
  Streptococcus pneumoniae
  Staphylococcus aureus
  Streptococcus pyogenes
Gram-positive bacilli
  Bacillus anthracis
  Rhodococcus equi
Gram-negative cocci
  Moraxella catarrhalis (Branhamella catarrhalis)
  Neisseria meningitides
Gram-negative rods
  Escherichia coli
  Klebsiella pneumoniae
  Pseudomonas aeruginosa
  Yersinia pestis
  Serratia and *Enterobacter* spp.
Gram-negative coccobacilli
  Haemophilus influenzae
  Legionella pneumophila
  Bordetella species
  Bartonella henselae and *Quintana*
  Francisella tularensis
Anaerobic bacteria

Mycobacteria
Mycobacterium tuberculosis
Mycobacterium bovis
Nontuberculous mycobacteria
  M. avium complex
  M. kansasii
  M. abscessus

Actinomyces
Nocardiosis
Actinomycosis

Fungi
Histoplasmosis
Coccidioidomycosis
North American blastomycosis
South American blastomycosis (paracoccidioidomycosis)
Cryptococcosis

Aspergillosis
  Invasive aspergillosis
  Semi-invasive aspergillosis
  Aspergilloma
Zygomycosis
Pneumocystis jiroveci (P. carinii) pneumonia

Mycoplasma, Chlamydia, and Rickettsiae pneumonias
Mycoplasma pneumoniae
Chlamydia
  C. trachomatis
  C. psittaci
  C. pneumoniae
Rickettsiae

RNA viruses
Influenza virus
Parainfluenza virus
Respiratory syncytial virus
Coronaviruses
Hantaviruses
Togaviruses (rubella)

DNA viruses
Herpesviruses
  Herpes simplex
  Varicella-zoster
Cytomegalovirus
Epstein-Barr virus
Adenoviruses

Parasites: protozoans, roundworms (nematodes), and flatworms
Amebiasis
Toxoplasmosis
Ascariasis
Strongyloidiasis
Dirofilariasis
Tropical eosinophilia
Toxocariasis (visceral larva migrans)
Paragonimiasis
Schistosomiasis
Echinococcosis (hydatid disease)
Cysticercosis

Staphylococcus aureus

Staphylococcus aureus is an uncommon cause of community-acquired pneumonia but an important cause of nosocomial pneumonia (Table 12-3). It possesses several virulence

TABLE 12.2   *Streptococcus pneumoniae*

Most common pneumonia associated with Gram-positive cocci
Most common pneumonia requiring hospitalization or resulting in death
Air-space (lobar) pneumonia often with air bronchograms
Multifocal consolidation consistent with a bronchopneumonia less common
Pleural effusion in <50%

factors that allow the organism to infect susceptible hosts. While *S. aureus* infection usually occurs via the tracheobronchial tree, hematogenous spread of organisms to the lungs from staphylococcal endocarditis or cellulitis is another common mode of pulmonary infection.

Staphylococcus aureus pneumonia uncommonly occurs in otherwise healthy outpatients, although it has a well-recognized propensity for occurring following influenza infection. When pneumonia occurs in these settings, abrupt onset of chest pain, fever, cough, and purulent sputum, occasionally with hemoptysis, is typical. Factors that place patients at risk for pneumonia include COPD and other chronic illnesses, advanced age, immunosuppression, and cystic fibrosis. Most commonly, *S. aureus* pneumonia is encountered in hospitalized patients and presents with fever and cough

FIG. 12.12. Pneumococcal pneumonia. Frontal chest radiograph shows homogenous right upper lobe consolidation (*arrows*) associated with air bronchograms.

TABLE 12.3 *Staphylococcus aureus*

Common cause of nosocomial pneumonia
Associated with influenza and hematogenous pulmonary dissemination from endocarditis
Usually bronchopneumonia with patchy lower lobe consolidation
Cavitation frequent
Pneumatoceles may be seen
Septic emboli
Pleural effusion in nearly 50%; empyema may result

productive of purulent, occasionally blood-streaked, sputum. The mortality rate associated with *S. aureus* pneumonia in hospitalized patients is often substantial.

Imaging Findings. S. aureus usually causes a bronchopneumonia, with homogeneous or patchy, often multifocal, consolidation (Fig. 12-14), often predominating in the lower lobes. Volume loss is common, but air bronchograms are not. Abscess formation with cavitation is frequent (see Fig. 9-48 in Chapter 9). Occasionally, pneumatoceles are seen, especially in children. Pneumatoceles, unlike abscesses, appear as thin-walled cystic structures that may contain air-fluid levels. The inner wall of a pneumatocele is usually thin and

regular, unlike that of a pulmonary abscess. Pneumatoceles tend to resolve spontaneously in weeks or a few months following infection.

On CT or HRCT, pneumonia usually appears as segmental consolidation often associated with centrilobular nodules or tree-in-bud opacity.

Pleural effusions occur in nearly 50% of patients with *S. aureus* pneumonia; empyema may complicate such effusions. The latter may be suggested when loculation is present, particularly when extensive pleural thickening (the "split-pleura" sign) is seen on CT.

Hematogenous dissemination (septic embolization) of *S. aureus* to the lungs, as may be encountered with intravenous drug abuse and bacterial tricuspid valve endocarditis, typically presents as multiple, poorly defined nodules that cavitate over a period of several days (Fig. 12-15A). These nodules are usually peripherally located and predominate in the lower lobes. CT may show the presence of cavitation (see Fig. 12-15B) to better advantage than radiography and may also reveal that the nodules are closely associated with pulmonary vessels; this association, termed the "feeding vessel sign," is typical of processes that are hematogenously

FIG. 12.13. Round pneumonia caused by pneumococcus. Frontal chest radiograph shows a round, mass-like opacity within the right upper lobe (*arrows*). Pneumococcus was recovered in the patient's sputum, and the opacity resolved following antibiotic therapy.

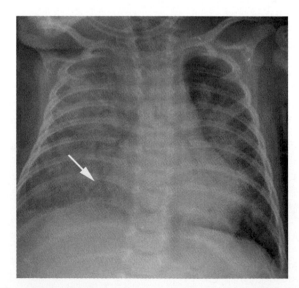

FIG. 12.14. Staphylococcal pneumonia. Frontal chest radiograph shows bilateral consolidation, associated with air bronchograms (*arrow*). Staphylococcal pneumonia was proven by blood and sputum cultures.

A   B

FIG. 12.15. Infective endocarditis with septic embolization. **A:** Frontal chest radiograph shows multiple, bilateral, peripheral nodules and cavities (*arrows*) representing septic emboli in a patient with *Staphylococcus aureus* infection of the tricuspid valve. **B:** Axial CT shows multiple, bilateral cavities (*arrows*) representing septic embolization.

disseminated to the lung. Wedge-shaped areas of peripheral consolidation, representing septic pulmonary infarction, are commonly seen in patients with septic embolization. Diffuse alveolar damage rarely follows septic embolization. The imaging manifestations of septic embolization are not specific to *S. aureus* and may be encountered with other bacterial pathogens, such as *S. epidermidis*.

Streptococcus pyogenes

Streptococcus pyogenes, a Gram-positive organism that is usually arranged in chains on smear, predominantly causes pneumonia in the very young and the elderly.

Pathologically, a bronchopneumonia pattern is usually observed with *S. pyogenes*. Much like *S. aureus*, *S. pyogenes* pneumonia frequently follows other respiratory infections, especially measles and whooping cough (*Bordetella pertussis*), although the frequency of these two infections has declined and *S. pyogenes* pneumonia is rarely seen.

Streptococcus pyogenes pneumonia usually presents with high fever, cough productive of purulent sputum, pleuritic chest pain, and shaking chills. The sputum may be blood streaked. Rarely, *S. pyogenes* pneumonia is accompanied by other *S. pyogenes* infections, such as scarlet fever and toxic shock syndrome.

Streptococcus pyogenes pulmonary infection typically causes patchy, segmental, multifocal consolidation that is often accompanied by pleural effusion. Unlike *S. aureus* pneumonia, pneumatocele formation is uncommon with *S. pyogenes* pneumonia, although lung abscesses may occur.

Other Gram-positive Cocci

Other Gram-positive cocci that rarely produce pulmonary infection include *S. viridans*, *S. faecalis* (*Enterococcus*), and

S. agalactiae. These organisms usually produce a bronchopneumonia pattern that is radiographically indistinguishable from *S. pyogenes* pneumonia or *S. aureus* pneumonia.

Gram-positive Bacilli

Bacillus anthracis

Bacillus anthracis is an encapsulated Gram-positive rod that forms spores (Table 12-4). The organism is most commonly found in agricultural areas, especially in Central and South America, Eastern and Southern Europe, Asia, the Middle East, and Africa. The spores are found in soil. Once they germinate, they are ingested by an animal, usually wild or domestic herbivores such as sheep, cattle, camels, and goats. Individuals who come in contact with these animals or their tissues may be exposed and become infected. Therefore, the highest-risk occupations include farmers, individuals who work with animal hides, and butchers.

Anthrax was largely unknown in the United States until October 2001, shortly following the terrorist attacks on the World Trade Center and Pentagon on September 11, 2001. From September 18 to November 20, 2001, 22 cases of

TABLE 12.4 *Bacillus anthracis*

Most common in agricultural areas (Central and South America, Eastern and Southern Europe, Asia, the Middle East, and Africa)
Contact with animals or their tissues
Three forms: cutaneous, gastrointestinal, and inhalational
Inhalational anthrax occurs when spore-containing dust is inhaled
Mediastinal widening, due to lymphadenopathy
Progressive pleural effusions

anthrax (11 inhalational, 11 cutaneous) occurred following exposure to mail contaminated with anthrax spores. Five of the 11 patients with inhalational anthrax died. In 2008, the Federal Bureau of Investigation identified a single perpetrator—a scientist in the biodefense industry—who committed suicide while awaiting prosecution.

Anthrax infection occurs in three forms: cutaneous, gastrointestinal, and inhalational. Humans usually become infected when they inhale spores after being exposed to infected animals or animal tissue. Rarely, infection is acquired through ingestion of undercooked meat from infected animals.

Inhaled anthrax spores are ingested by macrophages and are transported to the pulmonary lymphatics and eventually into the mediastinal and hilar lymph nodes. There the organisms may germinate and produce endotoxin, which results in hemorrhage and edema within the affected nodes. The organisms may then reach the bloodstream and cause sepsis.

Cutaneous anthrax occurs when the organism enters a host through an abrasion or laceration on the skin while an individual is handling infected animal tissue. This may be fatal if not treated, but treatment usually results in complete recovery.

Gastrointestinal anthrax occurs if infected animal tissue is ingested; it results in nausea, anorexia, vomiting, fever, and abdominal pain. Severe diarrhea is often present, and hematemesis is occasionally noted.

Inhalational anthrax occurs when spore-containing dust is inhaled. Symptoms of infection may initially resemble an upper respiratory tract viral infection, although an abrupt onset of high fever and chest pain occurs in some individuals. Inhalational anthrax often progresses to respiratory failure and shock. Inhalational anthrax is often fatal, although early antibiotic treatment may be curative for some patients.

Imaging Findings. Chest radiographic manifestations of anthrax include mediastinal widening, due to bulky lymphadenopathy, and progressively enlarging pleural effusions. Hilar lymphadenopathy may also be present. Lung opacity is usually minimal in comparison to the lymph node enlargement and pleural effusions. CT often shows high-attenuation lymphadenopathy and may also show peribronchiolar thickening resulting from lymphatic stasis.

Rhodococcus equi

Rhodococcus equi is a weakly acid-fast coccobacillus that has been primarily associated with pulmonary infection in immunocompromised individuals, particularly AIDS patients. The organism lives in soil, and human infection occurs via inhalation. Once a susceptible host inhales the organisms, they enter and replicate within alveolar macrophages. The presence of the organism induces an inflammatory response within the pulmonary parenchyma. Infection with *R. equi* is usually subacute in nature. Patients present with fever, productive cough, and chest pain. Infection with *R. equi* carries a high mortality rate. Imaging findings of *R. equi* pulmonary

infection include rounded areas of consolidation, often with cavitation.

Gram-negative Cocci

Moraxella catarrhalis (Branhamella catarrhalis)

Infection with *M. catarrhalis* usually occurs in patients with chronic illnesses such as COPD or patients on corticosteroid therapy. Other forms of immunocompromise may also place patients at risk for infection. *M. catarrhalis* is frequently found in the oral cavity. Upper and lower respiratory tract infection may occur in susceptible hosts. Patients present with fever and cough, usually mild. Infection with *M. catarrhalis* is usually mild, manifesting as a bronchopneumonia or bronchitis, and radiographic findings are nonspecific. Complications such as pleural effusion and empyema are uncommon.

Neisseria meningitides

Pulmonary infection with *N. meningitides* is uncommon and may occur with or without associated meningitis. Either lobar pneumonia or bronchopneumonia patterns may occur, occasionally with pleural effusion.

Gram-negative Rods

Gram-negative rods are an important cause of nosocomial pneumonia. Most ventilator-associated pneumonias are due to Gram-negative rods, and these infections are associated with high mortality. Gram-negative rod infection may also cause community-acquired pneumonia.

Escherichia coli

Escherichia coli is a normal inhabitant of the small and large bowel and may also be found within the oropharynx and nasopharynx following antibiotic treatment. Pulmonary infection occurs when the organism is aspirated into the lower respiratory tract. Gram-negative rods, including *E. coli*, typically cause a bronchopneumonia pattern.

Patients with *E. coli* pulmonary infection are usually either hospitalized or have chronic illnesses; they usually present with fever, cough productive of yellow sputum, shortness of breath, and pleuritic chest pain. When infection occurs in the outpatient setting, abrupt onset of fever, productive cough, pleuritic chest pain, and shortness of breath are the major presenting features.

The typical radiographic pattern of *E. coli* pulmonary infection is lower lobe bronchopneumonia. Pleural effusion is common.

Klebsiella pneumoniae

Although several *Klebsiella* species are known, *K. pneumoniae* is the most important organism from the point of view of human infection. *K. pneumoniae* classically affects older patients, particularly chronic alcoholics (Table 12-5).

TABLE 12.5 *Klebsiella pneumoniae*

Risk factors: old age, chronic alcoholism, chronic illness,
  chronic obstructive pulmonary disease (COPD)
Occurs with aspiration
Green sputum
Lobar pneumonia, sometimes bulging fissure sign
Abscesses common
Bronchopneumonia may be seen

TABLE 12.6 *Pseudomonas aeruginosa*

Nosocomial pneumonia, particularly in intensive care
  patients
Risk factors: chronic obstructive pulmonary disease,
  immunosuppression, mechanical ventilation, antibiotic
  use
Bronchopneumonia pattern, lower lobe involvement
Cavitation

Other chronic illnesses, such as diabetes mellitus and COPD, are associated with a higher prevalence of *K. pneumoniae* infection.

Klebsiella pneumoniae is occasionally a normal commensal in the human gastrointestinal tract. The organism may also colonize the upper airway in some patients, particularly those who are hospitalized. Lower respiratory tract infection may occur when oral secretions are aspirated. Bronchopneumonia and air-space pneumonia patterns may be observed, and tissue necrosis and abscess formation are common.

Klebsiella pneumoniae usually presents with rapid onset of fever, painful respiration, and shortness of breath. Cough productive of purulent green sputum is suggestive of *K. pneumoniae* infection, although occasionally the sputum is red and gelatinous ("currant jelly" sputum). Patients are usually quite ill and may even be hypotensive.

Imaging Manifestations. When *K. pneumoniae* presents with an air-space pattern, nonsegmental homogeneous consolidation resembling pneumococcal pneumonia is present. Air bronchograms are commonly seen. *K. pneumoniae* is known for its peculiar tendency to produce a large volume of consolidation, which causes expansion of a lobe, resulting in the bulging fissure sign (see Fig. 12-6). Pulmonary abscess formation is common, as are pleural effusion and empyema. A bronchopneumonia pattern may be seen with *K. pneumoniae* pulmonary infection, especially when the infection is hospital acquired.

Pseudomonas aeruginosa

Pseudomonas aeruginosa is typically found in soil and water but also in small numbers in the gastrointestinal tract of humans. *P. aeruginosa* is a common cause of nosocomial pneumonia, particularly in patients in the intensive care unit (Table 12-6). The organism typically lives within moist areas, such as showers, sinks, nebulizers, respiratory therapy equipment, and so forth. Infection with *P. aeruginosa* pneumonia is associated with numerous risk factors, including COPD, immunosuppression, mechanical ventilation, and prolonged antibiotic use.

Aspiration of organisms colonizing the upper respiratory tract is the usual cause of respiratory infection with *P. aeruginosa*. The organism elaborates a number of toxins and virulence factors that contribute to the ability to cause infection. The pattern of infection is bronchopneumonia,

with peribronchiolar microabscess formation, hemorrhage, and associated inflammation being common.

Patients usually present with fever, shaking chills, cough productive of purulent sputum (occasionally blood streaked), and shortness of breath. Mortality in ventilated patients or patients in the intensive care unit is high.

Imaging Findings. Chest radiographs show a pattern typical of bronchopneumonia, including segmental, often multifocal, patchy consolidation that favors the lower lobes. Pleural effusions may occur, as may empyema. Cavitation may also be seen (see Fig. 12-9). Tree-in-bud or centrilobular nodules may be seen on HRCT (see Fig. 10-28C in Chapter 10). The pattern of *P. aeruginosa* infection is insufficiently specific to distinguish it from other causes of bronchopneumonia.

Yersinia pestis

Yersinia pestis is the Gram-negative rod that causes plague. Historically, it has caused great epidemics, one of the largest of which occurred throughout Europe from 1347 to 1367, killing over one quarter of the population. While public health measures have largely controlled this disease, *Y. pestis* is still endemic in several areas of the world, including South America, China, parts of eastern and southern Africa, and the western United States. The disease usually occurs in the late spring through early fall. It affects men more commonly than women.

Yersinia pestis usually infects wild rodents (squirrels are the most important disease reservoir in the United States), although dogs and cats may become infected as well. In urban areas, rats are an important disease reservoir. The disease is transferred from animal to animal or animal to person by the bite of a tick or flea. Rare cases of plague occur following the inhalation of the organism from other infected patients.

Following a bite from an infected flea or tick, a local skin reaction occurs, after which regional lymphadenopathy develops. Infected lymph nodes are usually very enlarged and tender, and the skin overlying these lymph nodes is often discolored, giving rise to the "buboes" of **bubonic plague**. A septicemic phase may then occur, which affects the lungs and produces pneumonic plague. Person-to-person disease transmission may occur during this phase.

Yersinia pestis has several virulence factors that promote infection. The organism has a capsule that resists phagocytosis, and several surface antigens allow the organism to resist destruction and multiply within monocytes even if phagocytosed.

Pathologically, *Y. pestis* produces a severe bronchitis and bronchiolitis that rapidly evolve into severe bronchopneumonia. The air spaces may become filled with hemorrhage, edema, organisms, macrophages, and neutrophils, and alveolar necrosis is common.

Patients with pneumonic plague present with high fever, cough productive of bloody fluid, pleuritic chest pain, dyspnea, and cyanosis. Tender peripheral lymphadenopathy is often present. Prior to antibiotics, plague was uniformly fatal within 1 week of presentation. If antibiotic therapy is instituted in a timely fashion, recovery is the rule.

Pneumonic plague presents as severe, bilateral bronchopneumonia without cavitation, simulating ARDS. Pleural effusions may be present. Occasionally, regional lymph node enlargement is present, and this may be a clue to the diagnosis in endemic areas. Rarely, lymphadenopathy occurs without visible lung parenchymal abnormalities.

Serratia and *Enterobacter* Species

Both *Serratia* (*Serratia marcescens*) and *Enterobacter* spp. can cause pneumonia in debilitated, chronically ill patients, particularly those in the hospital. Bronchopneumonia patterns are typical. Pleural effusions are common with both organisms.

Gram-negative Coccobacilli

Haemophilus influenzae

Haemophilus influenzae is by far the most important human pathogen within the *Haemophilus* genus. This infection is particularly common in COPD patients (Table 12-7) and in children between the ages of 2 months and 3 years. Other risk factors include chronic illnesses such as diabetes, alcoholism, anatomic or functional asplenia, and immunodeficiency. *H. influenzae* also commonly afflicts young children and the elderly.

Haemophilus influenzae typically causes bronchitis in adults. In patients with viral respiratory infections, *H. influenzae* may cause a bronchopneumonia pattern; the air-space pneumonia pattern is less commonly observed. *H. influenzae* is a major cause of epiglottitis in both children and adults.

The clinical presentation of *H. influenzae* pneumonia consists of fever, cough productive of purulent sputum, and shortness of breath, usually superimposed on a background of chronic illness.

TABLE 12.7 *Haemophilus influenzae*

Risk factors: chronic obstructive pulmonary disease, chronic illness, alcoholism, immunodeficiency
Bronchitis and bronchopneumonia pattern
Lobar pneumonia less common

Imaging Findings. Chest radiography usually shows multifocal, bilateral patchy consolidation that favors the lower lobes. An air-space pneumonia pattern is occasionally encountered. Centrilobular nodules or tree-in-bud nodules may be seen on HRCT (see Fig. 10-28D in Chapter 10). Pleural effusions occur in about half of affected patients. Cavitation is uncommon.

Legionella pneumophila

Identified as the etiologic agent causing the pneumonia affecting the attendees of the National Convention of the American Legion in Philadelphia in 1976, *L. pneumophila* is recognized as the pathogen that causes the vast majority of cases of legionellosis. *Legionella* pneumonia is a fairly common cause of lower respiratory tract infection and is a frequent cause of nosocomial infection (Table 12-8). The organism is not part of the normal human flora; rather, *Legionella* resides in natural water sources. The organism is indigenous to freshwater lakes and streams, and human infection may occur when *Legionella* contaminates water systems, such as air conditioners and condensers. The organism may also contaminate showerheads and the like. Despite the frequency of *Legionella* nosocomial infection and the propensity of the organism to reside within sources of moisture, *Legionella* pneumonia is an uncommon cause of pulmonary infection in ventilator patients.

Legionella pneumonia usually affects older men, usually those with underlying chronic illnesses. Risk factors for infection include COPD, corticosteroid use, immunosuppression (including both AIDS and following organ transplantation), and malignancy.

Pathologically, *Legionella* causes a bronchopneumonia pattern of infection more commonly than an air-space pattern.

Legionella pneumonia may present with a wide range of severity, ranging from nearly asymptomatic to fulminant respiratory failure. On the mild end of the spectrum is the flu-like illness known as Pontiac fever, and on the severe end is respiratory failure with diffuse alveolar damage. The typical presentation is a middle-aged to elderly man with underlying chronic illness such as COPD, presenting with nonproductive cough, fever, headache, myalgia, mental status changes, and gastrointestinal symptoms, particularly diarrhea. As the disease progresses, shortness of breath and chest pain may occur, and the cough may become productive.

TABLE 12.8 *Legionella pneumophila*

Resides in natural water sources, contamination of water systems
Risk factors: old age, chronic obstructive pulmonary disease, steroid use, chronic illness, immunodeficiency
Bronchopneumonia or lobar pneumonia
Cavitation in immunosuppressed patients
Pleural effusion in 30%–60%

Central nervous system symptoms, gastrointestinal symptoms, and renal insufficiency are more commonly encountered in patients with *Legionella* pneumonia than other bacterial pneumonias. Electrolyte disturbances, such as hyponatremia, are also common.

Imaging Findings. *Legionella* pneumonia often causes peripheral focal consolidation that rapidly progresses to involve an entire lobe or perhaps several lobes on the side of initial presentation (see Fig. 2-13 in Chapter 2). Soon after, the consolidation becomes bilateral in the majority of patients, and this progression tends to occur even with proper antibiotic therapy. Cavitation is uncommon in immunocompetent patients but occurs frequently in immunocompromised patients. Pleural effusion is encountered in 30% to 60% of patients. Radiographic clearing of *Legionella* pneumonia is slow compared to other bacterial pneumonias.

Bordetella Species

Bordetella pertussis is by far the most important organism in the *Bordetella* genus to cause human disease. *B. pertussis* is the pathogen that causes the majority of cases of whooping cough. *B. pertussis* infection results in extensive mucous production, bronchitis, and bronchiolitis in infected patients. Infection can range from mild to quite serious, and bronchiectasis can result from severe infections.

Whooping cough classically presents in patients under the age of 2. The characteristic component of the infection is paroxysmal coughing that ends with a "whoop." Posttussive emesis may also occur. Adult infection is more common than previously recognized. Infection in adults may not follow the same pattern as in children, although the infection can be severe in some individuals.

Imaging Findings. The radiographic manifestations of *B. pertussis* infection include multifocal atelectasis and consolidation, occasionally accompanied by hilar lymphadenopathy. Radiographic abnormalities are most commonly found in the lower lobes, and central opacities obscuring the cardiac borders are common.

Bartonella henselae and quintana

Bartonella henselae and *quintana* are the causative agents of cat-scratch disease and bacillary angiomatosis in patients with AIDS.

Bartonella henselae and *quintana* pulmonary infections occur almost exclusively in patients with AIDS. Cat-scratch disease is an infection that primarily affects children and causes local lymphadenopathy. The mode of transmission of thoracic bacillary angiomatosis is unknown, but because cat-scratch disease is transmitted by animal-human contact, a similar mechanism may apply for thoracic bacillary angiomatosis.

Bartonella henselae and *quintana* infections produce extensive vascular proliferation, commonly involving the skin, mucous membranes, and internal organs, including the lungs.

Patients infected with *B. henselae* and *quintana* may present with fever, chest pain, weight loss, and night sweats. Hemoptysis has also been reported. Palpable lymphadenopathy may be evident on physical examination. The infection usually responds rapidly to antibiotic therapy.

Imaging Findings. Bacillary angiomatosis most commonly causes lung nodules. If large enough, the nodules may show intense enhancement. Large pleural effusions are often evident, and mediastinal lymphadenopathy is common. Enlarged lymph nodes often show extensive enhancement.

Francisella tularensis

Francisella tularensis is the cause of tularemia. This disease usually occurs in small animals, but human infection may occur when individuals come in contact with infected animals or insect vectors.

Infection is usually acquired by contact with infected animals, often through an open cut or skin abrasion while handling animal hides. Infection may also occur by ingesting contaminated meat or being bitten by infected insect vectors, such as ticks or deer flies. Infection is most frequently encountered in rural areas.

Several patterns of *F. tularensis* infection have been described. The most common patterns of pulmonary infection are the **typhoidal** and **ulceroglandular** forms of the disease. The typhoidal form of tularemia results from the ingestion of meat or water contaminated with organisms, whereas the ulceroglandular form of the disease results from direct patient skin inoculation through the handling of contaminated skins or hides. A rare pulmonary form of tularemia acquired by inhalation has been reported in laboratory employees working with *F. tularensis*.

The ulceroglandular form of tularemia causes ulcerated skin lesions and regional lymphadenopathy. The typhoidal form of the disease causes bacteremia. Clinical pneumonia develops in one third and three quarters of patients with the ulceroglandular and typhoidal forms of the disease, respectively. Patients present with high fever, weakness, and headaches, often with variable pharyngeal symptoms ranging from mild inflammation to ulcerative tonsillitis.

A nonspecific air-space pattern of pneumonia is most often encountered in patients with tularemia. Pleural effusion and hilar or mediastinal lymphadenopathy are also seen in nearly 50% of affected patients.

Anaerobic Bacteria

The major anaerobic bacteria implicated in human disease include organisms of the genus *Bacteroides, Fusobacterium, Porphyromonas,* and *Prevotella* (all Gram-negative bacilli); *Clostridium, Actinomyces,* and *Eubacterium* (Gram-positive bacilli); *Peptostreptococcus* and *Peptococcus* (Gram-positive cocci); and *Veillonella* (Gram-negative coccus).

TABLE 12.9 Anaerobic Bacteria

Organisms are normally found in the oral cavity
Risk factors: poor dental hygiene or gingivitis
Pneumonia occurs with aspiration
Few symptoms: foul-smelling sputum, fever, nonproductive
  cough
Involves gravitationally dependent regions
    Superior segments of lower lobes and posterior segments
      of upper lobes
    Right lower lobe more common than left lower lobe
Bronchopneumonia or lung abscess most common
Empyema may be associated

These organisms are normally found in the oral cavity, and they may result in disease when aspirated (Table 12-9). Therefore, conditions that favor the occurrence of aspiration, such as impaired consciousness, seizure, stroke, drug ingestion, and alcoholism, or conditions that impair the ability to clear aspirated secretions, such as obstructing endobronchial lesions or bronchostenoses, favor the development of anaerobic pulmonary infections. Additionally, factors that favor overgrowth of these organisms in the oral cavity, particularly poor dental hygiene or gingivitis, also predispose to the development of pulmonary anaerobic infections. Tonsillitis or chronic sinus infections are also associated with pulmonary anaerobic infections.

Pulmonary or pleural anaerobic infection begins with aspiration of infectious material from the oral cavity. Anaerobic bacterial infection produces a bronchopneumonia pattern, often associated with tissue necrosis; the latter produces radiographic evidence of cavitation.

Patients may initially present with fever and nonproductive cough and then develop foul-smelling sputum production once abscess formation occurs. Chest pain and hemoptysis may also occur. Quite often, anaerobic infection presents with few symptoms, making the infection difficult to diagnose.

Imaging Findings

Because anaerobic pulmonary infection is strongly related to aspiration, anaerobic bronchopneumonia most commonly involves the gravitationally dependent regions of lung: the superior segments of the lower lobes and the posterior segments of the upper lobes in the recumbent patient and the basal segments of the lower lobes in upright patients (Fig. 12-16). As a result of the relatively vertical orientation of the right main stem bronchus, the right lung is more commonly involved by aspiration events than is the left lung.

Bronchopneumonia in a basilar and dependent distribution is the most common radiographic abnormality in patients with aspiration-induced anaerobic infection. Pleural effusion commonly accompanies the lung parenchymal abnormalities. Occasionally, pleural effusion or empyema, without significant lung parenchymal abnormality, is the primary manifestation of anaerobic infection. Parenchymal cavitation is common and may evolve into a discrete lung abscess. Necrotizing pneumonia, manifesting as areas of consolidation with multiple areas of cavitation, is common. Lymphadenopathy may be present, and the radiographic appearance occasionally resembles pulmonary carcinoma. With treatment, cavities may slowly close, but residual scarring and bronchiectasis may occur.

A   B

FIG. 12.16. Aspiration pneumonia. **A:** Frontal chest radiograph shows bilateral, poorly defined opacities in the superior segments of both lower lobes (*arrows*). **B:** Axial CT image shows an air-space opacity within the superior segments of the lower lobes (*arrows*), associated with volume loss. The right lung is more abnormal than the left. The relatively vertical orientation of the right main stem bronchus predisposes the right lower lobe to aspiration pneumonia.

Mycobacteria

Mycobacteria are aerobic, non–spore-forming rods with unusually long doubling times. Numerous species of mycobacteria exist in nature, but the mycobacteria that cause human disease may be divided into two broad groups: the **tuberculosis complex** and the **nontuberculous**, or **atypical**, mycobacteria.

Another classification scheme for mycobacteria groups the organisms according to their rate of growth on solid medium: rapid growers usually show visible colonies within 7 days and slow growers require longer than 7 days to form visible colonies. Organisms classified as rapid growers that cause human pulmonary disease include *M. abscessus, M. fortuitum,* and *M. chelonae.* Organisms in the slow-growing group that cause pulmonary infection in humans include MTB, *Mycobacterium avium* complex (MAC), and *M. kansasii.* This classification scheme is useful from a clinical standpoint because rapid-growing mycobacteria are usually resistant to first-line antituberculosis drugs. Grouping mycobacteria into the tuberculosis complex and nontuberculous mycobacteria (NTMB) is more useful from an imaging standpoint.

The major organisms that cause human disease in the tuberculosis complex include MTB, *M. bovis, M. africanum,* and *M. microti.*

Mycobacterium tuberculosis

Tuberculosis has been an infection of importance throughout history. Although MTB infection rates had been steadily declining in the United States since the middle of the 19th century, worldwide MTB infection rates remain quite high. It has been estimated that at least 3 million people are infected with MTB throughout the world.

Numerous factors influence the likelihood of contracting tuberculosis. These include socioeconomic status, immune system integrity, age, general state of health, gender, and ethnicity. Patients with low socioeconomic status are at relatively higher risk for acquiring tuberculosis infection. Such patients often include those living in crowded housing conditions, individuals living in inner-city areas, homeless individuals, and drug abusers. Immunosuppressed patients, especially AIDS patients, are clearly at higher risk than the general population for the development of tuberculosis. Patients treated with corticosteroids or those who have undergone organ transplantation are also at increased risk for the development of MTB infection. Chronic illnesses, including diabetes mellitus, silicosis, and alveolar proteinosis, also place patients at increased risk for the development of tuberculosis. Very young and elderly patients are also at relatively increased risk for MTB infection, and men are more commonly affected than women. Finally, African American and Native American patients are at relatively higher risk for tuberculosis compared with other ethnic groups. In North America, immigrants from areas of the world that have a high prevalence of tuberculosis are at high risk for the development of infection.

MTB infection occurs with the inhalation of airborne respiratory droplets containing the organisms. Many factors influence the likelihood of contagion, including the presence of cavitation on imaging examinations, the burden of organisms, and the severity of cough. Person-to-person transmission is also more likely if exposure occurs in a poorly ventilated area or if contact with the infectious person is prolonged, such as occurs in relatively confined situations such as prisons, schools, and nursing homes.

Several different patterns of tuberculous infection have been described, differing in pathologic, clinical, and radiologic manifestations. These include primary MTB, progressive primary MTB, and postprimary MTB.

Primary Tuberculosis. Primary tuberculosis is said to occur when clinical infection occurs following the first exposure to the organism. Ultimately, the ability of MTB to cause human infection is related to the organism's ability to survive dormant within host macrophages for long periods of time and to incite a T-cell–mediated, delayed hypersensitivity response by the infected host. The host organism, under normal circumstances, will sequester the MTB organism by forming granulomas. Usually, these granulomas show **caseous necrosis**, a pattern characteristically, but not exclusively, associated with tuberculous infection. This initial infection has been termed the **Ghon focus** and usually heals by the development of a fibrous capsule around the focus of infection, which often calcifies. Shortly after the infection occurs, organisms may spread through the lymphatics to hilar and mediastinal lymph nodes, where a similar histopathologic reaction may occur. The combination of the lung parenchymal and lymph node MTB infection has been termed the **Ranke complex**. Organisms within the Ghon focus often gain access to the bloodstream and may disseminate to extrathoracic organs, but usually host defenses are sufficient to prevent overt infection from developing in extrathoracic sites. Although the pulmonary, lymphatic, and extrathoracic foci of infection are usually inactive at this point, organisms remain viable and may serve as the nidus for reactivation of disease when the circumstances are favorable.

Primary MTB infection in children is usually asymptomatic and may be detected only with the conversion of skin tests. When symptoms occur, cough and fever are most common. By contrast, adults with primary MTB infection are usually symptomatic and may present with weight loss, failure to thrive, fever, cough, and hemoptysis. Night sweats may also occur.

Imaging Findings. Patients with primary MTB most often show no radiologic abnormalities. If overt infection occurs, the pattern is usually one of air-space consolidation (Fig. 12-17), often involving an entire lobe. The right lung is more commonly affected than the left, although no definite zonal predominance is seen. Cavitation in primary MTB is unusual, and miliary dissemination is similarly uncommon.

Atelectasis is often encountered in children with primary MTB and may be related to airway compression by enlarged lymph nodes. Less commonly, rupture of an infected lymph node into an adjacent bronchus may cause endobronchial dissemination of infection associated with atelectasis. Adults with primary MTB uncommonly present with pulmonary atelectasis.

of disease resembling primary MTB infection. Such findings include consolidation associated with lymphadenopathy. Often, the lymphadenopathy is the dominant or only finding, and on CT, affected lymph nodes may show low central attenuation with peripheral enhancement following contrast administration (Fig. 12-25). HRCT commonly shows centrilobular nodules, often with tree-in-bud patterns. Pleural effusions may also occur. Normal radiographs are occasionally encountered in patients with AIDS and MTB, and extrapulmonary dissemination is also more frequent in this setting than in immunocompetent patients.

Mycobacterium bovis

The BCG (bacille Calmette-Guérin) vaccine, composed of an avirulent strain of *M. bovis*, is used to generate immunity against MTB in certain high-risk patients. BCG has also been used as an immune stimulant in the treatment of certain conditions, particularly carcinoma of the bladder. Although the organism used for this vaccine is not usually pathogenic in humans, in certain populations, particularly immunosuppressed patients, disseminated disease may develop, often manifesting as a miliary pattern on chest radiographs and HRCT.

Nontuberculous Mycobacteria

NTMB include at least 20 organisms that potentially cause human disease, although only a fraction of these organisms are important as a cause of thoracic infection. The NTMB have been subclassified according to Runyon criteria,

FIG. 12.25. Low-attenuation lymph nodes due to *Mycobacterium tuberculosis* infection in AIDS. Axial CT image shows low-attenuation lymphadenopathy anterior and posterior to the left brachiocephalic vein and superior vena cava (*arrows*).

based on their rate of growth and the presence or absence of pigment production: photochromogens (*M. kansasii*), scotochromogens (*M. szulgai* and *M. gordonae*), the nonphotochromogens (*M. avium* complex), and the rapid growers (*M. fortuitum* and *M. abscessus*). Most NTMB are inhabitants of natural water sources, such as lakes, rivers, and ponds, and some species may be found in soil or on animals. Infection may occur by various routes, including inhalation, ingestion, direct inoculation, or iatrogenic infection.

Many patients who develop NTMB infections are chronically ill. Risk factors include COPD, bronchiectasis, silicosis, cystic fibrosis, and AIDS. Other conditions associated with NTMB infection include diabetes mellitus, alcoholism, malignancy, and achalasia.

The pathologic patterns of most NTMB infections are similar to that of MTB infection. Pathologic features of NTMB infection include tissue destruction, necrosis, cavitation, and, occasionally, endobronchial spread of infection or miliary disease. Often, these disease patterns are superimposed on underlying chronic pulmonary abnormalities, complicating the pathologic appearance of NTMB infection.

For many patients, the symptoms of NTMB infection are indistinguishable from those of MTB pulmonary infection. One of the most common presenting symptoms is chronic cough.

Mycobacterium avium-intracellulare Complex. *M. avium-intracellulare* complex (MAC) is one of the most common human NTMB pathogens, and several patterns of infection in immunocompetent patients have been described (Table 12-12).

The first pattern resembles that of postprimary MTB, with upper lobe (often the apical and posterior segments) consolidation, cavities, scar formation, and small nodules suggesting endobronchial spread of infection. Pleural effusions and lymphadenopathy are relatively infrequent. This pattern of MAC infection is most often encountered in older men with some degree of mild underlying immunocompromise, such as COPD.

The second pattern of MAC infection consists of bronchiectasis and centrilobular nodules. The bronchiectasis and nodules may be found in all lobes, but they predominate in the right middle lobe and lingula (Fig. 12-26). Large nodules

TABLE 12.12 *Mycobacterium avium* **complex (MAC): Patterns of Disease**

MAC resembling postprimary *Mycobacterium tuberculosis*
    Most often in older men with mild immunocompromise or chronic obstructive pulmonary disease
MAC infection associated with bronchiectasis and nodules
    Usually women >60 years of age
    Often involves right middle lobe and lingula
    Patchy consolidation, bronchiectasis, nodules, and tree-in-bud
MAC with hypersensitivity pneumonitis
    Patchy ground-glass opacity or small nodules
    "Hot-tub lung"

FIG. 12.26. Spectrum of *Mycobacterium avium* complex (MAC) infection. **A:** Chest radiograph in a 72-year-old woman with MAC infection. Ill-defined nodular opacities (*large arrows*) are associated with bronchial wall thickening (*small arrows*) in the middle lobe and lingula. **B:** HRCT in a 70-year-old woman with MAC. Right middle lobe bronchiectasis (*large arrow*) is associated with centrilobular nodules (and tree-in-bud) (*small arrows*). **C:** HRCT of the right lung in an elderly woman with MAC. Small nodules and tree-in-bud opacities are visible (*small arrows*). Large nodules (*large arrow*) are also due to MAC. **D:** Axial HRCT image in a 67-year-old woman shows extensive right middle lobe and lingular bronchiectasis with centrilobular nodules and "tree-in-bud" opacities (*arrows*). **E:** Gross specimen shows centrilobular nodule (*arrow*) related to a dilated, irregular centrilobular bronchus (*double arrows*). (Image courtesy of Martha L. Warnock, MD, Professor Emerita, Department of Pathology, University of California, San Francisco.)

(more than 1 cm) are seen in some patients (see Fig. 12-26C). Patchy consolidations, representing foci of organizing pneumonia, are also seen. This pattern of infection most often affects older (more than 60 years of age) women.

A third pattern of MAC infection resembles hypersensitivity pneumonitis, with patchy ground-glass opacities and poorly defined ground-glass centrilobular nodules, and air trapping. MAC in this context is usually acquired via exposure to contaminated hot tubs, and the term "hot-tub lung" has been applied to this exposure (see Fig. 16-6 in Chapter 16).

Mycobacterium kansasii. The radiographic pattern of *M. kansasii* infection closely resembles that of postprimary MTB (Fig. 12-27). Several studies examining the differences in the radiographic abnormalities between these two infections have found no consistent feature that can distinguish the two infections, except that pleural effusions are very uncommon with *M. kansasii* infection.

Mycobacterium abscessus. *M. abscessus* pulmonary infection may be more common than previously thought. *M. abscessus* tends to cause bronchiectasis and centrilobular nodules, often with tree-in-bud morphology, predominating in the right middle lobe and lingula.

Nontuberculous Mycobacteria in AIDS. NTMB infection, especially MAC, is very common in patients with AIDS, and the incidence of infection rises as the CD4 cell count falls. Most patients with clinically overt MAC infection have CD4 cell counts below 50 cells/µL. Although MAC is often found in the sputum of patients with advanced AIDS, true pulmonary disease due to MAC is relatively uncommon. Clinically overt MAC infection in patients with AIDS often presents with small nodules, usually centrilobular in distribution, combined with air-space consolidation. Mediastinal lymph node enlargement may occur. Enlarged lymph nodes may show low attenuation, although this finding is more predictive of MTB than MAC infection. Occasionally, patients present with solitary pulmonary nodules resembling pulmonary carcinoma (Fig. 12-28). Hepatosplenomegaly is common.

Mycobacterium kansasii infection may also occur in patients with AIDS and most commonly present with consolidation and nodules located in the mid and lower lung zones; this presentation contrasts with the upper lobe cavitary pattern that often occurs in patients without HIV infection. When cavitation is present in these patients, it portends a worse outcome. Other concurrent infections are common.

Actinomyces

The actinomyces resemble fungi morphologically and are often classified with fungi, but they respond to antibiotics and are more appropriately considered bacteria. Disease is usually caused by *Nocardia* and *Actinomyces*.

Nocardiosis

The most important disease-causing *Nocardia* sp. is *N. asteroides*. Nocardiae are aerobic, Gram-positive, weakly acid-fast organisms that live in soil. Human disease is acquired via inhalation of the organism, although person-to-person transmission can occur (Table 12-13). *Nocardia* infection may occur in otherwise healthy patients but is most common in patients with underlying immunodeficiency, such as transplant recipients on immunosuppressive therapy, patients with connective tissue disease on corticosteroid therapy, patients with malignancy on cytotoxic therapy, or patients with AIDS. *N. asteroides* has a propensity for infecting patients with alveolar proteinosis.

FIG. 12.27. *Mycobacterium kansasii* infection. Frontal chest radiograph shows a left upper lobe cavity (*large arrow*) and numerous small nodules in the lower lobes (*small arrows*), representing endobronchial spread of infection.

FIG. 12.28. *Mycobacterium avium* complex infection in AIDS. Axial CT image shows a spiculated nodule (*arrow*) in the left upper lobe mimicking the appearance of carcinoma. Resection revealed that the nodule was caused by *M. avium* complex infection.

TABLE 12.13 Nocardiosis

Organisms live in soil
Acquired via inhalation of the organism; human-to-human
  spread less common
Immunodeficiency usually present
Bronchopneumonia pattern or multiple nodules
Cavitation may occur
Pleural effusion in 50%
Chest wall involvement may occur

Nocardia asteroides infection usually appears as either bronchopneumonia or multiple nodules, often accompanied by a neutrophilic exudate. Cough, chest pain, and fever are the most common presenting symptoms, and the course of the illness is often protracted. However, the disease course may be quite rapid in severely immunocompromised patients. In such patients, dissemination may occur, often affecting the brain.

Imaging Findings

Chest radiography or CT may show one or more areas of consolidation (i.e., bronchopneumonia) or a solitary pulmonary nodule or mass (Fig. 12-29), which may be cavitary (see Fig. 12-10). Multiple nodules, either large or small, may be seen, particularly in immunosuppressed patients (Fig. 12-30). Nodules are often sharply defined. Areas of decreased attenuation may be seen on CT within nodules or areas of consolidation due to necrosis. Pleural effusion or empyema occurs in nearly 50% of patients. Chest wall invasion is uncommon but may occur.

Actinomycosis

Among the various species within the genus *Actinomyces*, *Actinomyces israelii* is the most important cause of human infection. *A. israelii* is an anaerobic or microaerophilic organism that occasionally stains in a weakly Gram-positive fashion. The organisms uncommonly show minimal acid-fast staining characteristics if a weak decolorizing solution is used. *A. israelii* forms mycelia that, in tissue, may cluster to form sulfur granules. These granules are so named because of their yellow color, although they contain relatively little actual sulfur.

Actinomyces israelii is a normal inhabitant of the oropharynx. The organism causes disease when it is aspirated into the lungs or swallowed into the gastrointestinal tract. The organism is ubiquitous and no specific factors predisposing to infection are found in many patients, although alcoholics may be relatively predisposed to *A. israelii* infection due to their increased risk of aspiration and poor oral hygiene. The

A

B

FIG. 12.29. *Nocardia* infection. **A:** Chest radiograph in an immunosuppressed patient shows a cavitary mass in the right upper lobe (*arrows*). **B:** CT shows a cavity containing an air-fluid level.

FIG. 12.30. *Nocardia* infection in a patient with a heart transplant. CT shows multiple left lung nodules (*arrows*).

organism usually causes mandibular osteomyelitis following dental extraction, with gastrointestinal and thoracic diseases occurring less commonly.

When the organism reaches the lungs, it has a propensity for causing abscesses and sinus tracts. Acute and chronic inflammation, often with some degree of fibrosis, is present surrounding the sulfur granules.

Actinomyces israelii infection may start as a nonproductive cough that may become purulent over time, occasionally accompanied by hemoptysis. Fever may also be present. Pleuritic chest pain may occur if the infection involves the pleural space. If the infection remains untreated, patients may develop stigmata of chronic pulmonary disease, such as weight loss, and digital clubbing. As infection extends into the pleural space and then into the chest wall, bronchopleural-cutaneous fistulas and sinus tracts may develop. *A. israelii* infection may also invade the diaphragm and extend into the abdomen, into the mediastinum, or through the lung apex into the neck. Extrathoracic dissemination may occur.

Imaging Findings

Actinomyces israelii typically causes lower lobe peripheral air-space consolidation that may progress to abscess formation if proper therapy is not instituted in a timely fashion. On CT, foci of air-space consolidation may show areas of low attenuation, representing microabscess formation. If a frank abscess occurs, pleural effusion and empyema commonly develop, and chest wall invasion may also occur. The latter usually appears as a chest wall mass, often with periosteal reaction involving the ribs or frank rib destruction. A pattern particularly suggestive of *A. israelii* chest wall infection is wavy periosteal reaction affecting several contiguous ribs; this pattern may be seen in the absence of associated empyema. Although chest wall invasion has classically been associated with *A. israelii* infection, it is becoming very uncommon due to effective early antibiotic treatment.

Actinomyces israelii may present on chest radiography as a mass, often with cavitation, simulating lung carcinoma. Rare reported manifestations of thoracic *A. israelii* infection include endobronchial lesions, isolated pleural effusions, a miliary pattern, and biapical consolidation resembling pulmonary tuberculosis. For patients who develop chronic *A. israelii* pulmonary infection, extensive lung fibrosis and architectural distortion may occur.

Fungal Infections

Certain fungi—including *Histoplasma capsulatum*, *Coccidioides immitis*, North American blastomycosis, *Paracoccidioides brasiliensis*, and *Blastomyces dermatitidis*—are endemic to particular geographic areas and in these regions tend to affect otherwise healthy persons; these fungi are known as **endemic fungi**. These organisms typically live in soil as saprophytes and infect humans when their spores are inhaled.

Histoplasmosis

Histoplasma capsulatum is by far the most important *Histoplasma* species from a human disease perspective. Infection with *H. capsulatum* is usually asymptomatic, but clinically overt infection may result from overwhelming inoculation or infection in immunocompromised patients.

Histoplasma capsulatum normally lives in soil. The organism thrives in nitrogen-rich environments and is thus often found in soil contaminated with guano from bats or birds. Particularly high-risk environments include caves, pigeon roosts, chicken houses, or other environments where guano becomes concentrated.

Histoplasma capsulatum infection occurs most commonly in individuals living in the Ohio and Mississippi River valleys in the United States and less commonly in South America, Africa, Southeast Asia, and Europe. In these areas, infection is endemic, with 70% or more of the population showing positive histoplasmin skin tests.

Histoplasma capsulatum exists in a mycelial form in soil and may produce microconidia that may be inhaled by humans. The initial polymorphonuclear leukocytic response to the inhaled microconidia is ineffective in killing the organisms, and soon lymphocytes and macrophages are recruited. These cells are capable of killing the microconidia and the budding yeast into which microconidia transform. The recruitment of lymphocytes is part of the cell-mediated immunity that is important in the pathogenesis of *H. capsulatum* infection, and granulomatous inflammation very similar to tuberculosis is common. Early in the course of infection, spread to lymph nodes is ubiquitous, and extrathoracic dissemination, often to the liver, spleen, bone marrow, and lymph nodes, is also frequent. Healing with the formation of a fibrous capsule around the inflammatory focus usually occurs, often with calcification.

The vast majority of *H. capsulatum* infections are not associated with symptoms. When symptoms are associated with clinical evidence of infection, the term "acute histoplasmosis" is often used. Patients often present with fever, headache, chest pain, and cough, usually mild. Uncommonly, overwhelming exposures may produce severe infection, with hemoptysis, pericarditis, and even ARDS.

Imaging Findings

In the majority of patients with *H. capsulatum* infection, the chest radiograph appears normal. When findings are present, nonspecific multifocal areas of consolidation are often found. If infection is severe, the pattern may resemble bacterial air-space pneumonia. Lymphadenopathy is common, but pleural effusions are not.

In patients with large exposures, diffusely distributed, variably sized but usually small (occasionally small enough to resemble a miliary pattern) nodules may be seen, usually associated with lymphadenopathy. Such nodules may eventually undergo calcification when healing occurs (Fig. 12-31).

FIG. 12.31. Healed histoplasmosis with multiple calcified nodules. This appearance reflects the healing of diffuse nodular histoplasmosis.

The development of a solitary pulmonary nodule from *H. capsulatum* infection, or **histoplasmoma**, is a well-recognized pattern of disease. Such nodules are often circumscribed, measuring up to 3 cm and occasionally more (Fig. 12-32), and often contain central "bull's-eye" or "target" calcification (see Fig. 9-16 in Chapter 9). Adjacent satellite nodules may be present, and calcified lymph nodes are also common. Occasionally, histoplasmomas are multiple but usually not more than five in number.

Uncommonly, lymphadenopathy is the only abnormality seen on chest radiography. Enlarged lymph nodes may compress adjacent bronchi, causing atelectasis.

Chronic pulmonary histoplasmosis may appear as upper lobe fibrocavitary consolidation that closely resembles postprimary MTB. Often, these findings are superimposed on COPD, and air-fluid levels within bullae and increasing wall thickness of bullae may be seen. Over time, linear opacities develop, indicating the presence of fibrosis.

Histoplasma capsulatum infection of mediastinal lymph nodes may result in extensive necrosis and fibrosis of the affected lymph nodes (see Fig. 8-47 in Chapter 8). This pattern of infection may result in granulomatous or fibrosing mediastinitis, with venous obstruction, bronchial stenoses, and narrowing of the pulmonary arteries visible on CT scanning; the former is recognized by the formation of extensive mediastinal venous collateral vessels. Soft-tissue masses in the distribution of lymph node stations are present, and *H. capsulatum* may be assumed to be the cause when extensive calcifications of lymph nodes are seen. Esophageal obstruction and esophageal diverticula may occur.

Acute disseminated histoplasmosis usually occurs in very young children or in severely immunocompromised individuals, such as AIDS patients or transplant recipients. The typical radiographic appearance is a miliary pattern, and the liver, spleen, lymph nodes, adrenal glands, and bone marrow are often affected. The disease course may be fulminant (Table 12-14).

Coccidioidomycosis

Coccidioides immitis is a dimorphic fungus that exists in soil in a mycelial form. The mycelia produce arthrospores that may cause human infection when inhaled (Table 12-15). Once in tissue, the organisms exist as spherules and may undergo reproduction while in this form.

Coccidioides immitis infection is endemic in the Southwestern United States, Northern Mexico, and areas of Central and South America. Strong winds may carry infection beyond these areas, and travel through endemic areas may account for other cases that are noted outside endemic areas of the country. Within endemic regions, infection rates (often measured by conversion of skin tests) are high. Risk factors associated with *C. immitis* infection include living in

A   B

FIG. 12.32. Histoplasmoma. **A:** Chest radiograph shows a left upper lobe mass (*arrow*). **B:** CT shows ringlike calcification (*arrows*).

TABLE 12.14 **Histoplasmosis**

Organisms live in soil
Thrives in nitrogen-rich environments (soil contaminated
  with guano); high-risk environments: caves, pigeon
  roosts, and chicken houses
Ohio and Mississippi River valleys
Infection usually asymptomatic; if not, fever, headache,
  chest pain, cough
Radiographs may be normal
Radiographic findings:
  Patchy pneumonia
  Lymphadenopathy common
  Effusion uncommon
  Diffuse small nodules due to large exposure, may calcify
  Histoplasmoma, central "bull's-eye" or "target"
    calcification
  Chronic disease may mimic postprimary
    Mycobacterium tuberculosis
  Fibrosing mediastinitis
  Miliary spread, usually in children or
    immunocompromised patients

endemic areas and immunosuppression. It has been suggested that Filipinos, Native Americans, and African Americans are at relatively higher risk for infection than whites. Mini-epidemics have occurred in situations when soil has been disturbed in endemic areas, such as construction projects and earthquakes.

Coccidioides immitis infection has traditionally been divided into primary infection, persistent primary infection, and disseminated infection patterns. The primary infection pattern usually occurs at initial exposure. When inhaled, *C. immitis* arthrospores develop into sporangia, which induce pulmonary inflammation. Initially the pattern of inflammation resembles bronchopneumonia, but later granulomatous inflammation develops. In most patients, the inflammatory focus resolves without sequelae.

TABLE 12.15 **Coccidioidomycosis**

Organisms live in soil
Southwestern United States, Northern Mexico, Central
  and South America
Infection often asymptomatic
Primary infection pattern: usually occurs at initial exposure
  Resembles bronchopneumonia
  Unilateral consolidation
  Hilar lymphadenopathy may be present
  Resolves in most patients
Persistent primary infection: infection lasting >6 weeks
  Progressive pneumonia
  Development of nodular lesions, often with cavitation
  Cavities may be thin walled
  Calcification uncommon
Disseminated infection
  Male Filipino, Native American, African American, and
    immunocompromised patients
  Miliary pattern often with lymph node enlargement

In a few individuals, the initial site of inflammation progresses and necrosis develops. Such progressive disease may occupy an entire lobe or even a whole lung, and hilar and mediastinal lymph node involvement is common in this setting.

Persistent primary infection with *C. immitis* is said to be present when primary infection lasts longer than 6 weeks. This pattern of infection may result in progressive pneumonia or the formation of nodular lesions, often with central necrosis, residing within a fibrous capsule.

Disseminated infection tends to occur in male Filipino, African American, and immunocompromised patients. Using the lungs as an entry portal, *C. immitis* infection may disseminate to the brain and meninges, bones, skin, joints, and kidneys. Radiographic evidence of coincident pulmonary infection is usually present but occasionally is lacking. Miliary disease with *C. immitis* infection may occur and is usually accompanied by evidence of extrathoracic infection.

For most patients, primary *C. immitis* infection is asymptomatic. In some cases, flu-like symptoms are present, including fever, cough, headache, and chest pain. An erythematous rash may also be encountered. A syndrome known as "valley fever" has been noted with *C. immitis* infection; it consists of a flu-like constellation of symptoms in addition to erythema nodosum or erythema multiforme and arthralgias. Peripheral blood eosinophilia may be present in patients with valley fever.

Patients with persistent primary *C. immitis* pneumonia are often symptomatic, whereas those with nodular lesions are not.

Imaging Findings

When chest radiographic findings are present, primary *C. immitis* pulmonary infection usually manifests as unilateral air-space consolidation, often in the lower lobe (Fig. 12-33). The consolidation occasionally shows the tendency to resolve in one area and recur in another (phantom infiltrates). Lymphadenopathy is not uncommon, and pleural effusions, usually ipsilateral to the consolidation, are present in a few cases.

Progressive primary infection is associated with increasing multifocal pneumonia or the development of pulmonary nodules, either of which may cavitate. Occasionally, consolidation resolves into a peripheral nodule, which may then undergo progressive cavitation into a thin-walled (grape-skin) cyst, which then spontaneously resolves (Fig. 12-34). Such nodules are more commonly single than multiple, and they calcify in very few patients.

Similar to MTB and histoplasmosis, a progressive form of *C. immitis* infection has been described, variously referred to as chronic progressive coccidioidomycosis or progressive coccidioidal pneumonia. Radiographically, chronic progressive coccidioidomycosis appears as upper lobe consolidation associated with linear opacities and cavitation (Fig. 12-35) and therefore may closely resemble either postprimary MTB or chronic histoplasmosis.

Disseminated coccidioidomycosis occurs most frequently in immunocompromised patients, African Americans, or

A   **B**

FIG. 12.33. Primary coccidioidomycosis pulmonary infection proven by serology and bronchoscopy. **A:** Frontal chest radiograph shows homogenous left lower lobe consolidation (*arrow*). Left hilar enlargement reflects lymphadenopathy. **B:** Axial CT image shows homogenous left lower lobe mass-like opacity (*arrow*) without air bronchograms.

Filipinos. A miliary pattern is often present on chest radiographs or CT (Fig. 12-36), usually accompanied by hilar or mediastinal lymphadenopathy. Extrathoracic dissemination occurs frequently, often affecting the bones, brain and meninges, and spleen.

North American Blastomycosis

North American blastomycosis is caused by *B. dermatitidis*. This organism resides in soil but may assume a yeast form at body temperature.

Blastomyces dermatitidis is endemic in the central and southeastern United States and Canada (especially the Ohio and Mississippi River valleys, particularly Wisconsin) but may also be found in Central and South America and parts of Africa. Infection occurs by the inhalation of aerosolized fungal spores, often in previously healthy individuals, and has been associated with people living and working in wooded areas. Certain risk factors for *B. dermatitidis* have been identified, including immunosuppression and corticosteroid therapy. Similar to the other endemic fungi, disseminated disease is more likely in immunosuppressed patients.

Following inhalation of the organisms, bronchopneumonia occurs. The initial neutrophilic reaction is subsequently replaced with lymphocytes and macrophages and granulomatous inflammation, although caseous necrosis is uncommon.

Blastomyces dermatitidis infection may be asymptomatic, much like the other endemic fungi, but the frequency of asymptomatic primary infection may be less than the other endemic fungi. Symptomatic infection presents either as a flu-like illness or as an acute bronchopneumonia, with fever, chills, sputum production, and chest pain. Musculoskeletal symptoms and skin findings may be present.

Imaging Findings

Infection with *B. dermatitidis* may present as consolidation resembling other causes of bronchopneumonia. Occasionally, disease is rapidly progressive, with the development of multifocal bilateral air-space opacities or even ARDS. Miliary disease has been reported. Extrathoracic dissemination may occur, especially in immunocompromised patients, usually affecting the skin, musculoskeletal structures, and characteristically the genitourinary tract.

South American Blastomycosis (Paracoccidioidomycosis)

The causative agent of South American blastomycosis is the dimorphic fungus *P. brasiliensis*. Much like *B. dermatitidis*, *P. brasiliensis* exists in soil as a mycelial form but converts to a yeast form at body temperature.

Paracoccidioides brasiliensis is endemic in Central and South America, particularly Brazil. Patients outside these regions with *P. brasiliensis* infection usually have a history of travel to an endemic area. Asymptomatic infection may

A

B

FIG. 12.34. Progressive primary coccidioidomycosis pulmonary infection proven by percutaneous transthoracic biopsy. **A:** Frontal chest
radiograph at presentation shows a subpleural
left lower lobe nodule (*arrow*). **B:** Frontal chest
radiograph several months after presentation
shows cavitation (*arrow*). **C:** Frontal chest radiograph 1 year after presentation shows that the
left lower lobe nodule has evolved into a thin-
walled cavity (*arrow*), assuming the "grape-skin"
morphology characteristic of chronic pulmonary
coccidioidomycosis infection.

C

A   **B**

FIG. 12.35. Chronic progressive primary coccidioidomycosis pulmonary infection. **A:** Axial CT image shows thin-walled cavities (*arrows*) in the right upper lobe. **B:** Axial CT image obtained several months later, and after the initiation of antifungal therapy, shows persistence of the right upper lobe cavities (*large arrow*) and the development of nodular opacities in the left upper lobe (*small arrows*). Sputum examination was persistently positive for *Coccidioides immitis*.

show no gender predilection, but clinically apparent infection is far more common in men than women. Infection occurs following inhalation of the organisms, and dissemination may then occur. Patients at greatest risk for the development of infection are those who come in contact with soil in endemic regions, such as farmers and manual laborers.

Much like the other endemic fungi, cell-mediated immunity is important in the host response to *P. brasiliensis* infection. Patterns of infection include bronchopneumonia, nodules with or without cavitation, and miliary disease. A combination of granulomatous inflammation and a neutrophilic infiltrate may be seen pathologically.

Patients may be asymptomatic or present with a flu-like illness. Immunocompromised patients are at higher risk for developing disseminated disease and may present with hepatosplenomegaly, lymphadenopathy, and possibly central nervous system or gastrointestinal findings.

Imaging Findings

The imaging manifestations of *P. brasiliensis* pulmonary infection are similar to the other endemic fungi and include air-space consolidation and single or multiple nodules (Fig. 12-37) that may cavitate. Lymphadenopathy may occur, either alone or together with pulmonary parenchymal disease. The most commonly visible thoracic CT findings in patients with *P. brasiliensis* include focal, multifocal, or diffuse areas of consolidation and ground-glass opacity with variably sized nodules. Areas of low attenuation and interlobular septal thickening may also be evident. In the minority of patients, a "reversed halo" sign (the "atoll" sign) may

A   **B**

FIG. 12.36. Hematogenous dissemination of coccidioidomycosis pulmonary infection in AIDS. **A:** Frontal chest radiograph shows numerous bilateral small nodules, some of which are larger (*arrow*) than is typical for miliary *Mycobacterium tuberculosis* infection. **B:** Axial chest CT shows numerous, variably sized, randomly distributed nodules (*arrows*), consistent with hematogenous dissemination.

FIG. 12.37. Paracoccidioidomycosis proven by transthoracic needle biopsy. **A:** Frontal chest radiograph shows bilateral, poorly defined masses (*arrows*). **B:** Axial CT image shows poorly defined areas of nodular consolidation (*arrows*). Note the presence of air bronchograms within the left upper lobe opacity.

be encountered. Over time and following treatment, findings of fibrosis, including architectural distortion, traction bronchiectasis, peribronchovascular thickening, and irregular air-space enlargement, may be seen.

Cryptococcus

Cryptococcus neoformans is the most common etiologic agent resulting in cryptococcosis. Unlike the endemic fungi, *C. neoformans* exists only in a yeast form in both nature and when it infects humans. The organism often has a characteristic capsule that becomes visible with India ink preparations. Two variants of *C. neoformans* cause human disease: *C. neoformans* variant *neoformans* and *C. neoformans* variant *gattii*.

Cryptococcus neoformans is typically found in pigeon droppings, although it is unclear if contact with pigeons actually results in a demonstrably increased risk of developing cryptococcosis. *C. neoformans* variant *gattii* is found mostly in tropical regions and may infect otherwise healthy adults, whereas *C. neoformans* variant *neoformans* is found worldwide and primarily causes disease in immunocompromised patients.

Inhalation of the yeast provides the route for infection. It is likely that the capsule of the organism contributes to its ability to cause disease because organisms without a capsule are usually easily destroyed by neutrophils. Infection by *C. neoformans* may take the form of single or multiple nodules, bronchopneumonia, or miliary nodules. The pattern of inflammation is variable, occasionally with elements of a granulomatous response in some and a suppurative response in others. In patients with AIDS, there may be little inflammation associated with the organisms.

Cryptococcus neoformans infection in otherwise healthy patients is often asymptomatic. When symptoms occur, a flu-like illness is common. Patients with AIDS and *C. neoformans* infection may present with a variety of respiratory complaints as well as headache. The latter may indicate the presence of meningitis and may occur in the absence of radiographic evidence of pulmonary disease.

Imaging Findings

In healthy patients, cryptococcal infection usually manifests as one or more peripheral, circumscribed nodules, usually without cavitation. Less commonly, air-space consolidation is seen.

In patients with AIDS, a diffuse interstitial pattern, variously described as reticular or nodular, resembling *P. jiroveci* pneumonia (Fig. 12-38), may be seen. A miliary pattern may occur (Fig. 12-39), as may single (Fig. 12-40) or multiple

FIG. 12.38. Cryptococcosis in AIDS. Frontal chest radiograph shows bilateral linear and ground-glass opacity that resembles *Pneumocystis jiroveci* pneumonia. Bronchoscopy proved cryptococcal pneumonia.

FIG. 12.39. Cryptococcosis in AIDS. Frontal chest radiograph shows innumerable, bilateral, very small, and well-defined pulmonary nodules (*arrows*), consistent with a miliary pattern, proven to represent pulmonary cryptococcosis. Note the right paratracheal and bilateral hilar lymphadenopathy.

nodules (see Fig. 9-35B in Chapter 9), occasionally with cavitation (Fig. 12-41). Lymph node enlargement is uncommon, as is pleural effusion. Dissemination to extrathoracic structures is common in patients with AIDS, particularly to the brain and meninges.

Candida

Several species of *Candida* are capable of causing human disease, but *Candida albicans* is the most common and most important. *C. albicans* is found in the gastrointestinal

FIG. 12.40. Cryptococcosis in AIDS. Axial CT image shows an irregular left lower lobe nodule (*arrow*) with associated pleural reaction. Percutaneous biopsy recovered *Cryptococcus neoformans*.

tract and on the skin of normal individuals, but clinically overt pulmonary infection almost always occurs in the setting of immunosuppression. Such conditions include cytotoxic therapy for malignancy, AIDS, chronic antibiotic use, organ transplant recipients, chronic granulomatous disease of childhood, and patients with severe burns. As with other fungi, cell-mediated immunity is important for the prevention of *C. albicans* infection.

Candida albicans pulmonary infection usually occurs in the setting of multiorgan involvement in patients with disseminated disease. In this circumstance, the lungs show numerous small nodules with associated inflammation. Very rarely, *C. albicans* infection occurs as a result of aspiration of organisms from the oral cavity into the lungs. Symptoms of infection are nonspecific and include purulent cough and fever. Findings suggesting extrathoracic dissemination are often present.

The most common chest radiographic appearance of *C. albicans* pulmonary infection is focal or multilobar consolidation (Fig. 12-42), occasionally with linear abnormalities suggesting an interstitial component. Cavitation and lymphadenopathy are not features of *C. albicans* pulmonary infection. A miliary pattern may occur. HRCT may show multiple nodules with areas of ground-glass opacity and consolidation; the nodules may be poorly defined or circumscribed.

Aspergillus

Aspergillus species are ubiquitous fungi found throughout nature that may result in disease in susceptible hosts when inhaled. The most important *Aspergillus* species from a human infectious disease point of view is *A. fumigatus*. The organism exists in a mycelial form with hyphae that characteristically branch at 45-degree angles and may be found throughout nature. Other *Aspergillus* species, particularly *A. terreus*, are of growing importance as well.

Infections caused by *A. fumigatus* have traditionally been classified into four different forms: invasive aspergillosis, semi-invasive aspergillosis (also known as chronic necrotizing aspergillosis), allergic aspergillosis (including allergic bronchopulmonary aspergillosis [ABPA] and hypersensitivity pneumonitis; see Chapters 16 and 23), and aspergilloma. An uncommon manifestation of *A. fumigatus* infection that primarily affects AIDS patients, known as obstructing bronchial aspergillosis, also has been described.

Aspergillus infection may occur when a susceptible host inhales the organism. Various risk factors for the development of *A. fumigatus* infection exist, and each is related to a particular pattern of infection.

Invasive Aspergillosis

In normal hosts, inhaled *Aspergillus* organisms are rapidly destroyed by macrophages, with neutrophils providing additional immunity. The presence of granulocytopenia

A

B

C

FIG. 12.41. Cryptococcosis in AIDS. **A:** Frontal chest radiograph shows a poorly defined nodule in the right lung (*arrow*) associated with right hilar lymphadenopathy. **B:** Axial CT image photographed in lung windows shows a spiculated nodule (*arrow*) within the superior segment of the right lower lobe. **C:** Axial CT image photographed in soft-tissue windows shows that the nodule (*larger arrow*) is low in attenuation (necrotic) and contains a small amount of air due to cavitation. Right hilar lymphadenopathy (*smaller arrows*) is also present.

FIG. 12.42. Candidal pneumonia in a patient receiving steroids for collagen-vascular disease. Chest radiograph shows a focal left upper lobe pneumonia (*arrow*).

or neutropenia allows *Aspergillus* spores to germinate and develop into hyphae; the latter may invade tissues.

Aspergillus hyphae may invade the pulmonary vasculature, causing thrombosis, pulmonary hemorrhage, and infarction. This occurrence, termed **angioinvasive aspergillosis**, accounts for about 80% of cases of invasive aspergillosis (Table 12-16). *Aspergillus* within airways may invade the airway wall and peribronchial or peribronchiolar lung, a condition known as **airway invasive aspergillosis** or *Aspergillus* bronchopneumonia. This manifestation accounts for about 15% of cases of invasive aspergillosis. A third form of invasive aspergillosis, termed **acute tracheobronchitis**, results in more limited invasion of the trachea or bronchi; it accounts for about 5% of cases of invasive aspergillosis. Pathologically, ulcerated mucosa, fungal hyphae, mucus, and sloughed epithelial cells, combined with extensive submucosal inflammation, are present.

Invasive aspergillosis is primarily an infection of severely immunocompromised patients, such as hematopoietic stem

TABLE 12.16 Invasive Aspergillosis

Associated with granulocytopenia and neutropenia
Severely immunocompromised patients, transplant
   recipients, patients with hematologic malignancy, AIDS
Occurs in three forms:
   Angioinvasive aspergillosis
      80% of cases of invasive aspergillosis
      Results in thrombosis, pulmonary hemorrhage,
         infarction
      Patchy consolidations or multiple, ill-defined nodules
      Halo sign on CT in early disease
      Air-crescent sign after 2 weeks
   Airway invasive aspergillosis (*Aspergillus*
      bronchopneumonia)
         15% of cases of invasive aspergillosis
      Results in thrombosis, pulmonary hemorrhage,
         infarction
      Patchy air-space opacity
      Centrilobular nodules, centered on airways
      Tree-in-bud on HRCT
   Acute tracheobronchitis
      5% of cases of invasive aspergillosis
      Invasion of the walls of trachea or bronchi
      Radiographs often normal; CT may show plaques in
         airways

FIG. 12.43. Invasive aspergillosis in a bone marrow transplant patient. Axial CT image shows a left upper lobe nodule (*arrow*) with surrounding ground-glass opacity. This combination represents the halo sign.

cell transplant recipients, patients with hematologic malignancy, patients treated with high doses of corticosteroids, and patients with AIDS. Invasive aspergillosis is characterized by tissue invasion and destruction caused by *Aspergillus* organisms. Less commonly, invasive aspergillosis is seen in patients with milder forms of immunocompromise, such as obstructive lung disease and interstitial fibrosis. Rarely, invasive aspergillosis develops in patients with normal immune systems following massive inhalation of spores, a condition known as **primary invasive aspergillosis**.

Usually, the immune defect predisposing to invasive aspergillosis is known. Nonproductive cough, shortness of breath, and chest pain are some of the more common symptoms encountered. Fever may also occur, but often the febrile response is blunted in patients with severe immunodeficiency, especially those receiving high-dose corticosteroid therapy. The time course of angioinvasive aspergillosis following hematopoietic stem cell transplantation is frequently predictable. Infection is typically encountered at the point of most profound immunosuppression, generally about 15 to 25 days after induction chemotherapy or hematopoietic stem cell transplantation. Risk is maximal while the white blood cell count remains below 500 cells/mm³.

Imaging Findings. The imaging manifestations of invasive aspergillosis depend on the type of invasion present.

Angioinvasive Aspergillosis. Chest radiographs are often abnormal but nonspecific, revealing patchy segmental or lobar consolidations or multiple, ill-defined nodular opacities. Nodular opacities may show the "halo" sign on CT (Fig. 12-43; see also Fig. 9-7 in Chapter 9), a halo of ground-glass opacity

surrounding a denser central nodule; this finding correlates with the presence of hemorrhage (the halo) surrounding a region of septic infarction (the central nodule). As the patient's immune system recovers, about 2 weeks after the onset of infection, chest radiography or CT may demonstrate the "air-crescent" sign (see Fig. 9-27 in Chapter 9). The air-crescent sign consists of a nodular opacity that represents retracted, infarcted lung associated with crescentic or circumferential cavitation. Although this finding is not specific for angioinvasive aspergillosis, it is highly characteristic in the proper clinical setting. It is seen in nearly 50% of patients with invasive aspergillosis, particularly those in whom the initial lesion was consolidation or a mass.

Airway Invasive Aspergillosis (Aspergillus Bronchopneumonia). Radiographs usually show as patchy air-space opacity, often accompanied by small nodules. The radiographic appearance is nonspecific, and the differential diagnosis is extensive and includes pyogenic bronchopneumonia, pulmonary hemorrhage, noncardiogenic pulmonary edema, and other acute lung injury patterns. CT shows multifocal areas of air-space consolidation or nodules that may be peribronchiolar in distribution (Fig. 12-44). Small centrilobular nodules, indicative of bronchiolitis, may also be seen.

FIG. 12.44. Airway invasive aspergillosis in an immunosuppressed patient. Ill-defined nodules are visible bilaterally. A nodule on the right (*arrow*) surrounds a small bronchus.

Acute Tracheobronchitis. Chest radiography is unrevealing, but CT may reveal multifocal irregular plaques within the trachea, which are occasionally high in attenuation due to the ability of *Aspergillus* to fix calcium (see Fig. 12-1). Bronchoscopy is the procedure of choice for diagnosis and will reveal raised, white fungal plaques coating the airways.

Semi-invasive Aspergillosis

Semi-invasive aspergillosis, also known as chronic necrotizing aspergillosis, commonly occurs in patients with low-grade forms of immunocompromise, such as COPD, low-dose corticosteroid use, alcoholism, tuberculosis, diabetes mellitus, and collagen-vascular diseases (Table 12-17). Risk is compounded in those with preexisting structural lung disease, such as pneumoconioses or prior radiation treatment. Tissue invasion occurs following the inhalation of spores, but the time course of semi-invasive aspergillosis is different from that of angioinvasive aspergillosis. Tissue invasion and infarction occur over months with the former and over days or weeks with the latter.

Patients with semi-invasive aspergillosis present with low-grade fever and productive cough, often over a period of months. Hemoptysis may also occur. These symptoms may be superimposed on a background of chronic illness.

Imaging Findings. Semi-invasive aspergillosis mimics the appearance of active TB. It often presents with irregular upper lobe consolidation and pleural thickening that slowly progresses to cavitation over weeks or months. The upper lobe disease commonly contacts thickened pleura. The cavity may contain an internal opacity resembling an aspergilloma, largely consisting of fungus. Irregular strands may be seen extending from the intracavitary mass to the cavity wall (Fig. 12-45). Occasionally, regions of high attenuation are visible within the cavity on CT. This probably represents calcification occurring in relation to the fungus.

Aspergilloma

Aspergilloma, or mycetoma, is a saprophytic infection that occurs in patients with underlying structural lung disease.

TABLE 12.17 **Semi-invasive Aspergillosis**

Also known as chronic necrotizing aspergillosis
Associated with mild immunocompromise (chronic obstructive pulmonary disease, low-dose corticosteroid use, alcoholism, tuberculosis, diabetes, collagen-vascular diseases)
Low-grade fever, productive cough, often over a period of months
Mimics active *Mycobacterium tuberculosis* radiographically
  Progressive upper lobe consolidation
  Cavitation
  Pleural thickening
  Mass within the cavity due to fungus

A

B

FIG. 12.45. Semi-invasive aspergillosis in a patient with diabetes mellitus. **A:** Axial CT image through the lung apices shows an irregular left upper lobe cavity (*arrows*). Internal opacities reflect the presence of fungus. **B:** Gross specimen at autopsy shows the internal elements within the cavitary lesion.

Patients with mycetoma generally have normal immunity, although coexistent chronic diseases are often present. Pathologically, aspergilloma consists of a combination of fungal hyphae, cellular debris, and mucus within a cavity. The cavity wall commonly consists of fibrous tissue, inflammatory cells, and granulation tissue, the latter derived from the bronchial circulation. The most common cause of underlying structural lung disease in patients with aspergilloma is cavitary disease from prior TB. Structural lung disease due to sarcoidosis is the second most common condition predisposing to aspergilloma formation. Bullae, abscesses, and bronchiectasis are less common predisposing factors. The preexisting lung disease presumably impairs normal clearance of the organisms, allowing infection to occur. Characteristically, the fungus does not usually produce tissue invasion.

Often, patients with aspergilloma are asymptomatic. When symptoms are present, cough, weight loss, and hemoptysis are common. Hemoptysis may range from minor blood streaking to massive, life-threatening hemorrhage. The latter is commonly temporized with bronchial embolization, although pulmonary resection may be required. Although the overall prognosis of patients with aspergilloma is good, death from massive hemoptysis may occur, and rare cases of severe local parenchymal destruction and even dissemination have occurred.

Imaging Findings. Aspergilloma usually appears as a round or oval mass partially filling a cavity and creating the characteristic finding of the air-crescent sign (Fig. 12-46A). If the fungus ball completely fills the pulmonary cavity, the air-crescent sign may not be discernible. Aspergillomas often show mobility with decubitus imaging.

Aspergillomas are usually located in the upper lobes, adjacent to the pleura, which may be thickened. Aspergillomas rarely calcify, and they may diminish or remain unchanged in size over time. An air-fluid level is usually not present within the cavity. The cavity itself is usually thin walled, although thickening of the cavity walls before a discrete internal opacity is seen may indicate early infection.

CT shows a mobile, intracavitary mass (see Fig. 12-46B and C; see also Fig. 9-42 in Chapter 9) and may also reveal small fungal strands bridging the fungus ball and the cavity wall in cases when the air-crescent sign is not visible on chest radiographs. CT may also demonstrate foci of increased attenuation within the fungal ball, presumably reflecting calcium. As with chest radiography, CT may reveal thickening of the wall of a preexisting cavity before the fungus ball is evident.

Zygomycosis

Zygomycosis includes fungal infections caused by a variety of organisms, the most important of which include *Rhizopus, Rhizomucor,* and *Mucor.* Mucormycosis is probably the most common of these infections affecting the thorax.

The fungi that cause zygomycoses are found worldwide, usually in decaying matter. These organisms produce spores that may result in disease when inhaled. Disease almost always occurs in patients with impaired immunity, including patients with diabetes mellitus (especially in the context of ketoacidosis), corticosteroid therapy, AIDS (often when corticosteroid therapy is employed concomitantly), hematologic malignancy, lymphoma, and chronic renal failure. In particular, neutropenic patients are at risk for zygomycoses.

The pattern of infection caused by the zygomycotic fungi is variable, depending on the degree of underlying immunity. An extensive neutrophilic infiltrate may be present, but granulomatous inflammation is rare. Vascular invasion by the fungal organisms is common.

A

B

C

FIG. 12.46. Aspergilloma. **A:** Frontal chest radiograph shows biapical aspergillomas (*arrows*) in a patient with sarcoidosis. **B:** Axial supine HRCT image shows a dependent opacity (*arrow*) within the right upper lobe opacity. **C:** Axial prone HRCT image shows that the intracavitary opacity (*arrow*) is mobile.

A   **B**

FIG. 12.48. *Pneumocystis jiroveci* pneumonia in an AIDS patient. **A:** Chest radiograph shows perihilar ground-glass opacity, interstitial opacities, and poor definition of pulmonary vessels. **B:** HRCT shows perihilar ground-glass opacity and reticular opacities. The lung periphery is spared. Ground-glass opacity is always seen on HRCT in AIDS patients with *Pneumocystis* pneumonia.

characteristically thin-walled and are usually found in the upper lobes. The presence of these lesions may predispose to the development of pneumothorax.

Atypical chest radiographic manifestations of *P. jiroveci* infection include an upper lobe distribution, focal consolidation, single or multiple nodules, cavitation of a nodule, lymphadenopathy, and pleural effusions. A normal chest radiograph occurs uncommonly in patients with AIDS and *P. jiroveci* infection.

CT, in particular HRCT, shows multifocal ground-glass opacity predominantly in a perihilar distribution (see Figs. 12-47B and 12-48B); HRCT shows this finding in all AIDS patients with this infection. Smooth interlobular septal thickening may be present, and foci of consolidation are often encountered. Pneumatoceles and pneumothorax may also be evident (Fig. 12-49). Patients with a granulomatous

response to *P. jiroveci* infection may show small nodules in addition to ground-glass opacities. Rarely, evidence of fibrosis may be seen in patients who have recovered from *P. jiroveci* infection. Larger nodules or masses are occasionally seen (Table 12-18; see Fig. 9-35C in Chapter 9).

Mycoplasma, Chlamydia, and Rickettsiae Pneumonias

Mycoplasma pneumoniae

Mycoplasmas are the smallest free-living culturable organisms. They share some similarities with bacteria, but their lack of a cell wall and certain genetic features make them distinctly different than most bacteria. There are several distinct *Mycoplasma* spp., but *M. pneumoniae* is the most important from the human infectious disease standpoint.

Mycoplasma pneumoniae is a common cause of community-acquired pneumonia. *M. pneumoniae* pulmonary

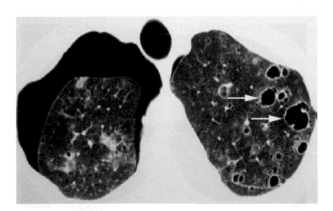

FIG. 12.49. *Pneumocystis jiroveci* pneumonia with pneumatoceles and pneumothorax in an AIDS patient with a low CD4 cell count. Axial HRCT image shows numerous thin-walled cysts (*arrows*), representing pneumatoceles, surrounded by ground-glass opacity. Pneumothorax is present on the right side, likely due to rupture of a pneumatocele.

TABLE 12.18 *Pneumocystis jiroveci (Pneumocystis carinii)*
Associated with AIDS, with transplant recipients on immunosuppression, low-dose corticosteroid therapy, cytotoxic therapy for malignancy
Associated with low CD4 count (<200)
Shortness of breath; dry, nonproductive cough; and high fever
Hypoxia, elevated lactate dehydrogenase level
Radiographs and HRCT
Perihilar ground-glass opacity
Air-space consolidation may be present
Effusion rare
Pneumatoceles may develop
May present with pneumothorax
HRCT is highly sensitive in AIDS patients
Ground-glass opacity visible in all patients

infection occurs mostly in younger patients, and infection is particularly common among military recruits. Infection is transmitted by person-to-person contact and respiratory droplets; infection rates peak in the fall and winter.

Mycoplasma pneumoniae causes infection by both direct cytotoxicity and damage incurred from the host inflammatory response. A peribronchiolar mononuclear cell infiltrate is one of the more common pathologic findings, although neutrophilic infiltration, chronic inflammatory cell infiltration, fibrosis, diffuse alveolar damage, organizing pneumonia, and pulmonary hemorrhage are additional reported pathologic features.

Upper respiratory tract infectious symptoms may precede overt *M. pneumoniae* infection. Patients develop nonproductive cough, headache, malaise, and fever, somewhat resembling a viral infection, although unlike viral infections, arthralgias and myalgias are usually absent. Rarely, infection is severe, resulting in hypoxemic respiratory failure, particularly in patients with sickle cell disease. Superimposed bacterial infection occurs rarely.

Patients with *M. pneumoniae* may develop extrathoracic disease manifestations, including aseptic meningitis, encephalitis, and transverse myelitis (among other neurologic syndromes); hemolysis, venous thrombosis, pericarditis, and myocarditis; and skin rashes.

Imaging Findings

The earliest chest radiographic findings are commonly interstitial in appearance, consisting of fine linear opacities followed by segmental air-space consolidation. Occasionally, these patterns are seen separately rather than sequentially. Pleural effusion occurs in fewer than 20% of patients, and lymphadenopathy is uncommon.

CT scanning typically shows patchy, segmental, and lobular consolidation or ground-glass opacity (Fig. 12-50),

FIG. 12.50. Mycoplasmal pneumonia. HRCT shows patchy, lobular areas of ground-glass opacity and consolidation (*white arrows*). Lobular lucencies (*black arrows*) reflect mosaic perfusion due to small airway abnormalities.

sometimes associated with thickening of the perihilar interstitium. Mosaic perfusion may be seen due to small airway obstruction. Air trapping may be present on expiratory scans.

Chlamydia

Chlamydia spp. are obligate intracellular organisms that possess their own cell walls and share some other characteristics with other bacteria. They exist in an extracellular form known as elementary bodies and then change to reticular bodies once they enter a cell. Three *Chlamydia* spp. are important in the pathogenesis of human disease: *Chlamydia trachomatis*, *C. psittaci*, and *C. pneumoniae*.

Chlamydia trachomatis

Chlamydia trachomatis infection usually causes a sexually transmitted disease, but an infant born through the birth canal of an infected patient may acquire pulmonary infection. Pathologically, *C. trachomatis* causes peribronchiolar inflammation, but few data regarding the pathologic appearance of *C. trachomatis* infection are available. Infants born to mothers infected with *C. trachomatis* may acquire pneumonia; such patients manifest disease shortly after birth, usually between 2 days and 2 weeks, and always by 6 months of age. Cough and tachypnea, often in the absence of significant fever, are common. Radiographs of infants infected with *C. trachomatis* often show multifocal air-space consolidation combined with interstitial opacities and areas of air trapping. Patchy areas of atelectasis are often seen.

Chlamydia psittaci

Chlamydia psittaci primarily infects birds. Humans usually acquire the disease from pigeons, parakeets, or poultry following inhalation of dried bird excrement containing the organisms. Peribronchiolar mononuclear inflammatory cell infiltration that eventually extends into the alveoli is one of the more common pathologic findings of *C. psittaci* pneumonia. Hyaline membrane formation may occur. Patients with *C. psittaci* pneumonia usually present with fever, nonproductive cough, headache, fever, and chills. The illness is usually mild, with cases of overwhelming infection with hypoxemic respiratory failure occurring rarely.

Chest radiographs in patients with *C. psittaci* pneumonia may show perihilar linear opacities, air-space consolidation, and multifocal or diffuse ground-glass opacities. Hilar lymph node enlargement has been reported as a common finding on the radiographs of patients infected with *C. psittaci*.

Chlamydia pneumoniae

Chlamydia pneumoniae is a fairly common cause of community-acquired pneumonia. The disease is rarely severe or fatal. Patients with *C. pneumoniae* pulmonary infection usually present with pharyngitis, fever, and nonproductive cough. The disease is usually self-limited.

The imaging appearances of *C. pneumoniae* pulmonary infection are nonspecific and include air-space consolidation, linear opacities simulating interstitial disease, or a combination of these findings. Pleural effusions occur in about one fifth of patients and may be moderate in size. The radiographic pattern of *C. pneumoniae* infection tends to progress to multilobar opacities over time.

Rickettsiae

Rickettsiae are small obligate intracellular organisms that cause disease when humans are bitten by the arthropods, often ticks, in which the organisms live. The *Rickettsia* that most commonly causes human pulmonary disease is *Coxiella burnetii*.

Coxiella burnetii causes Q fever. The organism usually lives in a variety of wild and domestic animals and insects, most notably ticks. Humans may acquire disease when bitten by the arthropod vector, although disease can be transmitted to humans by inhalation when humans come into contact with animals infected by the bacteria.

Few data regarding the pathologic appearance of Q fever are available. Interstitial and alveolar inflammation associated with hemorrhage, edema, and necrosis may occur.

Patients with Q fever present with fever, myalgia, malaise, headache, chills, nonproductive cough, and occasionally shortness of breath and chest pain. Extrathoracic disease manifestations, such as meningoencephalitis, myocarditis, venous thrombosis, and hepatitis, often occur.

Chest radiographs in patients with Q fever often show multifocal, bilateral, basilar predominant areas of consolidation that may be somewhat rounded. Segmental or lobar consolidation may also occur. Pleural effusions are uncommon. Areas of linear atelectasis may also be seen.

Viruses

The viruses that cause thoracic infection are usually transmitted from person to person by hand-to-hand contact, contact with infected surfaces, or aerosol transmission. Viral organisms may be deposited in the nasopharynx and cause upper respiratory infection only, although smaller organisms may be carried into the lungs, causing lower respiratory tract infections such as bronchitis, bronchiolitis, and pneumonia.

Viruses infect cells by interaction with various receptors on cell membranes. Once the virus enters the cell, the virus undergoes replication. This replication may kill the host cell, releasing more viruses to infect other cells. Alternatively, the viral replication may not kill the cell, but the virus continues to replicate within the cell and releases virions. In this situation, the infected cells may express viral antigens that may provoke a reaction from the host immune system. Lastly, viral infection may result in the virus incorporating itself into the DNA of the host cell, only to cause disease later upon reactivation of this latent infection.

Viral infections may be classified into the RNA virus group and the DNA virus group. RNA viruses that produce human infection include influenza virus, parainfluenza virus, hMPV, RSV, measles virus, coronaviruses, hantaviruses, togaviruses, reoviruses, picornaviruses, arenaviruses, and retroviruses. The DNA viruses that may result in human infection include herpesviruses, adenoviruses, papovaviruses, and poxviruses.

RNA Viruses

Influenza Virus

Influenza is responsible for up to 16 million excess respiratory illnesses per year in the United States among patients below the age of 20 years and up to 4 million excess respiratory illnesses among those 20 years and older. Each year, approximately 150,000 hospitalizations result from influenza, and as many as 35,000 deaths occur from influenza-related complications. Influenza occurs sporadically, in epidemics, and in worldwide pandemics. Transmission of influenza virus occurs by respiratory droplets, although direct transmission from animals to humans may occur.

Influenza outbreaks tend to occur in the winter. Patients at greatest risk for contracting disease include those with diabetes mellitus, COPD, chronic renal disease, cystic fibrosis, or heart disease; the elderly; immunocompromised patients; and cigarette smokers.

Influenza viruses are divided into types A, B, and C. Type A is most often responsible for serious illnesses, and both epidemics and pandemics are almost exclusively caused by influenza A. Influenza A virus includes several subtypes, the most important of which, from the human disease perspective, are H1N1—the virus that was responsible for the 1918 flu pandemic and the pandemic H1N1/09 virus (also known as the novel H1N1 virus) responsible for the 2009 "swine flu" pandemic, first recognized in April of 2009; H2N2—the "Asian flu" virus; H1N2—currently endemic, causing seasonal flu; H3N2—the cause of Hong Kong flu and seasonal flu; and the recently described H5N1 avian influenza virus, so-called "bird flu." Type B influenza tends to cause upper respiratory tract infections, and type C influenza causes sporadic, mild, lower respiratory tract infections. Influenza pulmonary infection causes hemorrhagic and edematous consolidation with diffuse alveolar damage and an associated mononuclear cell inflammatory infiltrate. Infection with influenza renders the host more susceptible to superinfection, usually with bacteria such as pneumococci and staphylococci. Such superinfection may prove fatal.

Influenza A H1N1 infection presents with dry cough, headache, myalgia, low-grade fever, and conjunctivitis. Young children may present with croup or otitis media. When overt pulmonary infection occurs, symptoms of bronchitis occur, followed shortly by signs of severe illness, including cyanosis, hypoxemia, shortness of breath, and chest pain. Bacterial superinfection may be heralded by the onset of purulent cough and worsening fever and chest pain, often in a patient who was improving.

From April 15 to July 24, 2009, a total of 43,771 cases of confirmed and probable swine flu infection were reported in the United States. Among these patients, 5,011 patients were hospitalized and 302 patients died. Many of the cases of influenza H1N1/09 requiring hospitalization or resulting in death occurred in individuals with underlying chronic illnesses or immunocompromise. However, early in the course of the swine flu epidemic it was recognized that swine flu causes a greater disease burden on patients under the age of 25 years compared with older patients.

The clinical features of influenza A H1N1/09 infection are similar to influenza A H1N1 infection, although vomiting and diarrhea may be more common among swine flu patients. Fever and cough are the most common symptoms, with shortness of breath, fatigue, weakness, chills, and myalgias occurring less commonly, in descending frequency. In contrast to seasonal flu (influenza A H1N1), in which the greatest fatality rate is seen in patients older than 65 years, the risk of death from swine flu is highest in younger patients, particularly those aged 25 to 49 years.

Chest radiography in patients with influenza A H1N1 often shows multifocal patchy consolidation that may be unilateral or bilateral. When unilateral, the pulmonary opacities may rapidly progress to bilateral disease. Pleural effusion is relatively uncommon. CT and HRCT may show multifocal, patchy air-space consolidation and ground-glass opacities. Imaging findings are usually nonspecific and resemble noncardiogenic pulmonary edema.

Few data regarding the imaging manifestations of patients infected with influenza A H1N1/09 (swine flu) are available at the time of this writing, although preliminary reports of small cohorts of patients infected with this virus suggest that chest radiography is often normal in these patients. Thoracic CT studies in patients infected with influenza A H1N1/09 have been reported to show patchy areas of rounded ground-glass opacity, even in patients with normal chest radiographs. Severely ill patients infected with influenza H1N1/09, particularly those admitted to the intensive care unit, may have an elevated prevalence of pulmonary embolism. Thoracic CT images from four patients with swine flu infection are shown in Figure 12-51. The images show a variable appearance for influenza A H1N1/09 respiratory infection, including patchy areas of ground-glass opacity, small poorly defined centrilobular nodules and bronchial wall thickening resembling other causes of bronchopneumonia, and areas of dense consolidation. It is possible that the thoracic imaging appearances of swine flu will be influenced by the presence or absence of other underlying medical conditions as well as the duration of infection prior to imaging.

Parainfluenza Virus

Parainfluenza viruses are classified into types 1 through 4. Types 1, 2, and 3 are responsible for the majority of human

FIG. 12.51. Thoracic CT findings of influenza A H1N1/09 (swine flu) respiratory infection in four patients. **A:** Patchy, faintly lobular ground-glass opacity and small solid nodules (*arrow*). **B:** Small, poorly defined ground-glass opacity centrilobular nodules (*arrowheads*) associated with airway thickening and peribronchial opacity, resembling other causes of community-acquired bronchopneumonia. **C:** More extensive disease, including areas of lobular and peribronchial ground-glass opacity (*double arrows*). **D:** Posterior dependent dense consolidation. (Images courtesy of Brett M. Elicker MD, Department of Radiology and Biomedical Imaging, University of California, San Francisco.)

disease. Parainfluenza virus types 1 and 2 usually cause outbreaks of croup or acute bronchiolitis in young children, usually in the fall and winter. Parainfluenza type 3 may cause pneumonia and acute bronchiolitis in children, often in the spring. Parainfluenza viral infections are usually self-limited.

Because parainfluenza viral infection is usually self-limited, little information regarding the pathologic characteristics of infection is available. Infection with parainfluenza virus does render the host more susceptible to bacterial superinfection.

In children, parainfluenza viral infection usually results in croup or, less commonly, acute bronchiolitis. Symptoms of parainfluenza viral acute bronchiolitis include coughing, dyspnea, and wheezing; physical examination may disclose crackles. Parainfluenza viral infection in adults usually causes tonsillitis and pharyngitis. Lower respiratory tract infection by a parainfluenza viral infection is rare in adults.

Radiographs in children with croup may show smooth subglottic tracheal narrowing, the so-called "steeple" sign. Acute bronchiolitis may manifest as a combination of multifocal atelectasis and areas of air trapping. HRCT may more effectively demonstrate these findings but is rarely indicated unless the patient is immunocompromised and the diagnosis is not straightforward. When parainfluenza virus pneumonia occurs, radiographs are often normal or may show only vague ground-glass opacity or interstitial prominence. HRCT reveals multifocal ground-glass opacity in many patients.

Respiratory Syncytial Virus

RSV is an important cause of both upper and lower respiratory tract diseases in infants and young children. Sporadic infection may occur, but outbreaks often occur in schools or nurseries. Infection is transmitted by respiratory droplets or hand-to-hand contact, often in the winter. Infants with congenital heart disease or pulmonary bronchodysplasia are at particularly high risk.

RSV may cause direct bronchiolar and pulmonary parenchymal damage, although hypersensitivity may also contribute to the pathogenesis of infection. The size of the viral inoculum may also play a role in the pathogenesis of RSV bronchiolar and pulmonary parenchymal infection. In children, RSV typically causes upper respiratory tract symptoms such as pharyngitis, rhinitis, and otitis media. Lower respiratory tract infection produces coughing, dyspnea, wheezing, and intercostal retractions. Physical examination may reveal crackles.

In adults, RSV usually causes symptoms of the common cold, and lower respiratory tract infection is rare. When the latter occurs, it usually affects chronically ill, debilitated, elderly, or immunocompromised patients and produces symptoms suggestive of pneumonia. Respiratory failure resulting from ARDS may occur.

Chest radiographs in patients with RSV infection commonly show perihilar linear opacities, bronchial wall thickening, patchy areas of consolidation, and areas of air trapping (see Fig. 12-2). Often, the radiographic findings seem unimpressive in comparison to the patient's clinical presentation. Hilar lymphadenopathy may occur in a few patients. HRCT may show patchy areas of ground-glass opacity and interstitial thickening (Fig. 12-52).

Human Metapneumovirus

hMPV is a negative-sense nonsegmented RNA virus of the pneumovirus subfamily, family Paramyxoviridae. hMPV is a recently recognized respiratory pathogen of the paramyxovirus family, although the virus has probably been responsible for human infection for at least 50 years. Initially described in infants in the Netherlands, hMPV is now recognized as a common cause of upper and lower respiratory tract infections worldwide, primarily in infants and young children and

FIG. 12.52. Respiratory syncytial virus pneumonia in an adult. HRCT shows patchy ground-glass opacity associated with interstitial thickening. Interlobular septal thickening is visible.

those greater than 65 years of age, but the virus may affect patients of practically any age. Patients with malignancy, COPD, and immunocompromised patients are at greater risk for hMPV respiratory infection. In children, additional risk factors for hMPV include congenital heart disease, chronic lung disease, organ or stem cell transplantation, and prematurity. hMPV infection is the second leading identifiable cause of lower respiratory tract infection in children of all age groups, second only to RSV.

The pathophysiology of respiratory infection with hMPV resembles RSV infection. The rate of infection with hMPV peaks in late winter and early spring in the United States, whereas peak infection rates in tropical regions occur during the spring and summer months.

The clinical features of hMPV infection range from asymptomatic to severe pneumonia. The clinical presentation of most symptomatic patients resembles RSV infection, with typical symptoms including rhinorrhea, cough, dyspnea, tachypnea, myalgia, fever, and wheezing. In severe cases, particularly immunosuppressed patients, hypoxemic respiratory failure may occur. Coinfection with other respiratory pathogens may occur, but it is unclear if disease severity is related to such coinfection.

The chest radiographic appearance of hMPV respiratory tract infection is indistinguishable from other forms of viral bronchitis or community-acquired pneumonia. Thoracic CT and HRCT may show multifocal, patchy, bilateral, ground-glass opacity and small nodular opacities. Air-space consolidation is present in less than half of patients.

hMPV infection can be difficult to identify during routine virologic procedures performed on nasal washes, swabs, endotracheal tube aspirates, or bronchoalveolar lavage fluid. Commercial tests to identify the presence of hMPV are available, including reverse transcriptase-polymerase chain reaction, enzyme-linked immunosorbent assays, and shell vial amplification.

Treatment of hMPV infection is supportive, including hydration, supplemental oxygen, and mechanical ventilation as necessary. Clinical trials of anti-hMPV monoclonal antibodies for the prevention of hMPV infection in high-risk infants are underway.

Measles (Rubeola) Virus

The incidence of measles infection has been dramatically reduced in recent years due to the introduction of immunization programs. Epidemics, particularly in underdeveloped countries, are still a problem. Adults may rarely contract the disease, possibly from lack of exposure to the infection during childhood.

Measles classically produces giant cell pneumonia, manifest as multinucleated giant cells containing viral inclusions, infiltrating the alveoli and bronchial epithelium. Giant cell pneumonia is characteristic of measles but may also be seen with parainfluenza and RSV infections.

Patients with measles viral infection initially usually present with fever, myalgia, headache, conjunctivitis, cough, and rhinorrhea, followed by the characteristic skin rash. Measles pneumonia develops either before or at the onset of the skin rash and presents with worsening cough and dyspnea. Bacterial superinfection may occur with measles infection, usually after the patient has begun to improve clinically, and presents with worsening purulent cough, fever, and chest pain.

Measles pneumonia usually manifests on chest radiography as bilateral patchy air-space consolidation associated with perihilar linear opacities, bronchial wall thickening, and small nodules. Radiographs in children may show lymph node enlargement, but radiographs in adults usually do not. CT of measles pneumonia may show multifocal ground-glass opacity and consolidation, often with small nodular opacities.

Coronaviruses

Until 2002, coronaviruses were considered relatively unimportant respiratory pathogens, causing only coryza and pharyngitis and other upper respiratory tract ailments. However, in the fall of 2002, a new respiratory illness, known as severe acute respiratory syndrome (SARS), began in southern China. The disease rapidly spread throughout Asia, Europe, and North America (especially Canada) over the ensuing months, eventually producing infection in 37 different countries. By spring 2003, over 4,400 worldwide cases of SARS had been reported, with 263 deaths as of April 23, 2003. Ultimately 8,096 known SARS cases occurred with 774 deaths, with a case fatality rate of just under 10%. By 2006, the SARS outbreak was declared contained, and, aside from one case of infection acquired in the laboratory in 2004, no additional reports of SARS infection have occurred since 2003 as of the time of this writing.

The World Health Organization defined SARS cases as either suspect or probable. A suspect case was defined as a patient presenting after November 1, 2002, with fever greater than 38°C; cough or dyspnea; close contact with a SARS patient; and history of travel to an affected area or residence within the affected area, all within 10 days prior to the onset of symptoms. A probable case was defined as a suspect case with radiographic evidence of opacities consistent with pneumonia or respiratory distress syndrome or autopsy results consistent with respiratory distress syndrome without an identifiable cause.

Patients presenting with SARS range from the second through seventh decades of life, and no definite gender predilection has been noted. Affected patients may either have underlying chronic illnesses or be previously healthy.

Viral isolation methods, histology, electron microscopy, and other sophisticated methods have shown that the causative agent of SARS is a coronavirus. The infection is transmitted by respiratory droplets or direct contact. The predominant pattern of the lungs found at autopsy is diffuse alveolar damage with hyaline membrane formation. Some of the tissue damage induced by SARS may be related to a cell-mediated host response.

The most common presenting symptoms of SARS include fever, dyspnea, nonproductive cough, malaise, chills or rigors, and myalgias. The disease course may be mild, or hypoxemic respiratory failure may occur. Factors associated with increased risk of death include advanced age, underlying chronic illness, elevated lactate dehydrogenase levels, and high absolute neutrophil count at presentation.

Imaging Findings. Radiographic abnormalities begin to appear about 12 days after viral exposure (range, 4–26 days) or about 5 days after the onset of fever. Patients may present with a normal chest radiograph, but abnormalities usually develop within a matter of a few days following an initially normal radiograph. Radiographic abnormalities in patients with SARS consist of poorly marginated consolidation that may start focally and remain unilateral until resolution, that may start focally and progress to bilateral multifocal opacities, or that may first be detected as multifocal bilateral opacities. When the progression of radiographic abnormalities occurs, it often does so rapidly, usually over a period of a few days. Radiographic abnormalities tend toward a lower lobe predominant location and peripheral distribution. Lymphadenopathy does not occur, and pleural effusions are quite rare in patients with SARS. Radiographic clearing may be delayed relative to clinical improvement. Volume loss and scarring have been reported in a few patients.

The HRCT findings of SARS include lower lobe predominant ground-glass opacity associated with thickening of the interlobular septa, occasionally with consolidation. In some patients, a peripheral distribution of the opacities is seen. Nearly half of patients who have undergone HRCT for SARS show some findings of fibrosis, including architectural distortion, traction bronchiectasis, and coarse linear opacities. Such changes may be more likely to occur in older men, patients admitted to the intensive care unit, patients with relatively higher peak levels of lactate dehydrogenase, and patients with more extensive radiographic abnormalities.

Hantaviruses

There are several antigenically different hantaviruses known to cause human disease, such as hemorrhagic fever with renal syndrome and the hantavirus pulmonary syndrome. The natural reservoir of hantaviruses is rodents, in particular the deer mouse. Hantavirus pulmonary syndrome is most commonly encountered in rural areas, especially in the Southwestern United States. Human disease is acquired by the inhalation of dried rodent excrement containing the virus.

Hantavirus infection causes both interstitial and air-space edema accompanied by lymphocytic infiltration, but with little evidence of vascular thrombosis or hyaline membrane formation.

Patients with hantavirus pulmonary syndrome present with fever, myalgia, and headache that progresses to worsening cough, shortness of breath, and then hypotension. Hypoxemic respiratory failure may occur. The death rate approaches 50%.

Chest radiographic findings of hantavirus pulmonary syndrome include peribronchiolar thickening, perihilar indistinctness, and interlobular septal thickening. Air-space consolidation may also be encountered. For patients who do not present with air-space consolidation on the initial chest radiograph, subsequent films may show developing consolidation. Pleural effusions occur in more than half of patients and may be large.

Togaviruses (Rubella)

Rubella is the only significant togavirus from a human respiratory infection viewpoint. Infants born to mothers infected with rubella during the first trimester may develop congenital anomalies. The teratogenic effects of congenital rubella infection include pulmonary abnormalities such as pulmonary artery stenoses and interstitial pneumonitis.

Infants born with pulmonary arterial stenoses from congenital rubella infection may be largely asymptomatic, or they may develop pulmonary hypertension and right heart failure. Interstitial pneumonitis related to congenital rubella infection may be mild or may produce fulminant respiratory failure.

DNA Viruses

Herpesviruses

Numerous antigenically different types of herpesviruses are known to exist, but herpesvirus types 1, 2, 6, 8, varicella-zoster virus, cytomegalovirus (CMV), and Epstein-Barr virus (EBV) are the most important from the standpoint of human disease.

Herpesviruses infect patients and incorporate themselves into the cell of the host, and there they may remain latent for the lifetime of the individual. On occasion, particularly when the host becomes immunocompromised, the herpes infection reactivates and causes clinically overt disease. While reactivation episodes are usually minor, they may become quite significant in immunocompromised patients.

Herpes Simplex. Herpes simplex virus type 1 (HSV-1) and herpes simplex virus type 2 (HSV-2) infections usually cause mucosal ulcerations following reactivation of latent infection.

HSV-1 infection is often acquired during childhood and usually affects the oral cavity. Following reactivation of latent disease, lower respiratory tract infection may occur if the organisms are transported into the trachea and bronchi, as could occur with aspiration or endotracheal intubation. However, overt oral cavity infection is not always present, implying that other mechanisms are operative. Patients with HSV-1 infection of the trachea and bronchi are often severely immunocompromised. Tracheobronchial involvement is suggested by the presence of fever and productive cough, occasionally in the presence of the oral ulcerative lesions. Symptoms of HSV-1 pneumonia are nonspecific. Chest radiographs may show multifocal consolidation due to bronchopneumonia. CT and HRCT also show patchy, multifocal ground-glass opacity and consolidation, often associated with small nodules.

HSV-2 pulmonary infection is acquired during birth as the fetus passes through the infected maternal birth canal. The newborn may present with fever, jaundice, seizure, and signs of pneumonia. Radiographs may show patchy air-space consolidation, usually without effusions.

HSV-6 causes roseola (a childhood skin infection). Pulmonary disease is exceedingly rare, usually occurring in immunocompromised patients.

HSV-8 (also called Kaposi's sarcoma–associated herpesvirus) has been implicated in the pathogenesis of both Kaposi's sarcoma and primary effusion lymphoma (previously known as body cavity–based lymphoma). Primary effusion lymphoma presents with fluid accumulation in body cavities, especially the pleural space and peritoneal cavity. Primary effusion lymphoma tends to present in patients with AIDS and a low CD4 cell count; shortness of breath is commonly present, and the pleural effusions may be quite large. Kaposi's sarcoma is discussed in Chapter 4.

Varicella-Zoster Virus. Hematogenous dissemination of the varicella virus develops soon after the organism is inhaled, and the organism subsequently invades the respiratory epithelium. Viral replication eventually results in a second viremic episode, which causes the skin eruption. If pneumonia occurs, the virus will induce diffuse alveolar damage and produce giant cell pneumonia.

Varicella represents the initial varicella-zoster infection in previously uninfected patients, also called chickenpox. Varicella is a very contagious skin infection that usually affects children. About one in six patients with skin infection caused by varicella develops coincident pulmonary infection; this figure is higher for patients ill enough to be admitted to the hospital or for immunocompromised patients. Zoster, also known as shingles, represents the reactivation of a latent herpes varicella-zoster infection. Pulmonary infection may occur with either form of herpes varicella-zoster, although it is more commonly seen with varicella. Varicella pneumonia presents as high fever that is usually rapidly followed by a painful skin rash. Chest pain, nonproductive cough, and shortness of breath are common. Radiographic abnormalities often persist after clinical improvement.

Varicella pneumonia appears on chest radiography as diffuse small nodules in the range of 5 to 10 mm that progress to air-space consolidation rather rapidly. Hilar lymphadenopathy is common, but pleural effusion is rare. Radiographic clearing of pulmonary opacities may take weeks or months. Some patients develop multiple, bilateral small calcified pulmonary nodules measuring 2 to 3 mm without hilar lymph node calcification.

Cytomegalovirus

Congenital CMV infection may occur by transplacental spread of the organism, or neonatal infection may occur when the fetus passes through an infected birth canal. Acquired infection with CMV is very common; infection is usually asymptomatic. Pulmonary infection with CMV is usually significant only in patients with impaired immunity. Cell-mediated immunity is particularly important in defense against CMV infection. Clinically overt CMV infection usually occurs as a result of reactivation of latent disease, although reinfection from an endogenous source can occur.

CMV infection may cause direct cellular damage, although the host reaction to infection also contributes to the infectious process. Nevertheless, it is clear that in most patients from whom CMV is isolated, the organism is not a primary pulmonary pathogen. When CMV infects cells, it often produces a characteristic pattern of intranuclear inclusions that fill most of the nucleus and are separated from the remaining nuclear membrane by a characteristic halo, resulting in the so-called owl-eye appearance.

Congenital CMV infection presents with hepatosplenomegaly, jaundice, chorioretinitis, microcephaly, seizures, and thrombocytopenic purpura; mental retardation often results. Neonatal CMV infection, acquired through maternal transmission from an infected birth canal, is often asymptomatic.

CMV infection acquired in childhood or adulthood is often asymptomatic or presents with low-grade fever, lymphadenopathy, and organomegaly.

In immunocompromised patients, CMV infection presents with nonproductive cough, fever, and shortness of breath. Diagnosis rests on demonstrating the presence of the organism and viral inclusions, usually with associated tissue damage, to prove that CMV is the culprit organism.

Imaging Findings. CMV infection usually occurs in the setting of impaired immunity. Chest radiographic findings associated with CMV infection include bilateral reticulation or interstitial opacities, diffuse ground-glass opacities, or multifocal consolidation; chest radiographs may be normal

(Fig. 12-53). Diffuse, small nodules are a less common pattern of infection with CMV, and lobar consolidation in CMV infection is uncommon. Bilateral opacities are more commonly encountered than unilateral disease.

CT may reveal multifocal, bilateral areas of ground-glass opacity and foci of air-space consolidation, occasionally accompanied by small centrilobular nodules (see Fig. 12-53; see also Fig. 10-31B in Chapter 10). Small pleural effusions are encountered in less than half of patients, and lymphadenopathy is infrequent.

Epstein-Barr Virus

EBV infects B lymphocytes and cells lining the pharynx. Direct person-to-person transmission is most common, although spread via blood transfusions may also occur.

EBV causes infectious mononucleosis, which presents as hepatosplenomegaly, lymphadenopathy, pharyngitis, and fever. When intrathoracic involvement occurs, lymphadenopathy is the most common manifestation; interstitial pneumonia may occur but is rare.

A

B

FIG. 12.53. Cytomegalovirus infection in an immunosuppressed patient. **A:** Chest radiograph is normal. **B:** Axial CT image shows multiple small centrilobular areas of ground-glass opacity.

Patients with infectious mononucleosis present with fever, malaise, weakness, a minimally productive cough, and pharyngitis. One of the most compelling physical examination findings of infectious mononucleosis is splenomegaly.

EBV is an important pathogen in the pathogenesis of lymphoproliferative disorders, especially Burkitt's lymphoma, lymphomas in patients with AIDS, and post-transplant lymphoproliferative disease.

Adenoviruses

Sporadic adenoviral infection is not an uncommon cause of respiratory infection in childhood. Epidemic outbreaks of adenoviral infection have been reported in military recruits and other situations in which the living quarters are close.

Adenoviral infection causes bronchitis and bronchiolitis that, in severe cases, progresses to hemorrhagic bronchopneumonia with edema and hyaline membranes.

Adenoviral infection usually presents with pharyngitis, fever, myalgia, malaise, and cough. Disease is usually mild, but rare cases of hypoxemic respiratory failure occur. As discussed previously, adenoviral infection may result in bronchiectasis and bronchiolitis obliterans, including Swyer-James syndrome.

Adenoviral pneumonia may present on chest radiography with multifocal, bilateral bronchopneumonia associated with air trapping. In one of the largest series detailing the chest radiographic appearance of adenoviral infection, lobar collapse was a common event; the right upper lobe was particularly commonly involved. Resolution of infection may be complete but occasionally results in pulmonary scarring, especially when infection occurs in patients under the age of 2 years.

Parasites: Protozoans, Roundworms (Nematodes), and Flatworms

Amebiasis

Amebiasis is caused by the protozoan *Entamoeba histolytica*. The organism usually causes amebic dysentery, with pulmonary disease occurring as a complication of colon or liver disease.

Amebic dysentery is most prevalent in underdeveloped countries, where transmission of the organism from person to person occurs by the fecal-oral route. In the United States, many cases of amebic dysentery occur in immigrants who have been in the United States for only a short time. Pulmonary amebiasis is far more common in men and usually occurs in young to middle-aged adults.

The life cycle of *E. histolytica* begins with the host ingesting cysts in contaminated food or water. The cyst form of the organism is acid resistant, so it is capable of passing through the stomach and into the small intestine unharmed. Once in the small intestine, *E. histolytica* excysts and forms trophozoites, which then migrate to the colon. From there, organisms may be passed in feces to complete the life cycle of the organism.

The organisms may be transported to the liver, where an amebic abscess may form; such abscesses are almost always located in the cranial portion of the liver, usually in the right lobe. From there, direct transdiaphragmatic spread of infection may cause pleural effusion or lung abscess formation. Very rarely, pulmonary or pleural infection forms in the absence of a liver abscess by extension of the organisms through the hemorrhoidal veins, the transdiaphragmatic lymphatics or the thoracic duct, or the hepatic veins.

Patients with pulmonary or pleural amebic abscesses usually present with right upper quadrant pain, fever, and cough. Chest pain may also be present. Patients may also expectorate the characteristic "anchovy paste" or "chocolate sauce" material that usually represents amebic abscesses. Rarely, biloptysis occurs. Gastrointestinal symptoms are often, but not invariably, present.

Amebic pulmonary infection usually presents as lower lobe air-space consolidation, usually on the right, often accompanied by a pleural effusion (Fig. 12-54). The latter may be quite large. Cavitation within the consolidation may occur. Amebic abscesses in the liver, uncomplicated by pulmonary abscesses, often cause elevation of the right diaphragm with basilar atelectasis; a small pleural effusion may be present.

Toxoplasmosis

Toxoplasmosis is caused by the protozoan *Toxoplasma gondii*. *T. gondii* is an intracellular protozoan that commonly causes human infection, although such infections are often not clinically apparent. *T. gondii* is distributed worldwide. Human infection is extremely common but usually asymptomatic.

The organism's definitive host is the cat, and mice or rats may serve as an intermediate host. Humans acquire disease when they ingest the oocyte form of the parasite in contaminated water or food or in undercooked meat. Once ingested, the oocyte excysts and forms trophozoites, which may cross the intestine and disseminate through the bloodstream. The trophozoites usually travel to the heart, skeletal muscle, and brain most commonly, where they may remain viable and cause infection when the host becomes immunocompromised. *T. gondii* can also be transmitted from women to their fetuses by the transplacental route.

Most infections caused by *T. gondii* are asymptomatic. When symptoms are present, they most often include low-grade fever and lymphadenopathy; the presentation somewhat resembles mononucleosis. Immunocompromised patients may develop disseminated disease; when *T. gondii* pneumonia occurs in this setting, fever, dry cough, and shortness of breath may be encountered. Neurologic symptoms, due to *T. gondii* brain infection, may occur.

Overt pulmonary infection in patients without impaired immunity is uncommon. Chest radiographs may show bilateral linear opacities suggesting an interstitial process, perhaps

A

B

FIG. 12.54. Amebic pneumonia and liver abscess. **A:** Frontal chest radiograph shows right lower lobe pneumonia and right pleural effusion (*arrows*), initially interpreted as community-acquired pneumonia and parapneumonic effusion. The patient's symptoms and the radiographic abnormalities failed to resolve with therapy directed toward community-acquired pneumonia. **B:** Axial CT image through the cranial aspect of the liver shows right lower lobe consolidation and a low-attenuation lesion within the liver (*arrow*).

accompanied by hilar lymphadenopathy. HRCT will reveal patchy areas of ground-glass opacity, possibly with some foci of consolidation.

Ascariasis

Ascaris lumbricoides is a nematode (roundworm) that causes the majority of cases of the infection known as ascariasis. *A. suum* may also cause this infection.

Ascaris lumbricoides infection is acquired by the ingestion of food or water contaminated by the worm's ova. The larval forms of the worm develop within the ovum inside the small intestine of the host. Once the larval forms hatch, they may burrow through the wall of the small intestine to reach the portal venous circulation. The larvae may then migrate to the pulmonary capillary circulation and then into the alveoli. From there, the larvae may migrate into the proximal airways and into the larynx, where they are swallowed. Eventually they reach the small intestine and develop into adult worms, where they may produce eggs that are passed in the feces to complete the worm's life cycle. *A. lumbricoides* infection is most commonly encountered in Southeast Asia, Africa, and Central and South America. However, infection does occur in the United States, especially in the southeastern region.

Although the worms can be comparatively large (often over 30 cm in length), *A. lumbricoides* infection is usually asymptomatic. Most patients who experience symptoms develop gastrointestinal complaints. As the worms migrate through the lungs, they can cause bronchopneumonia, producing symptoms of chest pain, shortness of breath, cough, and hemoptysis.

When pulmonary infection is present, air-space consolidation is usually encountered. Pneumonia may be caused by the migration of the larvae or by vomiting with aspiration. Often, the air-space opacities are transient.

Strongyloidiasis

Strongyloides stercoralis is the nematode (roundworm) that causes most cases of strongyloidiasis. *S. stercoralis* infection is endemic in tropical areas, although infection does occur in the United States. Immunocompromised patients, particularly those with AIDS, are at increased risk.

Human infection with *S. stercoralis* begins with larvae penetrating the skin of the human host, after which they travel to the lungs via the bloodstream. Once the larvae reach the lungs, they migrate through the airways into the larynx, then into the esophagus, and finally into the small intestine. There, the larvae develop into adult worms and lay eggs. The eggs may be passed in feces to perpetuate the life cycle, although eggs also have the ability to develop into larval forms while still in the intestine. Once larvae form in the intestine, they may directly penetrate the intestinal wall and migrate to the lungs and back to the gut. This ability is termed **autoinfection** and allows the organism to perpetuate infection within the host.

Most patients with *S. stercoralis* infection are asymptomatic. When symptoms occur, cough, shortness of breath, and hemoptysis may be seen.

Chest radiography in patients with *S. stercoralis* infection may show patchy areas of air-space consolidation. Other patterns, such as nodular consolidation, small nodules, or reticulation, have been reported. Pleural effusions occur in a few patients.

southern Europe (especially Switzerland and Germany), Alaska, Russia, and Canada.

The normal life cycle begins with the usual intermediate hosts ingesting the eggs, passed from definitive hosts, in contaminated food, water, or soil. The eggs develop into larvae in the gut of the intermediate host and eventually penetrate through the intestinal wall and migrate into the portal venous system and then to the liver. Many larvae are trapped in the liver, but some escape the liver and come to rest in the pulmonary circulation. Most larvae are killed, but some develop into cysts containing immature worms. The life cycle is completed when the definitive host feeds on the remains of the intermediate host, and the cysts develop into adult worms in the gut of the definitive hosts.

Humans acquire disease by the ingestion of food, water, or soil contaminated by intermediate-host feces containing the organisms (which usually live in the small intestine of the intermediate host). In this fashion, humans become an inadvertent intermediate host.

About 60% to 70% of cases of *E. granulosus* occur in the liver, and 15% to 30% occur in the lung parenchyma. The few remaining cases occur in a variety of other organs, including the brain, heart, and kidneys. Lung abnormalities are more common than liver findings in the sylvatic form of the disease.

The hydatid cysts that occur in intermediate hosts consist of an outer fibrotic capsule called the **pericyst**, an outer **exocyst**, and an inner **endocyst**. The endocyst produces fluid and gives rise to immature forms called **brood capsules**. Larval forms develop within these brood capsules. Daughter cysts may develop directly from the larval forms within the brood capsules or directly from the exocyst, creating the overall appearance of a multilocular cystic lesion on imaging studies.

Echinococcus multilocularis has a life cycle similar to *E. granulosus*. However, the structure of the cyst that forms in *E. multilocularis* is different than that of *E. granulosus*. In contrast to *E. granulosus*, the exocyst is rather poorly formed and the pericyst does not form at all.

Hydatid disease causes symptoms by the compression of adjacent structures or by rupture of a cyst with an ensuing host inflammatory response, although most patients remain asymptomatic. Cyst rupture may be heralded by the sudden onset of cough, hemoptysis, chest pain, fever, and systemic hypersensitivity. Purulent sputum production may occur with bacterial superinfection of hydatid cysts.

Imaging Findings

Chest radiographs in patients with echinococcosis often show a single, lower lobe, circumscribed nodule or mass of variable size, ranging from 1 cm to more than 15 cm (see Fig. 9-34 in Chapter 9). Multiple lesions are seen in 20% to 30% of patients. Pulmonary hydatid cysts grow slowly and, unlike their liver counterparts, usually do not calcify.

Pulmonary hydatid cysts may change shape with respiration and are often irregularly deformed by adjacent anatomy, such as vessels or mediastinal structures.

If the cyst acquires a communication with the tracheobronchial tree, several radiographic patterns may occur. If the pericyst ruptures, allowing air to gain access to the potential space between the pericyst and the exocyst, a meniscus or crescent sign may be observed. This sign is not very common overall and is practically seen only with the pastoral form of echinococcosis. If a communication develops between the tracheobronchial tree and the endocyst, an air-fluid level may form within the cyst, accompanied by surrounding pulmonary parenchymal consolidation that represents expelled cyst fluid. Additionally, once tracheobronchial communication with the cyst occurs, the cyst membrane may collapse and float on the resulting air-fluid level, creating an irregular contour to the air-fluid level, representing the characteristic "waterlily (camalote)" sign.

CT often shows that the rounded or oval lesions in patients with pulmonary echinococcosis have fluid attenuation. CT may also effectively show the collapsed cyst membranes as well as the configuration of daughter cysts. CT also effectively shows chest wall invasion or pleural extension by the cysts. In the uncommon patient in whom hydatid pulmonary disease results from extension of an infectious focus from the liver across the diaphragm, CT may show the cystic liver lesion in continuity with pulmonary and pleural disease.

Cysticercosis

The larval form of the tapeworm *Taenia solium* is the cause of cysticercosis. The adult *T. solium* tapeworms usually live asymptomatically in the intestine of the human definitive host. Cysticercosis is endemic in parts of Africa, Europe (especially Spain and Portugal), and Central America.

Humans acquire infection by ingesting undercooked meat containing cysticerci from an intermediate host, usually a pig. The ingested immature forms develop into adult worms within the human gut, shedding eggs in the feces, which are in turn eaten by the intermediate host, completing the organism's life cycle. Humans may also serve as both intermediate and definitive hosts, creating a pattern known as **autoinfection**. This occurs when humans ingest the eggs of the tapeworm directly or if the eggs are regurgitated back into the stomach. With autoinfection, the ingested eggs hatch into immature forms that migrate through the intestinal wall into the mesenteric veins and are then carried to various organs, such as the brain, eyes, and skeletal muscle, where they develop into cysticerci. Cysticercosis is often asymptomatic. Neurologic involvement may cause seizures, and respiratory muscle involvement may cause chest pain.

Cysticercosis may present as small calcified nodules, which may be oval or cigar-shaped and are often seen in the musculature of the thorax on chest radiographs.

SELECTED READING

Antonio GE, Wong KT, Hui DS, et al. Thin-section CT in patients with severe acute respiratory syndrome following hospital discharge: preliminary experience. Radiology 2003; 228:810–815.

Brecher CW, Aviram G, Boiselle PM. CT and radiography of bacterial respiratory infections in AIDS patients. AJR Am J Roentgenol 2003; 180:1203–1209.

Cattamanchi A, Nahid P, Marras TK, et al. Detailed analysis of the radiographic presentation of *Mycobacterium kansasii* lung disease in patients with HIV infection. Chest 2008; 133(4):875–880.

Erasmus JJ, McAdams HP, Farrell MA, Patz EF, Jr. Pulmonary nontuberculous mycobacterial infection: radiologic manifestations. Radiographics 1999; 19:1487–1505.

Franquet T, Müller NL, Gimenez A, et al. Spectrum of pulmonary aspergillosis: histologic, clinical, and radiologic findings. Radiographics 2001; 21:825–837.

Gotway MB, Dawn SK, Caoili EM, et al. The radiologic spectrum of pulmonary *Aspergillus* infections. J Comput Assist Tomogr 2002; 26:159–173.

Grinblat L, Shulman H, Glickman A, et al. Severe acute respiratory syndrome: radiographic review of 40 probable cases in Toronto, Canada. Radiology 2003; 228:802–809.

Gruden JF, Huang L, Turner J, et al. High-resolution CT in the evaluation of clinically suspected *Pneumocystis carinii* pneumonia in AIDS patients with normal, equivocal, or nonspecific radiographic findings. AJR Am J Roentgenol 1997; 169:967–975.

Kim EA, Lee KS, Primack SL, et al. Viral pneumonias in adults: radiologic and pathologic findings. Radiographics 2002; 22:S137–S149.

Leung AN. Pulmonary tuberculosis: the essentials. Radiology 1999; 210:307–322.

Leung AN, Brauner MW, Gamsu G, et al. Pulmonary tuberculosis: comparison of CT findings in HIV-seropositive and HIV-seronegative patients. Radiology 1996; 198:687–691.

Lieberman D, Ben-Yaakov M, Lazarovich Z, et al. *Chlamydia pneumoniae* community-acquired pneumonia: a review of 62 hospitalized adult patients. Infection 1996; 24:109–114.

Lieberman D, Porath A, Schlaeffer F, Boldur I. *Legionella* species community-acquired pneumonia. A review of 56 hospitalized adult patients. Chest 1996; 109:1243–1249.

Marom EM, Holmes AM, Bruzzi JF, et al. Imaging of pulmonary fusariosis in patients with hematological malignancies. AJR AM J Roentgenal 2008; 190:1605–1609.

McAdams HP, Rosado de Christenson ML, Lesar M, et al. Thoracic mycoses from endemic fungi: radiologic-pathologic correlation. Radiographics 1995; 15:255–270.

McAdams HP, Rosado de Christenson ML, Templeton PA, et al. Thoracic mycoses from opportunistic fungi: radiologic-pathologic correlation. Radiographics 1995; 15:271–286.

Porath A, Schlaeffer F, Pick N, et al. Pneumococcal community acquired pneumonia in 148 hospitalized adult patients. Eur J Clin Microbiol Infect Dis 1997; 16:863–870.

Reittner P, Muller NL, Heyneman L, et al. *Mycoplasma pneumoniae* pneumonia: radiographic and high-resolution CT features in 28 patients. AJR Am J Roentgenol 2000; 174:37–41.

Sanchez A, Larsen R. Emerging fungal pathogens in pulmonary disease. Curr Opin Pulm Med 2007; 13:199–204.

Saurborn DP, Fishman JE, Boiselle PM. The imaging spectrum of pulmonary tuberculosis in AIDS. J Thorac Imaging 2002; 17:28–33.

Sullivan KM, Monto AS, Longini IM, Jr. Estimates of the US health impact of influenza. Am J Public Health 1993; 83:1712–1716.

13

The Idiopathic Interstitial Pneumonias

W. RICHARD WEBB

The idiopathic interstitial pneumonias (IIPs) are a heterogeneous group of diffuse lung diseases occurring without known cause and associated with varying degrees of interstitial lung inflammation and fibrosis. The IIPs have been classified by a consensus committee of the American Thoracic Society and the European Respiratory Society into seven types, based on their histologic pattern, clinical features, and radiographic appearances (Table 13-1). Each of the IIPs is referred to using an acronym. Knowing these acronyms is appropriate, as they are in common usage.

In order of decreasing frequency, the IIPs are as follows:

1. Usual interstitial pneumonia (UIP) and idiopathic pulmonary fibrosis (IPF)
2. Nonspecific interstitial pneumonia (NSIP)
3. Cryptogenic organizing pneumonia (COP)
4. Acute interstitial pneumonia (AIP)
5. Respiratory bronchiolitis–interstitial lung disease (RB-ILD)
6. Desquamative interstitial pneumonia (DIP)
7. Lymphoid interstitial pneumonia (LIP)

In this classification, a distinction is made between the histologic pattern of the IIP and the idiopathic clinical syndrome associated with it. In several cases, these have different names (see Table 13-1).

Although the IIPs are designated as idiopathic, identical histologic patterns, radiographic appearances, and clinical symptoms may occur in association with specific diseases or exposures, including collagen-vascular disease, drug reactions, smoking, and infection (see Table 13-1). It is

TABLE 13.1 Idiopathic Interstitial Pneumonias: Classification and Differential Diagnosis

Histologic Pattern	Idiopathic Clinical Syndrome	Differential Diagnosis of the Histologic Pattern
Usual interstitial pneumonia (UIP)	Idiopathic pulmonary fibrosis (IPF)	Collagen-vascular disease, asbestosis, drug toxicity, radiation, chronic hypersensitivity pneumonitis, familial pulmonary fibrosis
Nonspecific interstitial pneumonia (NSIP)	Nonspecific interstitial pneumonia (NSIP)	Collagen-vascular disease, hypersensitivity pneumonitis, drug toxicity, infection, immunodeficiency
Organizing pneumonia (OP); also known as bronchiolitis obliterans organizing pneumonia (BOOP)	Cryptogenic organizing pneumonia (COP)	Infection, bronchial obstruction, aspiration, drug reactions, collagen vascular disease, toxic-fume inhalation, radiation pneumonitis, hypersensitivity pneumonitis
Diffuse alveolar damage (DAD)	Acute interstitial pneumonia (AIP)	Acute respiratory distress syndrome (ARDS) of known cause (e.g., sepsis, shock, infection, drug toxicity, toxic inhalations, trauma)
Respiratory bronchiolitis (RB)	Respiratory bronchiolitis–interstitial lung disease (RB-ILD)	Smoking (usually), inhalations
Desquamative interstitial pneumonia (DIP)	Desquamative interstitial pneumonia (DIP)	Smoking (usually), inhalations
Lymphoid interstitial pneumonia (LIP)	Lymphoid interstitial pneumonia (LIP)	Collagen-vascular diseases (particularly Sjögren's syndrome, rheumatoid arthritis, and lupus), immunologic disorders (e.g., Hashimoto's thyroiditis, autoimmune hemolytic anemia, myasthenia gravis, pernicious anemia, chronic active hepatitis), infection, immunodeficiency (e.g., AIDS), drug toxicity

helpful to think of the histologic patterns seen in the IIP as having a differential diagnosis, with one of the possible causes being an idiopathic syndrome (see Table 13-1). Since the radiographic appearances of the IIP parallel their histologic patterns, this approach allows the appropriate radiographic or high-resolution CT (HRCT) differential diagnosis to be suggested.

USUAL INTERSTITIAL PNEUMONIA AND IDIOPATHIC PULMONARY FIBROSIS

IPF is the idiopathic disease associated with the histologic pattern termed *usual interstitial pneumonia.*

Histologically, UIP is characterized by a heterogeneous pattern with different parts of the biopsy showing normal lung, interstitial inflammation, fibroblastic proliferation, interstitial fibrosis, and honeycombing; in other words, the biopsy shows *spatial heterogeneity.* Histologic abnormalities appear to represent different stages in the temporal evolution of fibrosis, a combination of end-stage and more active lesions. This is termed *temporal heterogeneity.* Spatial and temporal heterogeneity is characteristic of UIP and is not seen in other IIPs. Lung involvement is patchy, although there is a predominance in the subpleural and basal lung regions (Table 13-2).

UIP may be associated with collagen-vascular disease, asbestosis, drug toxicity, radiation, chronic hypersensitivity pneumonitis, or familial pulmonary fibrosis. Idiopathic UIP is termed idiopathic pulmonary fibrosis. IPF accounts for about 70% of cases of UIP.

IPF occurs most frequently in patients older than 50 (see Table 13-2). Symptoms include progressive dyspnea, cough, weight loss, and finger clubbing; symptoms usually precede presentation by 6 months. Pulmonary function tests (PFTs) show restriction with a reduced diffusing capacity. Treatment is largely ineffective. IPF has a poor prognosis, with a mean survival of 3 to 4 years from the onset of symptoms. The 5-year survival rate is 25% to 40%. Lung transplantation may be required.

The diagnosis of IPF is limited to patients with histologic findings of UIP; in other words, if it is not UIP, it is not IPF. Histologic diagnosis requires an open lung biopsy; transbronchoscopic biopsy is not sufficient for diagnosis but may be used to exclude other causes of lung disease.

Based on a 2002 consensus of the American Thoracic Society and European Respiratory Society, a diagnosis of IPF in the absence of lung biopsy can be based on a combination of clinical, functional, and HRCT findings. Based on this consensus, IPF is considered to be likely if all four major criteria and three of four minor criteria are present (Table 13-3). These criteria outline common features of this disease.

In a 2010 revision of these criteria, the diagnosis of IPF has been simplified to a combination of

TABLE 13.2 Usual Interstitial Pneumonia (UIP) and Idiopathic Pulmonary Fibrosis (IPF): Histologic, Clinical, and HRCT Features

UIP: histologic pattern
Characteristics
    Spatial and Temporal inhomogeneity
    Dense fibrosis, often with honeycombing
    Fibroblastic foci
    Patchy lung involvement
    Subpleural and basal predominance
Differential diagnosis
    Idiopathic (IPF)
    Collagen-vascular disease
    Asbestosis
    Drug toxicity
    Radiation
    Chronic hypersensitivity pneumonitis
    Familial pulmonary fibrosis

IPF: idiopathic clinical syndrome
Age >50 years
Progressive dyspnea; duration of symptoms 3 months or more
Velcro rales
Pulmonary function tests: restriction and impaired gas exchange
Treatment largely ineffective
5-year survival rate 25%–40%
HRCT findings highly accurate in diagnosis
    Honeycombing
    Reticulation
    Subpleural and basal predominance
    Little ground-glass opacity

1. A UIP pattern on HRCT or histopathology
2. The absence of an alternative etiology (e.g., collagen-vascular disease, asbestos exposure, drug treatment, hypersensitivity pneumonitis) after careful clinical evaluation (i.e., history, physical examination, pulmonary function testing, and laboratory assessment)

TABLE 13.3 Criteria for a Clinical Diagnosis of Idiopathic Pulmonary Fibrosis (2002)

Major criteria
Exclusion of known causes of infiltrative lung disease such as exposures, drugs, and connective tissue disease
Abnormal pulmonary function tests with evidence of restriction and impaired gas exchange
HRCT findings of bibasilar reticulation with minimal ground-glass opacity
Transbronchial lung biopsy or bronchoalveolar lavage showing no evidence of another disease
Minor criteria
Age >50 years
Insidious onset of dyspnea on exertion
Duration of illness of ≥3 months
Bibasilar inspiratory crackles (so-called Velcro rales)

FIG. 13.10. Nonspecific interstitial pneumonia. **A:** Chest radiograph shows a subtle increase in opacity at the lung bases. **B–D:** HRCTs at three levels show an increase in ground-glass opacity and reticular opacities, which is predominant at the lung bases and in the lung periphery.

Other findings in patients with OP/COP include small pleural effusions, present in 30% to 35% of cases, irregular linear opacities, mild honeycombing, and "crazy paving," with a superimposition of ground-glass opacity and interlobular septal thickening.

ACUTE INTERSTITIAL PNEUMONIA

AIP is a fulminant disease of unknown cause, usually occurring in a previously healthy person. It is associated with the histologic pattern of *diffuse alveolar damage (DAD)* with alveolar hyaline membranes and diffuse, active interstitial fibrosis (Table 13-6). The appearance of DAD in AIP is indistinguishable from DAD in patients with acute respiratory distress syndrome (ARDS) caused by sepsis, shock, infection, drug toxicity, toxic inhalations, trauma, or other insults.

The mean age at presentation is 50. A prodromal illness associated with symptoms of a viral upper respiratory infection is often present, followed by rapidly increasing dyspnea

and respiratory failure. Patients with AIP usually require mechanical ventilation within 1 to 2 weeks of the onset of symptoms. Fifty percent or more die within 6 months of presentation.

Because of its acute presentation and a histologic pattern identical to that of ARDS, AIP has been referred to as idiopathic ARDS. It was formerly known as *Hamman-Rich syndrome*.

Radiographic Findings

Chest radiographs show bilateral air-space consolidation or ground-glass opacity that is diffuse (50%) or may predominate in the upper (25%) or lower (25%) lung zones (Figs. 13-25 to 13-27). Honeycombing may be seen late in the disease. Findings are similar to other causes of ARDS.

HRCT Findings

There is little reason to obtain HRCT in a patient with AIP. Findings are similar to those of any patient with ARDS.

(text continues on page 442)

FIG. 13.11. Nonspecific interstitial pneumonia. **A:** Chest radiograph shows a subtle increase in ground-glass opacity at the lung bases. Supine (**B**) and prone (**C**) HRCTs show subpleural reticulation and ground-glass opacity.

FIG. 13.12. Nonspecific interstitial pneumonia with ground-glass opacity. Supine HRCTs show ground-glass opacity with superimposed fine reticulation. Abnormalities predominate at the lung bases. There is sparing of the immediate subpleural lung. Biopsy showed cellular nonspecific interstitial pneumonia.

FIG. 13.18. HRCT in cryptogenic organizing pneumonia/bronchiolitis obliterans organizing pneumonia (COP/BOOP). The classic appearance of COP/BOOP is patchy subpleural and peribronchial consolidation. In this patient, subpleural consolidation predominates.

FIG. 13.19. Subpleural and peribronchial consolidation in cryptogenic organizing pneumonia/bronchiolitis obliterans organizing pneumonia. HRCT shows irregular nodular areas of consolidation, many occurring in relation to bronchi. Air bronchograms are visible within the opacities. An example of the "atoll" or "reversed halo" sign is visible in the mid lung (*arrow*). The opacities have irregular margins.

FIG. 13.20. Patchy ground-glass opacity in cryptogenic organizing pneumonia/bronchiolitis obliterans organizing pneumonia. **A:** Chest radiograph shows an increase in lung opacity. **B:** HRCT shows patchy areas of ground-glass opacity.

A   B

FIG. 13.21. Consolidation and ground-glass opacity in cryptogenic organizing pneumonia/ bronchiolitis obliterans organizing pneumonia. **A:** CT through the upper lobes shows ground-glass opacity in the left upper lobe and a ring-shaped opacity surrounding ground-glass opacity (*arrows*). This represents the "atoll" or "reversed halo" sign. **B:** CT shows patchy areas of consolidation and ground-glass opacity with a subpleural predominance.

A   B

FIG. 13.22. Irregular nodular opacities in cryptogenic organizing pneumonia/bronchiolitis obliterans organizing pneumonia. **A:** CT shows irregular nodular opacities. A subpleural area of consolidation is visible in the posterior left lower lobe. **B:** At a lower level, multiple irregular nodular opacities are visible, many occurring in relation to bronchi. Some of the small nodules (*arrows*) in the left lower lobe appear centrilobular in location.

TABLE 14.7 Sjögren's Syndrome

Primary or secondary (associated collagen disease)
Triad of
   keratoconjunctivitis sicca
   xerostomia
   parotid swelling
More common in women
Lymphoid interstitial pneumonia (LIP) and follicular
  bronchiolitis
   Lung cysts characteristic
Lung disease with pattern of NSIP, IP, OP/BOOP
   HRCT similar to other collagen diseases
Tracheobronchial gland inflammation
Pleuritis with or without effusion
Focal lymphoid hyperplasia and lymphoma
   Lung nodules or masses

A

B

FIG. 14.23. Sjögren's syndrome (SS) with lung cysts. **A** and **B:** Multiple thin-walled cysts are visible. These are characteristic of SS and represent lymphoid interstitial pneumonia.

patients ranging from 40 to 70 years of age and is much more common in women.

Pleuropulmonary manifestations are relatively common and include lymphoid interstitial pneumonitis (LIP), follicular bronchiolitis, NSIP, UIP, OP/BOOP, tracheobronchial gland inflammation, and pleuritis with or without effusion. Focal lymphoid hyperplasia and lymphoma have an increased incidence in SS.

The frequency of reported radiographic abnormalities ranges from 2% to 30%. The most common radiographic finding consists of a reticular or reticulonodular pattern, usually with a basal predominance. This pattern may be caused by LIP, interstitial fibrosis, or occasionally lymphoma.

HRCT findings are largely nonspecific, including ground-glass opacity, fibrosis, and bronchiectasis, typically present in the lower lobes.

A characteristic appearance is that of multiple lung cysts occurring as an isolated abnormality (Fig. 14-23; see Fig. 13-34 in Chapter 13) or in association with ground-glass opacity. These reflect the presence of LIP, which is common in this disease. The HRCT manifestations of LIP in SS are similar to those seen in LIP associated with other conditions, although multiple lung cysts are most typical (see Chapter 13).

Lymphoma in patients with SS may result in diffuse interstitial infiltration or multiple nodules. Focal lymphoid hyperplasia may present as solitary or multiple lung nodules (see Fig. 5-31 in Chapter 5).

ANKYLOSING SPONDYLITIS

Upper lobe and apical lung fibrosis is seen in less than 1% of patients with ankylosing spondylitis, usually 10 years or more after the onset of the disease. Histologic abnormalities include nonspecific inflammation, fibrosis, and sometimes bronchiolitis obliterans or lipoid pneumonia (Table 14-8).

Radiologically, the process begins as apical pleural thickening; an apical infiltrate characteristically develops and progresses to cystic lung destruction. It may be unilateral or bilateral. The chest radiographic findings may closely mimic those of tuberculosis (Fig. 14-24). Symptoms are usually absent, but the cavities become secondarily infected, most commonly by *Aspergillus fumigatus*. HRCT more commonly shows abnormalities than do chest radiographs. The most common findings are apical fibrosis, bronchiectasis, paraseptal emphysema, and pleural thickening.

TABLE 14.8 Ankylosing Spondylitis

Upper lobe fibrosis in 1%
Apical pleural thickening
Cystic lung destruction, bronchiectasis, paraseptal emphysema
Associated aspergilloma

FIG. 14.24. Upper lobe fibrosis in ankylosing spondylitis. There is upward retraction of the hila with fibrosis in both apices.

SELECTED READING

Aquino SL, Webb WR, Golden J. Bronchiolitis obliterans associated with rheumatoid arthritis: findings on HRCT and dynamic expiratory CT. J Comput Assist Tomogr 1994; 18:555–558.

Arroliga AC, Podell DN, Matthay RA. Pulmonary manifestations of scleroderma. J Thorac Imag 1992; 7:30–45.

Bankier AA, Kiener HP, Wiesmayr MN, et al. Discrete lung involvement in systemic lupus erythematosus: CT assessment. Radiology 1995; 196:835–840.

Bhalla M, Silver RM, Shepard JO, McLoud TC. Chest CT in patients with scleroderma: prevalence of asymptomatic esophageal dilatation and mediastinal lymphadenopathy. AJR Am J Roentgenol 1993; 161:269–272.

Fenlon HM, Casserly I, Sant SM, Breatnach E. Plain radiographs and thoracic high-resolution CT in patients with ankylosing spondylitis. AJR Am J Roentgenol 1997; 168:1067–1072.

Fenlon HM, Doran M, Sant SM, Breatnach E. High-resolution chest CT in systemic lupus erythematosus. AJR Am J Roentgenol 1996; 166:301–307.

Franquet T, Giménez A, Monill JM, et al. Primary Sjögren's syndrome and associated lung disease: CT findings in 50 patients. AJR Am J Roentgenol 1997; 169:655–658.

Fujii M, Adachi S, Shimizu T, Kono M. Interstitial lung disease in rheumatoid arthritis: assessment with high-resolution computed tomography. J Thorac Imaging 1993; 8:54–62.

Gamsu G. Radiographic manifestations of thoracic involvement by collagen vascular diseases. J Thorac Imaging 1992; 7:1–12.

Kim JS, Lee KS, Koh EM, et al. Thoracic involvement of systemic lupus erythematosus: clinical, pathologic, and radiologic findings. J Comput Assist Tomogr 2000; 24:9–18.

Lee HK, Kim DS, Yoo B, et al. Histopathologic pattern and clinical features of rheumatoid arthritis-associated interstitial lung disease. Chest 2005;127:2019–2027.

Mino M, Noma S, Taguchi Y, et al. Pulmonary involvement in polymyositis and dermatomyositis: sequential evaluation with CT. AJR Am J Roentgenol 1997; 169:83–87.

Prakash UB. Respiratory complications in mixed connective tissue disease. Clin Chest Med 1998; 19:733–746.

Primack SL, Müller NL. Radiologic manifestations of the systemic autoimmune diseases. Clin Chest Med 1998; 19:573–586.

Remy-Jardin M, Remy J, Cortet B, et al. Lung changes in rheumatoid arthritis: CT findings. Radiology 1994; 193:375–382.

Remy-Jardin M, Remy J, Wallaert B, et al. Pulmonary involvement in progressive systemic sclerosis: sequential evaluation with CT, pulmonary function tests, and bronchoalveolar lavage. Radiology 1993; 188: 499–506.

Schurawitzki H, Stiglbauer R, Graninger W, et al. Interstitial lung disease in progressive systemic sclerosis: high-resolution CT versus radiography. Radiology 1990; 176:755–759.

Schwarz MI. Pulmonary and cardiac manifestations of polymyositis-dermatomyositis. J Thorac Imaging 1992; 7:46–54.

Souza AS, Jr, Müller NL, Marchiori E, et al. Pulmonary abnormalities in ankylosing spondylitis: inspiratory and expiratory high-resolution CT findings in 17 patients. J Thorac Imaging 2004; 19:259–263.

Tanaka N, Newell JD, Brown KK, et al. Collagen vascular disease-related lung disease: high-resolution computed tomography findings based on the pathologic classification. J Comput Assist Tomogr 2004; 28:351–360.

Tanaka N, Kim JS, Newell JD, et al. Rheumatoid arthritis-related lung diseases: CT findings. Radiology 2004;232:81–91.

Tanoue LT. Pulmonary involvement in collage vascular disease: a review of the pulmonary manifestations of the Marfan syndrome, ankylosing spondylitis, Sjögren's syndrome, and relapsing polychondritis. J Thorac Imaging 1992; 7:62–77.

Taorimina VJ, Miller WT, Gefter WB, Epstein DM. Progressive systemic sclerosis subgroups: variable pulmonary features. AJR Am J Roentgenol 1981; 137:277–285.

Tazelaar HD, Viggiano RW, Pickersgill J, Colby TV. Interstitial lung disease in polymyositis and dermatomyositis: clinical features and prognosis as correlated with histologic findings. Am Rev Respir Dis 1990; 141: 727–733.

Wiedemann HP, Matthay RA. Pulmonary manifestations of systemic lupus erythematosus. J Thorac Imaging 1992; 7:1–18.

Sarcoidosis

W. RICHARD WEBB

S arcoidosis is a systemic disorder of unknown cause, characterized by the presence of noncaseating granulomas. It may involve almost any organ, but most morbidity and mortality result from pulmonary disease. Pulmonary manifestations are present in 90% of patients. Approximately 25% of patients have respiratory symptoms at diagnosis, usually dyspnea; also common are weight loss, fatigue, and sometimes fever or night sweats. Erythema nodosum is common.

Pulmonary lesions may resolve spontaneously or progress to fibrosis; 20% to 25% of patients have permanent functional impairment. Hilar and mediastinal lymph node enlargement is a common finding.

STAGING OF SARCOIDOSIS BASED ON PLAIN RADIOGRAPHS

Sarcoidosis has been described as occurring in stages based on plain radiographic findings:

Stage 0: No visible abnormalities (10% of cases)
Stage 1: Hilar or mediastinal lymph node enlargement not associated with visible lung disease (50% of cases)
Stage 2: Hilar or mediastinal lymph node enlargement associated with visible lung disease (30% of cases)
Stage 3: Diffuse lung disease without lymph node enlargement (10% of cases)
Stage 4: This designation is sometimes used to refer to end-stage fibrosis.

The utility of this staging system is limited, although there is some correlation between the stage and the course of disease. Radiographic abnormalities resolve in 65% of stage 1 patients, 50% of stage 2 patients, and 20% of stage 3 patients. However, patients in one stage need not progress to the next. This staging system is not used with CT, which is much more sensitive than radiographs in detecting both lymph node enlargement and lung disease.

LYMPH NODE ABNORMALITIES

Mediastinal lymph node enlargement is very common with sarcoidosis, occurring in 60% to 90% of patients at some stage in their disease. Less than half of patients with lymph node enlargement also show findings of lung disease on plain radiographs. A greater percentage of patients with lymph node enlargement show evidence of lung disease on CT.

Typically, node enlargement involves the hilar and mediastinal nodes, and lymph node masses usually appear bilateral and symmetrical on chest radiographs. The combination of (1) right paratracheal, (2) right hilar, and (3) left hilar node enlargement, termed the 1-2-3 pattern, is typical of sarcoidosis (Fig. 15-1; see also Figs. 8-44 and 8-45 in Chapter 8). Aortopulmonary window lymph node enlargement may also be seen, a finding sometimes referred to as the 1-2-3-4 pattern (see Fig. 15-1A).

In patients with enlarged nodes, chest radiographs show abnormalities, in order of decreasing frequency, in the hila (85% to 95%), right paratracheal region (75%), aortopulmonary window (50% to 75%), subcarinal space (20%), and anterior mediastinum (10% to 15%; Fig. 15-2; Table 8-20). The presence of hilar lymph node enlargement is so typical of sarcoidosis that the absence of this finding in a patient with mediastinal lymphadenopathy should lead you to question the diagnosis. Enlarged internal mammary, paravertebral, and retrocrural lymph nodes can also be seen but are much less common. Unilateral hilar lymph node enlargement is seen in less than 5% of cases. Lymph nodes may show dense, stippled, or eggshell calcification.

On CT, lymph node enlargement is visible in more than 80% of patients with sarcoidosis, with most showing both hilar and mediastinal lymph node enlargement (see Fig. 15-1B,C; see also Figs. 8-44 and 8-45 in Chapter 8). The frequency of visible involvement of specific node groups is somewhat different on CT, as compared to plain radiographs. Specifically, hilar lymph node enlargement is not invariably seen on CT in patients with mediastinal adenopathy. In patients with enlarged nodes, CT shows abnormalities, in order of decreasing frequency, in the right paratracheal space (100%), aortopulmonary window (95%), hila (90%), subcarinal space (65%), prevascular space (50%), and posterior mediastinum (15%). Symmetry, or bilateral node involvement, is visible more often on CT than on radiographs.

Lymph node masses in sarcoidosis may be quite large. Lymph node calcification is visible on CT in 25% to 50% of cases and may be hazy or dense or show a stippled or eggshell

FIG. 15.1. The 1-2-3 pattern of lymph node enlargement in sarcoidosis. **A:** On a chest radiograph, lymph node enlargement is visible in the right paratracheal mediastinum (*1*), right hilum (*2*), and left hilum (*3*). The presence of aortopulmonary window lymph node enlargement (*apw*) makes it a 1-2-3-4 pattern. **B** and **C:** On CT, lymph node enlargement is visible in the right paratracheal mediastinum (*1*), right hilum (*2*), and left hilum (*3*). Aortopulmonary window (*apw*) and subcarinal (*subc*) lymph node enlargement is also visible.

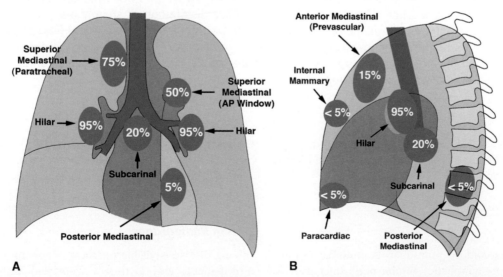

FIG. 15.2. Frequency of lymph node enlargement in patients with sarcoidosis as shown on posteroanterior (**A**) and lateral (**B**) radiographs.

FIG. 15.3. Pulmonary nodules in sarcoidosis. **A:** Detail view of the left upper lobe shows small, well-defined nodules. The lower lobes appeared normal. Left hilar enlargement is also seen. Most patients with lung nodules visible on radiographs also show lymph node enlargement. **B:** HRCT through the upper lobes shows a patchy perilymphatic distribution of sharply marginated nodules a few millimeters in diameter. The nodules involve the pleural surfaces and fissures (*small arrows*) and the peribronchovascular regions (*large arrows*). **C:** At a lower level, the nodules are less numerous, indicating an upper lobe predominance. **D:** Hilar lymph node enlargement with calcification (*arrows*) is visible using a soft-tissue window.

appearance (Fig. 15-3D; see also Figs. 8-38A and 8-45 in Chapter 8). Rarely nodes appear necrotic or low in attenuation or enhance on CT.

LUNG DISEASE

Nodules

In patients with sarcoidosis, pulmonary granulomas are found in relationship to lymphatics in the peribronchovascular interstitial space, subpleural interstitial space, and, to a lesser extent, the interlobular septa. This is termed a *perilymphatic*

distribution (see Figs. 10-20 and 10-21 in Chapter 10). Although sarcoid granulomas are microscopic in size, they often coalesce to form macroscopic nodules several millimeters or more in diameter.

Plain Radiographs

Lung disease is visible on chest radiographs in about 40% of patients and is usually associated with lymph node enlargement (i.e., stage 2). Lung abnormalities are often bilateral and symmetrical as seen on radiographs, with an upper lobe predominance in up to 80% of cases and a diffuse distribution in most others. A lower lobe predominance is unusual.

A nodular pattern is most common on chest radiographs, being seen in about half of the cases (see Figs. 15-3A and 15-6A). Nodules may appear well-defined or ill-defined and fuzzy and usually range from a few millimeters to 1 cm in diameter; a reticulonodular pattern is seen in an additional 25%.

Radiographs are relatively insensitive in showing lung abnormalities. In patients with radiographic stage 1 disease (i.e., no visible lung disease), 80% to 90% have lung lesions visible on high-resolution CT (HRCT) or on transbronchial biopsy.

HRCT

HRCT can show a variety of findings in patients with sarcoidosis (Table 15-1).

HRCT typically shows small nodules in patients with active disease. Nodules are as small as a few millimeters in diameter; they tend to be sharply defined despite their small size.

TABLE 15.1 HRCT Findings of Lung Disease in Sarcoidosis

Small sharply defined nodules
Typical of active lung disease
Perilymphatic distribution of nodules in most patients
  Parahilar and peribronchovascular
  Adjacent to fissures
  Subpleural in the lung periphery
  Interlobular septal nodules in some
  Centrilobular peribronchovascular nodules in some
Patchy upper lobe predominance in most
Calcification may occur

Large nodules and masses
  15%–25% of patients
  Due to confluence of small granulomas
With or without air bronchograms
Commonly parahilar (peribronchvascular)
Associated with satellite nodules (i.e., *the galaxy sign*)

Ground-glass opacity
  Uncommon
  Due to numerous very small granulomas
  Small nodules may be associated

Reticular opacities and fibrosis
  Develops in 15% of patients
  Peribronchovascular fibrosis with traction bronchiectasis
  Upper lobe volume loss
  Air-filled cysts
  Honeycombing in some
  Mycetoma may develop

Bronchial or bronchiolar abnormalities
  Endobronchial granulomas
  Atelectasis in some
  Mosaic perfusion and air trapping

In most cases, a perilymphatic distribution of small nodules is recognizable on HRCT (see Figs. 15-3B and C, and 15-4 to 15-6; see also Figs. 10-20 and 10-21 in Chapter 10). Sarcoid granulomas frequently predominate in relation to (1) the parahilar peribronchovascular interstitium (i.e., vessels and bronchi), (2) interlobar fissures, and (3) the peripheral subpleural regions. A distribution of nodules in relation to these three regions is highly suggestive of sarcoidosis. Interlobular septal thickening or nodules occurring in relation to septa may also be seen (see Figs. 15-5 and 15-6B), but this is not usually a predominant feature. Also, peripheral peribronchovascular nodules may appear centrilobular in location (see Fig. 15-6C). In occasional patients with extensive disease, nodules appear diffuse and "random" in distribution (see Fig. 10-23 in Chapter 10).

An upper lobe predominance of nodules is common but not invariable (see Figs. 15-3, 15-4, and 15-6). Sarcoid often appears patchy in distribution, with some lung regions being very abnormal while others appear normal. In up to 50% of patients, nodules may be few or focal (Fig. 15-7), being localized to small areas in one or both lungs.

Nodules may calcify (Fig. 15-8). These may be associated with calcified hilar or mediastinal lymph nodes.

Large Nodules and Masses

Large ill-defined opacities with or without air bronchograms, having the appearance of consolidation, can be seen on chest radiographs and CT in patients with sarcoid. These may be peripheral in location or parahilar (see Figs. 15-6A and B, 15-9, and 15-10). Although these opacities have been referred to as *alveolar sarcoidosis*, they result from the confluence of large numbers of interstitial granulomas.

(text continues on page 472)

FIG. 15.4. Perilymphatic distribution of nodules on HRCT. Nodules are small, well-defined, and several millimeters in diameter. They are located in relation to the subpleural interstitium in relation to the major fissures (*small arrows*) and the peribronchovascular interstitium adjacent to central vessels (*large arrows*), giving them a knobby appearance. Their distribution is patchy.

A   B

FIG. 15.5. Perilymphatic nodules on HRCT in sarcoidosis predominating in relation to interlobular septa. **A:** A scan at the lung base shows numerous thickening septa containing nodules (*arrows*). The pleural surfaces are also abnormal. **B:** At a higher level, nodules are visible involving the fissure (*arrows*).

A   B

FIG. 15.6. Perilymphatic nodules in sarcoidosis. **A:** Chest radiograph shows many lung nodules, having an upper lobe predominance. Some confluence is visible in the upper lobes. Elevation of the hila indicates some upper lobe volume loss, likely due to superimposed lung fibrosis. **B:** HRCT through the upper lobes shows multiple small lung nodules involving the lungs in a patchy fashion. Subpleural nodules (*black arrows*) and septal thickening (*white arrows*) are visible. Confluence of multiple peribronchovascular nodules is noted in the posterior lungs. **C:** HRCT at a lower level shows fewer lung nodules (*arrows*). The distribution is patchy. Subpleural nodules and peribronchovascular nodules are both seen. Some of the peripheral peribronchovascular nodules appear centrilobular in location.

C

A   B

FIG. 15.7. Subtle perilymphatic nodules in sarcoidosis. **A:** HRCT shows a few nodules in relation to the major fissure (*small arrows*). Peribronchovascular nodules in relation to small peripheral vessels (*large arrows*) are also seen. **B:** Hilar and mediastinal lymph node enlargement is also visible.

A   B

FIG. 15.8. Lung nodule calcification in sarcoidosis. **A:** HRCT shows a perilymphatic distribution of nodules. **B:** Soft-tissue window scan shows mediastinal lymph node enlargement. A left lung nodule is densely calcified (*arrow*).

FIG. 15.9. Confluent sarcoid granulomas resulting in a mass. HRCT shows a perilymphatic distribution of nodules involving the pleural surfaces and fissure (*small arrows*) and peribronchovascular interstitium (*large arrows*). Confluence of peribronchovascular nodules on the left (∗) results in a mass. Discrete satellite nodules are visible on the edge of the mass, resulting in the galaxy sign.

A   B

FIG. 15.10. Confluent sarcoid granulomas resulting in a mass. **A:** Confluence of peribroncho-vascular nodules on the left (∗) results in a large mass. Discrete satellite nodules are visible on the edge of the mass. Air bronchograms (*arrows*) are visible within the mass. This appearance has been termed alveolar sarcoidosis. **B:** At a lower level, a patchy perilymphatic distribution of nodules is visible.

Large nodules or masses (1 to 4 cm in diameter) are seen in 15% to 25% of patients on CT (see Figs. 15-6B, 15-9, and 15-10). These rarely cavitate. On CT, small nodules (i.e., satellite nodules) are often visible at the periphery of these masses (see Figs. 15-9 and 15-10). This appearance has been termed the "galaxy sign." It is often seen in patients with masses related to sarcoid but may be seen in other granulomatous diseases and some patients with neoplasm.

Ground-glass Opacity

Patients with sarcoidosis sometimes show patchy areas of ground-glass opacity on HRCT, which may be superimposed on a background of interstitial nodules (Fig. 15-11).

FIG. 15.11. Ground-glass opacity in sarcoidosis. HRCT shows clusters of many very small nodules with superimposed ground-glass opacity.

This finding usually reflects the presence of numerous very small granulomas. It is similar in etiology to alveolar sarcoidosis.

Reticular Opacities and Fibrosis

In many patients with stage 2 and 3 disease, radiographic abnormalities resolve with time. A persistent reticular pattern is seen on chest radiographs in 15% of cases; it is indicative of fibrosis and may be associated with honeycombing. Because active disease in sarcoidosis is typically patchy in distribution, areas of fibrosis also tend to be patchy.

Reticular opacities usually have an upper lobe predominance. Parahilar masses, usually in the upper lobes, may be visible due to peribronchial fibrosis. Upper lobe volume loss with upward retraction of the hila is common (see Figs. 15-6A and 15-12A). Areas of emphysema or air-filled cysts may also be seen in the peripheral lung.

The most common early HRCT finding of fibrosis is posterior displacement of the main and upper lobe bronchi associated with irregular reticular opacities (see Figs. 15-12 and 15-13). Progressive fibrosis leads to masses of peribronchovascular fibrous tissue with central conglomeration of parahilar bronchi and vessels, typically most marked in the upper lobes (Fig. 15-14). This finding is frequently associated with traction bronchiectasis; the only other diseases that commonly result in this appearance are silicosis and talcosis.

Honeycombing with lung cysts can be present in patients with sarcoidosis but is relatively uncommon. The honeycombing seen in patients with sarcoidosis usually involves the middle and upper lung zones, with relative sparing of the lung bases (Fig. 15-15); it may also involve central or

A

B

C

FIG. 15.12. Conglomerate masses and early lung fibrosis in sarcoidosis. **A:** Chest radiograph shows upward retraction of the hila associated with masslike opacities in the upper lobes (*arrows*). **B:** Masses with air bronchograms are visible in the upper lobes on HRCT. **C:** Posterior displacement of the upper lobe bronchi (*large arrow*) is an early sign of fibrosis. Distortion of lung architecture with displacement of the fissures (*small arrows*) and curving of pulmonary vessels also indicate volume loss and fibrosis.

A

B

C

FIG. 15.13. Lung fibrosis in sarcoidosis. **A** and **B:** HRCT scans show posterior displacement of the hila and upper lobe bronchi, associated with irregular reticular opacities and traction bronchiectasis. **C:** Extensive traction bronchiectasis is visible in the upper lobes, with areas of subpleural emphysema (*arrows*).

FIG. 15.14. Lung fibrosis in sarcoidosis. HRCT shows peribronchovascular masses of fibrous tissue (*arrows*) with central conglomeration of bronchi and traction bronchiectasis. The right upper lobe bronchi are displaced posteriorly. Other patchy areas of fibrosis are also visible.

peribronchovascular lung, a finding atypical of idiopathic pulmonary fibrosis (IPF). Rarely, the honeycombing may involve mainly the lower lung zones and mimic the appearance seen in IPF.

CT is helpful in assessing the presence and extent of some complications of sarcoidosis. Even though true cavitary sarcoidosis is rare, cystic lesions representing emphysema, bullae, or traction bronchiectasis are common in patients with extensive fibrosis (see Figs. 15-13C and 15-16 to 15-18). Superimposed mycetoma (aspergilloma) can be readily detected with CT and is very common, being present in as many as 10% of patients with end-stage sarcoidosis (see Figs. 15-17 and 15-18).

Bronchial and Bronchiolar Abnormalities

Airway involvement is common in sarcoidosis. Bronchial abnormalities have been reported in as many as 65% of patients, primarily consisting of nodular bronchial wall thickening or small endobronchial lesions (Fig. 15-19). HRCT may show small endobronchial granulomas. Obstruction of lobar or segmental bronchi by endobronchial granulomas or enlarged peribronchial lymph nodes may result in atelectasis; the right middle lobe is commonly affected (Fig. 15-20).

Small airway involvement by granulomas or fibrosis may result in obstruction, manifested on HRCT as mosaic perfusion on inspiratory scans (Fig. 15-21A) and air trapping on expiratory scans (see Fig. 15-21B).

A   B

FIG. 15.15. Honeycombing in sarcoidosis. **A:** Honeycombing is visible in the upper lobes. Central or peribronchovascular lung fibrosis is also present. **B:** Prone HRCT at the lung base shows interlobular septal thickening and findings of lung fibrosis, but honeycombing is absent. This distribution would be very unusual with idiopathic pulmonary fibrosis.

A   B

FIG. 15.16. End-stage sarcoidosis with fibrosis and cystic lesions. **A:** Chest radiograph shows reduced lung volume, upward retraction of the hila, and cystic lesions in the left upper lobe. **B:** HRCT shows extensive lung fibrosis with traction bronchiectasis and multiple cystic lesions in the left upper lobe. Enlargement of the hila represents pulmonary hypertension.

FIG. 15.17. End-stage sarcoidosis with an aspergilloma. HRCT shows upper lobe fibrosis, traction bronchiectasis, and emphysema. An aspergilloma (*arrow*) is present within a left upper-lobe cyst.

A   B

FIG. 15.18. End-stage sarcoidosis with an aspergilloma. **A:** Chest radiograph shows extensive left upper lobe fibrosis with volume loss and cystic abnormalities. **B:** HRCT shows a fungus ball (*arrow*) within a left upper lobe cyst.

FIG. 15.19. Airway involvement in sarcoidosis. HRCT shows nodular narrowing of the right upper lobe bronchus (*arrows*).

PLEURAL DISEASE

About 1% of patients with sarcoidosis develop pleural abnormalities, either pleural effusion or pleural thickening. These may reflect pleural involvement by sarcoidosis.

CARDIAC ABNORMALITIES

Sarcoidosis commonly involves the heart and may result in cardiomyopathy, arrhythmias, valvular lesions, and heart

FIG. 15.20. Right middle lobe collapse due to sarcoidosis. Narrowing of the right middle lobe bronchus (*arrow*) is associated with middle lobe atelectasis (*).

A

B

FIG. 15.21. Small airway involvement with sarcoidosis. **A:** Inspiratory scan shows heterogeneous lung attenuation because of mosaic perfusion. **B:** Expiratory scan shows air trapping.

failure. Cardiomegaly is sometimes seen and may be a clue to the diagnosis. Pulmonary hypertension may occur in patients with lung fibrosis.

SELECTED READING

Brauner MW, Grenier P, Mompoint D, et al. Pulmonary sarcoidosis: evaluation with high-resolution CT. Radiology 1989; 172:467–471.

Brauner MW, Lenoir S, Grenier P, et al. Pulmonary sarcoidosis: CT assessment of lesion reversibility. Radiology 1992; 182:349–354.

Hamper UM, Fishman EK, Khouri NF, et al. Typical and atypical CT manifestations of pulmonary sarcoidosis. J Comput Assist Tomogr 1986; 10:928–936.

Hansell DM, Milne DG, Wilsher ML, Wells AU. Pulmonary sarcoidosis: morphologic associations of airflow obstruction at thin-section CT. Radiology 1998; 209:697–704.

Kirks DR, McCormick VD, Greenspan RH. Pulmonary sarcoidosis: roentgenographic analysis of 150 patients. AJR Am J Roentgenol 1973; 117:777–786.

Lee KS, Kim TS, Han J, et al. Diffuse micronodular lung disease: HRCT and pathologic findings. J Comput Assist Tomogr 1999; 23:99–106.

Lenique F, Brauner MW, Grenier P, et al. CT assessment of bronchi in sarcoidosis: endoscopic and pathologic correlations. Radiology 1995; 194:419–423.

Lynch DA, Webb WR, Gamsu G, et al. Computed tomography in pulmonary sarcoidosis. J Comput Assist Tomogr 1989; 13:405–410.

McLoud TC, Epler GR, Gaensler EA, et al. A radiographic classification for sarcoidosis: physiologic correlation. Invest Radiol 1982; 17:129–138.

Müller NL, Kullnig P, Miller RR. The CT findings of pulmonary sarcoidosis: analysis of 25 patients. AJR Am J Roentgenol 1989; 152:1179–1182.

Müller NL, Mawson JB, Mathieson JR, et al. Sarcoidosis: correlation of extent of disease at CT with clinical, functional, and radiographic findings. Radiology 1989; 171:613–618.

Nakatsu M, Hatabu H, Morikawa K, et al. Large coalescent parenchymal nodules in pulmonary sarcoidosis: "sarcoid galaxy" sign. AJR Am J Roentgenol. 2002; 178:1389–1393

Nishimura K, Itoh H, Kitaichi M, et al. Pulmonary sarcoidosis: correlation of CT and histopathologic findings. Radiology 1993; 189:105–109.

Padley SP, Padhani AR, Nicholson A, Hansell DM. Pulmonary sarcoidosis mimicking cryptogenic fibrosing alveolitis on CT. Clin Radiol 1996; 51:807–810.

Patil SN, Levin DL. Distribution of thoracic lymphadenopathy in sarcoidosis using computed tomography. J Thorac Imaging 1999; 14:114–117.

Remy-Jardin M, Beuscart R, Sault MC, et al. Subpleural micronodules in diffuse infiltrative lung diseases: evaluation with thin-section CT scans. Radiology 1990; 177:133–139.

Remy-Jardin M, Giraud F, Remy J, et al. Pulmonary sarcoidosis: role of CT in the evaluation of disease activity and functional impairment and in prognosis assessment. Radiology 1994; 191:675–680.

Traill ZC, Maskell GF, Gleeson FV. High-resolution CT findings of pulmonary sarcoidosis. AJR Am J Roentgenol 1997; 168:1557–1560.

Allergic Lung Diseases: Hypersensitivity Pneumonitis and Eosinophilic Lung Disease

W. RICHARD WEBB

HYPERSENSITIVITY PNEUMONITIS

Hypersensitivity pneumonitis (HP), also known as extrinsic allergic alveolitis, is an allergic lung disease caused by the inhalation of antigens contained in a variety of organic dusts. Farmer's lung, the best-known HP syndrome, results from the inhalation of fungal organisms (thermophilic actinomycetes) growing in moist hay. Many other HP syndromes have been reported, and the list continues to grow. As with farmer's lung, HP syndromes are usually named after the setting in which exposure occurs or the organic substance involved. These include bird fancier's lung (bird proteins), mushroom worker's lung (thermophilic actinomycetes), malt worker's lung (*Aspergillus* species), maple bark disease (*Cryptostroma* species), bagassosis (thermophilic actinomycetes in sugarcane fibers), building-associated HP, and hot-tub lung (mycobacteria). In about 50% of cases, the responsible antigen cannot be determined despite a careful history and environmental assessment.

Acute exposure of susceptible individuals to an offending antigen produces fever, chills, dry cough, and dyspnea; long-term exposure can produce progressive shortness of breath with few or minimal systemic symptoms. Recurrent acute episodes are common with recurrent exposure.

Although the mechanisms by which HP occurs are unclear, it is associated with circulating antibodies (IgG and IgM). These, however, are not specific to HP, as they are commonly present in exposed individuals who are asymptomatic. There is a reduced incidence of HP in tobacco smokers.

The prognosis of patients with HP is good if the patient is removed from the antigenic environment. If not, progressive fibrosis can lead to significant respiratory disability and death.

The clinical, radiographic, and pathologic abnormalities occurring in patients with HP are similar regardless of the organic antigen responsible. These abnormalities can be classified into acute, subacute, and chronic stages. Often manifestations of more than one stage coexist.

Acute Stage

Exposure to large amounts of antigen in susceptible individuals may result in acute lung injury with dyspnea (Table 16-1).

The acute stage of HP is characterized by alveolar filling by a neutrophilic inflammatory exudate and pulmonary edema or hemorrhage due to diffuse alveolar damage.

Radiographs typically show ill-defined air-space consolidation, predominantly in the middle and lower lung zones, but they may be normal even in the face of marked symptoms. Ill-defined air-space nodules can also be seen with acute exposure. High-resolution CT (HRCT) in this stage may show bilateral air-space consolidation and small, ill-defined, centrilobular nodules.

Subacute Stage

Continued exposure to the antigen leads to progressive symptoms over a period of weeks or months. This is termed the subacute stage of HP. This stage of HP is characterized by alveolitis; interstitial infiltrates; small, irregular, poorly defined granulomas; and cellular bronchiolitis. Histologic abnormalities are usually most severe in a peribronchiolar distribution.

Radiographic Findings

After resolution of the acute abnormalities, which may take several days, or between episodes of acute exposure, a poorly defined nodular pattern or an ill-defined increase in lung density with obscuration of vascular margins (i.e., ground-glass opacity) may be visible on radiographs (Fig. 16-1). As in patients with acute disease, radiographs may be normal in the face of symptoms and an abnormal biopsy (Table 16-2).

HRCT Findings

HRCT is often first performed in the subacute stage of HP, weeks to months following first exposure to the antigen.

TABLE 16.1 Acute Hypersensitivity Pneumonitis

Exposure to large amounts of antigen
Acute dyspnea
Acute lung injury with diffuse alveolar damage, edema, or hemorrhage
Air-space consolidation on radiographs and HRCT

FIG. 16.1. Subacute hypersensitivity pneumonitis (HP). **A:** Chest radiograph shows reduced lung volumes and ill-defined increased lung opacity at the lung bases. **B:** HRCT shows patchy ground-glass opacity typical of subacute HP. Pneumomediastinum and subcutaneous emphysema are also present.

HRCT is more sensitive than chest radiographs in HP and may show typical features when chest films are normal. Typical HRCT findings include patchy ground-glass opacity (75% to 90%; see Figs. 16-1B, 16-2, and 16-3) and small ill-defined centrilobular nodules of ground-glass opacity, usually 3 to 5 mm in diameter (40% to 60%; see Figs. 16-2 and 16-4 to 16-6). These findings reflect the typical histologic abnormalities of HP; patchy ground-glass opacity correlates with the presence of alveolitis, while centrilobular nodules correlate with ill-defined peribronchiolar granulomas. These abnormalities are often seen in conjunction and may be diffuse or most marked in the middle or lower lung zones. The presence of ground-glass opacity nodules or patchy ground-glass opacity in a patient with known antigen exposure and typical symptoms is usually diagnostic in clinical practice.

Another common manifestation of subacute HP is the presence of focal areas of decreased attenuation (mosaic perfusion) on inspiratory HRCT (75% to 85%; see Figs. 16-2B,

16-7, and 16-8) or air trapping on expiratory HRCT (90%; see Figs. 16-8 and 16-9). These areas usually have sharply defined margins and a configuration consistent with involvement of single or multiple adjacent pulmonary lobules. The areas of decreased attenuation and air trapping result from the bronchiolitis seen in patients with HP. In some patients with HP, evidence of expiratory air trapping is seen in the absence of inspiratory scan abnormalities.

A combination of increased lung attenuation (ground-glass opacity) and decreased lung attenuation (mosaic perfusion) on inspiratory scans is termed the "headcheese sign" because it resembles a sausage of the same name (see Figs. 16-2B, 16-7, and 16-8). The headcheese sign is common in HP and is suggestive of the diagnosis.

In about 10% of patients with HP, thin-walled lung cysts are visible, ranging in size from a few millimeters to more than 2 cm in diameter. In most patients, fewer than five cysts are visible. The cysts are randomly distributed and often associated with ground-glass opacity or mosaic perfusion. They likely result from bronchiolitis and bronchiolar obstruction.

Findings of subacute HP usually resolve within weeks to months if exposure to the antigen is ended or the patient is treated. If exposure is ongoing or repeated exposure occurs, radiographic findings of fibrosis often develop (Fig. 16-10), being superimposed on the nodular opacities or ground-glass opacity typical of subacute disease.

Chronic Stage

The chronic stage of HP is characterized by the presence of fibrosis, which may develop months or years after the initial exposure (Table 16-3).

TABLE 16.2 Subacute Hypersensitivity Pneumonitis

Ongoing or recurrent exposure to antigen
Interstitial infiltrates, poorly defined granulomas, cellular
 bronchiolitis
HRCT
 Patchy ground-glass opacity
 Centrilobular nodules
 Mosaic perfusion
 "Headcheese" sign
 Air trapping
 Lung cysts
May progress to fibrosis

(text continues on page 482)

A   B

FIG. 16.2. Subacute hypersensitivity pneumonitis (HP) in a bird fancier. **A:** HRCT through the upper lobes shows patchy areas of ground-glass opacity and ill-defined nodular opacities with a centrilobular predominance. **B:** HRCT at the lung base shows patchy ground-glass opacities. Focal areas of relatively lucency represent mosaic perfusion. The combination of patchy ground-glass opacity and areas of lucency is termed the headcheese sign and is typical of HP.

A   B

FIG. 16.3. Subacute hypersensitivity pneumonitis with patchy ground-glass opacity. Scans through the upper and lower lobes show patchy areas of ground-glass opacity.

A

FIG. 16.4. Subacute hypersensitivity pneumonitis with diffuse centrilobular nodules. **A:** Scan through the upper lobes show diffuse centrilobular nodules. **B:** Detail view of the left upper lobe. The nodules do not involve the fissures or peripheral pleural surface. This appearance correlates with the presence of peribronchiolar infiltrates and ill-defined granulomas.

B

FIG. 16.5. Subacute hypersensitivity pneumonitis in a bird fancier, with ill-defined centrilobular nodules of ground-glass opacity. The nodules surround small vessels and spare the pleural surfaces. The chest radiograph in this patient was normal.

FIG. 16.6. Subacute hypersensitivity pneumonitis with diffuse centrilobular nodules, representing "hot-tub lung." Small, ill-defined nodules are visible.

FIG. 16.7. Subacute hypersensitivity pneumonitis with the headcheese sign. HRCT shows patchy ground-glass opacity and consolidation. Also, areas of lucency (*arrows*) containing small vessels represent mosaic perfusion. The combination of ground-glass opacity and mosaic perfusion constitutes the headcheese sign. It reflects lung infiltration (the ground-glass opacity) and bronchiolar obstruction with air trapping (areas of decreased attenuation).

A

B

FIG. 16.8. Subacute hypersensitivity pneumonitis with air trapping. **A:** Inspiratory scan shows diffuse ground-glass opacity and centrilobular nodules, with numerous focal, lobular areas of lucency (*arrows*) due to mosaic perfusion. The combination of ground-glass opacity and mosaic perfusion constitutes the headcheese sign. **B:** Expiratory scan at the same level shows air trapping in the lucent lung regions.

A

B

FIG. 16.9. Subacute hypersensitivity pneumonitis with air trapping. **A:** Inspiratory scan shows a fine nodular appearance and subtle mosaic perfusion. **B:** Expiratory scan shows patchy air trapping with geographic areas of lucency. Anterior bowing of the posterior tracheal membrane indicates a good expiration.

A

B

FIG. 16.10. Progression of subacute hypersensitivity pneumonitis to fibrosis in a bird fancier. **A:** HRCT shows diffuse ground-glass opacity and ill-defined ground-glass opacity nodules. Focal fibrosis is present in the left upper lobe (*arrows*) with early honeycombing. **B:** HRCT 15 months later shows progression of honeycombing and reticulation due to fibrosis (*arrows*). Ground-glass opacity has diminished.

Radiographic Findings

On chest radiographs, radiographic findings of fibrosis include irregular reticular opacities that predominate in the middle lung or lower lung zones and may be parahilar, peribronchovascular, or peripheral in distribution (Fig. 16-11A). A patchy distribution is common. In some cases, fibrosis in HP can mimic the appearance of idiopathic pulmonary fibrosis (IPF) with honeycombing.

HRCT Findings

On HRCT, chronic HP is characterized by fibrosis, although findings of subacute disease are often superimposed (Figs. 16-11 to 16-13). CT scans show irregular reticular opacities that may be associated with patchy bilateral areas of ground-glass opacity (90%), small ill-defined nodules (60%), areas of reduced lung attenuation due to mosaic perfusion, and air trapping on expiratory scans. In HP, fibrosis is often patchy in distribution or parahilar (see Fig. 16-13), lacking the subpleural predominance of IPF; in

some cases it is predominantly subpleural. Honeycombing is not common (20% of cases), but unlike IPF, it may be upper lobe in distribution or often appears patchy or peribronchovascular rather than subpleural (Fig. 16-14).

TABLE 16.3 Chronic Hypersensitivity Pneumonitis

Fibrosis
HRCT
 Irregular reticular opacities
 Traction bronchiectasis
 Honeycombing
 Distribution usually different than idiopathic pulmonary fibrosis
 Often appears patchy and parahilar rather than subpleural
Superimposed findings of subacute hypersensitivity pneumonitis may be present

A

B

C

FIG. 16.11. Chronic hypersensitivity pneumonitis with fibrosis. **A:** Chest radiograph shows marked reduction in lung volume with poorly defined reticular opacities at the lung bases. **B:** HRCT through the upper lobes shows findings of fibrosis with irregular reticular opacities and traction bronchiectasis. Some superimposed ground-glass opacity is also visible. Focal lucencies (*arrows*) reflect mosaic perfusion and the headcheese sign. **C:** HRCT at the lung bases shows similar findings. Traction bronchiectasis is visible in both lower lobes.

Findings of fibrosis in patients with chronic HP most often show a mid-lung or lower lung zone predominance or are evenly distributed throughout the upper, middle, and lower lung zones. Relative sparing of the lung bases, seen in many patients with chronic HP, allows distinction of this entity from IPF, in which the fibrosis usually predominates in the lung bases (Fig. 16-15).

A

B

FIG. 16.12. Chronic hypersensitivity pneumonitis with fibrosis. **A:** HRCT through the upper lobes shows ground-glass opacity, the headcheese sign, and irregular reticular opacities indicating early fibrosis. **B:** At the lung bases, irregular reticular opacities indicative of fibrosis, and areas of mosaic perfusion predominate.

A

B

FIG. 16.13. Chronic hypersensitivity pneumonitis with fibrosis. **A:** HRCT through the upper lobes shows patchy irregular reticular opacities. Traction bronchiectasis is visible bilaterally, with a patchy and parahilar predominance (*arrows*). **B:** At the lung bases, areas of fibrosis (*arrows*) are patchy and lack the subpleural predominance of idiopathic pulmonary fibrosis. Lobular lucencies are also visible.

A

B

FIG. 16.14. Chronic hypersensitivity pneumonitis with fibrosis. **A:** HRCT through the upper lobes shows irregular reticular opacities, traction bronchiectasis, and honeycombing (*arrows*). **B:** At the lung bases, patchy areas of fibrosis (*arrows*) are visible.

A

B

FIG. 16.15. End-stage chronic hypersensitivity pneumonitis with fibrosis and honeycombing. **A:** HRCT at the lung bases shows extensive lung fibrosis with mild subpleural honeycombing, traction bronchiectasis, and irregular reticulation. **B:** Similar findings are noted in the upper lobes.

TABLE 16.4 Classification of Eosinophilic Lung Disease

Idiopathic eosinophilic lung disease
Simple pulmonary eosinophilia
Chronic eosinophilic pneumonia
Acute eosinophilic pneumonia
Hypereosinophilic syndrome
Churg-Strauss syndrome
Bronchocentric granulomatosis
Idiopathic eosinophilic lung disease and angiitis
Wegener's granulomatosis
Polyarteritis
Collagen-vascular diseases
Eosinophilic lung disease with a known cause
Drugs
Parasitic disease and tropical pulmonary eosinophilia
Fungi
Bronchocentric granulomatosis

EOSINOPHILIC LUNG DISEASE

The term *eosinophilic lung disease* describes a group of entities characterized by an abundant accumulation of eosinophils in the pulmonary interstitium and air spaces. Peripheral blood eosinophilia is commonly present. Diagnostic criteria include (1) radiographic or CT findings of lung disease in association with peripheral eosinophilia, (2) biopsy-confirmed lung tissue eosinophilia, and (3) increased eosinophils at bronchoalveolar lavage.

The disorders can be classified into those of unknown cause and those with a known cause (Table 16-4). Some overlap exists between these categories.

IDIOPATHIC EOSINOPHILIC LUNG DISEASE

Common idiopathic eosinophilic lung diseases include (1) simple pulmonary eosinophilia, (2) chronic eosinophilic pneumonia, (3) acute eosinophilic pneumonia, (4) hypereosinophilic syndrome, and (5) Churg-Strauss syndrome. These conditions reflect a spectrum, being associated with symptoms ranging from mild to severe and radiographic abnormalities ranging from focal to diffuse.

Other idiopathic diseases also may be associated with blood or tissue eosinophilia and may be considered in the differential diagnosis of eosinophilic lung disease. Vasculitis is typically present. These diseases include Wegener's granulomatosis (see Chapter 19), polyarteritis, and collagen-vascular diseases such as rheumatoid arthritis, scleroderma, CREST syndrome, polymyositis-dermatomyositis, and Sjögren's syndrome (see Chapter 14). They are sometimes included in a category of eosinophilic lung disease with angiitis.

TABLE 16.5 Simple Pulmonary Eosinophilia (Loeffler's Syndrome)

Idiopathic
Blood eosinophilia
Mild dyspnea
History of asthma or atopy often present
Focal consolidation, usually transient or fleeting
May be self-limited

Simple Pulmonary Eosinophilia (Loeffler's Syndrome)

Simple pulmonary eosinophilia, also known as Loeffler's syndrome, is characterized by blood eosinophilia and radiographic findings of focal areas of consolidation, which are usually transient (Table 16-5). Although similar findings can be seen in association with a number of etiologic agents, particularly parasites and drugs, use of the term *simple pulmonary eosinophilia* should be limited to cases in which the cause is unknown. Approximately one third of patients with this pattern have idiopathic disease. The disease may be self-limited.

Patients typically have cough and mild shortness of breath; often a history of asthma or atopic disease is present. Pathologically, eosinophils and histiocytes accumulate in the alveolar walls and alveoli.

The radiographic manifestations are characteristic and consist of patchy transient (fleeting) and migratory areas of consolidation that usually clear spontaneously within 1 month. These may be single or multiple and usually have ill-defined margins. On radiographs and HRCT, the areas of consolidation often have a predominantly peripheral distribution. On HRCT, areas of ground-glass opacity, focal areas of consolidation, or large nodules may be seen.

Chronic Eosinophilic Pneumonia

Chronic eosinophilic pneumonia is an idiopathic condition characterized by extensive infiltration of the alveoli and interstitium by a mixed inflammatory infiltrate consisting primarily of eosinophils (Table 16-6). Chronic eosinophilic pneumonia is usually associated with increased eosinophils in the peripheral blood. Clinically, patients present with fever, cough, weight loss, malaise, and shortness of breath.

TABLE 16.6 Chronic Eosinophilic Pneumonia

Idiopathic
Blood eosinophilia
Fever, weight loss, dyspnea, often severe
Patchy peripheral consolidation, often persistent
Patchy ground-glass opacity
Mimics organizing pneumonia (BOOP), but usually shows an upper lobe predominance
Rapid resolution with steroids

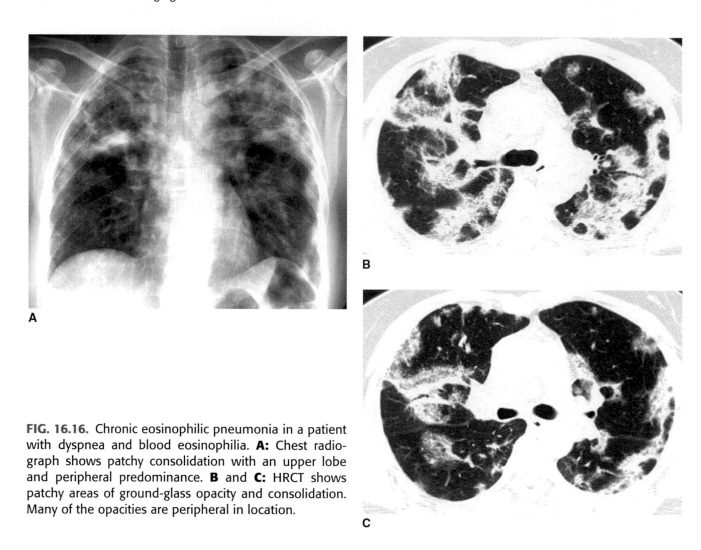

FIG. 16.16. Chronic eosinophilic pneumonia in a patient with dyspnea and blood eosinophilia. **A:** Chest radiograph shows patchy consolidation with an upper lobe and peripheral predominance. **B** and **C:** HRCT shows patchy areas of ground-glass opacity and consolidation. Many of the opacities are peripheral in location.

FIG. 16.17. Chronic eosinophilic pneumonia. **A:** Chest radiograph shows patchy peripheral consolidation. **B:** Following steroid treatment, the abnormalities have resolved.

FIG. 16.18. Chronic eosinophilic pneumonia. HRCT shows patchy areas of consolidation involving the peripheral lung.

FIG. 16.19. Chronic eosinophilic pneumonia. HRCT shows patchy ground-glass opacity in the peripheral right upper lobe. Similar abnormalities were visible at other levels.

Symptoms are often severe and last 3 months or more. Life-threatening respiratory compromise may occur, but this is unusual.

Radiographically, chronic eosinophilic pneumonia is characterized by the presence of homogeneous peripheral air-space consolidation, "the photographic negative of pulmonary edema" (Figs. 16-16 and 16-17; see also Fig. 2-9A in Chapter 2). Consolidation may be patchy. This pattern can remain unchanged for weeks or months unless steroid therapy is given; chronic eosinophilic pneumonia responds promptly to the administration of steroids. An upper lobe predominance is common (see Fig. 16-17).

The combination of blood eosinophilia, peripheral consolidation visible on radiographs, and rapid response to steroid therapy is often sufficiently characteristic to obviate the need for lung biopsy. However, this classic radiologic picture is seen in only about 50% of cases. The diagnosis may be difficult in patients with minimal blood eosinophilia or those in whom the peripheral distribution of infiltrates is not apparent.

On CT, chronic eosinophilic pneumonia is characterized by (1) consolidation, often peripheral and patchy in distribution (90%; Figs. 16-16, 16-18, and 16-19); (2) patchy or peripheral ground-glass opacity (80%), sometimes associated with "crazy-paving"; (3) linear or bandlike opacities (Fig. 16-20), usually seen during resolution (5%); and (4) an upper lobe predominance of abnormalities.

An appearance identical to that of chronic eosinophilic pneumonia can be seen in patients with simple pulmonary eosinophilia or Loeffler's syndrome. Simple pulmonary eosinophilia, however, is usually self-limited and associated with pulmonary infiltrates that are transient or fleeting. With simple pulmonary eosinophilia, areas of consolidation can appear and disappear within days; chronic eosinophilic pneumonia has a more protracted course, and areas of consolidation remain unchanged over weeks or months.

The presence of peripheral air-space consolidation can be considered suggestive of chronic eosinophilic pneumonia in the appropriate clinical setting (i.e., in patients with eosinophilia). An identical appearance of peripheral air-space consolidation can be seen in organizing pneumonia (OP/BOOP) although OP/BOOP often involves the lower lung zones to a greater degree.

A   B

FIG. 16.20. Chronic eosinophilic pneumonia. HRCTs at two levels show patchy consolidation in the peripheral lung. A bandlike opacity is visible (*arrow* in **B**), paralleling the pleural surface. This appearance mimics that of organizing pneumonia/bronchiolitis obliterans organizing pneumonia.

TABLE 16.7 Acute Eosinophilic Pneumonia

Idiopathic
Eosinophilia on bronchoalveolar lavage
Rapidly progressing respiratory failure
Radiographic findings resemble pulmonary edema

Acute Eosinophilic Pneumonia

Acute eosinophilic pneumonia is an acute febrile illness associated with rapidly increasing shortness of breath and hypoxemic respiratory failure (Table 16-7). The diagnosis is based on clinical findings of acute respiratory failure and the presence of markedly elevated numbers of eosinophils in bronchoalveolar lavage fluid. Response to steroids is prompt and the prognosis is good, with no residual disability.

The radiographic manifestations are similar to those of pulmonary edema. The earliest radiographic manifestation is reticular opacities, frequently with Kerley B lines. This progresses over a few hours or days to bilateral interstitial opacities and air-space consolidation involving mainly the lower lung zones. Small bilateral pleural effusions are present in most patients.

The HRCT findings of acute eosinophilic pneumonia include bilateral areas of ground-glass opacity, smooth interlobular septal thickening, small pleural effusions, and occasionally areas of consolidation (Fig. 16-21). The combination of ground-glass opacity and septal thickening may result in the appearance of "crazy paving."

FIG. 16.21. Acute eosinophilic pneumonia. HRCT shows extensive ground-glass opacity and consolidation with a lower lobe predominance. Interlobular septal thickening in also seen (*arrows*). Pneumomediastinum and right Pneumothorax are present and a right chest tube is in place. The patient had rapidly progressive respiratory failure and was intubated. Bronchoalveolar lavage revealed numerous eosinophils.

TABLE 16.8 Hypereosinophilic Syndrome

Idiopathic
Blood eosinophilia
Multiorgan infiltration by eosinophils
Pulmonary and pleural involvement in 40%
Ground-glass opacity or areas of consolidation
Cardiac involvement: cardiomegaly, pulmonary edema,
  pleural effusion
Poor prognosis

Hypereosinophilic Syndrome

Hypereosinophilic syndrome is characterized by blood eosinophilia present persistently for at least 6 months, associated with multiorgan tissue infiltration by mature eosinophils (Table 16-8). An underlying cause may or may not be evident. The main causes of morbidity and mortality are cardiac and central nervous system involvement. Pulmonary and pleural involvement occur in approximately 40% of cases. Pulmonary symptoms include cough, wheezing, and shortness of breath.

The radiographic manifestations are nonspecific and consist of transient hazy ground-glass opacity or areas of consolidation. Cardiac involvement eventually leads to cardiomegaly, pulmonary edema, and pleural effusion. The prognosis is poor.

The predominant HRCT finding is bilateral pulmonary nodules, 1 cm or less in diameter, mainly involving the peripheral lung regions. Nodules may show the halo sign.

Churg-Strauss Syndrome

Churg-Strauss syndrome (also known as Churg-Strauss granulomatosis or allergic granulomatosis and angiitis) is a multisystem disorder characterized by the presence of (1) necrotizing vasculitis, (2) extravascular granuloma formation, and (3) eosinophilic infiltration of various organs, particularly the lungs, skin, heart, nerves, gastrointestinal tract, and kidneys. Not all of these three findings need be present (Table 16-9).

Patients with this syndrome are usually middle-aged (average onset 40 to 50 years) and often have a history of allergic diseases, including asthma, nasal polyps, or sinusitis. Criteria for diagnosis include (1) asthma, (2) blood eosinophilia greater than 10%, (3) a history of allergy, (4) neuropathy, (5) migratory or transient pulmonary opacities visible radiographically, (6) sinus abnormalities, and (7) extravascular eosinophilia on biopsy. The presence of four or more of these criteria is 85% sensitive and nearly 100% specific for Churg-Strauss syndrome. Churg-Strauss syndrome may be associated with antineutrophil cytoplasmic antibody (ANCA), usually P-ANCA (perinuclear pattern).

TABLE 16.9 **Churg-Strauss Syndrome**

Idiopathic
Multisystem disorder
  Necrotizing vasculitis
  Extravascular granulomas
  Eosinophilic infiltration
History of atopy
Neuropathy
Sinus disorders
Renal involvement
P-ANCA
Three phases
  Allergic phase with rhinitis, sinusitis and asthma
  Eosinophilic phase
    Blood and tissue eosinophilia
    Findings of simple pulmonary eosinophilia or
     chronic eosinophilic pneumonia
  Systemic or small vessel vasculitis phase
Heart, kidney, musculoskeletal, and nervous systems involved
  Nodules or masses; may cavitate
Responds well to steroids

Cough and hemoptysis are common, but symptoms may reflect the involvement of various organs; these include skin rash, diarrhea, neuropathy, and congestive heart failure.

Patients usually respond well to treatment with steroids, but without treatment they may die within months. With treatment, the 5-year survival rate is good, up to 80%. Associated renal failure is associated with a poor prognosis.

Churg-Strauss syndrome may evolve in three phases:

1. An *allergic phase* with rhinitis, sinusitis, and asthma as the primary features
2. An *eosinophilic phase* associated with blood and tissue eosinophilia, usually involving the lung and gastrointestinal tract. Lung abnormalities usually resemble simple pulmonary eosinophilia or chronic eosinophilic pneumonia.
3. A *systemic or small-vessel vasculitis phase* in which other organs (heart, skin, musculoskeletal system, nervous system, and kidney) are also involved. This may occur years after the development of eosinophilia.

Radiographic abnormalities are common. Pulmonary opacities have been identified in 50% to 70% of patients in the eosinophilic or vasculitic phases of the disease, often consisting of transient multifocal areas of consolidation indistinguishable from simple pulmonary eosinophilia or chronic eosinophilic pneumonia. Pulmonary nodules or masses, hemorrhage, pulmonary edema, and pleural effusions may be present. In 40% of cases, pulmonary radiographic abnormalities precede the development of systemic vasculitis. Involvement of the heart may result in cardiomegaly with findings of congestive heart failure; otherwise, pleural effusion is uncommon.

HRCT findings are variable and nonspecific, reflecting the different pulmonary manifestations of this disease. Findings include (1) consolidation or ground-glass opacity (60%), which may have a peripheral distribution or be patchy and geographic; (2) pulmonary nodules or masses (20%) ranging from 0.5 to 3.5 cm in diameter, which may appear centrilobular or may contain air bronchograms (Fig. 16-22); (3) bronchial wall thickening or bronchiectasis (35%); and (4) interlobular septal thickening due to pulmonary edema (5%). Although cavitation of nodules or masses may occur, it is much less common than with Wegener's granulomatosis, which it may resemble clinically and radiographically. The absence of cavitation is helpful in distinguishing Churg-Strauss syndrome from Wegener's granulomatosis.

A   **B**

FIG. 16.22. Churg-Strauss syndrome. A and B: HRCT shows ill-defined focal regions of consolidation and ground-glass opacity. The nodular opacities contain air bronchograms.

EOSINOPHILIC LUNG DISEASE HAVING A SPECIFIC ETIOLOGY

Known causes of eosinophilic lung disease include drugs, parasites, and fungi.

Drug-related Disease

Drugs are an important cause of eosinophilic lung disease. Many drugs have been reported to be associated with eosinophilic lung disease; implicated drugs include antibiotics, nonsteroidal anti-inflammatory agents, and cytotoxic drugs. Reactions range from those similar to simple pulmonary eosinophilia to those imitating acute eosinophilic pneumonia (see Chapter 17, Table 17-5).

Parasitic Infestations

Parasites most commonly result in findings similar to simple pulmonary eosinophilia. Most cases are due to roundworms such as *Ascaris lumbricoides, Toxocara, Ancylostoma,* and *Strongyloides stercoralis.*

Tropical pulmonary eosinophilia is caused by the worms *Wuchereria bancrofti* and *Brugia malayi,* with most cases being reported in India, Africa, South America, and Southeast Asia. In the Far East, the lung fluke *Paragonimus westermani* is typically responsible. Symptoms are nonspecific but include fever, weight loss, dyspnea, cough, and hemoptysis. CT findings reported in paragonimiasis include patchy lung consolidation, cystic lesions filled with air or fluid, pneumothorax, and pleural effusion.

Fungal Disease

The primary fungal disease associated with pulmonary eosinophilia is allergic bronchopulmonary aspergillosis (ABPA), characterized by asthma, peripheral eosinophilia, central bronchiectasis, mucus plugging, and an allergic reaction to *Aspergillus fumigatus*. It is described in detail in Chapter 23. However, other patterns of disease may result from exposure to fungus, including HP, eosinophilic pneumonia, and bronchocentric granulomatosis.

Bronchocentric Granulomatosis

The characteristic histologic abnormality seen in patients with bronchocentric granulomatosis is necrotizing granulomatous inflammation centered around bronchioles and small bronchi (Table 16-10). It may be associated with complete destruction of the airway mucosa and filling of the airway lumen with necrotic material. In asthmatic subjects, bronchocentric granulomatosis is most commonly associated with *Aspergillus,* and fungal hyphae are often present within these lesions. Bronchocentric granulomatosis may

TABLE 16.10 Bronchocentric Granulomatosis

Necrotizing granulomas centered on bronchioles and bronchi
Hypersensitivity reaction
Peripheral eosinophilia
History of asthma in one third
Associated with *Aspergillus,* mycobacteria, inflammatory diseases
Nodules, masses, focal consolidation, mucoid impaction
Upper lobe predominance

also be seen in patients with mycobacterial infection or noninfectious inflammatory diseases such as rheumatoid arthritis and in immunosuppressed patients.

Bronchocentric granulomatosis is generally considered a hypersensitivity reaction. Patients are usually young; one third have a history of asthma; and peripheral eosinophilia is seen in half of cases. Tissue eosinophilia is also present in asthmatic patients. This process may be associated with ABPA in asthmatic patients, but abnormalities in bronchocentric granulomatosis tend to be more focal than those seen with ABPA. Symptoms are often mild, with fever, cough, chest pain, and hemoptysis.

Chest radiographs may show a nodule or focal area of consolidation. CT findings include a spiculated mass lesion or lobar consolidation with associated mild volume loss. Mucoid impaction may be present. The abnormalities predominantly involve the upper lobes. Masses and consolidation represent necrotic tissue associated with consolidation or eosinophilic pneumonia.

SELECTED READING

Adler BD, Padley SP, Müller NL, et al. Chronic hypersensitivity pneumonitis: high-resolution CT and radiographic features in 16 patients. Radiology 1992; 185:91–95.

Allen JN, Davis WB. Eosinophilic lung diseases. Am J Respir Crit Care Med 1994; 150:1423–1438.

Arakawa H, Webb WR. Air trapping on expiratory high-resolution CT scans in the absence of inspiratory scan abnormalities: correlation with pulmonary function tests and differential diagnosis. AJR Am J Roentgenol 1998; 170:1349–1353.

Bain GA, Flower CD. Pulmonary eosinophilia. Eur J Radiol 1996; 23:3–8.

Buschman DL, Waldron JA, Jr, King TE, Jr. Churg-Strauss pulmonary vasculitis: high-resolution computed tomography scanning and pathologic findings. Am Rev Respir Dis 1990; 142:458–461.

Cheon JE, Lee KS, Jung GS, et al. Acute eosinophilic pneumonia: radiographic and CT findings in six patients. AJR Am J Roentgenol 1996; 167:1195–1199.

Ebara H, Ikezoe J, Johkoh T, et al. Chronic eosinophilic pneumonia: evolution of chest radiograms and CT features. J Comput Assist Tomogr 1994; 18:737–744.

Gaensler EA, Carrington CB. Peripheral opacities in chronic eosinophilic pneumonia: the photographic negative of pulmonary edema. AJR Am J Roentgenol 1977; 128:1–13.

Hansell DM, Moskovic E. High-resolution computed tomography in extrinsic allergic alveolitis. Clin Radiol 1991; 43:8–12.

Hansell DM, Wells AU, Padley SP, Müller NL. Hypersensitivity pneumonitis: correlation of individual CT patterns with functional abnormalities. Radiology 1996; 199:123–128.

Kang EY, Shim JJ, Kim JS, Kim KI. Pulmonary involvement of idiopathic hypereosinophilic syndrome: CT findings in five patients. J Comput Assist Tomogr 1997; 21:612–615.

Kim Y, Lee KS, Choi DC, et al. The spectrum of eosinophilic lung disease: radiologic findings. J Comput Assist Tomogr 1997; 21:920–930.

King MA, Pope-Harman AL, Allen JN, et al. Acute eosinophilic pneumonia: radiologic and clinical features. Radiology 1997; 203:715–719.

Lynch DA, Newell JD, Logan PM, et al. Can CT distinguish hypersensitivity pneumonitis from idiopathic pulmonary fibrosis? AJR Am J Roentgenol 1995; 165:807–811.

Mindell HJ. Roentgen findings in farmer's lung. Radiology 1970; 97: 341–346.

Primack SL, Müller NL. Radiologic manifestations of the systemic autoimmune diseases. Clin Chest Med 1998; 19:573–586.

Remy-Jardin M, Remy J, Wallaert B, Müller NL. Subacute and chronic bird breeder hypersensitivity pneumonitis: sequential evaluation with CT and correlation with lung function tests and bronchoalveolar lavage. Radiology 1993; 198:111–118.

Silver SF, Müller NL, Miller RR, Lefcoe MS. Hypersensitivity pneumonitis: evaluation with CT. Radiology 1989; 173:441–445.

Ward S, Heyneman LE, Flint JD, et al. Bronchocentric granulomatosis: computed tomographic findings in five patients. Clin Radiol 2000; 55:296–300.

Webb WR. Thin-section CT of the secondary pulmonary lobule: anatomy and the image—the 2004 Fleischner lecture. Radiology 2006; 239: 322–338.

Winn RE, Kollef MH, Meyer JI. Pulmonary involvement in the hypereosinophilic syndrome. Chest 1994; 105:656–660.

Worthy SA, Müller NL, Hansell DM, Flower CD. Churg-Strauss syndrome: the spectrum of pulmonary CT findings in 17 patients. AJR Am J Roentgenol 1998; 170:297–300.

Iatrogenic Lung Diseases: Drug-Induced Lung Disease and Radiation Pneumonitis

W. RICHARD WEBB

DRUG-INDUCED LUNG DISEASE

Many drugs, both therapeutic and illicit, can be associated with lung disease. However, drug-induced lung disease is manifested in a limited number of ways. Specific pathologic reactions occurring with pulmonary drug toxicity include the following:

1. Hydrostatic and increased permeability pulmonary edema
2. Diffuse alveolar damage (DAD) and the acute respiratory distress syndrome (ARDS)
3. Pulmonary hemorrhage
4. Organizing pneumonia (OP/BOOP)
5. Eosinophilic pneumonia and hypersensitivity reactions
6. Chronic interstitial pneumonitis with fibrosis
7. Systemic lupus erythematosus (SLE)
8. Pulmonary vasculitis and pulmonary hypertension
9. Bronchiolitis obliterans

Each of these patterns is characteristically associated with a different group of drugs, although many drugs can result in more than one type of lung reaction, and some overlap between these patterns is common. In most cases, the radiographic appearances of a drug-related lung disease are nonspecific and the diagnosis must be based on observing a temporal relationship between the administration of a drug and the development of pulmonary abnormalities.

Because of the large number of drugs associated with drug reactions and the variety of patterns possible, a high degree of suspicion must be maintained when evaluating patients with unexplained lung disease, regardless of what it looks like or what drug treatment is being employed. Prompt recognition of drug-induced lung disease is important because early abnormalities may resolve completely if the drug is discontinued or appropriate therapy is instituted.

Radiographic abnormalities associated with drug-related lung injury vary with the histologic pattern present, and with a few exceptions, the appearance of each pattern appears the same regardless of the drug involved. High-resolution CT

(HRCT) is more sensitive than chest radiography in defining the radiographic abnormalities.

Pulmonary Edema

Hydrostatic pulmonary edema may result from drugs affecting the heart or systemic vasculature (Table 17-1). An example would be cocaine. Radiographic and HRCT findings are typical of any cause of hydrostatic edema. Pleural effusion may be present.

Increased permeability pulmonary edema also may occur. Onset is usually sudden. Increased permeability pulmonary edema occurring without DAD results in typical findings of pulmonary edema, including interlobular septal thickening (Kerley's lines; see Fig. 11-11 in Chapter 11), ground-glass opacity (see Fig. 11-13 in Chapter 11), and to a lesser extent, consolidation. This occurrence is typical of interleukin-2,

TABLE 17.1 Drugs Associated with Pulmonary Edema

Aspirin and salicylates
BCNU
Cocaine
Chlordiazepoxide
Codeine
Cyclophosphamide
Cytosine arabinoside
Heroin
Hydrochlorothiazide
Interleukin-2
Lidocaine
Methadone
Methotrexate
Nitrofurantoin
Nonsteroidal anti-inflammatory drugs
OKT3
Propoxyphene
Tocolytics (ritodrine and terbutaline)
Trimethoprim-sulfamethoxazole
Tricyclic antidepressants

but many other drugs are capable of causing increased permeability pulmonary edema. These include aspirin, nitrofurantoin, heroin, and cytotoxic agents such as methotrexate, cyclophosphamide, and BCNU. Unlike with hydrostatic edema, pleural effusion is typically absent. Prompt resolution may occur with appropriate treatment.

Diffuse Alveolar Damage

DAD with ARDS can be caused by a variety of drugs, most typically cytotoxic agents (e.g., bleomycin, busulfan, and cyclophosphamide), nitrofurantoin, and amiodarone (Table 17-2). As with pulmonary edema, onset is usually sudden and occurs within a few days of the onset of chemotherapy.

DAD reflects a more serious lung and capillary endothelial injury than occurs with increased permeability pulmonary edema. The acute or exudative stage of DAD occurs in the first week after injury and is characterized by necrosis of alveolar pneumocytes, edema, hemorrhage, and hyaline membrane formation. Radiographs and CT typically show extensive bilateral parenchymal consolidation, usually most marked in the dependent lung regions; interlobular septal thickening and Kerley's lines are typically absent (Fig. 17-1). Other than a temporal relationship to chemotherapy, there are no clinical or CT findings that allow this appearance to be distinguished from other causes of ARDS. The reparative stage of DAD, characterized by cellular hyperplasia and fibrosis, occurs after 1 to 2 weeks. Depending on the severity of the lung injury, abnormalities may regress, stabilize, or progress to fibrosis and honeycombing.

TABLE 17.2 Drugs Associated with Diffuse Alveolar Damage
Amiodarone
BCNU
Bleomycin
Busulfan
Chlorambucil
Cyclophosphamide
Cytosine arabinoside
Gold
Methotrexate
Mitomycin
Melphalan
Nitrofurantoin
Oxygen
Penicillamine
Tricyclic antidepressants
Vinblastine and vinca alkaloids

Pulmonary Hemorrhage

Drug-related diffuse pulmonary hemorrhage is uncommon. Typical causes include anticoagulants, cyclophosphamide, and penicillamine. Hemoptysis may or may not be present (Table 17-3). Radiographic and HRCT findings are typical of pulmonary hemorrhage, with bilateral patchy ground-glass opacity or consolidation (see Chapter 19). Pleural effusion is typically absent.

A

B

FIG. 17.1. Diffuse alveolar damage resulting from treatment with doxorubicin (Adriamycin). **A:** Chest radiograph coned to the right lung shows basilar consolidation. **B:** HRCT shows ground-glass opacity and consolidation with a basal and dependent predominance.

TABLE 17.3 Drugs Associated with Pulmonary Hemorrhage

Anticoagulants
Amphotericin B
Crack cocaine
Cyclophosphamide
Cytosine arabinoside
Penicillamine
Quinidine

TABLE 17.4 Drugs Associated with Organizing Pneumonia/Bronchiolitis Obliterans Organizing Pneumonia

Amiodarone
Bleomycin
Busulfan
Cyclophosphamide
Gold
Interferon
Methotrexate
Nitrofurantoin
Penicillamine
Sulfasalazine

Organizing Pneumonia/Bronchiolitis Obliterans Organizing Pneumonia

Organizing pneumonia/bronchiolitis obliterans organizing pneumonia (OP/BOOP) has been described with methotrexate, gold, penicillamine, nitrofurantoin, amiodarone, bleomycin, and busulfan (Table 17-4). Symptoms include progressive cough, dyspnea, and fever. Like other causes of OP/BOOP (see Chapter 13), this pattern is characterized by consolidation or ground-glass opacity that may have a patchy or nodular distribution and may predominate in a peribronchial or subpleural location (Figs. 17-2 and 17-3). Lung nodules with or without the "atoll sign" or "reversed halo sign" may be present (Figs. 17-2A and 17-3). OP/BOOP tends to predominate in the lower lobes (see Fig. 17-3).

Hypersensitivity Reactions and Eosinophilic Pneumonia

Hypersensitivity reactions can be attributed to a large number of drugs but are most commonly due to methotrexate, nitrofurantoin, bleomycin, procarbazine, BCNU, cyclophosphamide, nonsteroidal anti-inflammatory drugs, and sulfonamides; their presence is unrelated to the cumulative drug dose (Table 17-5).

Hypersensitivity reactions may have features of simple eosinophilia (Loeffler's syndrome), chronic eosinophilic pneumonia, or acute eosinophilic pneumonia. Cough and dyspnea, with or without fever, can be acute in onset or progress over a period of several months following institution of treatment. A peripheral eosinophilia is present in up to 40%. These reactions are characterized on chest radiographs and HRCT by patchy areas of consolidation or ground-glass opacity, which may be chronic or relatively acute, transient, and fleeting. A peripheral and subpleural distribution may be seen.

Chronic Interstitial Pneumonitis and Fibrosis

Both usual interstitial pneumonia (UIP) and nonspecific interstitial pneumonia (NSIP) have been associated with drug injury; in some cases the pattern may overlap that of OP/BOOP or DAD. The clinical and radiographic presentations are often identical to those of idiopathic pulmonary fibrosis. A long list of drugs has been implicated in the development of chronic pneumonitis, but this pattern is

A

B

FIG. 17.2. Organizing pneumonia/bronchiolitis obliterans organizing pneumonia (OP/BOOP) occurring in association with chemotherapy for breast carcinoma. **A.** CT through the lung apex shows ground-glass opacity in the left upper lobe and a ring of ground-glass opacity in the right upper lobe (*arrows*), representing the atoll sign of OP/BOOP. **B:** CT shows patchy subpleural areas of consolidation and ground-glass opacity typical of OP/BOOP.

A

B

C

FIG. 17.3. Nodular organizing pneumonia/bronchiolitis obliterans organizing pneumonia related to chemotherapy for Ewing's sarcoma. **A:** CT through the right lower lobe shows scattered nodules. Some have a dense rim and a ground-glass opacity center, the so-called atoll sign (*arrows*). **B:** HRCT at the same level. **C:** HRCT at a different level shows bilateral nodules of soft-tissue attenuation and ground-glass opacity visible in both lower lobes. Some nodules show the atoll sign.

TABLE 17.5 Drugs Associated with Eosinophilic Pneumonia and Hypersensitivity Reactions

BCNU
Bleomycin
Cyclophosphamide
Diphenylhydantoin
Erythromycin
Ethambutol
Fluoxetine
Gold
Imipramine
Isoniazid
Methotrexate
Nitrofurantoin
Nonsteroidal anti-inflammatory drugs
Paraaminosalicylic acid
Penicillamine
Penicillin
Procarbazine
Sulfasalazine
Tetracycline

most commonly the result of cytotoxic chemotherapeutic agents such as bleomycin, busulfan, methotrexate, doxorubicin, and carmustine (BCNU; Table 17-6). Nitrofurantoin, amiodarone, gold, and penicillamine are noncytotoxic drugs that can also result in this type of reaction.

Plain radiographs in patients with chronic pneumonitis and fibrosis typically show a mixture of reticulation and consolidation; abnormalities are usually bilateral and symmetric, with a predominant lower lung zone involvement.

The most common pattern seen on HRCT in patients with chronic pneumonitis and fibrosis includes irregular reticular opacities (Fig. 17-4), honeycombing (Fig. 17-5), architectural distortion, and traction bronchiectasis, with or without associated consolidation; ground-glass opacity may be seen in early cases (see Figs. 17-4 to 17-8). As on chest radiographs, HRCT abnormalities are usually bilateral and symmetric, with a predominant lower lung zone involvement. A peripheral and subpleural distribution of abnormalities is common, particularly in patients with bleomycin toxicity. Patchy fibrosis may be seen in patients receiving nitrofurantoin. The extent of abnormalities depends on

TABLE 17.6 Drugs Associated with Chronic Pneumonitis and Fibrosis

Adriamycin
Amiodarone
BCNU
Bleomycin
Busulfan
Chlorambucil
Cyclophosphamide
Gold
Methotrexate
Mitomycin
Nitrofurantoin
Penicillamine
Sulfasalazine
Tocainide

FIG. 17.4. Interstitial pneumonia with fibrosis following chemotherapy. Prone HRCT shows subpleural ground-glass opacity and fine reticular opacities. This appearance is consistent with a nonspecific interstitial pneumonia pattern or early usual interstitial pneumonia pattern.

the severity of lung damage. Mild damage is often limited to the posterior subpleural lung regions of the lower lung zones. In patients with more severe abnormalities, there is greater involvement of the remaining lung parenchyma.

Systemic Lupus Erythematosus

SLE related to drug treatment is indistinguishable clinically and radiographically from idiopathic SLE (Table 17-7). Pleural effusions and pericardial effusions are the most common manifestations.

Pulmonary Vasculitis and Pulmonary Hypertension

The use of various drugs may result in acute or chronic abnormalities of small vessels within the lung, with histologic abnormalities including pulmonary vasculitis, plexogenic arteriopathy, and pulmonary venoocclusive disease (Table 17-8).

The radiographic appearances of these vary with the specific abnormalities present. Pulmonary vasculitis may result in an appearance similar to that of pulmonary edema or pulmonary hemorrhage, with patchy or diffuse consolidation or ground-glass opacity. Plexogenic arteriopathy shows findings of pulmonary hypertension, with enlargement of central pulmonary arteries. Pulmonary venoocclusive disease mimics hydrostatic edema, but with normal heart size.

A   B

FIG. 17.5. Interstitial pneumonia with fibrosis following chemotherapy with methotrexate. **A:** HRCT through the upper lobes shows irregular reticular opacities and traction bronchiectasis. **B:** HRCT through the lung bases shows honeycombing with a subpleural predominance. This appearance is that of usual interstitial pneumonia and is indistinguishable from that of idiopathic pulmonary fibrosis.

FIG. 17.6. Amiodarone treatment with organizing pneumonia/bronchiolitis obliterans organizing pneumonia (OP/BOOP). **A:** Chest radiograph shows cardiomegaly, a pacemaker, and patchy lung consolidation. **B:** HRCT shows patchy areas of consolidation and ground-glass opacity in the lung periphery. This appearance is typical of OP/BOOP. The presence of a small left pleural effusion is not typical of OP/BOOP but may reflect heart failure. **C:** HRCT with a soft-tissue window shows the areas of lung consolidation to be denser than soft tissue (*arrows*). This is common in patients with amiodarone toxicity. However, dense lung may be seen in any patient on long-term amiodarone treatment who has lung consolidation; dense lung does not imply toxicity. **D:** CT through the upper abdomen shows the liver to be dense.

FIG. 17.7. Amiodarone treatment with lung fibrosis. **A:** Chest radiograph shows a pacemaker and streaky areas of fibrosis in the peripheral lungs. **B:** HRCT shows irregular reticular opacities, traction bronchiectasis, and nodular areas of consolidation in the lung periphery. This appearance resembles a combination of organizing pneumonia/bronchiolitis obliterans organizing pneumonia and lung fibrosis. The left pleural effusion is likely related to heart failure.

FIG. 17.8. Amiodarone treatment with lung fibrosis. Prone HRCT shows peripheral reticular opacities representing nonspecific interstitial pneumonia or usual interstitial pneumonia. The presence of subpleural sparing suggests NSIP.

Bronchiolitis Obliterans

The least common lung reaction to drugs is bronchiolitis obliterans, a finding described primarily in association with penicillamine therapy for rheumatoid arthritis (Table 17-9). However, the role of penicillamine is controversial, as bronchiolitis obliterans can be seen in patients with rheumatoid arthritis who have not been treated with this drug. Bronchiolitis obliterans has also been seen in patients treated with sulfasalazine. Chest radiographs may show large lung volumes. The abnormalities seen on HRCT consist of bronchial wall thickening and a pattern of mosaic perfusion, similar to that seen with other causes of bronchiolitis obliterans (see Figs. 10-36 and 10-38 in Chapter 10 and Figs. 23-24 and 23-25 in Chapter 23); air trapping on expiratory scans is typically present.

TABLE 17.7 Drugs Associated with Systemic Lupus Erythematosus

Anticonvulsants
Beta blockers
Digitalis
Gold
Hydralazine
Isoniazid
Levodopa
Nitrofurantoin
Nonsteroidal anti-inflammatory drugs
Penicillamine
Penicillin
Phenothiazines
Procainamide
Quinidine
Streptomycin
Sulfonamides
Thiouracil

TABLE 17.8 Drugs Associated with Pulmonary Vasculitis and Pulmonary Hypertension

Amphetamines (pulmonary hypertension)
Anorectic drugs such as fenfluramine and phenformin (pulmonary hypertension)
Anticonvulsants
Cocaine (pulmonary hypertension)
Hydralazine
Busulfan
Penicillin
Phenothiazines
Quinidine
Sulfonamides
Thiouracil

REACTIONS TO SPECIFIC DRUGS

Drug reactions may occur during treatment with a wide variety of agents. The highest incidence of adverse effects occurs with cytotoxic agents: up to 10% of patients receiving cytotoxic chemotherapeutic agents develop an adverse reaction. Some of the more common drugs to result in significant pulmonary disease are described below. Commonly used illicit drugs also are responsible for drug reactions, but lung abnormalities resulting from illicit drug use may also reflect injection of particulate matter (i.e., talc) or inhalation of toxic substances.

Amiodarone

Amiodarone is an iodinated drug used in the treatment of refractory cardiac tachyarrhythmias. It accumulates in the liver and lung, where it becomes entrapped in macrophage lysosomes. It results in pulmonary toxicity in 5% of patients.

Pathologic reactions to amiodarone include DAD, OP/BOOP (see Fig. 17-6), and chronic pneumonitis with fibrosis (see Figs. 17-7 and 17-8). The radiographic patterns of pulmonary reaction to amiodarone vary and include focal or diffuse areas of consolidation, reticular opacities, and less commonly ill-defined nodules or masses (see Fig. 17-6).

Regions of consolidated lung in patients with amiodarone-related lung toxicity appear denser than soft tissue on unenhanced CT because of their high iodine content (see Fig. 17-6C). However, dense lung may also be seen

TABLE 17.9 Drugs Associated with Bronchiolitis Obliterans

Gold
Penicillamine
Sulfasalazines

in any patient on long-term amiodarone treatment who develops lung consolidation or collapse. Patients with amiodarone pulmonary toxicity almost always show increased liver attenuation on CT (see Fig. 17-6D), although this finding is also present in patients treated with amiodarone who do not have drug toxicity.

Aspirin and Salicylates

As many as 5% of asthmatics are sensitive to aspirin; use causes bronchospasm. This may be related to inhibition of prostaglandin synthesis.

Salicylate-induced increased permeability pulmonary edema can occur when the blood salicylate level exceeds 40 mg/dL, particularly in the elderly or in smokers. This may represent a direct toxic effect on capillary permeability. Treatment may require mechanical ventilation; resolution within a week is typical.

Bleomycin

Bleomycin is a cytotoxic drug used in the treatment of lymphomas and some carcinomas. Bleomycin pulmonary toxicity is the most common pulmonary disease related to chemotherapy, with an incidence of about 4%. Toxicity is related to cumulative doses exceeding 400 mg. Associated risk factors for development of lung disease include recent radiation, oxygen therapy, renal disease, and advanced age.

A wide variety of reactions to bleomycin have been reported, including pulmonary edema (see Fig. 11-11 in Chapter 11), DAD with respiratory failure, chronic pneumonitis with fibrosis, OP/BOOP, and hypersensitivity reactions. Radiographic and CT appearances vary accordingly.

Pneumonitis with pulmonary fibrosis typically presents 1 to 2 months after the onset of treatment with progressive dyspnea and cough. Chest radiographs show reticulation, ground-glass opacity, and sometimes consolidation with a predominant subpleural and lower lobe predominance. With severe or progressive disease, more diffuse involvement of the lower, middle, and upper lungs is typically visible. HRCT is more sensitive than radiographs in detecting early disease. Some abnormalities resolve following cessation of treatment in patients with early disease.

A unique manifestation of bleomycin-related lung toxicity is the presence of multiple pulmonary nodules mimicking the appearance of metastases and having histologic characteristics of OP/BOOP.

Busulfan

Busulfan is an alkylating agent used in treating chronic myeloproliferative diseases, and clinically recognized lung toxicity occurs in about 5% of cases. It usually results in findings of chronic pneumonitis and fibrosis, OP/BOOP, or DAD. Radiographic and HRCT findings include patchy or diffuse consolidation or reticulation.

Cocaine and Crack

Use of sympathomimetic agents such as cocaine (or its derivative crack), either by injection or inhalation, may cause hydrostatic pulmonary edema by inducing ischemia-related transient myocardial dysfunction, severe peripheral vasoconstriction with transient left ventricular failure, cardiac arrhythmia, or frank myocardial infarction. Cocaine or crack may also cause acute lung injury with increased permeability pulmonary edema (see Fig. 11-13 in Chapter 11), pulmonary hemorrhage, or pulmonary hypertension. HRCT commonly reveals multifocal ground-glass opacities, occasionally centrilobular in distribution, associated with interlobular septal thickening. Because pulmonary edema, pulmonary hemorrhage, and acute lung injury may be radiographically indistinguishable and may occur in combination, the development of respiratory failure after cocaine or crack use, associated with evidence of bilateral air-space opacities, clearing rapidly following cessation of drug use has been termed "crack lung."

Cyclophosphamide (Cytoxan)

Cyclophosphamide is an alkylating agent used in the treatment of a variety of malignancies and autoimmune diseases and is commonly used in combination with other therapeutic agents; pulmonary toxicity occurs in less than 1% of cases. Histologic findings associated with lung injury are similar to those seen in patients with bleomycin toxicity and include chronic pneumonitis and fibrosis, OP/BOOP, DAD, pulmonary edema, and hypersensitivity reactions. Radiographic appearances vary accordingly.

Heroin and Narcotics

Use of heroin or other narcotics may result in increased permeability pulmonary edema. Possible mechanisms include a toxic effect on the alveolar capillary membrane, effects on the central nervous system with neurogenic edema, hypoxemia, and hypersensitivity. Symptoms of dyspnea typically occur from minutes to a few hours after injection. Radiographs show typical findings of increased permeability edema, with parahilar ground-glass opacity or consolidation, but the appearance may be complicated by associated aspiration. Hemorrhage may also be present. Resolution often occurs within 1 to 2 days.

Interleukin-2

Interleukin-2 is a T-cell growth factor used as an immune system stimulator for treating cancers, particularly melanoma and renal cell carcinoma. It may cause increased permeability pulmonary edema by a direct toxic effect on the capillary endothelium. Symptoms typically begin within 2 to 8 days of the onset of treatment. Radiographs show typical findings of interstitial or air-space edema. Pleural effusion, an unusual finding with increased permeability edema, is common. Clearing occurs within days of drug cessation.

Methotrexate

Methotrexate is a folate antagonist used in the treatment of malignancies and inflammatory diseases. Pulmonary toxicity occurs in 5% to 10% of cases and is unrelated to the duration of treatment or the cumulative dose.

In contrast to many other cytotoxic agents, methotrexate often results in reversible abnormalities. Symptoms usually develop within weeks of the onset of treatment and include fever, cough, and dyspnea. In most cases, the histologic appearance resembles hypersensitivity pneumonitis or less often OP/BOOP or DAD; peripheral eosinophilia is present in half of the cases. Chest radiographs show ill-defined reticular opacities, ground-glass opacity, or consolidation. A basal predominance is typical. HRCT usually shows ground-glass opacity as the predominant abnormality. Radiographic abnormalities usually regress following discontinuation of the drug. Some residual fibrosis may be seen. However, fibrosis and honeycombing may result (see Fig. 17-5).

Nitrofurantoin

Nitrofurantoin is an antibiotic used for treatment of urinary tract infections. It may result in either acute or chronic reactions; acute reactions are much more common, accounting for 90% of cases of toxicity. SLE related to nitrofurantoin has also been reported.

Acute nitrofurantoin toxicity is a hypersensitivity reaction and usually begins from 1 day to 2 weeks after initiation of therapy. Symptoms include fever, cough, and dyspnea; peripheral eosinophilia is present in most patients. Chest radiographs show an interstitial abnormality with Kerley's lines (i.e., pulmonary edema) or consolidation, which may be symmetric or asymmetric. Pleural effusion, usually small and unilateral, is present in one third of cases. Discontinuation of the drug results in clearing, usually within days.

Chronic nitrofurantoin reaction occurs from 2 months to years after the beginning of continuous treatment. It is unrelated to acute toxicity. Insidious cough and dyspnea are most common; fever is absent and eosinophilia is uncommon. Radiographs and HRCT show a diffuse reticular abnormality with a basal predominance due to chronic pneumonitis and fibrosis. The appearance closely resembles idiopathic pulmonary fibrosis (Fig 17-9). Discontinuing the drug should result in some improvement over a period of months. Steroid treatment may also be effective, but mortality is 10%.

Nonsteroidal Anti-inflammatory Drugs

These drugs have been associated with a hypersensitivity reaction with acute onset of dyspnea, cough, low-grade fever, and eosinophilia. They may also be associated with SLE.

A

B

C

FIG. 17.9. Chronic nitrofurantoin treatment with pulmonary fibrosis. **A:** Chest radiograph shows decreased lung volumes and reticular opacities at the lung bases. **B:** HRCT through the mid lungs shows peripheral reticulation. **C:** Honeycombing is visible at the lung bases. This is a UIP pattern.

OKT3

OKT3 is a monoclonal antibody directed against T cells that is used to treat rejection of solid organ transplants. Pulmonary edema is a common complication in patients who are fluid overloaded prior to the institution of treatment. Consequently, chest radiographs are routinely obtained before treatment begins to exclude preexisting pulmonary edema or heart failure.

Tocolytic Drugs

Tocolytic drugs used to treat premature labor (e.g., ritodrine and terbutaline) result in increased permeability pulmonary edema in about 1% of cases. Onset is typically 2 to 3 days after treatment. Increased risk is associated with overhydration, twin gestation, and use of steroids. Rapid recovery is typical.

Tricyclic Antidepressants

Overdose of tricyclic antidepressants may be associated with increased permeability pulmonary edema or DAD with development of ARDS as a direct toxic effect.

RADIATION PNEUMONITIS AND FIBROSIS

Following external-beam thoracic radiotherapy, approximately 40% of patients develop radiographic abnormalities and 7% develop symptomatic radiation pneumonitis.

The development and appearance of radiation lung injury depend on a number of factors, including (1) the volume of lung irradiated, (2) the shape of the radiation fields, (3) the radiation dose, (4) the number of fractions of radiation given, (5) the time period over which the radiation is delivered, (6) prior irradiation, (7) whether chemotherapy is also employed, (8) corticosteroid therapy withdrawal, (9) preex-

isting lung disease, (10) the type of radiation used, and (11) individual susceptibility.

Generally speaking, radiation is best tolerated by the patient if given in smaller doses, over a long period of time, and to a single lung or a small lung region. For unilateral radiation with fractionated doses, radiographic findings of radiation pneumonitis are seldom detected with doses below 3,000 cGy, are variably present with doses between 3,000 and 4,000 cGy, and are nearly always visible at doses of 4,000 cGy. Its likelihood is increased by a second course of radiation, the withdrawal of corticosteroid treatment, and the use of concomitant chemotherapy. Radiographic findings of radiation pneumonitis are usually not associated with symptoms, although low-grade fever, cough, and dyspnea are present in some patients.

Radiation Pneumonitis

Pulmonary abnormalities related to radiation injury have been divided into early and late manifestations. The early stage of radiation lung injury, referred to as radiation pneumonitis, occurs within 1 to 3 months after radiation therapy is completed and is most severe 3 to 4 months following treatment. Radiation pneumonitis is associated with histologic findings of DAD, intra-alveolar proteinaceous exudates, and hyaline membranes. Depending on the severity of lung injury, these abnormalities may resolve completely, but more often they undergo progressive organization, leading eventually to fibrosis.

Radiation Fibrosis

The late stage of radiation-induced lung injury, termed radiation fibrosis, develops gradually in patients with radiation pneumonitis when complete resolution does not occur. Radiation fibrosis evolves within the previously irradiated field 6 to 12 months following radiation therapy and usually becomes

A

B

FIG. 17.10. Acute radiation pneumonitis. **A:** Patchy areas of ground-glass opacity are visible in a paramediastinal distribution following mediastinal radiation. **B:** The areas of abnormality are nonanatomic but have straight margins corresponding to the radiation ports (*arrows*). Little volume loss is present at this stage.

stable within 2 years of treatment. Histologically, dense fibrosis with obliteration of lung architecture and traction bronchiectasis are present. Patients can present with radiation fibrosis without a previous history of acute pneumonitis.

Radiographic and CT Findings

The hallmark of radiation pneumonitis on radiographs or CT is homogeneous or patchy ground-glass opacity or consolidation corresponding closely to the location of the radiation ports (Fig. 17-10). Abnormalities are typically nonanatomic and do not tend to respect normal lung boundaries such as lobar fissures or lung segments. Volume loss can be seen; this is due to obstruction of bronchioles by inflammatory exudate, loss of surfactant, or both. Large airways are patent, and air bronchograms are commonly visible. Pleural thickening is sometimes seen adjacent to irradiated areas.

Although findings of radiation pneumonitis are characteristically confined to areas of irradiated lung, relatively mild abnormalities (ground-glass opacity or consolidation) are detected outside the radiation portal in as many as 20% of cases, perhaps related to a hypersensitivity reaction or OP/BOOP (Table 17-10).

Persistence or progression of radiographic or CT abnormalities more than 9 months after treatment likely indicates fibrosis (Fig. 17-11). The development of radiation fibrosis can be recognized by the appearance of streaky opacities, progressive volume loss, progressive dense consolidation (see Figs. 17-11 and 17-12), traction bronchiectasis (see Figs. 17-11B and 17-12), or pleural thickening within the irradiated lung. Fibrosis and volume loss typically result in

TABLE 17.10 Radiation Pneumonitis and Fibrosis
Occurrence is multifactorial
Seldom occurs below 3,000 cGy
Nearly always visible above 4,000 cGy
Radiation pneumonitis
1–3 months after radiation is completed
Most severe 3–4 months after radiation
Diffuse alveolar damage
Radiographs and HRCT
Homogeneous or patchy ground-glass opacity or consolidation
Edges correspond to radiation ports
Abnormalities outside of ports in 20%
Radiation fibrosis
6–12 months after radiation is completed
Unchanging after 2 years
Fibrosis and traction bronchiectasis
Radiographs and HRCT
Persisting abnormalities after 9 months
Dense consolidation
Edges correspond to radiation ports
Traction bronchiectasis typical
Honeycombing
Ipsilateral volume loss

a sharper demarcation between normal and irradiated lung regions than is seen in patients with radiation pneumonitis (see Figs. 17-11 and 17-12). This gives the abnormal lung regions a characteristically straight and sharply defined edge. Occasionally, the appearance of lung fibrosis mimics honeycombing (Fig. 17-13), although the distribution is related to the radiation ports and is quite different from that of

A   **B**

FIG. 17.11. Radiation fibrosis 12 months following axillary radiotherapy. **A, B:** CTs at two levels show consolidation in the peripheral lung. The abnormal areas have a straight edge (*white arrows*) due to the port used. Dense consolidation is typical of fibrosis. Traction bronchiectasis (*black arrow,* **B**) indicates that fibrosis is present.

FIG. 17.12. End-stage radiation fibrosis. HRCT shows dense paramediastinal fibrosis with a sharp edge (*white arrows*). Traction bronchiectasis (*black arrows*) is extensive. The ipsilateral hemithorax is reduced in volume compared with the opposite side.

FIG. 17.13. Paramediastinal fibrosis following radiation for Hodgkin's disease. HRCT shows paramediastinal reticulation, traction bronchiectasis, and honeycombing (*arrows*).

idiopathic pulmonary fibrosis. The adjacent lung may appear hyperinflated and may show bullae. The ipsilateral hemithorax may be reduced in volume (see Fig. 17-12).

Although pleural thickening is a common manifestation of radiation, pleural effusions are uncommon. Effusion related to radiation typically develops within 6 months of treatment, in conjunction with radiation pneumonitis, and resolves spontaneously. Rapid accumulation of fluid suggests malignancy.

Mediastinal lymph node calcification, particularly after radiation of lymphomas, the development of thymic cysts, pericarditis, and cardiomyopathy may also be seen.

SELECTED READING

Aquino SL, Webb WR, Golden J. Bronchiolitis obliterans associated with rheumatoid arthritis: findings on HRCT and dynamic expiratory CT. J Comput Assist Tomogr 1994; 18:555–558.

Aronchick JM, Gefter WB. Drug-induced pulmonary disorders. Semin Roentgenol 1995; 30:18–34.

Bellamy EA, Husband JE, Blaquiere RM, Law MR. Bleomycin-related lung damage: CT evidence. Radiology 1985; 156:155–158.

Bush DA, Dunbar RD, Bonnet R, et al. Pulmonary injury from proton and conventional radiotherapy as revealed by CT. AJR Am J Roentgenol 1999; 172:735–739.

Cooper JA, Jr. Drug-induced lung disease. Adv Intern Med 1997; 42:231–268.

Cooper JAD, White DA, Matthay RA. Drug-induced pulmonary disease, part 1: cytotoxic drugs. Am Rev Respir Dis 1986; 133:321–340.

Cooper JAD, White DA, Matthay RA. Drug induced pulmonary disease, part 2: noncytotoxic drugs. Am Rev Respir Dis 1986; 133:488–503.

Davis SD, Yankelevitz DF, Henschke CI. Radiation effects on the lung: clinical features, pathology, and imaging findings. AJR Am J Roentgenol 1992; 159:1157–1164.

Gotway MB, Marder SR, Hanks DK, et al. Thoracic complications of illicit drug use: an organ system approach. Radiographics 2002; 22:119–135.

Kuhlman JE. The role of chest computed tomography in the diagnosis of drug-related reactions. J Thorac Imaging 1991; 6:52–61.

Kuhlman JE, Teigen C, Ren H, et al. Amiodarone pulmonary toxicity: CT findings in symptomatic patients. Radiology 1990; 177:121–125.

Libshitz HI. Radiation changes in the lung. Semin Roentgenol 1993; 28:303–320.

Logan PM. Thoracic manifestations of external beam radiotherapy. AJR Am J Roentgenol 1998; 171:569–577.

Movsas B, Raffin TA, Epstein AH, Link CJ, Jr. Pulmonary radiation injury. Chest 1997; 111:1061–1076.

Padley SPG, Adler B, Hansell DM, Müller NL. High-resolution computed tomography of drug-induced lung disease. Clin Radiol 1992; 46:232–236.

Pietra GG. Pathologic mechanisms of drug-induced lung disorders. J Thorac Imaging 1991; 6:1–7.

Rosenow EC, Myers JL, Swensen SJ, Pisani RJ. Drug-induced pulmonary disease: an update. Chest 1992; 102:239–250.

Rossi SE, Erasmus JJ, McAdams HP, et al. Pulmonary drug toxicity: radiologic and pathologic manifestations. Radiographics 2000; 20:1245–1259.

Saxon RR, Klein JS, Bar MH, et al. Pathogenesis of pulmonary edema during interleukin-2 therapy: correlation of chest radiographic and clinical findings in 54 patients. AJR Am J Roentgenol 1991; 156:281–285.

Pneumoconioses

W. RICHARD WEBB

T he term *pneumoconiosis* refers to the presence of lung disease related to dust inhalation. Inhaled dusts may be toxic, resulting in fibrosis and disability (e.g., asbestosis and silicosis), or may be relatively inert, associated with radiographic abnormalities but causing little dysfunction (e.g., stannosis and baritosis). Inhalation of organic dusts results in hypersensitivity pneumonitis (see Chapter 16).

RADIOGRAPHIC CLASSIFICATION OF PNEUMOCONIOSES

The International Labour Office (ILO) has classified the plain radiographic abnormalities occurring in patients with dust exposure for the purpose of comparative epidemiological studies. This system provides a semiquantitative method for assessing the type and extent of abnormalities present. Classifications using this system are nonspecific, however, and it has little role in diagnosis. Furthermore, this system is complicated and difficult to remember unless used on a regular basis. However, limited familiarity with ILO system is appropriate (Table 18-1).

A combination of letters and numbers is used to indicate the type and extent (profusion) of opacities present.

Opacity Type

The type of opacity, either small or large, is indicated by a letter, either small or large.

Small rounded opacities are well circumscribed and nodular. They are indicated as p, q, or r, depending on their diameter. Nodules up to 1.5 mm in diameter are "p," opacities 1.5 to 3 mm are "q," and those between 3 and 10 mm are "r."

Small irregular opacities are linear or reticular in appearance and are indicated as s, t, or u according to their thickness. Opacities up to 1.5 mm in thickness are "s," those 1.5 to 3 mm are "t," and those 3 to 10 mm are "u."

Large opacities are larger than 10 mm. These are classified as "A" if a single lesion or cluster of several opacities is more than 10 mm, but 5 cm or less in diameter. "B" indicates one or more opacities larger or more numerous than those defined in A, with a combined area not exceeding that of the right upper lung zone. "C" is used for opacities larger than B.

Profusion

The number of small rounded or irregular opacities is indicated by the term *profusion*. Profusion is graded using four numbers with the following definitions, most easily determined by comparison to a standard reference set of radiographs:

0: Small opacities absent or less profuse than indicated by 1
1: Small opacities definitely present but few in number (normal lung markings are still visible)
2: Numerous small opacities (normal lung markings partially obscured)
3: Very numerous small opacities (normal lung markings usually obscured)

These four profusion grades may be further subdivided. If in interpreting a radiograph, more than one of these four grades

TABLE 18.1 International Labour Office Classification of Pneumoconioses

Opacity type	
Small rounded opacities (diameter)	
p	≤1.5 mm
q	>1.5–3 mm
r	>3–10 mm
Small irregular opacities (thickness)	
s	≤1.5 mm
t	>1.5–3 mm
u	>3–10 mm
Large opacities (diameter)	
A	One or a cluster of several opacities >10 mm to 5 cm
B	Larger or more numerous than A, not larger than the right upper lobe
C	Larger than B
Profusion (of small opacities)	
0	Absent or less profuse than 1
1	Definitely present but few in number (normal lung markings are still visible)
2	Numerous small opacities (normal lung markings partially obscured)
3	Very numerous small opacities (normal lung markings usually obscured)

was seriously considered but was determined not to be the profusion present, it is indicated following the final classification and separated from it by a slash. For example, if a patient is determined to have a profusion of 1, but 2 was also considered, this is indicated as 1/2. If no alternative was considered, the number is listed twice (e.g., 1/1). This leads to the following possibilities for profusion:

0/0	1/0	2/1	3/2
0/1	1/1	2/2	3/3
	1/2	2/3	

Also, 0/− may be used to indicate an obvious lack of small opacities, while 3/+ indicates a profusion much higher than 3/3.

Extent

In patients with large opacities, the lung is divided equally into three zones (upper, middle, and lower) using horizontal lines.

Accuracy of the ILO System

The National Institute of Occupational Safety and Health (NIOSH) has established a course and examination for the purpose of certifying physicians in the use of the ILO classification system. Completion of the course establishes the physician as an "A reader." Passing an examination confers "B reader" status. B readers must be recertified every 4 years. Trained readers show less interobserver variability in interpreting pneumoconiosis radiographs than untrained physicians.

ILO categories are nonspecific and an abnormal classification need not indicate lung disease or the presence of pneumoconiosis. Approximately 5% of subjects without occupational exposure have radiographs interpreted as having a 1/0 profusion of small opacities, a classification usually considered to be abnormal and consistent with pneumoconiosis.

ASBESTOSIS AND ASBESTOS-RELATED DISEASE

Asbestos is a silicate mineral composed of various amounts of magnesium, iron, calcium, and sodium. Asbestos is found in nature in the form of thin fibers and is classified as amphibole or serpentine, depending on its fiber type.

The toxicity of asbestos appears to be related to the fiber form of the mineral and its durability after inhalation. *Amphibole* asbestos has fibers that are thin and straight, allowing them to penetrate deeply into the lung, and is most likely to result in disease. Amphiboles important in industry and often responsible for asbestos-related disease include crocidolite, amosite, and tremolite. *Serpentine* asbestos fibers are curved. Chrysotile is the only commonly used serpentine asbestos; it is less likely to result in disease than the amphiboles.

Asbestos has a variety of uses, particularly in the construction industry. Asbestos exposure may occur in the mining of asbestos, in the production of asbestos products and their installation during construction, and during repair or removal of asbestos-containing materials.

Asbestos-related abnormalities include asbestosis, asbestos-related rounded atelectasis, and asbestos-related pleural disease. A significantly increased incidence of mesothelioma, lung cancer, and extrathoracic neoplasms (e.g., peritoneal mesothelioma and gastrointestinal, renal, oropharyngeal, and laryngeal carcinomas) is also associated with asbestos exposure. Most patients with asbestos-related abnormalities have no symptoms.

Asbestosis

The lung disease associated with asbestos fiber inhalation is known as asbestosis (Table 18-2). Asbestosis is defined as interstitial pulmonary fibrosis associated with the presence of intrapulmonary *asbestos bodies* or asbestos fibers. Asbestos bodies are visible on microscopy and consist of translucent asbestos fibers coated with protein and iron. Amphiboles are usually responsible for asbestos bodies. Uncoated asbestos fibers are much more numerous in the lung than asbestos bodies.

Asbestosis results from inflammation associated with inhaled asbestos fibers. The development of asbestosis depends on the duration and intensity of exposure, although host-related factors such as tobacco smoking are

TABLE 18.2 Lung Disease in Asbestos Exposure

Asbestosis
Interstitial lung fibrosis due to asbestos exposure
Asbestos bodies within the lung
Related to length and intensity of exposure, other factors
Correlation with severity of pleural disease
20–30 years after start of exposure
Radiographs
  ILO s, t, or u
  Shaggy heart sign
  Honeycombing
HRCT
  Findings of usual interstitial pneumonia
  Appearance mimics idiopathic pulmonary fibrosis
  Associated pleural disease visible in most
Rounded atelectasis
Does not necessarily indicate "asbestosis"
Related to visceral or parietal pleural thickening
Seen in 10%
May be preceded by parenchymal bands or crow's foot
Typical CT findings
  Round or oval
  Abutting the pleura
  Comet-tail sign
  Ipsilateral pleural disease
  Volume loss
Atypical findings common

also involved. There is a significant correlation between the presence and severity of pleural disease and the presence and severity of asbestosis.

Symptoms of asbestosis include dyspnea and finger clubbing, usually occurring 20 to 30 years after the start of exposure. Symptoms are progressive even without continued exposure. Pulmonary function tests show restrictive abnormalities. Associated findings of airway obstruction may reflect associated smoking-related disease (i.e., emphysema) or asbestos-related bronchiolar fibrosis. Longstanding exposure may result in significant respiratory dysfunction leading to cor pulmonale and death. Risk of death is related to the severity of fibrosis determined clinically, functionally, or radiographically.

After inhalation, asbestos fibers are first deposited in the respiratory bronchioles and alveolar ducts, but deposition becomes diffuse with longer and more extensive exposure. In patients with asbestosis, the earliest changes of fibrosis are peribronchiolar. As fibrosis progresses, it involves alveolar walls throughout the lobule and interlobular septa. Honeycombing can be seen in advanced cases. Visceral pleural thickening often overlies areas of parenchymal fibrosis. In asbestosis, abnormalities are usually most severe in the lower lungs, in the posterior lungs, and in a subpleural location.

The diagnosis of asbestosis usually is based on indirect evidence, including a combination of chest radiographic abnormalities, restrictive abnormalities on pulmonary function tests, appropriate physical findings, and known exposure to asbestos. These findings are limited in accuracy, however, being both nonspecific and insensitive in early disease.

Many cases of asbestosis have resulted from exposure before, during, or in the years after World War II. The incidence of asbestosis is decreasing, and new cases with obvious findings are uncommon.

Radiographic Findings

Asbestosis usually results in irregular reticular opacities (ILO classification s, t, or u) on chest radiographs. In its earliest stages, asbestosis appears as a fine reticulation in the lung bases, often best seen posteriorly on the lateral view (Fig. 18-1A and B). As it progresses, reticulation becomes coarser and more obvious, partially obscuring the heart borders (known as the "shaggy-heart sign"). In more advanced stages, honeycombing may be visible and abnormalities become more extensive, involving the mid-lungs. Radiographic findings of asbestosis are not usually detected until 10 years after exposure, and the latent period is sometimes as long as 40 years. Also, as many as 10% to 15% of patients with proven asbestosis have normal chest films.

The combination of pulmonary abnormalies with typical pleural abnormalities should suggest the diagnosis (see Fig. 18-1). However, plain film findings of pleural disease are absent in about 20% of patients with radiographic evidence of asbestosis.

High-Resolution CT Findings

Asbestosis can result in a variety of High-resolution CT (HRCT) findings, depending on the severity of the disease. In general, HRCT findings reflect the presence of interstitial fibrosis and are similar to those seen in patients with usual interstitial pneumonia and idiopathic pulmonary fibrosis. Although no findings is specific for asbestosis, the presence of parietal pleural thickening in association with lung fibrosis is highly suggestive (see Fig. 18-1C to E).

Thickening of interlobular septa, fine reticulation (intralobular interstitial thickening), traction bronchiectasis, architectural distortion, subpleural lines, and findings of honeycombing can all be seen, depending on the severity of disease. Honeycombing, common in advanced asbestosis, typically predominates in the peripheral and posterior lung bases (Figs. 18-1 to 18-3).

Patients with asbestosis usually show a number of HRCT findings indicative of lung fibrosis, and the abnormalities are usually bilateral and often somewhat symmetrical (see Figs. 18-1 to 18-3). The presence of focal or unilateral HRCT abnormalities should not be considered sufficient for making this diagnosis.

Parenchymal bands, linear opacities 2 to 5 cm in length, often extending to the pleural surface, are common in patients with asbestosis and asbestos exposure (Fig. 18-4). These often reflect coarse scars or areas of atelectasis adjacent to pleural plaques or areas of visceral pleural thickening. Several parenchymal bands occurring in the same location may give the appearance of a *crow's foot*; this abnormality is often related to overlying visceral or parietal pleural thickening and may precede the development of rounded atelectasis. The presence of parenchymal bands does not necessarily indicate asbestosis.

Rounded Atelectasis and Focal Fibrotic Masses

The term *rounded atelectasis* refers to the presence of focal lung collapse, with or without folding of the lung parenchyma (see Table 18-2). It is typically associated with pleural disease and thus is common in asbestos exposure. Focal masslike lung opacities reflecting the presence of rounded atelectasis or focal subpleural fibrosis are seen in 10% of patients with significant asbestos exposure; they are usually related to adjacent visceral pleural fibrosis and measure 2 cm to more than 5 cm in diameter. It is important to distinguish these masses from lung cancer, which has an increased incidence in asbestos-exposed individuals.

Plain films show a focal mass in association with pleural thickening, often contacting the pleural surface. Rounded atelectasis may be associated with curving of pulmonary vessels or bronchi into the edge of the lesion, the so-called *comet-tail sign* (see Fig. 2-42 in Chapter 2). CT is more accurate in making this diagnosis (see Chapter 2).

Rounded atelectasis is most common in the posterior lower lobes and is sometimes bilateral or symmetrical. It may have acute or obtuse angles where it contacts the pleura.

A

B

C

D

E

FIG. 18.1. Asbestos-related pleural plaques and asbestosis. **A:** Chest radiograph shows irregular, geographic areas of calcification (*arrows*) corresponding to pleural plaques seen en face. An increase in reticular opacities is visible at the lung bases. **B:** Lateral chest radiograph shows slight posterior displacement of the major fissures (*white arrow*) resulting from fibrosis and volume loss in the posterior lung bases. An increase in reticular opacities (*black arrows*) is visible posteriorly. **C:** CT with soft-tissue window setting shows calcified pleural plaques and areas of pleural thickening (*arrows*). **D:** CT with a lung window setting shows irregular reticular opacities in the lung periphery. Mild honeycombing is likely present. **E:** CT at the lung bases shows extensive reticulation consistent with fibrosis. This abnormality in association with pleural plaques makes asbestosis likely.

FIG. 18.2. Asbestosis. HRCT shows pleural plaques (*large white arrow*) at the peripheral pleural surface. Irregular nodular opacities (*small arrows*) at the lung base represent pleural plaques on the surface of the diaphragm, projecting into the lung. Irregular reticular opacities, thickening of interlobular septa, and a subpleural line (*black arrow*) are visible at the lung bases. Subpleural lines may reflect underlying pleural disease.

If the criteria for rounded atelectasis listed in Table 18.2 and described in detail in Chapter 2 are met, a confident diagnosis can usually be made. However, atypical cases are frequently encountered in patients with asbestos exposure, having appearances best described as lenticular, wedge-shaped, or irregular, and often are separated from the thickened pleura by aerated lung (see Figs. 2-45 and 2-46 in Chapter 2). If these lesions can be shown to be unchanged in size over several years, they are likely benign; if not, needle

FIG. 18.3. Asbestosis with honeycombing. In a patient with asbestos exposure and pleural thickening, HRCT shows honeycombing (*arrows*) with a peripheral and basal predominance. Except for the presence of pleural thickening, this appearance is identical to that of IPF.

biopsy may be necessary to distinguish them from cancer. FDG-PET scanning may also be of value; round atelectasis does not show the intense activity typical of cancer.

Asbestos-related Pleural Disease

Pleural disease is the most frequent thoracic manifestation of asbestos exposure (Table 18-3). Manifestations include pleural plaques, asbestos-related pleural effusion, and diffuse pleural thickening. Mesothelioma, a tumor commonly associated with asbestos exposure, is discussed in Chapter 26.

A

B

FIG. 18.4. Diffuse pleural thickening in asbestos exposure with parenchymal bands. **A:** HRCT shows diffuse (concentric) pleural thickening (*arrows*). **B:** Lung window at the same level shows coarse linear opacities (*arrows*) extending to the abnormal pleural surface. These are termed parenchymal bands; when grouped together they resemble a crow's foot. These need not represent asbestosis but usually represent coarse scars or areas of atelectasis. They may precede the development of rounded atelectasis.

TABLE 18.3 Asbestos-Related Pleural Disease

Pleural plaques
10–20 years after the onset of exposure
Nearly always parietal pleural
Overlie ribs
Most often posterolateral and domes of diaphragms
Spare apices and costophrenic angles
Radiographs
    Calcified in 10%–15% of cases
    Irregular and "geographic"
CT
    Mesa shaped
    Often appear as high attenuation
    Calcified in 15%–20% of cases
    Parietal pleural thickening may be seen without plaques

Visceral pleural thickening
Lateral lower lobes
May be associated with rounded atelectasis

Benign exudative pleural effusion
Early finding
First 10 years after exposure
3% of exposed individuals
Small, unilateral or bilateral

Diffuse pleural thickening
5% of patients
Related to prior benign pleural effusion
Radiographs and CT
    One fourth of the chest wall
    May involve costophrenic angles

Pleural Plaques and Parietal Pleural Thickening

Pleural plaques are localized areas of pleural thickening. They are the most common and the most characteristic feature of asbestos exposure. They develop 10 to 20 years after the onset of exposure. They are composed of dense fibrous tissue and contain asbestos fibers, and calcification is common. Plaques nearly always involve the parietal pleural surfaces and are frequently seen overlying ribs in the posterolateral thorax and in relation to the domes of the diaphragms. They tend to spare the apices and costophrenic angles. Plaques have "square shoulders" and appear mesa-shaped in cross section. They range from 2 to 10 mm in thickness.

Thin areas of focal parietal pleural thickening without thick plaques may be seen early in the course of disease in patients with asbestos exposure.

Visceral Pleural Thickening

Visceral pleural thickening may occur, usually along the lateral pleural surface of the lower lobes. Overlying rounded atelectasis may be seen.

Benign Exudative Pleural Effusion

Benign exudative pleural effusion can be an early manifestation of asbestos exposure, being the only finding present in the first 10 years after exposure; it occurs in 3% of exposed individuals.

Effusions may be associated with pleuritic pain and are often serosanguineous. Asbestos-related pleural effusions can be unilateral or bilateral and may be persistent or recurrent. They are usually less than 500 mL. Diagnosis is by exclusion; malignant mesothelioma must be considered in the differential diagnosis.

Diffuse Pleural Thickening

Diffuse pleural thickening is seen in up to 5% of patients with pleural disease. Diffuse pleural thickening usually represents a synthesis and fusion of thickened visceral and parietal pleural layers, and it is usually related to the presence of prior asbestos-related benign pleural effusion.

Radiographic Findings of Pleural Disease

Although plain radiographs may be diagnostic of asbestos-related plaques in some patients, they are only about 10% to 40% sensitive in detecting pleural plaques.

Pleural plaques are usually visible in the lower half of the thorax and may be seen en face or in profile along the lateral pleural surfaces (see Figs. 18-1 and 18-6; also see Fig. 26-10 in Chapter 26), most numerous between the sixth and tenth ribs, or in relation to the domes of the hemidiaphragms; they tend to spare the costophrenic angles. Because they are often posterolateral in location, bilateral oblique views are often advantageous in demonstrating their presence.

In profile, they are often visible internal to ribs, up to 1 cm in thickness, and sharply contrasted with adjacent normal pleura. They are calcified in 10% to 15% of cases; diaphragmatic plaques are most often calcified. When seen en face, plaques appear round or irregular and "geographic" in shape. En face plaques are difficult to recognize as such unless calcified and may mimic lung nodules. Focal or diffuse thickening of the fissures may also be seen, indicative of visceral pleural disease, but is less common. Plaques are usually bilateral.

Pleural effusion occurring as a result of asbestos exposure has no distinguishing characteristics. It may or may not be associated with plaques.

Diffuse pleural thickening appears as a diffuse or concentric increase in pleural thickness. It is often considered to be present if pleural disease continuously involves at least one quarter of the chest wall. It may affect the costophrenic angles, an uncommon occurrence with plaques.

Collections of extrapleural fat may mimic asbestos-related pleural thickening. These occur in a distribution similar to that of plaques, involving the lower portion of the posterolateral thorax, but are usually longer, have tapering margins, are smooth and symmetrical, and are sometimes seen as lower in attenuation than soft tissue.

CT and HRCT Findings of Pleural Disease

CT and HRCT are considerably more sensitive than chest radiographs in detecting pleural abnormalities. On HRCT, parietal pleural thickening is easiest to see internal to visible rib segments (Fig. 18-5; also see Fig. 26-10 in Chapter 26).

A   **B**

FIG. 18.5. Asbestos-related pleural thickening. **A:** Coned CT of the left hemithorax shows focal areas of pleural thickening and pleural plaques (*large arrows*). Pleural thickening may be diagnosed most easily internal to ribs. A thin layer of fat may separate the thickening pleura from the rib. A similar linear density seen between the ribs (*small arrows*) is normal and represents the innermost intercostal muscle. **B:** CT at a different level shows plaques and concentric areas of pleural thickening (*arrows*).

Thickened pleura measuring as little as 1 to 2 mm can be readily diagnosed in this location. Pleural thickening is also easy to recognize in the paravertebral regions. In the paravertebral regions, the intercostal muscles are anatomically absent, and any distinct stripe of density indicates pleural thickening.

Asbestos-related pleural thickening appears smooth and sharply defined. Early pleural thickening is discontinuous. Plaques are usually bilateral (see Fig. 18-5B), although they appear unilateral in up to one third of cases. The presence of bilateral pleural plaques or focal pleural thickening is

strongly suggestive of asbestos exposure, particularly when calcification is also seen. Pleural calcification is visible on HRCT in about 15% to 20% of patients. Often, even when not grossly calcified, asbestos-related areas of pleural thickening appear denser than adjacent intercostal muscles, likely because of their mineral content.

Since the dome of the diaphragm lies roughly in the plane of the CT scan, the detection of uncalcified pleural plaques on the diaphragmatic surface can be difficult (see Figs. 18-2 and 18-6). In some patients, however, diaphragmatic pleural

A   **B**

FIG. 18.6. Asbestos-related pleural thickening. **A:** Chest radiograph shows geographic opacities (*small arrows*) overlying the lung bases, representing pleural plaques. Pleural plaques are also visible at the domes of the hemidiaphragms (*large arrows*). **B:** CT shows plaques (*arrows*) on the surface of the diaphragm.

FIG. 18.7. Asbestos-related pleural plaques, rounded atelectasis, and pleural effusion due to mesothelioma. Extensive pleural thickening with calcification is visible. A right pleural effusion (*black arrow*) is also visible. It is unusual to see benign pleural effusion with such marked pleural thickening, and in this case the pleural effusion reflects mesothelioma. Rounded atelectasis is visible in the adjacent lung (*white arrows*).

TABLE 18.4 Silicosis
Dust containing silicon dioxide
Heavy-metal mining and hard-rock mining
10–20 years after the onset of exposure
Silicotic nodule
Peribronchiolar
Laminated connective tissue
Upper lobes and parahilar regions
Progression after exposure—progressive massive fibrosis
Silicoproteinosis
Acute silicosis with alveolar proteinosis

plaques are visible deep in the posterior costophrenic angle, below the lung base; in this location, the pleural disease can be localized with certainty to the parietal pleura because only parietal pleura is present below the lung base. Pleural plaques along the mediastinum have been considered unusual in patients with asbestos-related pleural disease but are visible on CT scans in about 40% of patients. Paravertebral pleural thickening is also common.

On CT, diffuse pleural thickening is defined by the presence of a sheet of thickened pleura 8 cm in a craniocaudal dimension and 5 cm along the surface of the lung as seen in cross section (see Fig. 18-4); extensive calcification is uncommon. Diffuse pleural thickening may be associated with significant impairment of pulmonary function.

Benign pleural effusion is an early finding of asbestos-related pleural disease. Although it may be seen in association with pleural plaques, it is unusual in patients with extensive pleural disease. Pleural effusion may also indicate the presence of mesothelioma (Fig. 18-7).

SILICOSIS AND COAL-WORKER'S PNEUMOCONIOSIS

Silicosis and coal-worker's pneumoconiosis (CWP) result from the inhalation of different inorganic dusts, have different histology, and should be considered distinct diseases. However, their radiographic and HRCT appearances are quite similar, and they cannot be easily or reliably distinguished in individual cases.

Silicosis

Silicosis is caused by inhalation of dust containing silica (silicon dioxide or SiO_2) (Table 18-4). Heavy-metal mining and hard-rock mining are the occupations most frequently associated with chronic silicosis. Pathologically, the primary pulmonary lesion seen in patients with silicosis is a centrilobular, peribronchiolar nodule consisting of layers of laminated connective tissue, termed a *silicotic nodule*. The nodules measure from 1 to 10 mm in diameter, and although diffuse, they are usually most numerous in the upper lobes and parahilar regions. Focal emphysema (also known as focal-dust emphysema) surrounding the nodule is common.

The diagnosis of silicosis requires the combination of an appropriate history of silica exposure and characteristic findings on the chest radiograph. The risk of silicosis is dose-related. It usually becomes evident 10 to 20 years after the onset of exposure. Progression of disease both radiographically and clinically may occur for years after exposure has ended. Large conglomerate masses of silicotic nodules, so-called progressive massive fibrosis, may result.

A unique manifestation of acute exposure to large amounts of silica (e.g., in sand blasting) is termed *acute silicosis* or *silicoproteinosis*; except for the presence of inhaled silica, it is indistinguishable from idiopathic pulmonary alveolar proteinosis.

Coal-worker's Pneumoconiosis

CWP results from inhalation of coal dust containing little if any silica; exposure to other carbonaceous materials, such as graphite (pure carbon), may result in a similar disease (Table 18-5). As with silicosis, a history of 10 years or more of exposure is necessary to consider the diagnosis. The characteristic lesion of CWP is the *coal macule*, a 1- to 5-mm focal accumulation of coal dust surrounded by a small amount of fibrous tissue. As in patients with silicosis, these abnormalities tend to surround respiratory bronchioles and are therefore primarily centrilobular in location. With progression, coal macules are surrounded by small areas of focal emphysema.

TABLE 18.5 Coal-Worker's Pneumoconiosis

Dust containing coal or carbon
Coal mining
10–20 years after the onset of exposure
Coal macule
    Peribronchiolar
    Coal dust and small amount fibrosis
    Upper lobes and parahilar regions
Progression to conglomerate masses

Radiographic and HRCT Findings

Small Lung Nodules

The earliest and most characteristic plain radiographic finding in patients with both silicosis and CWP consists of small well-circumscribed nodules, usually measuring 2 to 5 mm in diameter but up to 10 mm in patients with silicosis (Table 18-6). These may be diffuse but mainly involve the upper and posterior lung zones (Fig. 18-8). These nodules

FIG. 18.8. Small lung nodules in silicosis. Small nodules are visible in the upper lobes. Hilar enlargement is also visible. Calcification of a lymph node or nodule is visible in the left upper lobe (*arrow*).

TABLE 18.6 Radiographic and HRCT Findings in Silicosis and Coal-Worker's Pneumoconiosis (CWP)

Simple or uncomplicated silicosis and CWP
Well-circumscribed nodules usually measuring 2 to 5 mm
Predominate in the posterior upper lungs
ILO p, q, or r
Centrilobular and subpleural distribution on HRCT
Nodules in silicosis
    May be up to 10 mm
    Better defined
    More likely to calcify (10%–20%)

Complicated silicosis/CWP
Large opacities and conglomerate masses
Worsening symptoms, particularly in silicosis
Silicosis
    Termed progressive massive fibrosis
    Numerous aggregated nodules associated with dense fibrous tissue
CWP
    Amorphous black mass of dust surrounded by some fibrous tissue
Masses may cavitate (ischemia, tuberculosis, bacterial infection)
ILO A, B, C
Lenticular masses in upper lobes
    Upper lobe nodules decrease in number
    Satellite nodules
    Calcification common
    Adjacent emphysema may be present

Lymph node enlargement
Hilar and mediastinal node enlargement in 30%–40%
Calcification common
Eggshell calcification typical of silicosis

indicate *simple or uncomplicated silicosis or CWP*. They are indicated as p, q, or r, in the ILO system.

The nodules of silicosis tend to be better defined than those of CWP and are more likely to calcify. Calcification of nodules is eventually visible on radiographs in 10% to 20% of patients with silicosis and tends to involve the entire nodule. Calcification in CWP may first involve the center of individual nodules.

HRCT is superior to both conventional CT and chest radiography in the detection of small nodules in patients with silicosis and CWP. Simple silicosis or simple CWP is characterized by small nodules that tend to be centrilobular and subpleural. Most typically, nodules show a distinct predominance in the posterior upper lobes and appear symmetrical (Fig. 18-9). Calcification of the nodules is seen in up to 30% of cases on HRCT. More severe silicosis or CWP is characterized on CT by an increase in the number and size of nodules.

Large Opacities and Conglomerate Masses

The appearance of large opacities (by definition more than 1 cm), also known as *conglomerate masses*, indicates the presence of *complicated silicosis or CWP*. Large opacities tend to develop with time and progression of the disease. They are indicated as A, B, or C in the ILO system.

In patients with silicosis, these masses represent a conglomeration of numbers of silicotic nodules associated with dense fibrous tissue (*progressive massive fibrosis*); in CWP, they consist of an amorphous dust-containing mass surrounded by some fibrous tissue. In both silicosis and CWP, these masses can undergo necrosis and cavitation. Cavitation

FIG. 18.9. HRCT of silicosis. Multiple small well-defined lung nodules are visible. The nodules are bilateral and symmetrical and show a posterior and upper lobe predominance. This distribution is characteristic. (Courtesy of Luigia Storto.)

is related to ischemia, tuberculosis (which has an increased incidence in both silicosis and CWP), or anaerobic bacterial infection.

On plain radiographs, these masses are first seen in the midportion or periphery of the upper lung zones and migrate toward the hila with time, leaving emphysematous spaces between them and the pleural surface. On the lateral radiograph, these masses may appear lenticular in shape, often oriented posteriorly, paralleling the major fissure (Fig. 18-10; also see Fig. 9-32 in Chapter 9).

Small nodules may also be visible. However, because these masses develop from conglomeration of small nodules, their appearance is associated with a corresponding decrease in the number of small nodules visible. Although usually bilateral, they may be unilateral or asymmetrical. Progressive massive fibrosis may also occur in the lower lobes, but it is less common in this location.

On CT, conglomerate masses are usually seen to be associated with a background of small nodules (Fig. 18-11). Conglomerate masses are usually oval and often have irregular borders. Apical scarring and adjacent bullae may be seen and are more conspicuous in patients with silicosis than in those with CWP. Calcification in association with conglomerate masses is common (see Fig. 18-11B). Areas of necrosis, visible as low attenuation, with or without cavitation may be present. Increased reticular opacities are not a prominent feature of silicosis or CWP, but honeycombing is occasionally visible.

Although simple silicosis and simple CWP cause few symptoms and little clinical impairment, the development of complicated silicosis or CWP is associated with symptoms and a deterioration of lung function. Patients with silicosis usually have greater respiratory impairment for a given degree of radiographic abnormality than do patients with CWP. Furthermore, the complicated form of silicosis has a poorer prognosis than does simple silicosis, but this is not necessarily the case with CWP. In patients with silicosis, the size of the conglomerate masses is often related to the severity of symptoms.

A

B

FIG. 18.10. Progressive massive fibrosis in silicosis. Posteroanterior (**A**) and lateral (**B**) radiographs show typical irregular masses (*arrows*) in both upper lobes, associated with volume loss.

A

B

C

FIG. 18.11. Progressive massive fibrosis in silicosis. **A:** HRCT shows bilateral upper lobe masses associated with distortion of lung architecture. This appearance is typical of progressive massive fibrosis. Small (satellite) nodules are seen adjacent to the larger mass. **B:** Soft-tissue window shows calcification within the masses, common in silicosis. **C:** Lung window scan at a lower level shows multiple small nodules typical of silicosis. Hilar enlargement is visible.

Caplan's Syndrome

Caplan's syndrome in patients with CWP or silicosis and rheumatoid arthritis may also be seen, with large necrobiotic nodules superimposed on small nodules. Caplan's syndrome (see Chapter 14) is more common with CWP than silicosis.

Lymph Node Enlargement

On plain radiographs, hilar lymphadenopathy is visible in many patients (see Fig. 18-8). The lymph nodes are often calcified. Characteristic peripheral "eggshell" calcification is seen in about 5% of cases of silicosis (Fig. 18-12) and is almost pathognomonic of this entity in a patient with exposure. Calcification of mediastinal lymph nodes may also be seen. Eggshell calcification is not typical of CWP; when it is seen in a patient with CWP, it reflects the presence of silica in the coal dust. On CT, hilar or mediastinal lymph node enlargement is visible in 30% to 40% of patients with silicosis or CWP.

FIG. 18.12. Eggshell calcification in silicosis. Right hilar lymph node enlargement with typical eggshell calcification is visible (*arrows*). An ill-defined upper lobe mass reflects progressive massive fibrosis.

TALCOSIS

Talc is magnesium silicate occurring in thin sheets. Talcosis, or lung disease related to talc, may result from inhalation or intravenous injection. However, talc is less pathogenetic than asbestos or silica.

Inhalation of talc may result in pneumoconiosis similar to asbestosis, although milder in degree. Findings include pleural thickening or calcification, sometimes associated with interstitial fibrosis. However, mined talc or commercially available talc is often contaminated with other minerals, such as asbestos or silica. If this is the case, the resulting pneumoconiosis may more closely resemble asbestosis or silicosis (talco-asbestosis and talco-silicosis, respectively).

Talcosis secondary to intravenous injection of talc is seen almost exclusively in drug users who inject medications intended for oral use, which contain talc as an inert ingredient. When drug users inject a solution of crushed tablets, numerous talc particles become trapped within pulmonary arterioles and capillaries. The particles result in small granulomas composed of multinucleated giant cells surrounded by a small amount of fibrous tissue.

The initial radiologic manifestations of injection talcosis consist of numerous discrete nodules 1 mm or less in diameter. Follow-up chest radiographs show gradual coalescence of the nodules toward the parahilar regions of the upper lobes. Eventually talcosis results in conglomerate masses in the upper lobes, which closely resemble the progressive massive fibrosis seen in silicosis (Fig. 18-13A). On HRCT, the small nodules may appear centrilobular. The confluent parahilar masses may be seen to contain high-attenuation material representing talc (see Fig. 18-13B).

MISCELLANEOUS SILICA AND SILICATE PNEUMOCONIOSES

Exposure to a variety of other substances containing varying amounts of silica (as in silicosis) and silicates (as in asbestosis) can result in a pneumoconiosis resembling one or both of these, or a mixture of the two. However, radiographic and clinical abnormalities are usually less profound than in silicosis or asbestosis.

INERT DUST PNEUMOCONIOSIS

Some dusts are not fibrogenic when inhaled. They result in few symptoms because of the absence of fibrosis but may result in significant radiographic abnormalities.

Siderosis results from inhalation of dust containing iron. The most common occupations involved are electric-arc welders and oxyacetylene welders, who may inhale

A

B

FIG. 18.13. Talcosis with progressive massive fibrosis. **A:** Chest radiograph shows ill-defined upper lobe masses similar to those seen in silicosis (*arrows*). **B:** On HRCT, the masses contain high-attenuation talc.

fine particles of iron oxide during their work. Little fibrosis results, but the particles accumulate in macrophages aggregated in relation to peribronchiolar and peribronchial lymphatics. Plain radiographs show small nodules with a parahilar predominance that may appear dense; these may clear with time. HRCT shows small centrilobular nodules, some of which have a fine branching appearance. Focal areas of consolidation may appear very high in attenuation due to the presence of iron.

Stannosis results from inhalation of tin, often by miners or refiners. The tin accumulates in macrophages surrounding small airways. Ill-defined nodules or thin, dense branching opacities may be seen, which may be very dense (Fig. 18-14).

A B

FIG. 18.14. Stannosis in a tin miner. **A:** Chest radiograph shows numerous small very dense nodules predominating in the middle lung zones. **B:** Coned-down view shows the very dense nodules. These represent accumulations of tin but result in little fibrosis.

Other such pneumoconioses with a similar appearance include *baritosis* (barium), *argyrosiderosis* (silver and iron), antimony, and rare earth exposure.

BERYLLIOSIS

Exposure to beryllium can occur in the ceramics industry, in nuclear weapons production, or in fluorescent lamp manufacture. Acute berylliosis results from massive exposure and has the appearance of acute lung injury with pulmonary edema or acute respiratory distress syndrome. Chronic berylliosis is a systemic granulomatous lung disease resulting from occupational exposure to beryllium over a period of years. A latent period of years between exposure and presentation is typical. Chronic berylliosis is indistinguishable from sarcoidosis histologically and radiographically, although a history of exposure and hypersensitivity to beryllium allows the diagnosis to be made. It may have a poor prognosis.

ALUMINUM

Inhalation of dusts containing metallic or oxidized aluminum has been associated with pulmonary fibrosis, granuloma formation, desquamative interstitial pneumonia, and alveolar proteinosis, but pneumoconiosis related to aluminum dust is rare. HRCT may show subpleural or diffuse honeycombing resembling idiopathic pulmonary fibrosis, centrilobular nodules resembling those seen in silicosis, or irregular reticulation.

HARD-METAL PNEUMOCONIOSIS

Hard metal is an alloy of tungsten carbide and cobalt, sometimes mixed with other metals. Exposure to hard metal results in interstitial inflammation with fibrosis and lung destruction, which may develop within a few years of exposure. Radiographic and CT findings include coarse reticular opacities, consolidation, architectural distortion, and subpleural bullae. On CT, traction bronchiectasis may be seen. The distribution may be patchy or with a lower lobe predominance.

SELECTED READING

Aberle DR, Balmes JR. Computed tomography of asbestos-related pulmonary parenchymal and pleural diseases. Clin Chest Med 1991; 12: 115–131.

Akira M. Uncommon pneumoconioses: CT and pathologic findings. Radiology 1995; 197:403–409.

Akira M, Yamamoto S, Yokoyama K, et al. Asbestosis: high-resolution CT-pathologic correlation. Radiology 1990; 176:389–394.

Akira M, Yokoyama K, Yamamoto S, et al. Early asbestosis: evaluation with high-resolution CT. Radiology 1991; 178:409–416.

Akira M. High-resolution CT in the evaluation of occupational and environmental disease. Radiol Clin North Am 2002; 40:43–59.

Akira M, Kozuka T, Yamamoto S, et al. Inhalational talc pneumoconiosis: radiographic and CT findings in 14 patients. AJR Am J Roentgenol 2007; 188:326–333.

Antao VC, Pinheiro GA, Terra-Filho M, et al. High-resolution CT in silicosis: correlation with radiographic findings and functional impairment. J Comput Assist Tomogr 2005; 29:350–356.

Balaan MR, Weber SL, Banks DE. Clinical aspects of coal workers' pneumoconiosis and silicosis. Occup Med 1993; 8:19–34.

Chong S, Lee KS, Chung MJ, et al. Pneumoconiosis: comparison of imaging and pathologic findings. Radiographics 2006; 26:59–77.

Copley SJ, Wells AU, Sivakumaran P, et al. Asbestosis and idiopathic pulmonary fibrosis: comparison of thin-section CT features. Radiology 2003; 229:731–736.

Gamsu G, Salmon CJ, Warnock ML, Blanc PD. CT quantification of interstitial fibrosis in patients with asbestosis: a comparison of two methods. AJR Am J Roentgenol 1995; 164:63–68.

Gevenois PA, de Maertelaer V, Madani A, et al. Asbestosis, pleural plaques and diffuse pleural thickening: three distinct benign responses to asbestos exposure. Eur Respir J 1998; 11:1021–1027.

Henry DA. International Labor Office Classification System in the age of imaging: relevant or redundant. J Thorac Imaging 2002; 17:179–188.

Kim KI, Kim CW, Lee MK, et al. Imaging of occupational lung disease. Radiographics 2001; 21:1371–1391.

Mossman BT, Churg A. Mechanisms in the pathogenesis of asbestosis and silicosis. Am J Respir Crit Care Med 1998; 157:1666–1680.

Newman LS, Buschman DL, Newell JD, Lynch DL. Beryllium disease: assessment with CT. Radiology 1994; 190:835–840.

Remy-Jardin M, Degreef JM, Beuscart R, et al. Coal worker's pneumoconiosis: CT assessment in exposed workers and correlation with radiographic findings. Radiology 1990; 177:363–371.

Savranlar A, Altin R, Mahmutyazicioglu K, et al. Comparison of chest radiography and high-resolution computed tomography findings in early and low-grade coal worker's pneumoconiosis. Eur J Radiol 2004; 51:175–180.

Sette A, Neder JA, Nery LE, et al. Thin-section CT abnormalities and pulmonary gas exchange impairment in workers exposed to asbestos. Radiology 2004; 232:66–74.

Shida H, Chiyotani K, Honma K, et al. Radiologic and pathologic characteristics of mixed dust pneumoconiosis. Radiographics 1996; 16:483–498.

Staples CA. Computed tomography in the evaluation of benign asbestos-related disorders. Radiol Clin North Am 1992; 30:1191–1207.

Ward S, Heyneman LE, Reittner P, et al. Talcosis associated with IV abuse of oral medications: CT findings. AJR Am J Roentgenol 2000; 174: 789–793.

CHAPTER

19

Diffuse Pulmonary Hemorrhage and Pulmonary Vasculitis

W. RICHARD WEBB

DIFFUSE PULMONARY HEMORRHAGE

Making a specific diagnosis of pulmonary hemorrhage based on radiographic findings is difficult. Lung consolidation visible radiographically in association with hemoptysis and anemia strongly suggests the diagnosis. However, chest radiographic and CT findings are often nonspecific (Fig. 19-1), and hemoptysis may be lacking even in patients with sufficient hemorrhage to result in anemia.

For the purposes of differential diagnosis, diffuse pulmonary hemorrhage should be distinguished from focal pulmonary hemorrhage occurring as a result of abnormalities such as bronchiectasis, chronic bronchitis, active infection (e.g., tuberculosis), chronic infection, neoplasm, pulmonary embolism, or other vascular abnormalities such as arteriovenous fistula.

Diffuse pulmonary hemorrhage can result from a variety of diseases (Table 19-1). The differential diagnosis of diffuse pulmonary hemorrhage includes (1) anti–glomerular basement membrane disease (Goodpasture's syndrome), (2) idiopathic pulmonary hemosiderosis (IPH), (3) Large vessel vasculitis (including Behçet's disease), (4) small vessel vasculitis

associated with antineutrophilic cytoplasmic antibody or ANCA (Wegener's granulomatosis, Churg-Strauss syndrome, microscopic polyangiitis), (5) immune complex–related vasculitis (collagen-vascular diseases, Henoch-Schönlein purpura, mixed cryoglobulinemia), (6) drug reactions, (7) anticoagulation, and (8) thrombocytopenia (see Fig. 19-1).

Goodpasture's syndrome, vasculitis syndromes, and collagen-vascular diseases are often associated with the combination of pulmonary hemorrhage and renal abnormalities and may be termed *pulmonary-renal syndromes*.

Radiographic Findings of Diffuse Pulmonary Hemorrhage

Radiographic findings in diseases causing diffuse pulmonary hemorrhage may be identical. In general, radiographs and high-resolution CT (HRCT) show patchy or diffuse consolidation or ground-glass opacity in the presence of acute hemorrhage (see Figs. 19-1 to 19-5). Ill-defined centrilobular nodules may be seen and predominate in some patients; these are sometimes visible on radiographs but are easiest to see on HRCT (see Figs. 19-2 and 19-5). Chest radiographs

A **B**

FIG. 19.1. Pulmonary hemorrhage associated with leukemia and thrombocytopenia. **A:** Chest radiograph shows ill-defined increased lung opacity. **B:** HRCT shows patchy areas of ground-glass opacity. The appearance is nonspecific and could also reflect pulmonary edema or infection. A left pleural effusion is also present.

TABLE 19.1 Causes of Diffuse Pulmonary Hemorrhage

Goodpasture's syndrome
Idiopathic pulmonary hemosiderosis
Large vessel pulmonary vasculitis
   Behçet's syndrome
Small vessel pulmonary vasculitis with ANCA
   Wegener's granulomatosis
   Churg-Strauss granulomatosis
   Microscopic polyangiitis
Immune complex–related vasculitis
   Collagen-vascular diseases
   Henoch-Schönlein purpura
   Mixed cryoglobulinemia
Drug reactions
Anticoagulation and coagulation disorders
Thromocytopenia
Diffuse alveolar damage
Elevated pulmonary venous pressure
Pulmonary venoocclusive disease
Pulmonary capillary hemangiomatosis
Lymphangiomyomatosis

may be normal or show very subtle abnormalities in patients with pulmonary hemorrhage.

Opacities may be diffuse with uniform lung involvement (see Fig. 19-3) or may show a central and perihilar predominance with relative sparing of the apices, lung periphery, and costophrenic angles (Fig. 19-4). Pleural effusions are not generally associated with pulmonary hemorrhage, although they may be seen in patients with coincident renal failure.

FIG. 19.2. Centrilobular nodules in pulmonary hemorrhage. CT scan in a patient with SLE and pulmonary hemorrhage shows ill-defined centrilobular nodules (*arrows*).

Within a few days of an acute episode of hemorrhage, hemosiderin-laden macrophages begin to accumulate in the interstitium. This occurrence is manifested on chest radiographs by the presence of Kerley's lines, which may be seen in isolation or in conjunction with residual consolidation or ground-glass opacity. On HRCT, interlobular septal thickening may replace or be seen in association with ground-glass opacity (Fig. 19-5). Unless further hemorrhage occurs,

A   B

FIG. 19.3. Diffuse pulmonary hemorrhage in idiopathic pulmonary hemosiderosis **A:** Interstitial opacities are visible bilaterally. The appearance is nonspecific. **B:** HRCT in a different patient with pulmonary hemorrhage shows diffuse ground-glass opacity.

FIG. 19.4. Pulmonary hemorrhage in SLE with a parahilar predominance. Patchy ground-glass opacities and consolidation are visible.

complete clearing of air-space and interstitial opacities usually occurs within 10 days to 2 weeks of an acute episode of hemorrhage. This is considerably slower than clearing of pulmonary edema, which hemorrhage may closely resemble.

In patients with recurrent episodes of pulmonary hemorrhage, a persistent reticular abnormality may be seen between episodes of bleeding. This reflects interstitial hemosiderin deposition and mild lung fibrosis and has been termed *pulmonary hemosiderosis*. It may be seen in any cause of recurrent hemorrhage but is particularly common in patients with IPH, as described below.

GOODPASTURE'S SYNDROME

Anti–glomerular basement membrane disease (Goodpasture's syndrome) most typically occurs in patients aged 20 to 30; men are affected four times as commonly as women (Table 19-2). Hemoptysis, usually mild, and anemia are present in 90%.

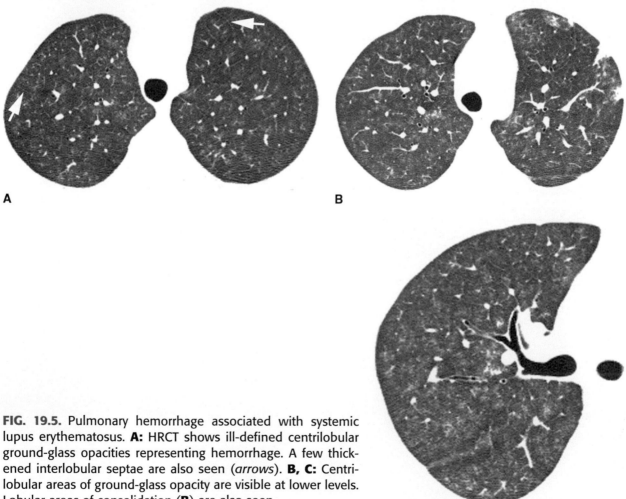

FIG. 19.5. Pulmonary hemorrhage associated with systemic lupus erythematosus. **A:** HRCT shows ill-defined centrilobular ground-glass opacities representing hemorrhage. A few thickened interlobular septae are also seen (*arrows*). **B, C:** Centrilobular areas of ground-glass opacity are visible at lower levels. Lobular areas of consolidation (**B**) are also seen.

TABLE 19.2 Goodpasture's Syndrome

Anti–glomerular basement membrane antibodies in 95%
Glomerulonephritis
Age 20–30 years
Four times more common in men than women
Hemoptysis and anemia in 90%
Consolidation or ground-glass opacity

Other symptoms include cough, dyspnea, and weakness. Findings of renal disease are usually but not always present, including hematuria, proteinuria, and renal failure. Anti–glomerular basement membrane antibodies are almost always (95%) present in the serum. These antibodies are directed against type IV collagen and cross-react with alveolar basement membrane. A pulmonary capillaritis is present. Renal biopsy shows glomerulonephritis with linear deposition of IgG in the glomeruli.

Although plain radiographs may be normal, they usually show diffuse air-space consolidation or ground-glass opacity, typically bilateral and symmetrical and often with a perihilar predominance (Figs. 19-6A and 19-7). HRCT usually

FIG. 19.7. Goodpasture's syndrome. Chest radiograph shows ill-defined parahilar and lower lobe opacities. The heart appears enlarged because of renal failure and fluid overload, and a dialysis catheter is in place.

A

B

FIG. 19.6. Goodpasture's syndrome. **A:** Chest radiograph shows a subtle increase in lung opacity. **B:** HRCT shows patchy ground-glass opacity.

shows consolidation or ground-glass opacity and may be abnormal in the face of subtle plain film findings or normal radiographs (see Fig. 19-6B).

After an acute episode of hemorrhage, the air-space opacities tend to resolve, being superseded by an interstitial abnormality or septal thickening.

IDIOPATHIC PULMONARY HEMOSIDEROSIS

IPH is a disease of unknown origin characterized by recurrent episodes of diffuse pulmonary hemorrhage without associated glomerulonephritis or a serologic abnormality (Table 19-3). Pathologic findings include alveolar hemorrhage, hemosiderin-laden macrophages, and a variable degree of interstitial fibrosis in longstanding cases. IPH most commonly occurs in children under the age of 10 or young adults. In adults, men are affected twice as often as women. IPH is sometimes associated with cow's milk allergy, thyroid disease, or immunoglobulin A gammopathy. It has recently been reported in infants with exposure to toxic mold (*Stachybotrys*). Symptoms include cough, hemoptysis, dyspnea, and anemia. The diagnosis is usually made by exclusion. About a quarter of patients die as a result of respiratory insufficiency or cor pulmonale.

Plain radiographic and HRCT findings are similar to those of Goodpasture's syndrome. Predominant findings in

TABLE 19.3 Idiopathic Pulmonary Hemosiderosis

No serologic abnormalities
No glomerulonephritis
Children or young adults
Associated with exposure to toxic mold, other conditions

TABLE 19.4 Classification of Pulmonary Vasculitis

Large vessel vasculitis
Giant-cell (temporal) arteritis
Takayasu's arteritis
Behcet's disease
Medium-sized vessel vasculitis
Polyarteritis nodosa
Kawasaki's disease
Small vessel vasculitis
Antineutrophilic cytoplasmic antibody (ANCA) associated
   Wegener's granulomatosis
   Churg-Strauss granulomatosis
   Microscopic polyangiitis
Immune complex vasculitis
   Goodpasture's syndrome
   Collagen-vascular diseases
   Behçet's disease
   Henoch-Schönlein purpura
   Antiphospholipid syndrome
   IgA nephropathy
   Mixed cryoglobulinemia

the acute phase of disease include diffuse ground-glass opacity (Fig 19-3). On HRCT ill-defined centrilobular nodular opacities may also be seen. Hemosiderosis and fibrosis may develop with recurrent episodes of hemorrhage.

PULMONARY VASCULITIS

Pulmonary hemorrhage may be associated with vasculitis. Systemic vasculitis syndromes are classified into three groups based on the size of vessels primarily involved (Table 19-4): large vessel vasculitis, medium-sized vessel vasculitis, and small vessel vasculitis. These are briefly reviewed, with emphasis on those associated with pulmonary or intrathoracic abnormalities. Small vessel vasculitis is most important as a cause of pulmonary hemorrhage. Although Goodpasture's syndrome does not result in a systemic vasculitis, it may be classified as a small vessel vasculitis because pulmonary capillaritis is present.

LARGE VESSEL VASCULITIS

Giant Cell (Temporal) Vasculitis

Temporal arteritis is relatively common. Affected patients are generally over 50 years of age. Arteries of the head and neck are typically involved, and the most common symptoms are headache and tenderness in the region of the temporal artery.

Large and medium-sized pulmonary arteries are rarely involved in this disease. Although upper respiratory symptoms such as cough and hoarseness occur in up to 10% of cases, radiographic correlates are lacking. Some patients show nonspecific radiographic abnormalities such as pleural effusion and diffuse reticular opacities, but what these are due to is unclear.

Takayasu's Arteritis

Takayasu's arteritis affects large and medium-sized arteries, most often the aorta and its branches. Women, usually under the age of 40, are affected in 90% of cases. In early disease, pathology shows vessel inflammation and poorly defined necrotizing and nonnecrotizing granulomas; in later lesions, vascular fibrosis and destruction of elastic tissue are present. Pulmonary arteries are involved in 50% of patients. Pulmonary hypertension may occur in late-stage disease, but is seldom severe.

Radiographic abnormalities usually reflect aortic involvement, with aortic contour abnormalities, such as dilatation of the arch, a wavy-appearing descending aorta, and premature aortic calcification. CT and MRI show concentric aortic wall thickening and narrowing of the aortic lumen.

Central pulmonary artery dilatation may be seen on chest radiographs due to pulmonary hypertension but is relatively uncommon. On CT or MRI, stenosis or obstruction of segmental or smaller pulmonary arteries is often seen in late-stage cases. This may be associated with a patchy decrease in the attenuation of peripheral lung parenchyma (i.e., mosaic perfusion), a finding that sometimes is also recognized on chest films. Regional decrease in lung perfusion may be shown using $\dot{V}/\dot{Q}$ scintigraphy.

Behçet's Disease

Behçet's disease is a rare systemic large and small vessel vasculitis likely due to deposition of immune complexes. It is associated with recurrent oral aphthous ulcers, genital ulcers, uveitis, and skin lesions such as erythema nodosum. Other organs and sites are commonly involved, including the joints (arthritis), heart, kidney, gastrointestinal system, and lung.

Behçet's disease is most common in young adults (20 to 35 years) and is particularly common in the Middle East (most notably Turkey) and the Far East (Japan). A familial incidence suggests hereditary factors, including HLA-5. The vasculitis of Behçet's disease results in vessel thrombosis, vascular obstruction, aneurysms, and sometimes vessel rupture. Involvement of the lung or intrathoracic vessels occurs in about 5% to 10% of cases.

Pulmonary artery aneurysms, otherwise an uncommon entity, are frequent in Behçet's disease involving the thorax. These appear as one or more, unilateral or bilateral, rounded hilar or perihilar opacities measuring up to several centimeters in diameter. On CT, these may opacify with contrast, may contain thrombus, or may not opacify because of thrombosis (Fig 19-8). Poor definition of an aneurysm may be associated with surrounding hemorrhage. Hemoptysis may occur due to leakage or rupture of an aneurysm and may be massive and life threatening. Pulmonary artery aneurysm is thus associated with a poor prognosis.

FIG 19.8. Behçet's disease in a 25 year old man with pulmonary artery aneurysms, pulmonary hemorrhage, and frank hemoptysis. **A:** Large left pulmonary artery aneurysm (*arrow*) is partially lined by thrombus, and is densely opacified on a volumetric HRCT. **B:** Surface display reconstruction shows two left sided pulmonary artery aneurysms (*arrows*). **C:** At a different level, an aneurysm is thrombosed (*arrow*). **D:** Lung window scan at the level of (**A**) shows poor definition of the aneurysm because of surrounding hemorrhage. Patchy and centrilobular hemorrhage is also visible in the right lower lobe. **E:** Lung window scan at the level of (**C**) shows right lower lobe hemorrhage. Vessels in the right lower lobe appear smaller than those in the anterior lung. This may be related to thrombosis shown in (**C**). This patient subsequently died as a result of aneurysm rupture.

Pulmonary artery thrombosis and occlusion may be associated with infarctions or focal pulmonary hemorrhage. Diffuse or patchy consolidation may also be seen, likely related to multiple areas of pulmonary hemorrhage.

Thrombosis of the superior vena cava and brachiocephalic veins may occur, resulting in superior vena cava syndrome, mediastinal edema, and widening of the mediastinum, as seen on chest radiographs. Pleural fluid may be seen, representing (1) effusion associated with pulmonary infarction, (2) hemothorax due to rupture of a pulmonary artery aneurysm, or (3) chylothorax due to great vein obstruction.

Hughes-Stovin syndrome, described in the 1950s, is characterized by pulmonary artery aneurysms, superior vena cava thrombosis, and thrombophlebitis. It likely represents Behçet's disease or a variant of Behçet's disease.

MEDIUM-SIZED VESSEL VASCULITIS

Polyarteritis Nodosa

Classic polyarteritis nodosa (PAN) typically affects small to medium systemic arteries, resulting in a necrotizing vasculitis. Involvement of arterioles, venules, and capillaries is absent, as is glomerulonephritis. Such abnormalities indicate the presence of microscopic polyangiitis, described below, which may otherwise resemble PAN. Pulmonary artery involvement is rare. Pulmonary hemorrhage reported to occur in PAN may represent microscopic polyangitis.

SMALL VESSEL VASCULITIS ASSOCIATED WITH ANCA

Wegener's Granulomatosis

Wegener's granulomatosis is a multisystem disease of unknown cause associated with involvement of the upper respiratory tract (nasal, oral, or sinus inflammation), lower respiratory tract (airway or lung), and kidney. Upper respiratory tract involvement occurs in nearly all patients; lung involvement occurs in 90%; glomerulonephritis occurs in 80% (Table 19-5).

Lung disease associated with Wegener's granulomatosis is characterized by granulomatous inflammation and necrotizing vasculitis. Limited Wegener's granulomatosis, involving only the lung, may occur.

Wegener's granulomatosis most commonly affects patients between the ages of 30 and 60 years. Most patients have symptoms of sinus disease at presentation (Fig. 19-9). Cough and hemoptysis are also common. Renal disease associated with hematuria, proteinuria, and renal failure is often absent at presentation but develops in most patients. Musculoskeletal symptoms occur in about 30% of patients, usually consisting of arthralgia or arthritis. Neurologic manifestations occur in 20% to 35% of patients. Ocular or skin involvement may also occur.

TABLE 19.5 Wegener's Granulomatosis
Multisystem disease
Upper respiratory tract involved in nearly all patients
Lung involvement occurs in 90%
Glomerulonephritis occurs in 80%
Ages 30–60 years
C-ANCA in 90%
Chest radiographs abnormal in 75% at presentation
Multiple nodules and masses
Usually 2–4 cm
Cavitation common
Cavities become thin walled with treatment
Lung consolidation due to hemorrhage
Tracheobronchial involvement
Tracheal wall thickening
Subglottic trachea most often involved
Luminal narrowing

The presence of C-ANCA is characteristic, being seen in 90% of cases; it is less often present in patients with disease limited to the lung. Lung biopsy is usually more helpful in diagnosis than renal biopsy, which may be nonspecific.

Untreated Wegener's granulomatosis is associated with a poor prognosis, with death usually occurring within 6 months of the onset of renal failure. However, there is a high remission rate following treatment with cyclophosphamide and steroids. Recurrence may be precipitated by infection.

At presentation, chest radiographic abnormalities are visible in 75% of patients with Wegener's granulomatosis.

Lung Nodules and Consolidation

Multiple lung nodules or masses are most common, being visible in more than half of patients at presentation (see Figs. 19-9 and 19-10). Typically, there are fewer than a dozen nodules visible. In most cases, the nodules are bilateral and widely distributed without predominance in any lung region. A solitary nodule or mass may be seen, but this is less common. Masses usually range from 2 to 4 cm in diameter but may be much larger. Masses are round or oval and may be well defined or poorly defined. Calcification of the masses does not occur.

With progression of disease, nodules and masses tend to increase in size and number. With treatment, nodules usually resolve over a period of months. Complete resolution may occur.

Cavitation occurs in approximately 50% of cases (see Figs. 19-9 and 19-10). Cavities are usually thick walled, with an irregular inner margin. Air-fluid levels may be present. Typically, cavitary nodules and masses become thin walled (see Fig. 19-10) and decrease in size with treatment.

FIG. 19.9. Wegener's granulomatosis. **A:** Chest radiograph shows bilateral cavitary lung masses. **B:** Sinus CT shows soft-tissue thickening in the left maxilla with thickening and poor definition of the maxillary wall (*arrows*). **C, D:** Cavitary mass and solid soft-tissue masses are visible on CT.

Air-space consolidation or ground-glass opacity is the second most common radiographic finding in Wegener's granulomatosis and may occur with or without associated lung nodules or masses. These areas of consolidation usually represent pulmonary hemorrhage. They may be focal, diffuse, or patchy (Figs. 19-11 and 19-12).

Tracheobronchial Involvement

Tracheobronchial lesions occur in approximately 15% to 25% of patients with Wegener's granulomatosis. Concentric airway wall thickening due to inflammation, with narrowing of the airway lumen, is present. Involvement of the subglottic trachea is most typical (see Fig. 22-16 in Chapter 22), with variable involvement of the vocal cords, distal trachea, and proximal mainstem bronchi (see Fig. 22-17 in Chapter 22). Segmental, lobar, or lung atelectasis may result.

Abnormalities may be focal or diffuse. They are described in detail in Chapter 22.

Other Findings

Hilar or mediastinal lymph node enlargement may be seen, but this is uncommon and never an isolated finding. Pleural effusions occur in about 10% of cases.

Churg-Strauss Granulomatosis

Churg-Strauss granulomatosis is also associated with ANCA, usually P-ANCA (perinuclear pattern). It is typically manifested by findings of simple pulmonary eosinophilia (i.e., fleeting consolidation), chronic eosinophilic pneumonia (i.e., peripheral areas of consolidation), or pulmonary edema due to cardiac involvement with heart failure.

FIG. 19.10. Wegener's granulomatosis with progression. **A:** CT shows two small lung nodules. **B:** Chest radiograph 1 year later shows a right upper lobe mass containing an air-fluid level. Other ill-defined nodules are also visible. **C:** Two weeks after (**B**), there was an increase in the size of the right upper lobe mass with progressive cavitation. The cavity is thin-walled and an air-fluid level is again seen. **D:** CT 2 months after (**B**) shows an irregular cavitary mass. **E:** Radiograph 3 months after (**B**) shows a large thin-walled cavity. **F:** CT 5 months after (**B**) shows a persisting thin-walled cavity.

FIG. 19.11. Focal pulmonary hemorrhage in Wegener's granulomatosis. Focal consolidation is visible in the right lower lobe.

Uncommonly, it results in pulmonary hemorrhage. It is described in Chapter 16.

Microscopic Polyangiitis

Microscopic polyangiitis results in systemic necrotizing small vessel vasculitis. Although the histology is similar to classic PAN, involvement of arterioles, venules, and capillaries distinguishes it from PAN. Also, ANCA (usually P-ANCA) is present in 80%; ANCA is rare in PAN.

Microscopic polyangiitis typically occurs in middle-aged adults; men are more commonly involved. Glomerulonephritis develops in 90% of patients, and other organs may

be involved. Pulmonary hemorrhage related to capillaritis occurs in 25%, associated with dyspnea and hemoptysis. Radiographic findings are typical of pulmonary hemorrhage. Pleural effusion and pulmonary edema are seen in about 10%, likely related to renal disease. Progression to pulmonary fibrosis is rare. Treatment with cyclophosphamide and steroids often results in remission.

IMMUNE COMPLEX SMALL VESSEL VASCULITIS

Deposition of immune complexes in the walls of small vessels and capillaries occurs in a number of systemic vasculitis syndromes, resulting in capillaritis and pulmonary hemorrhage. Diseases associated with circulating immune complexes include Goodpasture's syndrome, collagen-vascular diseases, Henoch-Schönlein purpura, mixed cryoglobulinemia, antiphospholipid syndrome, IgA nephropathy, and others. Typically, these diseases are not included in the classification of pulmonary vasculitis.

Collagen-Vascular Diseases

Diffuse pulmonary hemorrhage may occur with many collagen diseases, probably associated with circulating immune complexes and small vessel vasculitis. Systemic lupus erythematosus (SLE) is most common (see Figs. 19-2, 19-4, 19-5, and 19-13). Hemoptysis often occurs and may be massive. Radiographic and HRCT findings are similar to other causes of diffuse pulmonary hemorrhage. The pulmonary manifestations of the collagen diseases are described in Chapter 14.

Henoch-Schönlein Purpura

Henoch-Schönlein purpura is characterized by purpura, abdominal pain, gastrointestinal hemorrhage, arthralgia, and glomerulonephritis, although not all are typically present

FIG. 19.12. Patchy pulmonary hemorrhage in Wegener's granulomatosis. Patchy ground-glass opacity is visible on HRCT (*arrows*).

FIG. 19.13. Pulmonary hemorrhage in lupus. Patchy ground-glass opacity is visible on HRCT.

and glomerulonephritis occurs in only 20%. It is usually seen in young children and often follows a respiratory tract infection. Relapses are common, but the prognosis is good. Chronic renal failure develops in a few patients. Diffuse or patchy consolidation may result from capillaritis and pulmonary hemorrhage. Hemoptysis is often associated. Pleural effusion may be seen.

Mixed Cryoglobulinemia

This disease is characterized by purpura, arthralgia, glomerulonephritis, hepatosplenomegaly, and lymph node enlargement. Serum globulins that precipitate with cold are present. Many cases are related to hepatitis C infection; others are associated with other infections, lymphoma, lymphoproliferative disease, or collagen-vascular diseases. Pulmonary disease is uncommon and difficult to characterize. A diffuse reticular pattern may be present, but what this represents is unclear.

SELECTED READING

Aberle DR, Gamsu G, Lynch D. Thoracic manifestations of Wegener granulomatosis: diagnosis and course. Radiology 1990; 174:703–709.

Cheah FK, Sheppard MN, Hansell DM. Computed tomography of diffuse pulmonary haemorrhage with pathological correlation. Clin Radiol 1993; 48:89–93.

Collard HR, Schwarz MI. Diffuse alveolar hemorrhage. Clin Chest Med 2004; 25:583–592.

Connolly B, Manson D, Eberhard A, et al. CT appearance of pulmonary vasculitis in children. AJR Am J Roentgenol 1996; 167:901–904.

Cordier JF, Valeyre D, Guillevin L, et al. Pulmonary Wegener's granulomatosis. A clinical and imaging study of 77 cases. Chest 1990; 97:906–912.

Hoffman GS, Kerr GS, Leavitt RY, et al. Wegener granulomatosis: an analysis of 158 patients. Ann Intern Med 1992; 116:488–498.

Ioachimescu OC, Sieber S, Kotch A. Idiopathic pulmonary haemosiderosis revisited. Eur Respir J 2004; 24:162–170.

Jennette JC, Falk RJ, Andrassy K, et al. Nomenclature of systemic vasculitides. Proposal of an international consensus conference. Arthritis Rheum 1994; 37:187–192.

Lee KS, Kim TS, Fujimoto K, et al. Thoracic manifestation of Wegener's granulomatosis: CT findings in 30 patients. Eur Radiol 2003; 13:43–51.

Marten K, Schnyder P, Schirg E, et al. Pattern-based differential diagnosis in pulmonary vasculitis using volumetric CT. AJR Am J Roentgenol 2005; 184:720–733.

Mayberry JP, Primack SL, Müller NL. Thoracic manifestations of systemic autoimmune diseases: radiographic and high-resolution CT findings. Radiographics 2000; 20:1623–1635.

Ozer C, Duce MN, Ulubas B, et al. Inspiratory and expiratory HRCT findings in Behcet's disease and correlation with pulmonary function tests. Eur J Radiol 2005; 56:43–47.

Primack SL, Miller RR, Müller NL. Diffuse pulmonary hemorrhage: clinical, pathologic, and imaging features. AJR Am J Roentgenol 1995; 164:295–300.

Primack SL, Müller NL. Radiologic manifestations of the systemic autoimmune diseases. Clin Chest Med 1998; 19:573–586.

Reuter M, Schnabel A, Wesner F, et al. Pulmonary Wegener's granulomatosis: correlation between high-resolution CT findings and clinical scoring of disease activity. Chest 1998; 114:500–506.

Seely JM, Effmann EL, Müller NL. High-resolution CT of pediatric lung disease: imaging findings. AJR Am J Roentgenol 1997; 168:1269–1275.

Seo JB, Im JG, Chung JW, et al. Pulmonary vasculitis: the spectrum of radiological findings. Br J Radiol 2000; 73:1224–1231.

Tunaci A, Berkmen YM, Gokmen E. Thoracic involvement in Behcet's disease: pathologic, clinical, and imaging features. AJR Am J Roentgenol 1995; 164:51–56.

Weir IH, Müller NL, Chiles C, et al. Wegener's granulomatosis: findings from computed tomography of the chest in 10 patients. Can Assoc Radiol J 1992; 43:31–34.

Witte R, Gurney J, Robbins R, et al. Diffuse pulmonary alveolar hemorrhage after bone marrow transplantation: radiographic findings in 39 patients. AJR Am J Roentgenol 1991; 157:461–464.

Diffuse Lung Disease Associated with Lipid: Exogenous Lipid Pneumonia and Alveolar Proteinosis

W. RICHARD WEBB

ENDOGENOUS LIPOID PNEUMONIA

Lipoid pneumonia (lung consolidation containing lipids) may be endogenous or exogenous. Endogenous lipoid pneumonia may occur due to bronchial obstruction with accumulation of lipid-rich cellular debris distal to the obstructing lesion; this is sometimes termed "golden pneumonia" because of its yellow color at gross pathology. The term "postobstructive pneumonia" usually suffices for this condition.

EXOGENOUS LIPOID PNEUMONIA

Exogenous lipoid pneumonia results from the chronic aspiration or inhalation of animal, vegetable, or petroleum-based oils or fats (Table 20-1). Petroleum-based oil (mineral oil) aspiration is most common, usually associated with its use as a laxative. Responsible animal-based oils (e.g., cod-liver and shark-liver oils, clarified butter) and vegetable-based oils are usually aspirated during ingestion or because of esophageal motility abnormalities with reflux.

TABLE 20.1 Exogenous Lipoid Pneumonia

Chronic aspiration of animal, vegetable, or petroleum-based oils or fats
Esophageal dysmotility or reflux
Variable fibrosis and inflammation
Consolidation or masses
Usually dependent or lower lobe
CT
  Well-defined or ill-defined masses
  Variable amounts of low attenuation fat (−35 to −75 HU)
  Necrosis or cavitation
  Patchy ground-glass opacity or crazy paving

Acute aspiration results in an aspiration pneumonia. Chronic aspiration results in lipoid pneumonia associated with variable fibrosis and inflammation. The degree of lung inflammation or fibrosis associated with the aspirated oil is related to the amount of free fatty acid present. Animal fats generally result in more inflammation and fibrosis than vegetable or mineral oils because they are hydrolyzed by lung lipases, releasing fatty acids.

A large quantity of oily material must usually be aspirated over a period of time before symptoms develop. Symptoms include cough, mild fever, and chest discomfort; they are least common with mineral oil aspiration. Fat may be identified in the sputum in some patients.

Radiographic and CT Findings

Consolidation, ill-defined masses, or sometimes findings of fibrosis are seen on chest radiographs (Figs. 20-1A, 20-2A, and 20-3A). A lower-lobe distribution is typical but not always present. Opacities may be bilateral or unilateral. The radiographic appearance is nonspecific.

CT shows masses that may be well-defined or ill-defined, or areas of consolidation. As on chest radiographs, these areas tend to have a lower-lobe predominance and are often bilateral. A dependent location is also typical. Bronchi may be seen leading to the abnormal areas.

If a large amount of lipid has been aspirated, CT can show areas of low-attenuation consolidation (−35 to −75 HU) or low-attenuation regions within larger masses (see Figs. 20-1B to E and 20-2B); this appearance is most common in patients with chronic mineral oil aspiration. Because inflammation or fibrosis accompanies the presence of the lipid material, the CT attenuation of the consolidation or mass need not be low, but often small areas of low-attenuation oil are visible (see Figs. 20-1D and E, and 20-2B). In some patients, necrosis and cavitation are present.

FIG. 20.1. Exogenous lipoid pneumonia resulting from chronic mineral oil aspiration. **A:** Chest radiograph shows irregular masses (*arrows*) in both lungs. **B:** CT shows an irregular mass (*white arrow*) in the posterior right upper lobe. This mass is dependent in location, and the posterior segmental bronchus of the right upper lobe (*black arrow*) leads to it. Several other nodular opacities are also seen. **C:** An ill-defined area of consolidation is visible in the superior segment of the left lower lobe (*white arrow*). It is dependent, and branches of the superior segment bronchus (*black arrow*) lead to it. **D** and **E:** Soft-tissue window scans at the same levels as (**B**) and (**C**) show low attenuation (−75 HU; *arrows*) within these masses.

A   **B**

FIG. 20.2. Exogenous lipoid pneumonia resulting from chronic mineral oil aspiration. **A:** Chest radiograph shows irregular consolidation (*arrows*) in both lower lobes. **B:** CT shows irregular masses (*large arrows*) in both lower lobes. The left lower-lobe mass shows low attenuation (−100 HU; *small black arrow*) within the mass, although most of the mass appears to be of soft-tissue attenuation.

In patients with less severe abnormalities, ground-glass opacity or crazy paving (ground-glass opacity in association with interlobular septal thickening) or centrilobular nodules may also be seen on CT (see Fig. 20-3B). Subpleural pulmonary fibrosis and honeycombing are occasionally encountered. Some resolution of abnormalities is possible with time.

PULMONARY ALVEOLAR PROTEINOSIS

Pulmonary alveolar proteinosis (PAP) is a disease characterized by filling of the alveolar spaces with a PAS-positive proteinaceous material, rich in lipid. The lung interstitium is largely normal, although the lipoprotein may also accumulate within interlobular septa.

A   **B**

FIG. 20.3. Exogenous lipoid pneumonia resulting from mineral oil aspiration. **A:** Chest radiograph shows patchy parahilar consolidation. **B:** HRCT shows ill-defined parahilar consolidation and ground-glass opacity.

Three clinically distinct forms of this disease have been described: *congenital PAP*, due to mutations in genes encoding surfactant B or C or the βc chain of the receptor for granulocyte-macrophage colony-stimulating factor (GM-CSF); *secondary PAP*, occurring in association with a wide variety of disorders, including inhalation of silica (acute silicosis or silicoproteinosis) (Fig 20-6), infection (e.g., *Pneumocystis jiroveci*), and hematologic and lymphatic malignancies; and an acquired form of the disease unassociated with other conditions (*idiopathic PAP*).

Idiopathic PAP accounts for nearly 90% of cases. Idiopathic PAP is an autoimmune disease in which IgG antibodies to GM-CSF result in interference with the degradation or clearance of intra-alveolar surfactant. The result is a disruption in surfactant homeostasis (Table 20-2).

Men with PAP outnumber women by the ratio 4:1. Patients range in age from a few months to more than 70 years, with two thirds of patients being between 30 and 50 years old. Symptoms are usually mild and of insidious onset. They include nonproductive cough, fever, and mild dyspnea on exertion. About 30% of patients are asymptomatic.

Radiographic and HRCT Findings

Radiographic manifestations of PAP include bilateral, patchy, diffuse, or parahilar air-space consolidation or hazy ground-

---

TABLE 20.2 Pulmonary Alveolar Proteinosis

PAS-positive lipoproteinaceous material fills alveoli
May be idiopathic, secondary, or congenital
Idiopathic PAP
  90% of cases
  Autoimmune disease: antibodies to granulocyte-
    macrophage colony-stimulating factor
  Decreased degradation or clearance of surfactant
Secondary PAP
  Acute silicosis, immunodeficiency, malignancies,
    chemotherapy
Symptoms mild and insidious
Superimposed infection with Nocardia, Mycobacterium
  avium-intracellulare, and *P. jiroveci* (*P. carinii*)
Treated with bronchoalveolar lavage
Radiographs show ill-defined opacity, consolidation
  uncommon
HRCT
  Bilateral, patchy, and geographic ground-glass opacity
  "Crazy paving" typical
  Abnormalities decrease after lavage

---

glass opacity, which is usually most severe in the lung bases (Figs. 20-4A and 20-5A); dense consolidation and air bronchograms are rare. Although reticular opacities may be seen, they are usually mild. The radiographic appearance often resembles that of pulmonary edema, except for the absence of cardiomegaly and pleural effusion.

High-resolution CT (HRCT) findings (see Figs. 20-4 to 20-6) in patients with PAP include the following:

1. Bilateral areas of ground-glass opacity
2. Smooth interlobular septal thickening in lung regions showing ground-glass opacity (i.e., crazy paving)
3. Consolidation
4. A patchy or geographic distribution

In many patients, areas of ground-glass opacity or consolidation are sharply demarcated from the surrounding normal parenchyma. In some of these cases, sharply marginated lung opacities appear to represent lobules. The distribution of disease is variable, sometimes being mainly central and sometimes peripheral. It is typically bilateral but may be asymmetrical.

The combination of a geographic distribution of areas of ground-glass opacity with smoothly thickened interlobular septa resulting in a crazy paving appearance, is suggestive of alveolar proteinosis in patients with subacute or chronic symptoms (see Figs. 20-4B to D to 20-6). However, this appearance can be seen in other chronic lung diseases, including eosinophilic pneumonia, organizing pneumonia (BOOP), and lipoid pneumonia, and in acute diseases such as pneumonia, pulmonary edema, and pulmonary hemorrhage.

Superimposed infection, often by *Nocardia asteroides*, is a common complication of alveolar proteinosis, resulting in focal areas of dense consolidation or abscess formation (see Fig. 20-6B). *Mycobacterium avium-intracellulare* complex (MAC) and *P. jiroveci* (*P. carinii*) infections have also been reported in patients with PAP.

Bronchoalveolar lavage is used to wash out the intra-alveolar material. Successful treatment is associated with a reduction in the severity of ground-glass opacity, although septal thickening may persist, at least temporarily (see Fig. 20-4E). Prior to the advent of bronchoalveolar lavage, about 30% of patients died of respiratory insufficiency or superimposed infection, but the prognosis has improved considerably. After lavage, many patients remain in remission, but others relapse; patients who relapse require retreatment every 6 to 24 months, and a few become refractory to treatment. Inoccasional cases, interstitial fibrosis develops.

(text continues on page 535)

FIG. 20.4. Pulmonary alveolar proteinosis in a patient with progressive dyspnea. **A:** Chest radiograph shows an ill-defined increase in opacity at the lung bases. Frank consolidation and air bronchograms are absent. **B–D:** HRCT shows patchy and geographic areas of ground-glass opacity. Interlobular septal thickening is visible within the areas of ground-glass opacity. This appearance is termed "crazy paving." It is typical of pulmonary alveolar proteinosis but nonspecific. **E:** HRCT at the same level as (**D**), following bronchoalveolar lavage. Interlobular septal thickening remains visible, but there is a considerable decrease in ground-glass opacity.

FIG. 20.5. Pulmonary alveolar proteinosis in a 40-year-old woman. **A:** Chest radiographs show patchy lung opacity. **B–D:** Patchy areas of ground-glass opacity and associated interlobular septal thickening (i.e., crazy-paving) are visible. Intervening lung appears normal.

FIG. 20.6. Pulmonary alveolar proteinosis in a patient with severe exposure to silica dust (i.e., acute silicosis). **A:** HRCT shows patchy and geographic ground-glass opacity with crazy paving. **B:** A focal area of consolidation in the right lung (*arrow*) is due to *Nocardia* infection. Crazy paving is evident.

SELECTED READING

Franquet T, Giménez A, Bordes R, et al. The crazy-paving pattern in exogenous lipoid pneumonia: CT-pathologic correlation. AJR Am J Roentgenol 1998; 170:315–317.

Godwin JD, Müller NL, Takasugi JE. Pulmonary alveolar proteinosis: CT findings. Radiology 1988; 169:609–613.

Hugosson CO, Riff EJ, Moore CC, et al. Lipoid pneumonia in infants: a radiological-pathological study. Pediatr Radiol 1991; 21:193–197.

Johkoh T, Itoh H, Müller NL, et al. Crazy-paving appearance at thin-section CT: spectrum of disease and pathologic findings. Radiology 1999; 211:155–160.

Lee KN, Levin DL, Webb WR, et al. Pulmonary alveolar proteinosis: high-resolution CT, chest radiographic, and functional correlations. Chest 1997; 111:989–995.

Lee KS, Müller NL, Hale V, et al. Lipoid pneumonia: CT findings. J Comput Assist Tomogr 1995; 19:48–51.

Prakash UBS, Barham SS, Carpenter HA, et al. Pulmonary alveolar phospholipoproteinosis: experience with 34 cases and a review. Mayo Clin Proc 1987; 62:499–518.

Trapnell BC, Whitsett JA, Nakata K. Pulmonary alveolar proteinosis. N Engl J Med 2003; 349:2527–2539

Wang BM, Stern EJ, Schmidt RA, Pierson DJ. Diagnosing pulmonary alveolar proteinosis: a review and an update. Chest 1997; 111:460–466.

Diffuse Lung Diseases Associated with Calcification

W. RICHARD WEBB

A wide variety of lung diseases may be associated with some degree of lung calcification, most notably granulomatous diseases such as sarcoidosis or tuberculosis (Table 21-1).

Several diffuse lung diseases are associated with extensive lung calcification as a common finding or as a primary manifestation of the disease. These are discussed in this chapter.

DIFFUSE PARENCHYMAL AMYLOIDOSIS

The term *amyloidosis* refers to a group of conditions characterized by extracellular deposition of abnormal fibrillar protein. Amyloidosis may be classified according to its etiology, the proteins involved, or its primary manifestation (Table 21-2). The first two of these categories overlap, are somewhat confusing, and are reviewed briefly. Classification according to its primary manifestation is most appropriate to the radiologic assessment of amyloidosis and is easiest to remember.

Classification by Etiology

An etiologic classification of amyloidosis includes (1) *primary amyloidosis* (i.e., associated with a plasma cell disorder or idiopathic); (2) *secondary amyloidosis* (i.e., associated with chronic inflammatory disorders or neoplasms such as Hodgkin's disease); (3) *heredofamilial amyloidosis* (i.e., having a genetic basis); and (4) *senile amyloidosis*, which usually occurs in patients over the age of 70.

It may be subdivided into systemic forms (i.e., diffuse involvement of multiple organs) or localized forms (i.e., focal involvement largely limited to one organ).

Classification by Specific Proteins

When amyloidosis is classified according to the specific abnormal protein involved, the most important types producing lung disease are amyloid L and amyloid A.

Amyloid L (AL, or light chain amyloidosis) is the most common form of systemic amyloidosis. It may be either idiopathic or associated with plasma cell disorders (about 90% of cases). The lung is involved in 70% to 90% of patients with AL amyloidosis. Cardiomyopathy almost always is present if the lung is involved. Prognosis generally is poor. AL amyloidosis also may result in localized lung involvement. AL typically occurs in patients in their 50s or 60s.

Amyloid A (AA) occurs as secondary amyloidosis in patients with chronic inflammatory diseases (e.g., collagen vascular disease, infections, inflammatory bowel disease, and familial Mediterranean fever) and some neoplasms such as Hodgkin's disease. The lung is commonly involved to some degree, but deposits often are small or clinically insignificant. The prognosis is better than that for AL.

Among patients who have pulmonary involvement by amyloid, about 65% have primary systemic amyloidosis (systemic AL), 30% have localized amyloidosis (localized AL), and 5% have secondary amyloidosis (AA).

Classification by Manifestation

From a radiographic standpoint, it is most useful to classify amyloidosis on the basis of the abnormalities it produces. In general, pulmonary amyloidosis is classified

---

TABLE 21.1 Diffuse or Multifocal Lung Calcification

Infectious diseases
    Tuberculosis
    Histoplasmosis
    Healed varicella pneumonia
    Parasitic infections
Sarcoidosis
Silicosis and coal-worker's, pneumoconiosis
Calcified metastases
    Osteogenic and chondrosarcoma
    Mucinous adenocarcinoma
    Thyroid carcinoma
Pulmonary ossification with mitral stenosis
Lung fibrosis with dystrophic calcification
Amyloidosis
Alveolar microlithiasis
Metastatic calcification

TABLE 21.2 Classification of Amyloidosis

By etiology
Primary amyloidosis—plasma cell disorder or unassociated with underlying disease
Secondary amyloidosis—associated with chronic inflammatory disorders or neoplasm
Heredofamilial amyloidosis
Senile amyloidosis—usually in patients over 70
Systemic (diffuse involvement of multiple organs)
Localized (focal involvement largely limited to one organ)

By specific proteins
Amyloid L (AL; light-chain amyloidosis)
  Most common
  Usually primary amyloidosis
  Lung involved in 70%–90%, localized or diffuse
  Cardiac involvement
  Poor prognosis
Amyloid A
  Secondary amyloidosis
  Lung involved to a minor degree
  Better prognosis

By manifestation
Diffuse (alveolar septal) amyloidosis
  Usually primary systemic and AL
  Dyspnea due to lung or heart disease
  Small nodules or reticular opacities
  Consolidation
  Lymph node enlargement
  Calcification common
Localized nodular amyloidosis
  Usually primary localized and AL
  Usually asymptomatic
  Lung nodules, often calcified
  Nodules grow slowly
Localized tracheobronchial amyloidosis
  Usually primary localized and AL
  Tracheal and bronchial narrowing or masses
  Calcification common

into three types: (1) diffuse or alveolar septal amyloidosis, (2) localized nodular amyloidosis, and (3) tracheobronchial amyloidosis.

Diffuse (Alveolar Septal) Amyloidosis

Symptoms of respiratory insufficiency are common with diffuse or alveolar septal amyloidosis, and may be related to diffuse lung disease or associated cardiac involvement. This form of amyloidosis is most often related to primary systemic amyloidosis (systemic AL). Diffuse lung involvement is much less common and may be incidental with AA amyloidosis or senile amyloidosis. Occasionally, diffuse alveolar septal amyloidosis reflects localized rather than systemic disease.

The lung may be diffusely involved in the absence of a radiographic abnormality. If radiographs are abnormal, a reticular or reticulonodular pattern typically is seen, usually bilateral and diffuse or with a basal and subpleural predominance (Figs. 21-1 and 21-2A). Focal or patchy areas of consolidation also may be seen. The abnormal areas can calcify or, rarely, show frank ossification. Less often, a small nodular pattern mimicking sarcoidosis or miliary tuberculosis may be seen.

Hilar or mediastinal lymph node enlargement may be seen in patients with AL, either as an isolated finding or in association with interstitial disease. Cardiac infiltration with heart failure may result in pulmonary edema or pleural effusion.

On HRCT, the most common pulmonary manifestations of diffuse parenchymal amyloidosis consist of multiple small nodules, usually ranging from 2 to 4 mm in diameter (see Fig. 21-2B and C), interlobular septal thickening, fine reticular opacities, focal consolidation, foci of calcification within nodules or areas of consolidation (Fig. 21-3), and traction bronchiectasis. A subpleural and basal predominance may be seen.

Progression of the diffuse parenchymal disease typically occurs with time, with an increase in the reticular opacities, septal thickening, the size and number of nodules, the extent of consolidation, and the size and number of calcifications.

As on chest radiographs, other findings seen on CT include lymphadenopathy, lymph node calcification (Fig. 21-4), and pleural effusion. Lymph node enlargement occurs in up to 75% of cases.

FIG. 21.1. Diffuse alveolar septal amyloidosis. A diffuse reticulonodular pattern is visible, with the abnormality predominating at the lung bases. Lung and lymph node calcification is present, and the heart is enlarged.

A

B

C

FIG. 21.2. Diffuse alveolar septal amyloidosis. **A:** Coned-down view of a PA radiograph shows a reticular pattern within the left lung, with a basal predominance. **B** and **C:** HRCT shows a diffuse nodular abnormality, with nodules visible in relation to the fissures and interlobular septa.

A

B

FIG. 21.3. Diffuse alveolar septal amyloidosis. HRCTs at two levels show extensive lung consolidation and calcification. A tracheal stent (*arrow* in **A**) is in place because of airway involvement and narrowing.

FIG. 21.4. Lymph node enlargement and calcification in amyloidosis. Mediastinal lymph nodes (*arrows*) are densely calcified.

FIG. 21.5. Localized nodular amyloidosis. A large right lung nodule is visible. Small subpleural nodules or focal pleural thickening also are seen.

The prognosis of patients is usually related to the underlying disease or to involvement of other organs such as the kidney, liver, and heart. In some patients, lung involvement is severe enough to require lung transplantation.

Localized Nodular Amyloidosis

Patients with localized nodular amyloidosis (localized AL) usually are asymptomatic. Localized nodular amyloidosis may manifest as single or multiple lung nodules or masses,

usually well-defined and round, ranging from 0.5 to 5 cm in diameter (Fig. 21-5), with stippled or dense calcification in up to 50% of cases on CT and cavitation in a small percentage. Nodules may grow slowly or remain stable over several years.

Localized Tracheobronchial Amyloidosis

Localized AL may involve the larynx, trachea, and central bronchi; focal deposits of amyloid within the airway wall or diffuse wall infiltration may be present. Symptoms are common and include hoarseness, stridor, dyspnea, cough, hemoptysis, and recurrent infections. The trachea typically is involved, and concentric or nodular wall infiltration is most common. Calcification is common (Fig. 21-6; also see Fig. 22-20 in Chapter 22).

A   **B**

FIG. 21.6. Tracheobronchial amyloidosis. **A:** CT shows extensive bronchial calcifications (*large arrows*). Hilar lymph node calcification (*small arrow*) also is present. **B:** Airway calcification due to amyloid deposition also is visible more peripherally.

PULMONARY ALVEOLAR MICROLITHIASIS

Pulmonary alveolar microlithiasis is characterized by the presence of numerous minute calculi (so-called *microliths* or *calcispheres*) within alveoli (Table 21-3). It is very rare but has a characteristic radiographic appearance.

Histologically, the calcispheres are located largely within the alveolar lumen, although they probably are formed within the alveolar walls. They consist of concentric layers of calcium phosphate. In the early stages of disease, the alveolar walls appear normal, although fibrosis may occur late in the disease process. Emphysema also may be seen, particularly in the apices and subpleural regions.

Microlithiasis may be seen at any age, but most cases occur in patients from 20 to 50 years of age. Its etiology is unknown, but in about half of cases, the disease also occurs in family members, particularly siblings, suggesting autosomal recessive transmission. Environmental factors also are involved. Abnormalities of calcium metabolism are absent.

Patients typically are asymptomatic at diagnosis, despite spectacular radiographic abnormalities. There is a tendency for the abnormalities to progress slowly over a period of several years, although findings may remain stable. Dyspnea may develop with progression of the disease, with other symptoms including hemoptysis and finger clubbing. Although lung fibrosis and cor pulmonale may develop, the prognosis generally is good. There is no treatment.

Radiographs show characteristic findings. Despite their small size, the individual calcispheres may be visible as discrete, dense dots, less than 1 mm in diameter (Fig. 21-7). A basal predominance is typical (see Fig. 21-7). When limited in number, the calcispheres predominate in a subpleural location and in relation to vessels, bronchi, and interlobular septa. When myriad, they become confluent and appear very dense, obscuring the hemidiaphragm, heart, and

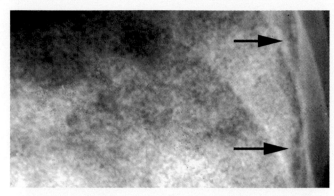

FIG. 21.7. Alveolar microlithiasis. Detail view of the left lower lobe in a patient with diffuse lung opacity. Individual dense calcispheres are visible. The subpleural lung appears relatively lucent (*arrows*). This is the so-called black pleural line.

mediastinal contours. If the lungs are sufficiently dense, the heart may appear relatively lucent, a very unusual finding. Another typical finding on chest radiographs, although it is not always seen, is the so-called *black pleural line*, a stripe of relative lucency at the pleural surface (see Fig. 21-7). Although this feature was thought to be due to sparing of the pleura by the calcispheres, it reflects small subpleural areas of emphysema.

High-resolution CT (HRCT) shows a posterior and lower lobe predominance of the calcifications with a high concentration in the subpleural parenchyma and in association with bronchi and vessels (Figs. 21-8 and 21-9). A perilobular and centrilobular distribution of the calcifications may be seen, or calcifications may be associated with interlobular septa. Intraparenchymal emphysema may be seen.

TABLE 21.3 Pulmonary Alveolar Microlithiasis
Calcispheres within alveoli (consist of calcium phosphate)
Very rare
20–50 years of age
Familial incidence in half
Often asymptomatic at diagnosis
Abnormalities progress slowly
Radiographs
Dense lungs
Basal predominance
Individual calcified nodules visible
Black pleural line
HRCT
Subpleural and perivascular predominance of calcified nodules
Black pleural line = emphysema

FIG. 21.8. HRCT in alveolar microlithiasis. Extensive lung calcification is present with a subpleural and perivascular predominance.

FIG. 21.9. HRCT in alveolar microlithiasis. Lung calcification is confluent in some regions and nodular in others. Small areas of emphysema (*arrows*) in the peripheral lung account for the black pleural line.

Subpleural paraseptal emphysema (i.e., the black pleural line) is common (see Fig. 21-9). In children or patients with early disease, ground-glass opacity or reticulation may be the predominant finding; calcifications may be difficult to detect.

Calcification of small interstitial nodules seen on HRCT has a limited differential diagnosis. Multifocal lung calcification, often associated with lung nodules, also has been reported in association with amyloidosis, infectious granulomatous diseases such as tuberculosis, sarcoidosis, silicosis and coal-worker's pneumoconiosis, talcosis, and metastatic calcification.

METASTATIC CALCIFICATION

The term *metastatic calcification* refers to the deposition of calcium in soft tissues due to abnormal calcium and phosphate metabolism (Table 21-4). It is associated with hypercalcemia and is most common in patients with chronic renal failure and secondary hyperparathyroidism and in those undergoing chronic hemodialysis.

Metastatic calcification commonly affects the lung; it typically is interstitial, involving the alveolar septa, bronchioles, and pulmonary arteries, and can be associated with secondary lung fibrosis. Patients may be asymptomatic or may have dyspnea. With appropriate treatment of the underlying abnormality, metastatic calcification may resolve.

Abnormalities typically predominate in the lung apices because they are more alkaline than the lung bases, increasing the likelihood of calcium salt precipitation in this region. A higher ratio of ventilation to perfusion in the apices

TABLE 21.4 Metastatic Calcification

Calcification due to abnormal calcium and phosphate metabolism
Hypercalcemia
Renal failure
Secondary hyperparathyroidism
Chronic hemodialysis
Commonly affects lung
Apices most often involved (more alkaline)
Radiographs
Nodular opacities or consolidation
HRCT
Opacities often centrilobular
May be ground-glass opacity
May or may not appear calcified
Radionuclide bone (^{99m}Tc-diphosphonate) scintigraphy useful
Opacities may resolve with treatment

results in a decrease in the partial pressure of CO_2 and a corresponding increase in pH.

Plain radiographs are relatively insensitive in detecting metastatic calcification. In some patients, ill-defined nodules or patchy areas of increased opacity may be seen (Figs. 21-10 and 21-11A). Nodules visible on chest films usually appear to be about 1 to 2 cm in diameter. They may or may not appear to be of calcium density. With progressive

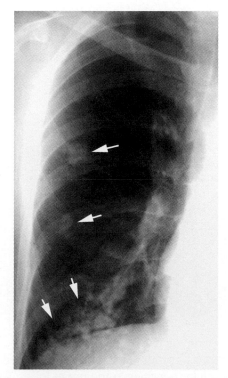

FIG. 21.10. Metastatic calcification in a patient with renal disease and secondary hyperparathyroidism. Dense nodular opacities (*arrows*) are visible in the right lung.

FIG. 21.11. Metastatic calcification in renal failure. **A:** Chest radiograph shows ill-defined nodular opacities (*arrows*) with an apical predominance. **B** and **C:** CT with a lung window setting shows nodular opacities in the peripheral upper lobes. These opacities appear lobular or centrilobular in distribution. **D:** Soft tissue window scan shows evidence of calcification.

FIG. 21.12. Metastatic calcification in renal failure. **A** and **B:** HRCTs with a lung window setting show nodular opacities in the upper lobes. These opacities appear centrilobular in distribution. They were not obviously calcified on soft tissue windows. (*Figure continues.*)

C

D

FIG. 21.12. (*continued.*) **C:** CT at the lung base shows dense subpleural calcification and calcification of consolidated lung (*arrows*). **D:** Radionuclide bone (⁹⁹ᵐTc-diphosphonate) scintigraphy shows extensive isotope uptake within both lungs.

disease, these opacities become confluent, mimicking pneumonia. An apical predominance of opacities is typical but not invariable (see Fig. 21-11A).

CT can show areas of ground-glass opacity, consolidation, or calcification in the absence of plain film abnormalities. Numerous fluffy and poorly defined nodules, measuring 3 to 10 mm in diameter, are typical, but opacities can appear focal, centrilobular, lobular, patchy, or diffuse (Figs. 21-11 to 21-13). Even with HRCT, these opacities

may not appear calcified. An apical predominance is common. Calcification of vessels in the chest wall may also be seen.

Radionuclide bone (⁹⁹ᵐTc-diphosphonate) scintigraphy (see Fig. 21-12D) is highly sensitive for the detection of metastatic calcification, and may show lung uptake when chest films are normal. It may serve to confirm the diagnosis when CT shows typical apical opacities without obvious calcification.

FIG. 21.13. Metastatic calcification in renal failure. HRCT shows centrilobular and lobular ground-glass opacities without obvious calcification. A dialysis catheter is in place.

SELECTED READING

Aylwin ACB, Gishen P, Copley SJ. Imaging appearance of thoracic amyloidosis. J Thorac Imaging 2005; 20:41–46.

Ayuso MC, Gilabert R, Bombi JA, Salvador A. CT appearance of localized pulmonary amyloidosis. J Comput Assist Tomogr 1987; 11:197–199.

Cluzel P, Grenier P, Bernadac P, et al. Pulmonary alveolar microlithiasis: CT findings. J Comput Assist Tomogr 1991; 15:938–942.

Deniz O, Ors F, Tozkoparan E, et al. High resolution computed tomographic features of pulmonary alveolar microlithiasis. Eur J Radiol 2005; 55:452–460.

Georgiades CS, Neyman EG, Barish MA, et al. Amyloidosis: review and CT manifestations. Radiographics 2004; 24:405–416.

Graham CM, Stern EJ, Finkbeiner WE, Webb WR. High-resolution CT appearance of diffuse alveolar septal amyloidosis. AJR Am J Roentgenol 1992; 158:265–267.

Hartman TE, Müller NL, Primack SL, et al. Metastatic pulmonary calcification in patients with hypercalcemia: findings on chest radiographs and CT scans. AJR Am J Roentgenol 1994; 162:799–802.

Helbich TH, Wojnarovsky C, Wunderbaldinger P, et al. Pulmonary alveolar microlithiasis in children: radiographic and high-resolution CT findings. AJR Am J Roentgenol 1997; 168:63–65.

Johkoh T, Ikezoe J, Nagareda T, et al. Metastatic pulmonary calcification: early detection by high-resolution CT. J Comput Assist Tomogr 1993; 17:471–473.

Korn MA, Schurawitzki H, Klepetko W, Burghuber OC. Pulmonary alveolar microlithiasis: findings on high-resolution CT. AJR Am J Roentgenol 1992; 158:981–982.

Kuhlman JE, Ren H, Hutchins GM, Fishman EK. Fulminant pulmonary calcification complicating renal transplantation: CT demonstration. Radiology 1989; 173:459–460.

Lachmann HJ, Goodman HJB, Gilbertson JA, et al. Natural history and outcome in systemic AA amyloidosis. N Engl J Med 2007; 356:2361–2371.

Pickford HA, Swensen SJ, Utz JP. Thoracic cross-sectional imaging of amyloidosis. AJR Am J Roentgenol 1997; 168:351–355.

Utz JP, Swensen SJ, Gertz MA. Pulmonary amyloidosis. The Mayo Clinic experience from 1980 to 1993. Ann Intern Med 1996; 124:407–413.

The Trachea

W. RICHARD WEBB

THE NORMAL TRACHEA

The trachea extends from the inferior aspect of the cricoid cartilage (at the level of the sixth cervical vertebra) to the carina (at the level of the fifth thoracic vertebra). It measures from 10 to 12 cm in length. The trachea is divided into extrathoracic and intrathoracic portions at the level it passes posterior to the manubrium; the extrathoracic trachea is 2 to 4 cm in length, while the intrathoracic trachea measures 6 to 9 cm in length. From 16 to 22 horseshoe-shaped bands of hyaline cartilage support the anterior and lateral tracheal walls. The incomplete posterior portion of these rings is bridged by a thin band of smooth muscle and fibrous tissue, the *posterior tracheal membrane* (Fig. 22-1).

The plain film appearance of the trachea is described in Chapter 7. On CT, the trachea usually is round or oval in shape, but it can appear horseshoe-shaped, triangular, or like an inverted pear in some normal patients. The tracheal wall is delineated by air in its lumen internally and by mediastinal fat externally, and is usually visible as a 1- to 2-mm soft tissue stripe. The posterior tracheal membrane appears thinner than the anterior and lateral tracheal walls, and is variable in shape due to its lack of cartilage; it can appear convex, concave, or flat. The tracheal cartilages may appear calcified or slightly denser than adjacent soft tissue. Calcification of cartilage is most common in older patients, and is particularly common in women (Fig. 22-2). In patients with calcified cartilage, little soft tissue is seen in the tracheal wall internal to the cartilage.

Tracheal diameter varies widely in normal subjects. In normal men, tracheal diameter averages 19.5 mm, with a range of 13 to 25 mm (mean ± 3 SD) in the coronal plane and 13 to 27 mm in the sagittal plane. In women, tracheal diameter is slightly smaller, averaging 17.5 mm and ranging from 10 to 21 mm in the coronal plane and 10 to 23 mm in the sagittal plane.

On CT performed during or after forced expiration, the posterior tracheal membrane bulges anteriorly, narrowing and, in some cases, nearly obliterating the tracheal lumen (Fig. 22-3). The mean anterior-posterior diameter of the trachea decreases by 30% to 40% during forced expiration due to anterior bulging of the posterior membrane; the transverse diameter decreases by 10% to 20%. The cross-sectional area of the trachea may diminish by more than 50% in normal subjects with forced expiration.

Tracheal Bronchus

A tracheal bronchus represents the origin of all or part (usually the apical segment) of the right upper lobe bronchus from the trachea; its incidence is about 0.1% (see Figs. 1-1 and 1-2 in Chapter 1). Left tracheal bronchus also occurs but is much less common.

ABNORMALITIES ASSOCIATED WITH TRACHEAL NARROWING

Focal tracheal narrowing may be seen with tracheal tumors, tuberculosis (TB), tracheal stenosis or stricture, tracheomalacia, or occasionally with saber sheath trachea, Wegener's granulomatosis, or amyloidosis. Diffuse or generalized tracheal narrowing may be seen with tracheomalacia, saber sheath trachea, Wegener's granulomatosis, amyloidosis, tracheobronchopathia osteochondroplastica, and relapsing polychondritis.

Tracheal Tumors

Tumors of the trachea are rare (Table 22-1). Symptoms often are absent or nonspecific (e.g., cough, dyspnea), and early diagnosis is difficult. Tracheal tumors tend to be inconspicuous on chest radiographs, and may become quite large before they are detected. CT is highly sensitive in detecting tracheal tumors and their extent of spread. Together, squamous cell carcinoma and adenoid cystic carcinoma account for more than 85% of tracheal tumors. Tumors of many other cell types, both epithelial and mesenchymal, may occur in the trachea but are much less common.

Squamous cell carcinoma is associated with smoking and is multifocal in 10% of cases, often involving the distal trachea; a main bronchus also may be involved (see Figs. 3-19 and 3-20 in Chapter 3). *Adenoid cystic carcinoma* originates from tracheal mucous glands and is most common in the upper trachea (Figs. 22-4 and 22-5). It is slightly less common than squamous cell carcinoma. Adenoid cystic carcinoma often arises from the posterolateral tracheal wall (Figs. 22-5 and 22-6B).

On CT, a primary malignant tracheal tumor may appear as a polypoid lesion, a focal sessile lesion, eccentric narrowing of the tracheal lumen, or circumferential wall thickening

A   **B**

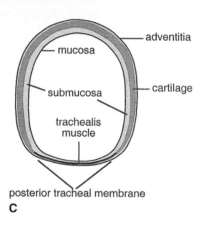

FIG. 22.1. The normal trachea. **A:** HRCT through the normal trachea. The tracheal wall (*arrow*) is outlined by mediastinal fat externally and usually is visible as a 1- to 2-mm soft-tissue stripe. The posterior tracheal membrane usually appears thinner than the anterior and lateral tracheal walls, and is variable in shape due to its lack of cartilage. At this level, it is partially obscured by the esophagus. **B:** At the level of the aortic arch, the tracheal wall (*arrows*) is outlined by mediastinal fat and the right lung in the region of the right paratracheal stripe. The tracheal wall appears thin. **C:** Diagrammatic representation of the normal components of the tracheal wall.

C

FIG. 22.2. Normal calcification of tracheal cartilage in an elderly woman. Discontinuous calcification of the tracheal wall reflects calcification of individual cartilage rings. The tracheal wall appears thin.

(see Fig. 22-5). Attachment to the tracheal wall may be either broad based (Fig. 22-5) or narrow and pedunculated. CT may underestimate the longitudinal extent of the tumor; submucosal spread may be difficult to see on CT. However, CT is superior to bronchoscopy in evaluating extraluminal spread and the trachea distal to an obstructing lesion.

Metastases to the trachea may occur via direct extension or by hematogenous spread. Direct extension to involve the trachea most often is secondary to a primary tumor of the lung, larynx, esophagus, or thyroid. These tumors may compress the trachea, displacing tracheal cartilage inward, or may invade the tracheal lumen, with tumor being seen as abnormal tissue internal to tracheal cartilage (Fig. 22-7; also see Fig. 3-38 in Chapter 3). Hematogenous metastases usually originate from melanoma, or from carcinomas of the breast, colon, or kidney. On CT, hematogenous metastases may appear as single or multiple, sessile or pedunculated endotracheal lesions (Fig. 22-8).

Squamous cell papilloma is the most common benign tracheal tumor. It represents an abnormal proliferation of squamous epithelium, and may appear sessile, papillary, lobulated, or polypoid. Solitary papilloma is associated with

A   **B**

FIG. 22.3. Normal expiratory CT. **A:** On inspiration, the trachea has a rounded appearance. **B:** During a dynamic forced expiratory scan, there is marked anterior bowing of the posterior tracheal membrane (*arrow*). This appearance is normal. Little side-to-side narrowing occurs because of the tracheal cartilage.

TABLE 22.1 Tracheal Tumors

Primary malignant
Most common (85% of cases)
   Squamous cell carcinoma
   Adenoid cystic carcinoma
Rare
   Other types of bronchogenic carcinoma
   Carcinoid tumor
   Sarcoma
   Lymphoma

Metastatic
Direct invasion most common
   Thyroid carcinoma
   Laryngeal cancer
   Lung cancer
   Esophageal cancer
Hematogenous metastases
   Melanoma
   Breast carcinoma
   Colon carcinoma
   Kidney carcinoma

Benign
Squamous cell papilloma
Papillomatosis
Hamartoma
Mesenchymal tumors

FIG. 22.4. Adenoid cystic carcinoma of the proximal trachea. An eccentric narrowing (*arrows*) of the tracheal lumen is caused by a sessile mass arising from the right tracheal wall.

A

B

FIG. 22.5. Adenoid cystic carcinoma of the trachea. **A:** A large mass (*large arrows*) in the upper trachea markedly narrows the tracheal lumen (*small arrow*) and invades the mediastinum. **B:** On a sagittal reconstruction, the mass (*arrows*) can be seen to arise from the posterior tracheal wall. This location is typical of adenoid cystic carcinoma.

smoking and is most common in adults. The condition of multiple papillomas (i.e., papillomatosis) usually begins in childhood with laryngeal involvement and is associated with human papillomavirus infection. On CT, a solitary papilloma appears as a well-circumscribed nodule that is confined to the tracheal wall and projects into the tracheal lumen; it often shows acute angles where it contacts the tracheal wall. Tracheal cartilage is unaffected. Papillomatosis is characterized by numerous nodules involving the entire length of the trachea (see Fig. 3-56 in Chapter 3) or diffuse thickening of the tracheal wall (Fig. 22-9). Other benign tracheal tumors include hamartoma and tumors of mesenchymal origin such as lipoma or chondroma.

polypoid   sessile

circumferential wall thickening

A   B

M

FIG. 22.6. CT appearances of primary tracheal tumor. **A:** Tracheal malignancies may appear polypoid, sessile, or circumferential. **B:** Adenoid cystic carcinoma results in a sessile mass (*M*) arising from the posterior tracheal wall and protruding into the tracheal lumen. The mass extends into the adjacent mediastinum (*arrows*).

FIG. 22.7. Esophageal carcinoma with tracheal invasion. Tumor has invaded the trachea and is seen as soft tissue (*small arrows*) internal to the calcified tracheal cartilage (*large arrows*). The tracheal lumen is narrowed.

A

B

C

FIG. 22.8. Tracheal metastasis. Tracheal metastases may result in tracheal compression with inward displacement of the tracheal wall, an endotracheal mass, or a combination of these findings. **A, B:** There is narrowing of the trachea with an endoluminal mass (*arrow*). **C:** Soft-tissue window at the same level as (**B**) shows a mass involving the right tracheal wall and mediastinal soft tissues (*arrows*).

FIG. 22.9. Tracheobronchial papillomatosis with tracheal wall thickening. **A:** Concentric thickening of the tracheal wall (*arrows*) is due to diffuse involvement by papillomas. The tracheal lumen is markedly narrowed. **B:** Multiple cystic pulmonary lesions may be seen in some patients with tracheobronchial papillomatosis.

Tracheomalacia

Tracheomalacia refers to weakness of the tracheal wall, usually due to abnormalities of the tracheal cartilage, associated with excessive collapsibility of the trachea on expiration (Table 22-2). It may be congenital and associated with deficient cartilage, but most often is acquired as a result of intubation injuries, tracheal compression by extrinsic masses or vascular lesions (e.g., aortic aneurysm), chronic infection, chronic obstructive pulmonary disease, or in association

TABLE 22.2 Non-Neoplastic Tracheal Diseases

Disease	Extent	Appearance	Associations
Tracheomalacia	Focal or diffuse	Collapse of tracheal wall with expiration	Congenital intubation, extrinsic masses, chronic infection, COPD, saber sheath trachea, polychondritis, tracheobronchomegaly
Tuberculosis	Distal trachea (and main bronchi)	Early: concentric wall thickening Late: stricture or distortion of cartilage	Mediastinal lymph node disease
Post intubation stenosis	Proximal trachea	Early: concentric wall thickening Late: stricture or distortion of cartilage	Malacia may be present
Saber-sheath trachea	Early: thoracic inlet Late: intrathoracic trachea	Side-to-side narrowing, sagittal diameter normal or increased	COPD, chronic cough; malacia may be present
Wegener's granulomatosis	Focal (subglottic trachea) or diffuse	Concentric wall thickening, cartilage destruction	Occurs in 15–25% of cases; malacia not often present
Amyloidosis	Focal (nodular) or diffuse	Concentric or nodular wall thickening	Calcification common; malacia is not present
Tracheobronchopathia osteochondroplastica	Diffuse	Calcified submucosal nodules adjacent to tracheal cartilage, nodules spare the posterior membrane	Malacia is not present
Relapsing polychondritis	Diffuse	Thickening of anterior and lateral wall, posterior membrane normal	Arthritis; malacia may be present
Tracheobronchomegaly (Mounier-Kuhn syndrome)	Diffuse	Increased tracheal diameter (>3 cm), tracheal wall normal or appears scalloped, tracheal diverticula	Cystic bronchiectasis often present; COPD, pulmonary fibrosis, Marfan's syndrome, cystic fibrosis, Ehlers-Danlos syndrome, cutis laxa

with saber-sheath trachea, relapsing polychondritis, or tracheobronchomegaly. It may be localized, or it may involve a long tracheal segment.

Abnormal flaccidity of the tracheal wall may result in inefficient cough, retention of secretions, and chronic airway infection and bronchiectasis. Symptoms include recurrent infection, dyspnea, and stridor.

Radiographs or CT on inspiration may show increased or decreased tracheal diameter in patients with tracheomalacia. The hallmark of tracheomalacia is a significant decrease in the tracheal diameter or collapse of the tracheal walls with expiration (see also Fig. 22-10). Tracheal collapse may be diffuse or side to side. A 50% decrease in tracheal diameter or cross-sectional area with expiration is usually considered indicative of tracheomalacia, but this degree of tracheal narrowing may be seen in normals. With forced expiration, invagination of the posterior tracheal membrane may result in near-complete obliteration of the tracheal lumen in some normal subjects (see Fig. 22-3). A diagnosis of tracheomalacia should generally be avoided in the absence of symptoms or pulmonary function findings of airway obstruction (Fig. 22-10).

Tuberculosis

TB typically involves both the distal trachea and the proximal main bronchi; isolated tracheal disease is rare. Active inflammation with granulation tissue causes irregular circumferential wall thickening with narrowing of the tracheal lumen. In many cases, tracheal infection results from spread from adjacent lymph nodes, and enlarged mediastinal nodes or increased density of mediastinal fat may be seen. Tracheal TB also may occur due to endobronchial spread of infection.

With treatment, wall thickening and tracheal narrowing usually are reversible, although in some patients stricture results, with narrowing of the tracheal lumen in the absence of wall thickening.

Bronchial strictures may be associated with tracheal narrowing. Strictures from TB most often involve the left main bronchus, perhaps because it is longer than the right. CT findings that help to differentiate TB stricture from carcinoma include a long segment of circumferential involvement and the absence of an intraluminal mass.

Tracheal Stenosis

Congenital tracheal stenosis may result from a ring-shaped tracheal cartilage. Acquired tracheal stenosis usually is due to prior intubation or tracheostomy. Progressive dyspnea following extubation typically is present. Inflammation and pressure necrosis of the tracheal mucosa most commonly occur at either the tracheostomy stoma or at the level of the tube balloon, 1 to 1.5 cm proximal to the tube tip; the stenosis usually involves 1.5 to 2.5 cm of the tracheal wall. The extrathoracic trachea most often is involved. Focal narrowing may be seen if the tube tip presses on one part of the tracheal wall, usually the anterior wall.

Acute postintubation stenosis results from edema of the tracheal wall or intraluminal granulation tissue. Plain films may show an eccentric or hourglass-shaped tracheal narrowing. On CT, this may be seen as eccentric or concentric soft tissue internal to normal-appearing tracheal cartilage (Fig. 22-11). The outer tracheal wall has a normal appearance, without evidence of deformity or narrowing. Dynamic expiratory images show little change in tracheal dimensions.

A   **B**

FIG. 22.10. Tracheomalacia in a patient with pulmonary function test findings of airway obstruction and "negative effort dependence" (the harder the patient tried to expire, the more obstruction there was). **A:** CT obtained on inspiration shows the trachea to be normal in caliber. There is a mild saber-sheath tracheal deformity (**B**). Following a forced expiration, there in marked narrowing of the lumen of the trachea with reduction in both its coronal and its sagittal diameters.

FIG. 22.11. Postintubation tracheal stenosis due to granulation tissue. **A:** Near the thoracic inlet, the trachea appears normal. **B:** Below the level shown in (**A**), focal narrowing of the tracheal lumen is associated with increased soft tissue (*white arrows*) within the tracheal lumen. The calcified tracheal cartilage (*black arrows*) appears normal, without evidence of deformity or collapse. **C:** Coronal reconstruction in a patient with an hourglass-shaped tracheal stenosis following intubation. The tracheal wall appears normal (*large arrows*), and granulation tissue is seen narrowing the tracheal lumen (*small arrows*). **D:** Diagrammatic representation of tracheal stenosis due to granulation tissue, compared to the appearance of a normal trachea. (From **Webb EM, Elicker BM, Webb WR.** Using CT to diagnose nonneoplastic tracheal abnormalities: appearance of the tracheal wall. AJR Am J Roentgenol 2000; 174:1315–1321.)

A

B

normal

tracheal stenosis
(cartilage deformity)

C

FIG. 22.12. Postintubation tracheal stenosis due to stricture. **A** and **B:** CT at two levels shows side-to-side narrowing of the tracheal lumen resulting from deformity of the tracheal cartilage (*arrows*). **C:** Diagrammatic representation of tracheal stenosis due to cartilage deformity, compared to the appearance of a normal trachea. (From **Webb EM, Elicker BM, Webb WR.** Using CT to diagnose nonneoplastic tracheal abnormalities: appearance of the tracheal wall. AJR Am J Roentgenol 2000; 174:1315–1321.)

With *chronic postintubation stenosis* or stricture, fibrosis usually is present with deformity of tracheal cartilage and collapse of the tracheal wall. On CT, thickening of the mucosa and submucosa is absent or mild, and deformity of the tracheal cartilage or posterior tracheal membrane accounts for narrowing of the lumen (Figs. 22-12 and 22-13). The area of narrowing may be thin and weblike or long and hourglass shaped. Dynamic expiratory images may or may not show significant malacia. Because of the focal nature of the stenosis, treatment with stenting is useful.

Acute and chronic stenosis may also result from sarcoidosis, histoplasmosis, Wegener's granulomatosis, and ulcerative colitis.

Saber-Sheath Trachea

Saber-sheath trachea is common and almost always is associated with chronic obstructive pulmonary disease. It is characterized by a marked decrease in the coronal diameter of the intrathoracic trachea associated with an increase in its sagittal diameter (Fig. 22-14); the extrathoracic trachea is normal. Although it may involve the entire intrathoracic trachea, in its earliest stages it is visible only at the thoracic inlet. It is thought to be due to chronic injury and malacia of tracheal cartilage due to coughing or increased intrathoracic pressure. The main bronchi are of normal size.

On frontal radiographs, a characteristic side-to-side narrowing of the tracheal lumen is visible beginning at the thoracic inlet (see Fig. 22-14). The right paratracheal stripe, primarily representing tracheal wall, appears normal or slightly increased in thickness. On the lateral radiograph, the tracheal diameter appears normal or slightly increased. If the tracheal diameter on the lateral film measures 1.5 times that seen on the frontal film, saber sheath trachea is considered to be present.

FIG. 22.13. Postintubation tracheal stenosis due to deformity of tracheal cartilage. **A:** CT shows side-to-side narrowing of the tracheal lumen resulting from deformity of the tracheal cartilage (*arrows*). The tracheal wall is outlined by mediastinal fat. **B:** Coronal reconstruction shows an hourglass-shaped stenosis, with inward collapse of the tracheal wall (*white arrows*). Calcified tracheal cartilage (*black arrow*) is displaced inward. **C:** Three-dimensional reconstruction shows the hourglass-shaped stenosis.

On CT, there is inward displacement of the lateral portions of the tracheal wall and tracheal cartilage with side-to-side narrowing of the tracheal lumen (Fig. 22-15). The tracheal wall usually is of normal thickness. During forced expiration, CT demonstrates further inward bowing of the tracheal walls in many patients.

Wegener's Granulomatosis

Wegener's granulomatosis is a systemic vasculitis. In 90% of cases, serum antineutrophil cytoplasmic antibodies characterized by a diffuse granular cytoplasmic immunofluorescent staining pattern (cytoplasmic antineutrophil cytoplasmic antibody [C-ANCA]) are present.

Tracheobronchial involvement occurs in about 15% to 25% of cases; symptoms are common and include hoarseness, cough, and stridor. Subglottic tracheal involvement is most typical (Fig. 22-16), with variable involvement of the vocal cords, distal trachea, and proximal mainstem bronchi. Abnormalities may be focal or diffuse. Pathologic findings include circumferential airway wall thickening and inflammation, and concentric narrowing of the tracheal lumen; mucosal ulceration and destruction of the cricoid or tracheal cartilage are less common. Tracheal involvement may be life threatening, but treatment with stents may be helpful.

Plain radiographs show tracheal narrowing on both the frontal and lateral radiographs; this narrowing may be localized or diffuse. Characteristic CT findings include focal or

FIG. 22.14. Saber-sheath trachea in a patient with chronic obstructive pulmonary disease. **A:** PA chest radiograph shows hourglass-shaped narrowing of the intrathoracic trachea (*black arrows*). The extrathoracic trachea (*white arrows*) appears normal. **B:** In the lateral projection, the tracheal diameter appears normal or increased (*arrows*).

circumferential thickening of the tracheal wall, an increase in the overall tracheal diameter due to wall thickening, and narrowing of the tracheal lumen (Fig. 22-17). Malacia is not typically seen, but may be present (Fig. 22-18). Proximal bronchi may be involved (Figs. 22-17C and 22-19).

Amyloidosis

Tracheobronchial amyloidosis is rare (see Chapter 21). Symptoms are common and include hoarseness, stridor, dyspnea, cough, hemoptysis, and recurrent infections.

Primary tracheobronchial amyloidosis is usually confined to the airways, with no evidence of concurrent parenchymal disease. Deposits are multifocal or diffuse, being submucosal in location, and involve the length of the trachea; the main bronchi also are commonly affected. On plain radiographs and CT, diffuse tracheobronchial amyloidosis usually leads to concentric or nodular thickening of the tracheal wall (Fig. 22-20). Calcification or ossification is common. Malacia is not present. Rarely, a single localized submucosal nodule is present, resulting in eccentric wall thickening. Multiple isolated lesions also may be seen. Atelectasis may be associated with bronchial involvement. Progression is typical, and bronchoscopic resection of focal lesions or airway stenting may be helpful in some cases.

Tracheobronchopathia Osteochondroplastica

Tracheobronchopathia osteochondroplastica is a rare, benign disease characterized by the development of cartilaginous and osseous nodules within the submucosa of the tracheal and bronchial walls. It is most typical in men older than 50, and usually is detected incidentally. In some patients, dyspnea, cough, hemoptysis, and wheezing may be present.

Nodules tend to be localized to the submucosa directly associated with the tracheal cartilage, sparing the posterior tracheal membrane (Figs. 22-21 and 22-22). The nodules may consist of cartilage or exostoses occurring in relation to the perichondrium of the tracheal cartilage, or they may be metaplastic, arising in elastic tissue.

Plain radiographs show extensive irregular tracheal and central bronchial calcification. CT findings include thickened cartilage with small irregular nodules along their inner aspect, protruding into the tracheal lumen (Figs. 22-21 and 22-22). The nodules typically measure between 3 and 8 mm in diameter and are usually calcified. The appearance is much more irregular than that seen with normal cartilage calcification. Similar central bronchial calcification also is seen in many patients. No significant decrease in tracheal diameter is seen with forced expiration.

FIG. 22.15. Saber-sheath trachea on CT. **A:** The extrathoracic trachea is normal. The tracheal cartilage is calcified and well seen. **B** and **C:** The intrathoracic trachea at two levels is markedly narrowed from side to side (*arrows*), associated with deformity of the tracheal cartilage. The sagittal tracheal diameter is increased. The tracheal wall is otherwise normal in appearance. **D:** Diagrammatic representation of saber-sheath trachea. (From **Webb EM, Elicker BM, Webb WR.** Using CT to diagnose nonneoplastic tracheal abnormalities: appearance of the tracheal wall. AJR Am J Roentgenol 2000; 174:1315–1321.)

A   B

FIG. 22.16. Subglottic tracheal stenosis in Wegener's granulomatosis. **A:** Excessive soft tissue (*arrows*) is visible internal to the cricoid cartilage. A tracheostomy is in place below this level. **B:** Coronal reconstruction in subglottic stenosis due to Wegener's granulomatosis. The focal narrowing (*large arrows*) is just below the level of the vocal cords (*small arrows*).

Relapsing Polychondritis

Relapsing polychondritis is a rare systemic disorder characterized by recurrent episodes of cartilage inflammation most commonly affecting the ear, nose, joints, and the laryngeal and tracheal cartilage. Nonerosive polyarthritis, nasal deformity, and auricular chondritis are characteristic, but need not be present in all cases. The upper airways are affected in more than 50% of cases, and recurrent pneumonia is the most common cause of death. Diffuse tracheal involvement, characterized by a dense inflammatory exudate, is limited to the cartilage and perichondrium, and does not affect the mucosa or submucosa. Histologic findings include edema, granulation tissue, cartilage destruction, and, eventually, fibrosis of the tracheal wall. Both the extrathoracic and intrathoracic portions of the trachea are involved. Treatment often requires the use of tracheal and bronchial stents to maintain airway patency.

Plain radiographs usually show cylindrical narrowing of the extrathoracic and intrathoracic trachea and main bronchi (Fig. 22-23). In most cases, CT shows thickening of the anterior and lateral tracheal walls, but the posterior membrane is of normal thickness (Figs. 22-24 and 22-25). Both the inner and outer margins of the thickened tracheal walls are smooth in contour. Collapse of tracheal cartilage may be seen in chronic disease. Narrowing of both the tracheal lumen and the main bronchi is often present. Tracheomalacia is often present (Fig. 22-26).

ABNORMALITIES ASSOCIATED WITH INCREASED TRACHEAL DIAMETER

Tracheal Diverticulum

Tracheal diverticulum represents a focal herniation of tracheal mucosa through the tracheal wall. Tracheal diverticulum may be seen in normal subjects, although it tends to be associated with chronic obstructive pulmonary disease. It usually is asymptomatic and is detected incidentally.

Tracheal diverticulum almost always occurs near the thoracic inlet, along the posterolateral right trachea, between the cartilaginous and muscular portions of the tracheal wall (Fig. 22-27). It can appear as an isolated paratracheal air cyst (Fig. 22-28), usually a few millimeters in diameter, or as an air-filled structure communicating with the tracheal lumen (see Fig. 22-27). Tracheal diverticulum is easily seen on CT, but is rarely visible on plain radiographs.

Mounier-Kuhn Syndrome (Tracheobronchomegaly)

Tracheobronchomegaly, also referred to as *Mounier-Kuhn syndrome*, is characterized by marked dilatation of the trachea and mainstem bronchi, often in association with tracheal diverticulosis, recurrent lower respiratory tract infections, and bronchiectasis, which is typically cystic in appearance (see Table 22-2). Tracheobronchomegaly is diagnosed most often in men in their third and fourth decades; it is much

(*text continues on page 565*)

FIG. 22.17. Tracheal and bronchial narrowing in Wegener's granulomatosis. **A:** Chest radiograph shows bilateral lung nodules (*arrows*). A tracheostomy is in place. **B:** CT shows tracheal narrowing associated with concentric thickening of the tracheal wall (*arrows*). **C:** At the level of the carina, bronchial wall thickening (*arrow*) also is seen. **D:** Diagrammatic representation of abnormalities in Wegener's granulomatosis. Concentric wall thickening is visible. (From **Webb EM, Elicker BM, Webb WR.** Using CT to diagnose nonneoplastic tracheal abnormalities: appearance of the tracheal wall. AJR Am J Roentgenol 2000; 174:1315–1321.)

A

B

FIG. 22.18. Tracheomalacia in Wegener's granulomatosis. **A:** CT on inspiration shows the tracheal lumen to be slightly reduced in diameter. **B:** CT during dynamic forced expiration shows marked reduction in the tracheal lumen. The patient was symptomatic.

A

B

FIG. 22.19. Bronchial narrowing in Wegener's granulomatosis. **A:** CT shows narrowing of the proximal left main bronchus, associated with thickening of its wall (*arrows*). **B:** Three-dimensional reconstruction shows left main bronchus narrowing (*arrows*). The distal trachea is slightly narrowed.

FIG. 22.20. Tracheobronchial amyloidosis. CTs through the proximal trachea using lung (**A**) and soft tissue (**B**) windows show eccentric thickening of the tracheal wall (*arrows*). **C:** CT shows nodular thickening and calcification of the walls of the right main and right upper lobe bronchi (*arrows*). **D:** Coronal reformation shows tracheal wall thickening (*large arrows*) and focal thickening and calcification of bronchial walls (*small arrows*). Lymph node calcification also is visible. **E:** Diagrammatic representation of the appearance of the trachea in amyloidosis. Concentric or nodular wall thickening is seen, sometimes with calcification.

FIG. 22.21. Tracheobronchopathia osteochondroplastica. **A** and **B:** CT at two levels shows nodular thickening and calcification of the anterior and lateral tracheal wall. The posterior tracheal membrane is normal in thickness and devoid of calcifications. **C:** Diagrammatic representation of the appearance of the trachea in tracheobronchopathia osteochondroplastica. Tracheal cartilages are thickened, with small irregular calcific nodules along their inner aspect, protruding into the tracheal lumen. (From **Webb EM, Elicker BM, Webb WR.** Using CT to diagnose nonneoplastic tracheal abnormalities: appearance of the tracheal wall. AJR Am J Roentgenol 2000; 174:1315–1321.)

A   B

C

FIG. 22.22. Tracheobronchopathia osteochon-droplastica. **A** and **B:** CT at two levels shows nodules arising from the anterior and lateral tracheal wall, projecting into the lumen. The nodules are uncalcified. **C:** Photograph at bronchoscopy shows nodules arising from tracheal cartilage. The posterior trachea is normal.

FIG. 22.23. Relapsing polychondritis. Chest radiograph shows cylindrical narrowing of the entire trachea (*arrows*).

FIG. 22.24. Relapsing polychondritis. A: CT shows tracheal narrowing. The anterior and lateral tracheal walls (i.e., the cartilaginous portions) are thickened (*large arrows*). The posterior tracheal membrane is of normal thickness (*small arrow*). This appearance is characteristic. **B:** Narrowing of the main bronchi also is seen. The anterior bronchial walls are thickened (*large arrows*), while the posterior wall of the bronchus appears normal (*small arrow*). **C:** Diagrammatic representation of relapsing polychondritis. The anterior and lateral tracheal walls are thickened; the posterior tracheal membrane is of normal thickness. (From **Webb EM, Elicker BM, Webb WR.** Using CT to diagnose nonneoplastic tracheal abnormalities: appearance of the tracheal wall. AJR Am J Roentgenol 2000; 174:1315–1321.)

A   B

C   D

FIG. 22.25. Relapsing polychondritis. **A** and **B:** CT shows marked narrowing of the tracheal lumen, with typical thickening of the anterior and lateral tracheal walls. **C:** Coronal reconstruction shows diffuse narrowing of the trachea with thickening of its lateral walls (*arrows*). **D:** Sagittal reformation shows diffuse narrowing of the trachea (*arrows*).

A   B

FIG. 22.26. Relapsing polychondritis with tracheomalacia. Expiratory CT (**B**) shows significant collapse of the tracheal lumen compared with an inspiratory scan (**A**).

FIG. 22.27. Tracheal diverticulum in a patient with chronic obstructive pulmonary disease. A defect in the right posterolateral tracheal wall (*small arrow*) communicates with a small diverticulum (*large arrow*). This location is characteristic.

less common in women. There may be a history of recurrent respiratory tract infection or chronic cough dating to childhood, but this is not seen in all patients.

Although tracheal enlargement is seen in some patients with chronic pulmonary fibrosis or chronic infection, tracheobronchomegaly most likely is congenital in origin. Histologic

examination of the trachea shows a deficiency of smooth muscle and elastic fibers. A cartilage abnormality undoubtedly is present as well, although this abnormality probably is acquired. Tracheomegaly also may occur in association with other congenital disorders such as Marfan's syndrome, cystic fibrosis, Ehlers-Danlos syndrome, and cutis laxa.

The diagnosis is based on radiographic findings of increased tracheal and bronchial diameter. Dilatation usually involves the intrathoracic trachea and the first few bronchial divisions (Fig. 22-29). Tracheobronchomegaly may be suggested in a man if the tracheal diameter measured on the frontal and lateral radiographs exceeds 25 and 27 mm, respectively; in a woman, it may be suggested if these measurements exceed 21 and 23 mm. The trachea tends to have a corrugated or scalloped contour (see Fig. 22-29) because of mucosa protruding between the tracheal cartilage. On the lateral view, this is visible anteriorly. Frank tracheal diverticula also may be present. Bronchiectasis commonly is present and tends to involve the central bronchi; peripheral airways appear normal.

On CT, a tracheal diameter greater than 3 cm (measured 2 cm above the aortic arch) and diameters of 2.4 and 2.3 cm for the right and left main bronchi have been used to make the diagnosis of tracheobronchomegaly (Figs. 22-30 and 22-31), although these measurements are more conservative than those proposed for use on chest radiographs. Tracheal scalloping is more difficult to see in cross section than on chest films. Diverticula, on the other hand, are more easily seen on CT, typically occurring along the posterolateral tracheal wall. Also common is the finding of a marked tracheal flaccidity or tracheomalacia on expiratory scans. Cystic bronchiectasis may be seen in the central or parahilar lung regions (Figs. 22-29 and 22-31).

A

B

FIG. 22.28. Tracheal diverticulum. **A:** A paratracheal air cyst is present in the upper mediastinum, representing a diverticulum (*arrow*). **B:** A defect in the right posterolateral tracheal wall (*arrow*) communicates with the diverticulum.

FIG. 22.29. Tracheobronchomegaly. A bronchogram shows tracheal dilatation (*arrows*), with the tracheal wall having a corrugated or scalloped contour. Central bronchiectasis also is visible.

FIG. 22.31. Tracheobronchomegaly with bronchiectasis. **A:** CT above the aortic arch shows tracheal dilatation. The trachea wall has a scalloped appearance. Central bronchiectasis is present, with bullae in the lung periphery. **B:** The left main bronchus has a scalloped appearance, and cystic bronchiectasis is present.

FIG. 22.30. Tracheobronchomegaly. CT above the aortic arch shows marked tracheal dilatation. The trachea measures 37 mm in diameter.

SELECTED READING

Boiselle PM, O'Donnell CR, Bankier AA, et al. Tracheal collapsibility in healthy volunteers during forced expiration: assessment with multidetector CT. Radiology 2009; 252:255–262.

Choplin RH, Wehunt WD, Theros EG. Diffuse lesions of the trachea. Semin Roentgenol 1983; 18:38–50.

Gamsu G, Webb WR. Computed tomography of the trachea and mainstem bronchi. Semin Roentgenol 1983; 18:51–60.

Goo JM, Im JG, Ahn JM, et al. Right paratracheal air cysts in the thoracic inlet: clinical and radiologic significance. AJR Am J Roentgenol 1999; 173:65–70.

Im JG, Chung JW, Han SK, et al. CT manifestations of tracheobronchial involvement in relapsing polychondritis. J Comput Assist Tomogr 1988; 12:792–793.

Kwong JS, Müller NL, Miller RR. Diseases of the trachea and main-stem bronchi: correlation of CT with pathologic findings. Radiographics 1992; 12:647–657.

Mariotta S, Pallone G, Pedicelli G, Bisetti A. Spiral CT and endoscopic findings in a case of tracheobronchopathia osteochondroplastica. J Comput Assist Tomogr 1997; 21:418–420.

Pickford HA, Swensen SJ, Utz JP. Thoracic cross-sectional imaging of amyloidosis. AJR Am J Roentgenol 1997; 168:351–355.

Roditi GH, Weir J. The association of tracheomegaly and bronchiectasis. Clin Radiol 1994; 49:608–611.

Screaton NJ, Sivasothy P, Flower CD, Lockwood CM. Tracheal involvement in Wegener's granulomatosis: evaluation using spiral CT. Clin Radiol 1998; 53:809–815.

Shin MS, Jackson RM, Ho KJ. Tracheobronchomegaly (Mounier-Kuhn syndrome): CT diagnosis. AJR Am J Roentgenol 1988; 150:777–779.

Stern EJ, Graham CM, Webb WR, Gamsu G. Normal trachea during forced expiration: dynamic CT measurements. Radiology 1993; 187:27–31.

Webb EM, Elicker BM, Webb WR. Using CT to diagnose nonneoplastic tracheal abnormalities: appearance of the tracheal wall. AJR Am J Roentgenol 2000; 174:1315–1321.

Airway Disease: Bronchiectasis, Chronic Bronchitis, and Bronchiolitis

W. RICHARD WEBB

AIRWAY MORPHOLOGY

Airways divide by dichotomous branching. There are approximately 23 divisions from the trachea to the alveoli.

Bronchi are conducting airways that contain cartilage in their walls. The anatomy of the lobar and segmental bronchi is described in Chapter 6.

Bronchioles are airways not containing cartilage. The largest bronchioles measure about 3 mm in diameter and have walls about 0.3 mm thick. A *terminal bronchiole* is the last purely conducting airway and does not participate in gas exchange. It is approximately 0.7 mm in diameter and gives rise to respiratory bronchioles. A *respiratory bronchiole* is the largest bronchiole with alveoli arising from its walls, and, thus, is the largest bronchiole that participates in gas exchange. It gives rise to alveolar ducts and alveoli.

BRONCHIECTASIS

Bronchiectasis is defined as localized, irreversible dilatation of the bronchial tree. Usually, this term is used to refer only to cartilage-containing airways, larger than 2 to 3 mm in diameter.

Etiology

Bronchiectasis has a wide variety of causes (Table 23-1), but in up to 40% of cases, the etiology cannot be determined. Bronchiectasis is commonly associated with acute, chronic, or recurrent infection, particularly infection with bacteria and mycobacteria. Also, bronchiectasis often is present in patients with bronchiolitis obliterans (BO) or the Swyer-James syndrome resulting from viral or mycoplasma infection. Immunodeficiency syndromes including acquired immunodeficiency syndrome (AIDS), abnormalities of mucociliary clearance, structural abnormalities of the bronchial wall, and chronic bronchial obstruction are associated with bronchiectasis, largely because they result in infection.

Noninfectious diseases that result in airway inflammation and mucous plugging also can result in bronchiectasis. These include allergic bronchopulmonary aspergillosis (ABPA), and, to a lesser extent, asthma. Bronchiectasis also is seen in patients with BO resulting from chronic rejection following lung transplantation or chronic graft-versus-host disease (GVHD) in patients with bone marrow transplantation.

Causes of bronchiectasis having a genetic basis include cystic fibrosis (CF); the dyskinetic cilia (Kartagener's) syndrome (Fig. 23-1); Young's syndrome; Williams-Campbell

TABLE 23.1 Causes of Bronchiectasis

Infection
Bacteria (*Pseudomonas, Staphylococcus, Bordetella pertussis*)
Mycobacteria (tuberculosis, *Mycobacterium avium-intracellulare* [MAC])
Virus
Mycoplasma

Immune deficiency states
Congenital (e.g., hypogammaglobulinemia)
Acquired (e.g., AIDS)

Mucociliary clearance abnormalities
Cystic fibrosis (abnormal mucus)
Dyskinetic cilia syndrome (abnormal cilia)
Young's syndrome

Bronchial obstruction
Congenital bronchial atresia
Endobronchial tumor
Bronchial compression by lymph nodes

Bronchial wall abnormalities
Tracheobronchomegaly
Williams-Campbell syndrome

Immune reactions
ABPA
Asthma
Lung transplant rejection
Graft-versus-host disease

Proteinase-antiproteinase imbalance
Alpha-1-antitrypsin deficiency

Systemic Diseases
Collagen-vascular disease
Inflammatory bowel disease

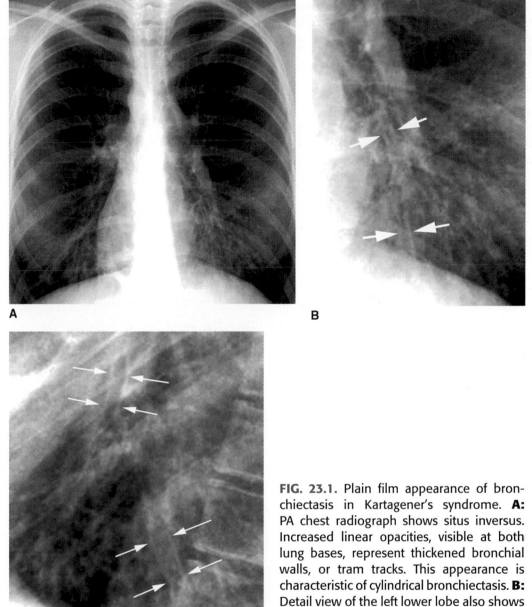

FIG. 23.1. Plain film appearance of bronchiectasis in Kartagener's syndrome. **A:** PA chest radiograph shows situs inversus. Increased linear opacities, visible at both lung bases, represent thickened bronchial walls, or tram tracks. This appearance is characteristic of cylindrical bronchiectasis. **B:** Detail view of the left lower lobe also shows tram tracks (*arrows*). **C:** Detail view of the lateral radiograph shows parallel lines, representing thickened bronchial walls, or tram tracks (*arrows*).

syndrome (congenital deficiency of the bronchial cartilage); Mounier-Kuhn syndrome (congenital tracheobronchomegaly); alpha-1-antitrypsin deficiency; immunodeficiency syndromes, including Bruton's hypogammaglobulinemia, IgA, and combined IgA-IgG deficiencies; and the yellow nail lymphedema syndrome (yellow nails, lymphedema, and pleural effusions).

Pathologic Abnormalities

Bronchiectasis usually is associated with bronchial wall thickening, inflammation, destruction of muscular and elastic elements of the bronchial wall, and bronchial and peribronchial fibrosis. Loss of muscular and elastic tissues allows the bronchi to dilate in response to the pull of adjacent tissues (i.e., the normal negative interstitial pressure). Ciliated epithelium is usually replaced by nonciliated or squamous epithelium. These structural abnormalities of the bronchial wall encourage infection, which, in turn, further damages the bronchi.

Inflammation and fibrosis also are associated with obliteration of small airways and a reduction in the number of bronchial branches, particularly when the disease occurs during childhood, when the lungs are growing.

The affected lung is typically reduced in volume and may be airless. Pulmonary arteries supplying the abnormal lung usually are reduced in number and size, and regional lung perfusion is decreased accordingly.

Clinical Diagnosis

In general, a clinical diagnosis of bronchiectasis is possible only in the most severely affected patients, and differentiation from chronic bronchitis may be difficult. Most patients present with purulent sputum production, recurrent pulmonary infections, fever, weight loss, and sometimes dyspnea. Hemoptysis also is common, occurring in up to 50% of cases, and may be the only clinical finding. Hemoptysis usually is associated with bronchial artery enlargement related to chronic inflammation. Sputum culture often reveals bacterial infection, with common organisms being *Streptococcus pneumoniae, Pseudomonas, Haemophilus influenzae,* and *Staphylococcus aureus. Aspergillus* species and mycobacteria also may be present.

Pulmonary function tests may show airflow obstruction. However, bronchitis, bronchiolitis, or emphysema often accompanies bronchiectasis and may predominate as the cause of obstructive abnormalities.

Classification

Traditionally, bronchiectasis has been classified into three morphologic types: *cylindrical, varicose,* and *cystic.* The severity of bronchial dilatation and anatomic abnormalities, and, to a lesser extent, functional abnormalities, correlate with these three types. Cylindrical bronchiectasis is associated with the least severe abnormalities, and cystic bronchiectasis is associated with the most severe. However, differentiating between the types of bronchectasis is less important in clinical practice than is a determination of its extent and distribution.

Cylindrical Bronchiectasis

Cylindrical bronchiectasis is characterized by mild bronchial dilatation. The dilated bronchi are of relatively uniform caliber and have roughly parallel walls. Often, smaller bronchi are plugged with purulent secretions. The number of bronchial divisions from the carina to the periphery is slightly reduced.

Varicose Bronchiectasis

With increasingly severe abnormalities of the bronchial wall and increasing bronchial dilatation, the bronchi may assume an irregular, beaded or bulbous configuration, referred to as *varicose bronchiectasis.* Usually, peripheral bronchi are obliterated by fibrous tissue. The number of bronchial divisions is reduced significantly.

Cystic Bronchiectasis

With severe bronchiectasis, airways appear ballooned or "cystic" or "saccular," often exceeding 2 cm in diameter. The typical branching appearance of bronchi in areas of bronchiectasis may be difficult to see. The cysts often appear isolated and are not associated with other abnormal airways. Cysts may be seen in a subpleural location. The number of bronchial divisions from the carina to the periphery is markedly reduced.

Bronchography

Although traditionally considered the gold standard for diagnosing bronchiectasis, bronchography has been replaced by CT. The same findings that were considered classic indicators of bronchiectasis on bronchography still can be used in interpreting CT. These include the following:

1. Proximal or distal bronchial dilatation
2. Abnormal bronchial contours
3. Lack of normal tapering of peripheral airways
4. Reduction in the number of bronchial branches (i.e., "pruning")
5. Luminal filling defects due to mucus.

Plain Radiograph Diagnosis

Plain radiographs are abnormal in 80% to 90% of patients with bronchiectasis, although findings are often nonspecific, and the diagnosis can be suggested in only about 40% of patients. The more severe the abnormality, the easier it is to see, and the more likely it is that an accurate diagnosis will be made.

Tram tracks, parallel line shadows representing thickened bronchial walls, are a common finding in bronchiectasis (see Figs. 23-1 and 23-2). They may be the only finding visible in patients with cylindrical bronchiectasis. However, tram tracks also may be seen with bronchial wall thickening in the absence of bronchiectasis, and thus are nonspecific. When seen in cross section, thick-walled bronchi appear as ring shadows (Fig. 23-2D).

Recognizing dilatation of bronchi on plain films is more difficult, unless the dilatation is significant or obvious contour abnormalities are present (e.g., in varicose bronchiectasis). The dilated bronchi may be visible as irregular, oval, or branching tubular air-filled structures (see Fig. 23-2). When seen in cross section, a dilated bronchus may appear larger than the artery adjacent to it. This is known as the *signet-ring* sign, and indicates that bronchial dilatation is present. Mucous plugs or fluid filling the bronchi sometimes is visible and may aid in recognizing them as dilated. Mucous plugs within dilated bronchi may be visible as oval ("finger in glove") or branching ("hand in glove") opacities.

Cystic bronchiectasis results in multiple, air-filled, cystic lesions, which may be thick- or thin-walled, and clustered, lobar, patchy, or diffuse in distribution. Multiple air-fluid levels often are seen because of infection or retained secretions (see Fig. 9-28 in Chapter 9). Because the cysts communicate with each other through the bronchial tree, air-fluid levels tend to be at about the same height in all the affected cysts, but with less fluid present in the upper lobe cysts than in lower lobe cysts (i.e., water flows downhill).

FIG. 23.2. Bronchiectasis in cystic fibrosis. **A:** Chest radiograph shows a number of examples of tram tracks and ring shadows in the upper lobes. **B:** Detail view of the right upper lobe shows tram tracks (*arrows*) due to cylindrical bronchiectasis. **C:** HRCT in this patient shows bilateral upper lobe bronchiectasis. **D:** In another patient with cystic fibrosis, ring shadows (*arrows*), indicate bronchiectasis.

Less specific radiographic findings often seen in bronchiectasis include (1) loss of definition of vascular markings in the affected lung, presumably secondary to peribronchial inflammation or fibrosis, (2) increased "lung markings" in the central lung regions, (3) volume loss in the affected lung or lobe, (4) decreased vessel size in the aerated bronchiectatic lung, (5) consolidation of abnormal lung, and (6) compensatory expansion of normal lung.

CT Diagnosis

HRCT with images spaced at 1 cm intervals or volumetric helical CT using thin collimation (3 cm or less)

is very accurate in the diagnosis of bronchiectasis with sensitivity and specificity values exceeding 95%. The use of appropriate and consistent window mean and width settings (−600 to 700/1,000 to 1,500 HU) is important. Excessively low or narrow window settings exaggerate bronchial wall thickness.

Specific findings of bronchiectasis indicate that bronchial dilatation is present (Table 23-2). Less specific findings include bronchial wall thickening (diagnosed subjectively or because bronchi are visible in the peripheral lung) and the presence of mucoid impaction or fluid within airways. Ancillary findings, commonly seen in bronchiectasis include volume loss, mosaic perfusion visible on inspiratory scans,

TABLE 23.2 HRCT Findings in Bronchiectasis

Specific findings of bronchial dilatation
Increased bronchoarterial ratio
   Internal bronchial diameter > adjacent pulmonary artery
   "Signet-ring" sign
Lack of tapering
Contour abnormalities
   Cylindrical bronchiectasis—"tram tracks"
   Varicose bronchiectasis—"string of pearls"
   Cystic bronchiectasis—"cluster of grapes"
Visibility of airways in peripheral 1 cm of lung

Common nonspecific findings
Bronchial wall thickening
Fluid- or mucus-filled bronchi

Ancillary findings
Volume loss
Mosaic perfusion
Air trapping
Tree-in-bud
Bronchial artery enlargement

focal air trapping identifiable on expiration scans, "tree-in-bud," and bronchial artery enlargement.

Bronchial Dilatation

Because bronchiectasis is defined by the presence of bronchial dilatation, recognition of increased bronchial diameter is key to the CT diagnosis of this entity. On CT, bronchial dilatation may be diagnosed by an increased bronchoarterial ratio, by detecting a lack of bronchial tapering, and by abnormal bronchial contours.

Increased Bronchoarterial Ratio

The diameter of a bronchus seen in cross section may be compared to that of the adjacent pulmonary artery by measuring the *bronchoarterial ratio* (the ratio of the internal diameter of a bronchus to that of the adjacent pulmonary artery) (Fig. 23-3A); the bronchoarterial ratio averages about 0.65 to 0.7 in normal subjects.

Bronchiectasis is generally considered to be present if the bronchoarterial ratio exceeds 1. However, this may sometimes be seen in the absence of bronchial wall abnormalities in a small percentage of normals, including elderly patients and in patients living at high altitudes (e.g., Denver). Usually, true bronchiectasis results in a bronchoarterial ratio

FIG. 23.3. Bronchoarterial ratio. A: Bronchoarterial (B/A) ratio equals the internal diameter of a bronchus, divided by the diameter of the adjacent pulmonary artery branch. As shown in this diagram, it measures 0.65–0.7 in normals. **B:** Appearances of a normal B/A ratio (0.70) and B/A ratios of 1.0 and 1.5. A B/A ratio greater than 1 may be seen in some normal patients. A B/A ratio of 1.5 is almost always due to true bronchiectasis. **C:** In a patient with bronchiectasis, HRCT through the left lower lobe shows a number of examples of the signet-ring sign. The signet-ring sign is present when a dilated bronchus (*large arrows*) is associated with a much smaller pulmonary artery (*small arrows*). Bronchial walls are thick.

greater than 1.5 (Fig. 23-3B). Unless dilatation is obvious, bronchiectasis should not be diagnosed on the basis of an increased bronchoarterial ratio alone. Fortunately, bronchial wall thickening and other abnormalities typically are present in patients with true bronchiectasis.

The association of a dilated bronchus with a smaller adjacent pulmonary artery branch has been termed the *signet-ring sign* (Figs. 23-3C and 23-4). This sign is valuable in recognizing bronchiectasis on CT and in distinguishing it from other cystic lung lesions. An increased bronchoarterial ratio not only reflects the presence of bronchial dilatation but also indicates some reduction in pulmonary artery size

as a consequence of decreased lung perfusion in the affected lung regions.

Lack of Bronchial Tapering

Lack of bronchial tapering may be important in the diagnosis of bronchiectasis, in particular subtle cylindrical bronchiectasis. For this finding to be present, the diameter of the airway should remain unchanged for at least 2 cm distal to a branching point (see Fig. 23-4A, C, and D). Accurate detection of this finding is difficult, however, in the absence of contiguous HRCT sections, especially for vertically or obliquely oriented airways.

A

C

B

D

FIG. 23.4. CT findings of bronchiectasis in four patients. **A:** CT shows several examples of the signet-ring sign in the lower lobe (*white arrows*). In the right middle lobe, bronchi are seen in the peripheral 1 cm of lung, do not taper, and have a cylindrical appearance (*black arrows*). Bronchial wall thickening is also visible. **B:** Numerous examples of the signet-ring sign (*arrows*) are visible. Note that the bronchus appears much larger than the adjacent artery. **C:** Cylindrical bronchiectasis with lack of bronchial tapering (*arrows*). Numerous thick-walled and dilated bronchi are visible, along with mucous plugging in the posterior right lower lobe. **D:** Bronchiectasis in a patient with cystic fibrosis. A dilated bronchus in the right upper lobe (*arrow*) shows a lack of tapering. Examples of the signet-ring sign are also visible.

Abnormal Bronchial Contours

Bronchiectasis may be classified as cylindrical, varicose, or cystic. Recognition of one of these abnormal contours is diagnostic.

Cylindrical bronchiectasis varies in appearance on CT, depending on whether the abnormal bronchi lie in the scan plane (see Fig. 23-4A, C, and D) or perpendicular to it (Fig. 23-4B). When in the plane of scan, bronchi fail to show normal tapering and are recognizable as "tram tracks."

Varicose bronchiectasis results in more irregular bronchial dilatation with a typical varicose appearance (Fig. 23-5A). The bronchial walls often are irregularly thickened. This diagnosis of varicose bronchiectasis can be made easily only when the involved bronchi course horizontally in the plane of scan. This appearance has been likened to a "string of pearls." When seen in cross section, the dilated bronchi are visible as thick-walled ring shadows indistinguishable from those of cylindrical bronchiectasis.

Cystic bronchiectasis is characterized by the presence of numerous cysts (see Fig. 23-5B). In general, the dilated airways in patients with cystic bronchiectasis are thick-walled; however, the cysts may be thin-walled. A clear-cut branching appearance of the dilated airways generally is lacking, and it may be difficult to make the distinction from cystic lung disease in some cases. This appearance has been described as similar to a "cluster of grapes." Air-fluid levels may be seen.

Bronchial Wall Thickening

Although bronchial wall thickening is a nonspecific finding, it usually is present in patients with bronchiectasis (see Figs. 23-3C, and 23-4A and C). Identification of bronchial wall thickening is largely subjective. Because bronchiectasis and bronchial wall thickening often are multifocal rather than diffuse and uniform, a comparison of one lung region to another can be helpful in making this observation (Fig. 23-6). It must be emphasized that using consistent window settings is very important in the diagnosis of bronchial wall thickening; bronchial walls can vary significantly in apparent thickness with different CT window settings.

Visibility of Peripheral Airways

In normal subjects, airways in the peripheral 2 cm of lung are uncommonly seen because their walls are too thin. Peribronchial fibrosis and bronchial wall thickening in patients with bronchiectasis, in combination with dilatation of the bronchial lumen, allow the visualization of small airways in the lung periphery. Bronchi visible within 1 cm of the costal pleural surfaces indicate bronchiectasis (see Figs. 23-4A, 23-5B, and 23-7), but bronchi may be seen within 1 cm of the mediastinal pleural surfaces in normal subjects.

Mucous Impaction and Air-Fluid Levels

The presence of mucus- or fluid-filled bronchi is nonspecific, but may be helpful in confirming a diagnosis of bronchiectasis (Figs. 23-5B and 23-8). The HRCT appearance of fluid- or mucus-filled airways is dependent on both their size and orientation relative to the scan plane. Larger, mucus-filled airways result in abnormal lobular or branching structures when they lie in the same plane as the CT scan. In cross section, impacted bronchi appear similar to vessels, but on contrast-enhanced scans they may be seen to be low in attenuation.

Patients with cystic bronchiectasis may show fluid levels within the abnormal bronchi (see Fig. 23-5B), due to retained secretions and chronic infection. Air-fluid levels within

A   **B**

FIG. 23.5. Contour abnormalities in bronchiectasis. **A:** Varicose bronchiectasis results in irregular bronchial dilatation (*arrow*). **B:** Cystic bronchiectasis. Air-fluid levels are visible within the abnormal bronchi (*arrows*). The dilated bronchi are visible in the lung periphery.

FIG 23.6. Bronchial wall thickening. CT shows several thick-walled bronchi (*large arrows*). Other bronchi show normal bronchial wall thickness (*small arrows*).

FIG 23.7. Visibility of a peripheral airway as an indication of bronchial wall thickening. In a patient with bronchiectasis, a bronchus (*arrow*) is visible in the peripheral lung. The fact that it is visible indicates that its wall is thickened.

the multiple cystic spaces are typical, and since they tend to communicate with each other through the bronchi, the air-fluid levels appear similar in height.

Mosaic Perfusion and Air Trapping

Many patients with bronchiectasis also show pathologic findings of small airway disease, either BO or infectious bronchiolitis. Consequently, HRCT findings of small airways disease, such as mosaic perfusion (on inspiratory scans) and

FIG. 23.8. Extensive mucous plugging in bronchiectasis. Numerous dilated, opacified bronchi are visible (*arrows*), both along their axis and in cross section.

focal air trapping (on expiratory scans) are often seen in patients with bronchiectasis.

Tree-in-Bud

The term *tree-in-bud* refers to the presence of nodular and Y-shaped branching structures which resemble a budding tree, in the lung periphery (Fig. 23-9; see also Fig. 10-28 in Chapter 10). This appearance reflects the presence of dilated, mucus- or pus-filled centrilobular bronchioles (the trunk and branches) associated with small nodular areas of bronchiolar dilatation or peribronchiolar inflammation (the buds) at the tips of the branches. This finding is common in patients with airway infection, and, therefore, is common in patients with various causes of bronchiectasis.

Bronchial Artery Enlargement

Enlarged bronchial arteries can be identified pathologically in most cases of bronchiectasis. This may result in massive and life-threatening hemoptysis. With multidetector CT using thin collimation and contrast infusion, abnormally enlarged bronchial arteries may be identified; bronchial arteriograms also may be used for diagnosis in patients with hemoptysis. Bronchial artery embolization may be curative in patients with hemoptysis due to bronchiectasis.

Severity of Bronchiectasis

Systems for grading the severity of bronchiectasis using CT have been developed but are not in common clinical use. However, the severity of bronchiectasis may be related to the diameter of the abnormal bronchi. Also, there is a significant correlation between the extent of bronchiectasis

FIG. 23.9. Tree-in-bud in bronchiectasis. **A:** Dilated thick-walled bronchi are visible, with areas of mucous plugging. Tree-in-bud is visible in the lung periphery (*arrows*). **B:** In another patient with bronchiectasis, thick-walled bronchi are visible in the right lower lobe. Peripheral bronchioles filled with fluid or pus (*arrows*) represent tree-in-bud.

and the forced expiratory volume in 1 second (FEV$_1$) and the forced vital capacity (FVC). Furthermore, patients with cystic bronchiectasis are more likely to have infection and purulent sputum than are patients with either cylindrical or varicose bronchiectasis.

Pitfalls in the Diagnosis of Bronchiectasis

Several potential pitfalls in the diagnosis of bronchiectasis should be avoided.

Artifacts due to cardiac or respiratory motion may cause ghosting that can very closely mimic the appearance of tram tracks. Observing other artifacts related to motion helps in identifying them appropriately.

Bronchiectasis is difficult to diagnose with certainty in patients with atelectasis. Normal bronchi dilate in the presence of atelectasis because the collapsed lung results in increased tension on the bronchial wall. Bronchi return to normal size when the collapse resolves. This phenomenon is known as "reversible bronchiectasis" (see Fig. 2-24 in Chapter 2); this term is an oxymoron, since part of the definition of bronchiectasis is that it is irreversible.

Consolidation may obscure vascular anatomy, making assessment of bronchoarterial ratios difficult or impossible.

Bronchiectasis may occur in association with fibrotic lung diseases (i.e., "traction" bronchiectasis). Traction bronchiectasis does not represent primary airways disease and is not associated with symptoms of chronic infection. The typical corkscrewed appearance of traction bronchiectasis and its association with obvious fibrosis are diagnostic.

SPECIFIC CAUSES OF BRONCHIECTASIS

In most instances, the radiographic appearance of bronchiectasis is nonspecific and does not allow a determination of its cause. However, a few diseases, discussed in the following sections, require special attention.

Cystic Fibrosis

CF is the most common cause of pulmonary insufficiency in the first three decades of life. It results from an autosomal recessive genetic defect in the structure of the CF transmembrane conductance regulator (CFTR), which leads to abnormal chloride transport across epithelial membranes (Table 23-3). The mechanisms by which this leads to lung disease are not entirely understood, but an abnormally low water content of airway mucus is at least partially responsible, resulting in decreased mucus clearance, mucous plugging of airways, and an increased incidence of bacterial airway infection. Bronchial wall inflammation progressing to secondary bronchiectasis is universal in patients with long-standing disease.

Although a single defect in CFTR is responsible for most cases, more than 100 genetic abnormalities may be associated with CF. These CF genotype variants often cause less severe disease and thus are more likely to be found in adults who first present with symptoms. Individuals who are carriers of the CF gene may have a selective advantage; they appear to be more resistant to typhoid fever than the general population.

Pulmonary abnormalities may be present within weeks of birth, with the earliest abnormalities being retention of mucus in small peripheral airways, mucous gland hyperplasia, and inflammation. The presence of airway infection is fundamental to the development of CF; the first organisms involved are *S. aureus, H. influenzae,* and mucoid *Pseudomonas* species. In adults with CF, *Pseudomonas aeruginosa* predominates (90% of cases), although *Aspergillus* (up to 50% of cases) species and mycobacteria (up to 20% of cases) also may be present. Bronchial wall damage and bronchiectasis occur largely as a result of infection.

Clinical Presentation

Clinical findings of chronic and recurrent infection in a child, associated with abnormal sweat chlorides, usually are

TABLE 23.3 Cystic Fibrosis (CF)

Autosomal-recessive genetic defect in CF transmembrane conductance regulator
Abnormal chloride transport resulting in abnormal mucus
Bronchiectasis and infection universal
  Pseudomonas (90%)
  Aspergillus (50%)
  Mycobacteria (20%)
Radiographic findings
Increased lung volumes
Small nodular opacities due to impaction of small airways
Bronchial wall thickening or bronchiectasis
Mucoid impaction
Right upper lobe predominance
Atelectasis
Cysts (bronchiectasis, abscess cavities, bullae)
Pneumomediastinum or pneumothorax
Hilar enlargement
HRCT findings
Bronchiectasis
  Central bronchi and upper lobes involved in all cases
  Typically severe (varicose and cystic) and widespread
Bronchial wall thickening
  Central and upper lobe distribution
  Right upper lobe first involved
Mucous plugging
Tree-in-bud
Large lung volumes
Atelectasis
Mosaic perfusion
Air trapping on expiration

diagnostic. Hemoptysis occurs in more than half of cases because of bronchial artery hypertrophy.

Radiographic Findings

Typical radiographic findings (see Figs. 23-2 and 23-10) can help confirm the diagnosis in patients with symptoms or may be suggestive in patients with an atypical presentation (e.g., young adults with CF variants).

Early in the course of disease, plain films are normal. Initial abnormalities include the following:

1. Increased lung volumes due to obstruction of small airways (i.e., increased retrosternal space, flattening of the hemidiaphragms).
2. Impaction of small airways, resulting in small nodular or reticular opacities in the lung periphery.
3. Accentuated linear opacities in the central or upper lung regions due to bronchial wall thickening or bronchiectasis.

The earliest abnormalities in patients with CF are in the right upper lobe. Consequently, early findings may include right upper lobe atelectasis or thickening of the wall of the right upper lobe bronchus, best seen on the lateral radiograph.

In older children and adults, bronchiectasis is typical, often involving bronchi in the central lung regions, i.e., *central bronchiectasis*. Dilated bronchi may be cylindrical, varicose, or cystic, depending on the duration and severity of disease. In adult patients and patients with chronic disease, additional abnormalities (see Figs. 23-2 and 23-10) can include the following:

1. Mucoid impaction with oval or branching opacities ("finger in glove" or "hand in glove")
2. Cysts or ring shadows in the upper lobes, representing cystic bronchiectasis, healed abscess cavities, or bullae
3. Atelectasis
4. Pneumothorax (up to 20% of cases)
5. Hilar enlargement due to lymphadenopathy or pulmonary hypertension
6. Pleural thickening (although pleural effusion is uncommon).

In most patients with an established diagnosis of CF, clinical findings and chest radiographs are sufficient for clinical management. A significant exacerbation of symptoms may occur with little visible radiographic change.

CT Findings

CT can demonstrate morphologic abnormalities in patients with early CF who are asymptomatic, have normal pulmonary function, or have normal chest radiographs. In patients with more advanced disease, HRCT also can show abnormalities not visible on chest radiographs, including bronchiectasis and mucous plugging.

On CT and HRCT, bronchiectasis is seen in all patients with advanced CF (Figs. 23-2C, 23-11 and 23-12). Proximal or parahilar bronchi always are involved when bronchiectasis is present, and bronchiectasis is limited to these central bronchi (i.e., *central bronchiectasis*) in about one third of cases. Typically, all lobes are involved, although early in the disease abnormalities often predominate in the upper lobes; often abnormalities are most severe in the right upper lobe. The differential diagnosis of central bronchiectasis also includes ABPA, tuberculosis, radiation fibrosis, Mounier-Kuhn syndrome (tracheobronchomegaly), and Williams-Campbell syndrome.

Cylindrical bronchiectasis is most common (95%) on HRCT; varicose and cystic bronchiectasis are visible in as many as one third of cases. *Cystic lesions* representing cystic bronchiectasis, abscess cavities, or bullae are visible in half of patients and typically predominate in the subpleural regions of the upper lobes.

Bronchial wall or peribronchial interstitial thickening also is commonly present in patients with CF. It usually is more evident than bronchial dilatation in patients who have early disease and may be seen independent of bronchiectasis. Thickening of the wall of the proximal right upper lobe bronchi often is the earliest abnormal feature visible on HRCT.

FIG. 23.10. Radiographic findings in adults with cystic fibrosis. **A** and **B:** PA chest radiograph in two different patients shows increased lung volumes. The hila are elevated because of upper lobe volume loss, and the minor fissure (*arrow*) is bowed upward. Increased markings in the upper lobes reflect bronchiectasis. **C:** In this patient, large lung volumes are associated with ring shadows and an increase in markings in the central lung regions, due to bronchiectasis. **D:** Large lung volumes are present. Upper lobe bronchiectasis is present, with ring shadows and branching mucous plugs.

FIG. 23.11. HRCT findings in cystic fibrosis. Parahilar (*central*) bronchiectasis is present (*arrows*), with a predominance in the right upper lobe. Patchy areas of lucency reflect mosaic perfusion. Some right upper lobe volume loss is apparent.

Mucous plugging is visible in one quarter to one half of cases and may be visible in all lobes. Volume loss, collapse, or consolidation can be seen in as many as 80% of patients.

Tree-in-bud (i.e., bronchiolar dilatation with associated infection or mucus impaction) often is visible and can be an early sign of disease in children.

Focal areas of decreased lung opacity, representing *mosaic perfusion,* are common (see Figs. 23-11 and 23-12). These may appear to surround dilated, thick-walled, or mucus-plugged bronchi. *Air trapping* often is seen on expiratory scans.

Lung volumes may appear increased on CT, although this diagnosis is rather subjective and may be better assessed on chest radiographs.

Hilar or mediastinal lymph node enlargement and pleural thickening also can be seen, largely due to chronic infection. Pulmonary artery dilatation resulting from pulmonary hypertension also can be seen in patients with long-standing disease.

Allergic Bronchopulmonary Aspergillosis

ABPA reflects a hypersensitivity reaction to *Aspergillus* organisms and characteristically is associated with eosinophilia, symptoms of asthma (e.g., wheezing), "central" or "proximal" bronchiectasis, mucoid impaction, atelectasis, and consolidation similar to that seen in patients with eosinophilic pneumonia (Table 23-4). ABPA typically occurs in young adults with a history of asthma or atopy, and in 2% to 10% of patients with CF. Asthma may be present for many years before the diagnosis of ABPA.

ABPA results from both type I (IgE-mediated hypersensitivity) and type III (IgG-mediated antigen-antibody complex reaction) immunologic responses to the endobronchial growth of fungal (e.g., *Aspergillus*) species.

The type I response results in immediate wheezing when the patient is exposed to *Aspergillus* antigens.

The type III reaction results in bronchial inflammation in response to fungi in the airway, which eventually leads to bronchiectasis. Bronchiectasis usually is varicose or cystic in appearance, central in location (i.e., central bronchiectasis), and associated with formation of mucous plugs that contain fungus and inflammatory cells.

Clinical Presentation

Symptoms of ABPA are similar to those of uncomplicated asthma, and include wheezing, cough, and dyspnea.

A **B**

FIG. 23.12. HRCT findings in cystic fibrosis. **A, B:** Central (*parahilar*) bronchiectasis and bronchial wall thickening are present. Mosaic perfusion results in patchy lung opacity with decreased vessel size in the lung periphery.

TABLE 23.4 Allergic Bronchopulmonary Aspergillosis

Hypersensitivity reaction to *Aspergillus*
History of asthma or atopy, cystic fibrosis
Type I (IgE-mediated) hypersensitivity results in wheezing
Type III (IgG-mediated antigen-antibody complex) reaction results in bronchiectasis

Radiographic findings
Consolidation (i.e., eosinophilic pneumonia)
Central bronchiectasis, upper lobe or widespread
Mucous plugging ("finger in glove")
Increased lung volume
Upper lobe volume loss or scarring

HRCT findings
Central bronchiectasis, widespread
Upper lobe predominance common
Mucous plugging; mucus plugs appear high-density
Tree-in-bud
Atelectasis
Peripheral consolidation or diffuse ground-glass opacity
Mosaic perfusion
Air trapping on expiration

Occasionally, fever, hemoptysis, and chest pain may be associated. Expectoration of mucous plugs containing fungus may occur.

The diagnosis of ABPA is a based on a combination of clinical, laboratory, and radiographic findings. The five essential criteria for diagnosis can be rememberd by the acronym *ASPER*, and include:

1. **A**sthma
2. **S**pecific **S**erum antibodies (IgE and IgG) to *Aspergillus*
3. **P**roximal (central) bronchiectasis
4. **E**levated IgE (greater than 1,000 ng/mL)
5. **R**eactive skin test (wheal-and-flare skin reaction to *Aspergillus* antigen)

If proximal (central) bronchiectasis is absent or undetected, a diagnosis of *seropositive ABPA* can be made in the presence of criteria 1, 2, 4, and 5.

Additional criteria, not required for diagnosis, include:

1. Blood eosinophilia
2. Serum precipitins to *Aspergillus* antigen
3. Pulmonary infiltrates on chest radiographs

ABPA typically is characterized by repeated exacerbations. Disease progression may be divided into five phases, although these are not invariable: (1) acute presentation; (2) resolution with clearing of pulmonary abnormalities and decline in serum IgE; (3) recurrence; (4) development of dependence on corticosteroids; leading in some cases to (5) pulmonary fibrosis.

Radiographic Findings

Patients presenting with an acute exacerbation of ABPA often show consolidation on chest radiographs. Some consolidations are patchy, resembling eosinophilic pneumonia. These may be peripheral or parahilar, surrounding abnormal bronchi. Segmental or lobar consolidation may reflect atelectasis resulting from bronchial obstruction by mucous plugs.

Bronchiectasis is commonly visible with acute or recurrent disease (Figs. 23-13 and 23-14). The abnormal bronchi often are lobar or segmental and, thus, central in location. They may have an oval or branching appearance or may appear round if seen in cross section. Mucous plugs may be seen within the bronchi, outlined by air, or may fill the bronchi, resulting in a "*finger in glove*" or "*hand in glove*" appearance (see Fig. 23-13). The presence of a dilated, thick-walled bronchus sometimes is termed a *bronchocele*, whereas a bronchocele containing a mucous plug may be referred to a *mucocele*. These tend to have an upper lobe predominance in patients with ABPA.

Lung distal to a mucous plug may be collapsed or may be aerated due to collateral ventilation. Aerated lung may appear hyperlucent and hypovascular due to air trapping. Lung volume may be increased.

The radiographic findings in ABPA (e.g., central bronchiectasis with an upper lobe predominance (see Figs. 23-13 and 23-14), mucous plugging, consolidation, large lung volumes) may mimic those of CF. In the later stages of disease, upper lobe scarring and volume loss may mimic prior tuberculosis.

CT Findings

HRCT is more sensitive than are plain radiographs in detecting airway abnormalities associated with ABPA. HRCT findings include central bronchiectasis (present in 85% of lobes), usually varicose or cylindrical (see Fig. 23-14B); bronchial occlusion due to mucous plugging (see Figs. 23-13C, D and 23-14B to D); and bronchial wall thickening. An upper lobe predominance for these abnormalities is common but not invariable. Ectatic airways sometimes may contain an air-fluid level or an aspergilloma.

In about 25% of cases, mucous plugs in ABPA are greater in attenuation than soft tissue (see Figs. 23-13E and 23-14D); these plugs may be quite dense, measuring more than 100 HU. This finding is strongly suggestive of ABPA and is thought to be due to concentration of calcium oxalate by the fungus. Dense mucous plugs also may be seen with bronchial atresia (see Chapter 1).

A tree-in-bud appearance resulting from mucus filling the bronchioles may be seen, but in most patients with ABPA, the peripheral airways appear normal.

Parenchymal abnormalities including consolidation, collapse, cavitation, and bullae may be identified in as many as 40% of cases, particularly in the upper lobes. Masslike foci of

FIG. 23.13. Allergic bronchopulmonary aspergillosis (ABPA). PA (**A**) and lateral (**B**) radiographs show parahilar mucous plugs within areas of central bronchiectasis (*arrows*). **C** and **D:** CT at two levels shows the branching mucous plugs within dilated central bronchi. **E:** CT at the same level as (**C**) shows the mucous plugs (*arrows*) to be denser than soft tissue and great vessels. This appearance is suggestive of ABPA.

eosinophilic pneumonia may be seen with acute exacerbation. Mosaic perfusion and air trapping may be seen.

Asthma

Asthma is characterized by airway inflammation, which is largely reversible (Table 23-5). Pathologically, patients with asthma show bronchial and bronchiolar wall thickening caused by inflammation, infiltration by eosinophils, smooth muscle hyperplasia, and edema, and excess mucus production, which can result in mucous plugging.

Bronchiectasis may be seen in some patients with long-standing asthma.

Pulmonary function tests show findings of airway obstruction (e.g., increased airway resistance, increased total lung volume, increased residual volume, and decreased FVC) during an asthma episode, but typically return to normal between attacks.

Radiographic Findings

Radiographic findings associated with asthma usually are subtle. They include increased lung volume (30% to 40%),

FIG. 23.14. Allergic bronchopulmonary aspergillosis. **A:** PA radiographs show a mucous plug in the central left upper lobe (*arrows*). **B:** HRCT shows multiple areas of central bronchiectasis and bronchial wall thickening (*arrows*) and a large central mucous plug (∗). **C:** HRCT slightly above (**B**) shows the branching mucous plug (*arrows*). **D:** CT at the same level as (**B**) shows the mucous plug (*arrow*) to be denser than soft tissue.

TABLE 23.5 Asthma

Reversible airway inflammation and obstruction
Radiographic findings subtle
  Increased lung volume (30%–40%)
  Increased lucency
  Mild bronchial wall thickening (50%)
  Mild hilar prominence
Radiographs most useful in diagnosing complications
  Pneumonia
  Atelectasis
  Pneumomediastinum and pneumothorax
HRCT used to diagnose complications, allergic bronchopul-
  monary aspergillosis, or emphysema
  Mild bronchial wall thickening or dilatation
  Mucous plugs or tree-in-bud (20%)
  Mosaic perfusion (20%–30%)
  Air trapping on expiration (50%)

increased lung lucency, mild bronchial wall thickening (50%), and mild prominence of hilar vasculature due to transient pulmonary hypertension (10%). Bronchiectasis is not usually recognized, but small mucous plugs sometimes can be seen. Associated complications of asthma, although uncommon, include pneumonia, atelectasis, pneumomediastinum, and pneumothorax. Pneumomediastinum is more common than pneumothorax. Radiographic abnormalities generally are more common and more severe in children with asthma.

Plain radiographs are not commonly used to make a diagnosis of asthma; radiographs often are normal, and visible abnormalities in this disease usually are nonspecific. Radiography also has limited usefulness in patients with an established diagnosis of asthma who suffer an acute attack. Correlation between the severity of radiographic findings and the severity and reversibility of an asthma attack usually is poor, and radiographs provide significant information that alters treatment in 5% or less of patients with acute asthma. Although it is difficult to generalize regarding the role of radiographs in adults and children with acute asthma, chest films often are used to exclude the presence of associated pneumonia or other complications when significant symptoms or appropriate clinical or laboratory findings are suggestive.

HRCT Findings

CT is not commonly indicated in the routine assessment of patients with asthma, but it sometimes is used when complications, particularly ABPA, are suspected, or in diagnosing emphysema in smokers with asthma.

HRCT shows mild bronchial wall thickening or dilatation of small bronchi (diagnosed by a bronchoarterial ratio slightly greater than 1) in about half of patients with uncomplicated asthma.

Mucoid impaction and tree-in-bud have been reported in as many as 20% of cases, and typically clear following treatment.

Mosaic perfusion or diffuse hyperlucency has been observed on inspiratory scans in 20% to 30% of cases. Expiratory CT can show evidence of patchy air trapping in as many as 50% of asthmatic patients.

Although asthma and ABPA can result in similar abnormalities, patients with ABPA have a higher frequency of bronchiectasis (95%, vs. 30% for asthma), a higher incidence of mucoid impaction, and more severe and extensive abnormalities.

Mycobacterium Avium-Intracellulare Complex Infection

Bronchiectasis predominantly involving the right middle lobe and lingua, in association with lung nodules and tree in bud, is characteristic of nontuberculous mycobacterial infection resulting from *Mycobacterium avium-intracellulare* complex (MAC) and is described in detail in Chapter 12. It typically is seen in women older than 60 years.

Dyskinetic Cilia Syndrome and Kartagener's Syndrome

Dyskinetic cilia syndrome (DCS) is characterized by abnormal ciliary structure and movement, resulting in abnormal mucociliary clearance and chronic infection (Table 23-6). Bronchiectasis and sinusitis are common manifestations. About half of patients with DCS also have situs inversus. The combination of bronchiectasis, sinusitis, and situs inversus is called *Kartagener's syndrome* (see Fig. 23-1).

DCS is an autosomal recessive genetic abnormality with an incidence of about 1 in 20,000 births. Men and women are equally affected. A variety of ultrastructural abnormalities of ciliary microtubules have been reported in association with this syndrome, although in some cases the cilia appear normal.

TABLE 23.6 Dyskinetic Cilia Syndrome and Kartagener's Syndrome

Autosomal-recessive defect
Abnormal ciliary structure and movement
Abnormal mucociliary clearance
50% have situs inversus: Kartagener's syndrome
Sinusitis common
Bilateral bronchiectasis, typically lower or middle lobe

In men, the syndrome may be associated with immotile spermatozoa and infertility; in women, fertility is not affected. Other congenital abnormalities also may be present. In patients with chronic infections and situs inversus, the diagnosis is not difficult. In the absence of situs inversus, criteria for attributing chronic infection to DCS may include immotile spermatozoa (in men), a family history of DCS, or abnormal cilia on biopsy.

Symptoms of recurrent bronchitis, pneumonia, and sinusitis often date from childhood. Radiographs and CT typically show bilateral bronchiectasis with a basal (lower or middle lobe) predominance. Cylindrical bronchiectasis is most common. Appropriate antibiotic treatment is associated with a normal life expectancy.

Young's Syndrome

Young's syndrome, also referred to as *obstructive azoospermia*, is characterized by male infertility caused by obstruction of the epididymis, bronchiectasis, and sinusitis. It may resemble DCS clinically, but ciliary abnormalities are absent. The cause is unknown. The radiographic appearance of the bronchiectasis is nonspecific.

Syndrome of Yellow Nails and Lymphedema

The syndrome of yellow nails and lymphedema is characterized by (1) slowly growing nails that are thickened, curved, and yellow-green in color; (2) lymphedema, usually of the lower extremities, due to lymphatic hypoplasia; and (3) exudative pleural effusions associated with pleural lymphatic dilatation. It is not necessary for all three manifestations to be present; pleural effusion is least common. Chronic sinusitis, airway infection, and bronchiectasis are present in about half of patients (Fig. 23-15). The syndrome typically presents in adulthood.

Tracheobronchomegaly (Mounier-Kuhn Syndrome)

Tracheobronchomegaly, also referred to as *Mounier-Kuhn syndrome*, is characterized by marked dilatation of the trachea and mainstem bronchi, recurrent lower respiratory tract infections, and bronchiectasis (see Figs. 22-29 and 22-31 in Chapter 22). It is most often diagnosed in men in their third and fourth decades; it is much less common in women. The finding of central bronchiectasis associated with dilatation of the trachea is diagnostic. It is described in detail in Chapter 22.

FIG. 23.15. Syndrome of yellow nails. HRCT shows tree-in-bud in the right lower lobe, as a manifestation of airway infection.

Williams-Campbell Syndrome

Williams-Campbell syndrome is a rare type of congenital cystic bronchiectasis due to defective cartilage in the fourth- to sixth-order (central) bronchi. Radiographs and HRCT may show areas of central cystic bronchiectasis with distal regions of abnormal lucency, probably related to air trapping or bronchiolitis (Fig. 23-16). Ballooning of the central bronchi on inspiration and collapse on expiration may occur. These findings are useful in differentiating Williams-Campbell syndrome from other causes of cystic bronchiectasis.

Alpha-1-Antitrypsin Deficiency

In addition to emphysema, bronchiectasis often (40%) is present in patients with alpha-1-antitrypsin deficiency. This correlates well with the fact that approximately 50% of patients with this deficiency manifest symptoms of airway disease—in particular, chronic sputum production. It is likely that bronchiectasis results from a proteinase-antiproteinase imbalance (also responsible for the emphysema), discussed in Chapter 24.

Bronchiectasis Associated with Systemic Diseases

Bronchiectasis may be an important finding in a number of systemic diseases. Of particular interest are the associations between bronchiectasis and collagen-vascular disease and inflammatory bowel disease.

FIG. 23.16. Williams-Campbell syndrome with cystic bronchiectasis. Marked cystic bronchiectasis (*arrows*) is visible in the central lung regions.

Collagen-Vascular Disease

Rheumatoid arthritis (RA) may be associated with a variety of parenchymal abnormalities, including pulmonary fibrosis, organizing pneumonia (OP/BOOP), respiratory tract infections, and necrobiotic nodules. Airway disease, including both bronchiectasis and bronchiolectasis, may also occur in association with RA (see Fig. 14-7 in Chapter 14). One hypothesis suggests that chronic bacterial infections may trigger an immune reaction in genetically predisposed individuals, leading to RA; bronchiectasis may precede RA by years. It has also been suggested that steroids or immunosuppressive therapy may lead to an increased incidence of respiratory infections.

On HRCT, bronchiectasis is seen in up to 35% of patients with this disease, even when chest radiographs are normal. Other findings include mosaic perfusion on inspiratory scans (20%) and air trapping on expiratory scans in (30%). Bronchiectasis may be identified in up to 20% of patients with systemic lupus erythematosus (SLE). A similarly high prevalence of airway pathology has also been noted in patients with primary Sjögren's syndrome.

Ulcerative Colitis and Inflammatory Bowel Disease

A wide range of airway abnormalities have been identified in patients with ulcerative colitis. In addition to OP/BOOP and diffuse interstitial lung disease, these include subglottic tracheal stenosis, chronic bronchitis, and chronic suppurative inflammation of both large and small airways (Fig. 23-17). Similar to what is seen in patients with RA, chronic suppurative airway disease may precede, coexist with, or follow the development of inflammatory bowel disease. Unlike other causes of bronchiectasis, chronic suppurative airway disease associated with ulcerative colitis often responds to treatment with inhaled steroids. Bronchiectasis also is associated with Crohn's disease.

Airway Disease Related to HIV and AIDS

An accelerated form of bronchiectasis may occur in patients with human immunodeficiency virus (HIV) infection and patients with AIDS. It is likely that bronchiectasis results from recurrent or chronic bacterial airway infection. A wide range of organisms may affect the airways in patients with AIDS, most commonly *H. influenzae, P. aeruginosa, S. viridans, S. pneumoniae,* mycobacteria, and fungi such as *Aspergillus* organisms.

HRCT findings include bronchial wall thickening, bronchiectasis, bronchial or bronchiolar impaction with tree-in-bud, consolidation, and air trapping (Fig. 23-18). A lower lobe predominance is typical, and both lower lobes usually are involved.

About 10% of all reported cases of aspergillosis in AIDS patients will affect the airways. *Aspergillus* infection typically occurs late in the course of HIV infection and usually is associated with corticosteroid use and granulocytopenia. There are several distinct types of airway aspergillosis, including necrotizing tracheobronchitis, airway invasive aspergillosis, and obstructing bronchopulmonary aspergillosis.

Necrotizing tracheobronchitis and airway invasive aspergillosis are discussed in Chapter 12.

Obstructing bronchopulmonary aspergillosis in AIDS patients typically presents with acute fever, dyspnea, and cough associated with the expectoration of fungal casts. It is characterized on CT by the presence of mucoid impaction, typically involving the lower lobe airways. It has been suggested that this form of disease is unique to patients with AIDS.

CT Diffezrentiation of Causes of Bronchiectasis

The reliability of radiographs and CT for distinguishing between different causes of bronchiectasis is limited. However, several general rules apply:

1. Lower lobe bronchiectasis is most typical of childhood infections and syndromes associated with impaired mucociliary clearance or immunodeficiency (see Figs. 23-18 and 23-19).
2. Bilateral upper lobe bronchiectasis is seen most commonly in patients with CF and ABPA (see Figs. 23-2C, and 23-11 to 23-14).

FIG. 23.17. Bronchiectasis in Crohn's disease. **A:** Chest radiograph shows large lung volumes, increased markings in the central lung, and evidence of bronchial wall thickening, particularly in the upper lobes. **B:** HRCT shows bronchiectasis and bronchial wall thickening (*arrows*).

Emphysema and Chronic Obstructive Pulmonary Disease

W. RICHARD WEBB

EMPHYSEMA

As defined by the American Thoracic Society, emphysema is "a condition of the lung characterized by permanent, abnormal enlargement of air spaces distal to the terminal bronchiole, accompanied by the destruction of their walls," but "without obvious fibrosis." Currently, it is estimated that 2 million people in the United States suffer from emphysema. It is a significant cause of morbidity and mortality.

PATHOGENESIS OF EMPHYSEMA

It is generally accepted that emphysema results from an imbalance in the dynamic relationship between elastolytic and antielastolytic factors in the lung, usually related to cigarette smoking or enzymatic deficiency. Abnormal or unopposed elastase activity is thought to lead to the tissue destruction that is the primary pathologic abnormality present in patients with this disease.

The proposed mechanisms in the development of emphysema in smokers are as follows:

1. Inhaled tobacco smoke attracts macrophages to distal airways and alveoli (referred to as respiratory bronchiolitis).
2. The macrophages, along with airway epithelial cells, release chemotactic substances that attract neutrophils and induce them to release elastases and other proteolytic enzymes. Macrophages also release proteases in response to tobacco smoke.
3. These elastases have the ability to cleave a variety of proteins, including collagen and elastin. Lung elastin normally is protected from excessive elastase-induced damage by alpha-1-protease inhibitors (alpha-1-antiprotease or alpha-1-antitrypsin) and other circulating antiproteinases.
4. Tobacco smoke tends to interfere with the function of alpha-1-antiprotease.
5. In combination, these interactions result in structural damage in the distal airways and alveoli, leading to emphysema.

Inherited deficiency in alpha-1-antiprotease similarly results in lung destruction and emphysema when neutrophils release elastases and other proteolytic enzymes in response to pulmonary infection.

CLASSIFICATION OF EMPHYSEMA

Emphysema usually is classified into three main subtypes, based on the anatomic distribution of the areas of lung destruction: (1) centrilobular, proximal acinar, or centriacinar emphysema; (2) panlobular or panacinar emphysema; and (3) paraseptal or distal acinar emphysema. The terms *centrilobular, panlobular,* and *paraseptal* are generally accepted and are used to describe these three types of emphysema in the remainder of this chapter. In their early stages, these three forms of emphysema can be easily distinguished morphologically. However, as the emphysema becomes more severe, distinguishing among the types becomes more difficult.

Centrilobular emphysema predominantly affects the respiratory bronchioles in the central portions of acini, and therefore involves the central portion of secondary lobules. It usually results from cigarette smoking and involves mainly the upper lung zones.

Panlobular emphysema involves all the components of the acinus more or less uniformly, and therefore involves entire secondary lobules. It is classically associated with alpha-1-protease inhibitor (alpha-1-antitrypsin) deficiency, although it also may be seen without protease deficiency in smokers, in elderly persons, distal to bronchial and bronchiolar obliteration, and associated with illicit drug use.

Paraseptal emphysema predominantly involves the alveolar ducts and sacs in the lung periphery, with areas of destruction often marginated by interlobular septa. It can be an isolated phenomenon in young adults, often associated with spontaneous pneumothorax, or can be seen in older patients with centrilobular emphysema.

Bullae can develop in association with any type of emphysema, but they are most common with paraseptal or centrilobular emphysema. A *bulla* is a sharply demarcated area of emphysema measuring 1 cm or more in diameter and possessing a wall less than 1 mm in thickness. In some patients with emphysema, bullae can become quite large, resulting in significant compromise of respiratory function; this syndrome is sometimes referred to as *bullous emphysema*. Bullae are most common in a subpleural location, representing foci of paraseptal emphysema associated with air trapping and progressive enlargement.

Irregular air-space enlargement is an additional type of emphysema that occurs in patients with pulmonary fibrosis; this form of emphysema also is referred to as *paracicatricial* or *irregular emphysema*. It commonly is found adjacent to localized parenchymal scars, diffuse pulmonary fibrosis, and in the pneumoconioses, particularly those pneumoconioses associated with progressive massive fibrosis.

DIAGNOSIS OF EMPHYSEMA AND CHRONIC OBSTRUCTIVE PULMONARY DISEASE

In patients with emphysema, pulmonary function tests usually show findings of chronic airflow obstruction and reduced diffusing capacity. Airflow obstruction in patients with emphysema is due to airway collapse on expiration, resulting largely from destruction of lung parenchyma and loss of airway tethering and support. Abnormal diffusing capacity is due to destruction of the lung parenchyma and the pulmonary capillary bed.

It is important to keep in mind that many patients with emphysema also have chronic bronchitis; both conditions are smoking-related diseases.

The term *chronic obstructive pulmonary disease* (COPD) often is used to describe patients with chronic and largely irreversible airway obstruction, most commonly associated with some combination of emphysema and chronic bronchitis. The term itself indicates some uncertainty as to the exact pathogenesis of the functional abnormalities present; it also may be used to refer to diseases usually associated with airway obstruction, such as emphysema and chronic bronchitis, even if no obstruction is demonstrated on pulmonary function tests.

Respiratory symptoms in patients with COPD usually include chronic cough, sputum production, and dyspnea. Although, cough and sputum production are largely manifestations of chronic bronchitis in patients with COPD, the relative contributions of airways disease and emphysema to respiratory disability often are difficult to determine. Typical pulmonary function abnormalities in emphysema include reductions in the ratio of forced expiratory volume in 1 second (FEV_1) to forced vital capacity (FVC), the FEV_1, and the diffusing capacity.

Radiographic Findings

Radiographic abnormalities in patients with COPD are largely the same as those of emphysema. These include increased lung volume and lung destruction (bullae or reduced vascularity). When both findings are used as criteria for diagnosis, a sensitivity as high as 80% has been reported for chest films, although the likelihood of a positive diagnosis depends on the severity of disease. When only findings of lung destruction are used for diagnosis, plain films are only about 40% sensitive.

Although the accuracy of chest radiographs in diagnosing emphysema is controversial, it can be reasonably concluded from the studies performed that moderate to severe emphysema can be diagnosed radiographically, whereas mild emphysema is difficult to detect.

The presence of increased lung volume, or overinflation, is important in making the diagnosis of emphysema on plain radiographs. However, overinflation is an indirect sign of this disease, and findings of increased lung volume are nonspecific. Such findings can be absent in some patients with emphysema but present in patients who have other forms of obstructive pulmonary disease.

Plain radiographic findings of overinflation (Figs. 24-1 and 24-2; Table 24-1) include the following:

1. Lung height of 29.9 cm or more, measured from the dome of the right diaphragm to the tubercle of the first rib
2. Flattening of the right hemidiaphragm on the lateral projection, with a height of less than 2.7 cm measured perpendicular to a line drawn from the anterior to posterior costophrenic angles
3. Flattening of the right hemidiaphragm on a posteroanterior (PA) radiograph, with the highest level of the dome of the right hemidiaphragm being less than 1.5 cm measured perpendicular to a line drawn between the costophrenic angle laterally and the vertebrophrenic angle medially
4. Increased retrosternal air space, measuring more than 4.4 cm at a level 3 cm below the manubrial-sternal junction
5. Right hemidiaphragm at or below the level of the anterior end of the seventh rib
6. Sternodiaphragmatic angle measuring 90 degrees or more

Blunting of the costophrenic angles or visible diaphragmatic slips (i.e., attachments of the diaphragm to the ribs) on the PA view are common findings in markedly increased lung volume; inversion of the hemidiaphragms may be seen on the lateral view (Fig. 24-2).

The presence of bullae on chest radiographs is the only specific sign of lung destruction caused by emphysema and usually means that paraseptal or severe centrilobular emphysema is present (Fig. 24-3). However, this finding is uncommon and may not reflect the presence of generalized disease. Bullae usually are visible in the lung periphery, have thin walls, appear lucent, and lung markings are not seen within them. Lung lucency may reflect the presence of bullae when they are not visible as discrete structures.

A reduction in the size of pulmonary vessels or vessel tapering in the lung periphery also can reflect lung destruction in patients with emphysema (see Fig. 24-2), but this finding lacks

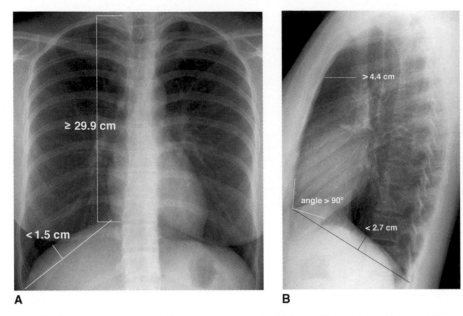

A   B

FIG. 24.1. Plain film measurements in emphysema. **A:** Plain radiographic findings of emphysema on the PA radiograph include a lung height of 29.9 cm or more, measured from the dome of the right diaphragm to the tubercle of the first rib and flattening of the right hemidiaphragm on a posteroanterior radiograph, with the highest level of the dome of the right hemidiaphragm less than 1.5 cm above a perpendicular line drawn between the costophrenic angle laterally and the vertebrophrenic angle medially. **B:** Findings of emphysema on the lateral radiograph include flattening of the right hemidiaphragm, with a height of less than 2.7 cm measured from anterior to posterior costophrenic angles; an increased retrosternal air space, measuring more than 4.4 cm at a level 3 cm below the manubriosternal junction; and a sternodiaphragmatic angle measuring 90 degrees or more.

A   B

FIG. 24.2. Chest radiographs in emphysema. **A:** PA radiograph shows increased lung height with flattening of the diaphragm. The dome of the right hemidiaphragm is below the level of the anterior right seventh rib (7). Blunting of the costophrenic angles is common in increased lung volumes, as are visible diaphragmatic slips (*arrow*) extending to the chest wall. The lungs appear lucent, and vessel size is reduced. Mild prominence of the hila likely reflects pulmonary hypertension. **B:** The lateral view shows increased depth and lucency of the retrosternal space. The diaphragms are flattened and appear inverted (i.e., their normal curvature is reversed).

TABLE 24.1 Radiographic Findings in Emphysema

Increased lung volume
PA view
  ≥29.9 cm from the dome of the right diaphragm to the first rib
  Flattening of the right hemidiaphragm with a height <1.5 cm
  Right hemidiaphragm at or below the level of the anterior seventh rib
  Blunting of the lateral costophrenic angles
  Visible diaphragmatic slips
Lateral view
  Flattening of the right hemidiaphragm with a height of <2.7 cm
  Increased retrosternal air space, measuring >4.4 cm
  Sternodiaphragmatic angle measuring 90 degrees or more
  Blunting of the posterior costophrenic angle

Lung destruction
Bullae
Lung lucency
Decreased vessel size

sensitivity and can be unreliable. Focal absence or displacement of vessels may reflect the presence of bullae (see Fig. 24-3).

On chest radiographs, centrilobular emphysema usually shows an upper lobe predominance of increased lucency and decreased vascularity (see Figs. 24-3 and 24-4). In panlobular emphysema, lucency and decreased vascularity usually appear to involve the lung uniformly or have a basal predominance (Fig. 24-5).

Pulmonary hypertension may develop in patients with emphysema and COPD as a result of destruction of the pulmonary vascular bed. In its early stages, this condition is manifested by dilatation of central pulmonary arteries (see Fig. 24-2). Later, the development of cor pulmonale may result in cardiomegaly and right ventricular enlargement.

HRCT Findings

CT with thick slices is inadequate for the diagnosis of emphysema, but high-resolution CT (HRCT) is highly accurate. On HRCT, emphysema is characterized by the presence of areas of abnormally low attenuation, which can be easily contrasted with surrounding normal lung parenchyma if a sufficiently low window mean (−600 to −700 HU) is used. HRCT

A

B

C

FIG. 24.3. Severe centrilobular emphysema. **A:** Chest radiograph shows lucency in the upper lobes, with vessels being invisible. This appearance is diagnostic of severe emphysema or bullae. Vessels appear displaced inferiorly (*arrows*). This is a common finding with severe emphysema or bullae. **B** and **C:** HRCTs at two levels show severe centrilobular emphysema with marked reduction in vessel size. Areas of emphysema have become confluent, having the appearance of panlobular emphysema.

FIG. 24.7. Severe centrilobular emphysema. Multiple focal lucencies are visible in the upper lobes, without visible walls.

In severe panlobular emphysema, the characteristic appearance of extensive lung destruction and the associated paucity of vascular markings are easily distinguished from normal lung parenchyma. On the other hand, mild

A

B

FIG. 24.8. Centrilobular emphysema with bullae. **A, B:** Centrilobular emphysema is visible in the upper lobes. Areas of emphysema larger than 1 cm are bullae. They often have visible walls. Areas of emphysema in an immediate subpleural location represent paraseptal emphysema.

TABLE 24.3 Panlobular Emphysema
Affects the entire lobule
Alpha-1-antitrypsin deficiency or cigarette smoking
Diffuse or lower lobe predominance
Diffuse decrease in lung attenuation
Focal areas of destruction or bullae usually absent
Reduction in vessel size
May be subtle in its early stages

and even moderately severe panlobular emphysema can be very subtle and difficult to detect. Diffuse panlobular emphysema unassociated with focal areas of lung destruction or bullae may be difficult to distinguish from diffuse small airway obstruction and air trapping resulting from bronchiolitis obliterans.

About 40% of patients with alpha-1-antitrypsin deficiency show bronchiectasis or bronchial wall thickening on HRCT. Patients with alpha-1-antitrypsin deficiency are more susceptible to airway damage during episodes of infection than are normal patients because of the same protease-antiprotease imbalance that leads to emphysema.

Paraseptal Emphysema

Paraseptal emphysema is characterized by the involvement of the distal part of the secondary lobule and, therefore, is most striking in a subpleural location (Table 24-4). Areas of subpleural paraseptal emphysema often have visible walls, but these walls are very thin and often correspond to interlobular septa (Fig. 24-11). Even mild paraseptal emphysema is easily detected by HRCT.

Areas of paraseptal emphysema larger than 1 cm in diameter are most appropriately termed *bullae* (see Fig. 24-11). Subpleural bullae often are considered to be manifestations of paraseptal emphysema, although they may be seen in all types of emphysema and also as an isolated phenomenon.

HRCT may be useful in the detection of apical subpleural bullae invisible on radiographs in patients with idiopathic spontaneous pneumothorax. This form of pneumothorax occurs most often in tall young adults and is thought to be due to rupture of a subpleural bulla. Apical subpleural emphysema is visible on CT in 80% to 90% of patients with spontaneous pneumothorax.

Although paraseptal emphysema may superficially mimic the appearance of honeycombing, several differences make it possible to distinguish between these entities. Paraseptal emphysema occurs in a single layer at the pleural surface (see Fig. 24-11B and C), whereas honeycombing may occur in multiple layers. Paraseptal emphysema is most severe in the apices (see Fig. 24-11); honeycombing is almost always most severe at the bases. Paraseptal emphysema often is associated with cystic spaces larger than 1 cm; such spaces are uncommon with honeycombing.

FIG. 24.9. Panlobular emphysema in alpha-1-antitrypsin deficiency (same patient shown in Fig. 24-5). HRCT scans through the upper (**A**) and lower (**B**) lobes both show a decrease in lung attenuation and vessel size. Focal lucencies, as seen in centrilobular emphysema, are not present.

Bullous Emphysema

The term *bullous emphysema* does not represent a specific pathologic entity but refers to the presence of emphysema associated with large bullae (Table 24-5). It usually is seen in patients with centrilobular or paraseptal emphysema (see Figs. 24-8 and 24-11). A syndrome of bullous emphysema, or *giant bullous emphysema*, has been described based on clinical and radiologic features and is also known as "vanishing lung syndrome" or "primary bullous disease of the lung." Giant bullous emphysema often is seen in young men and is characterized by the presence of large, progressive, upper lobe bullae, which occupy a significant volume of a hemithorax, and often are asymmetric (Figs. 24-12 and 24-13).

Arbitrarily, giant bullous emphysema is said to be present if bullae occupy at least one third of a hemithorax. Most patients with giant bullous emphysema are cigarette smokers, but this entity may also occur in nonsmokers.

Typically, bullae increase progressively in size over time. Rarely, bullae may spontaneously decrease in size or disappear, usually as a result of secondary infection or obstruction of the proximal airway. Spontaneous pneumothorax is common.

Quantitative Evaluation of Emphysema

Although routine axial HRCT images usually suffice for evaluating emphysema, minimum-intensity projection (MinIP)

FIG. 24.10. Panlobular emphysema in alpha-1-antitrypsin deficiency (right lung) in a patient with a left lung transplant. HRCT scans through the upper (**A**) and lower (**B**) lobes both show decreased lung attenuation and vessel size. The right lung is considerably larger than the (normal) left lung. The normal left lung attenuation, vascular size, and volume may be contrasted with that of the emphysematous lung.

TABLE 24.4 Paraseptal Emphysema

Affects subpleural lobules
Cigarette smoking or idiopathic
Upper lower predominance
May be associated with centrilobular emphysema
Focal subpleural lucencies marginated by interlobular septae
Bullae common

images may be used, especially in cases with subtle disease. Coronal reconstructions may be useful in showing the distribution of emphysema.

Emphysema may be quantitated visually or based on CT measurements. Usually, visual quantitation of emphysema as mild, moderate, or severe and a determination of its type and distribution are sufficient for clinical purposes.

Computer analysis of digital data obtained from HRCT also has been used to determine the severity of emphysema. The simplest method involves the use of a threshold value below which emphysema is considered to be present and a determination of the percentage of lung below that threshold; this is termed the "density mask" or "pixel index" technique. Normal lung attenuation usually varies from −770 to −875 HU; on HRCT, emphysema is considered to be present if attenuation measures less than −950 HU.

COMPLICATIONS AND EXACERBATION OF EMPHYSEMA AND COPD

Acute complications of COPD include pneumonia, infection of bullae, and pneumothorax.

Pneumonia may have a typical appearance with dense consolidation, but in patients with moderate or severe emphysema, and in patients with bullae, lung consolidation may be inhomogeneous with consolidation outlining areas of lung destruction or "holes." In this situation, the lung may have a cystic or "Swiss cheese" appearance; the appearance may mimic cavitation.

A

B

C

FIG. 24.11. Paraseptal and centrilobular emphysema in a smoker. **A:** HRCT at the lung apices shows extensive emphysema with bullae. The subpleural bullae represent paraseptal emphysema. **B:** At a lower level, more discrete areas of paraseptal emphysema and subpleural bullae are visible (*arrows*). Emphysema within the central upper lobes is centrilobular. **C:** At a level below that seen in (**B**), the areas of emphysema appear smaller and occur in a single layer.

TABLE 24.5 Bullous Emphysema

Emphysema associated with bullae
May be seen with paraseptal or centrilobular emphysema
Cigarette smoking or idiopathic
"Vanishing lung syndrome"
Large bullae
Often upper lobe
Often asymmetric
Compression of normal lung
Bullae increase or sometimes resolve

The presence of an air-fluid level in a preexisting bulla may indicate infection, hemorrhage, or neoplasm. Thickening of the wall of a bulla may be seen with chronic infection, particularly associated with *Aspergillus*, mycetoma, or neoplasm.

Pneumothorax may occur in patients with emphysema, particularly in the presence of paraseptal emphysema and bullae. COPD is the most common cause of secondary spontaneous pneumothorax (pneumothorax associated with a recognized disease). In some patients with emphysema, it may be difficult to distinguish pneumothorax and bullae on chest radiographs. CT may be valuable in this situation.

Exacerbation of symptoms in patients with COPD may be due to one of these complications. However, exacerbations more often are due to abnormalities not associated with distinct radiographic findings, such as worsening airway infection, increased mucous plugging, and obstruction of small airways. Only about 15% of patients with an exacerbation of COPD show significant abnormal radiographic findings and, based on these abnormalities, treatment is changed in only 5%. It has been recommended that chest radiographs be obtained in patients with an exacerbation of COPD only if there is a history of heart disease or congestive heart failure, intravenous drug abuse, seizures, immunosuppression, other pulmonary disease, or an elevated white blood cell count, fever, chest pain, or edema.

UTILITY OF HRCT IN THE DIAGNOSIS OF EMPHYSEMA AND COPD

HRCT is more sensitive and accurate than plain radiographs in diagnosing the presence, type, and extent of emphysema. Furthermore, HRCT has a high specificity for diagnosing emphysema; emphysema rarely is overdiagnosed in normal individuals or in patients with severe hyperinflation due to other causes.

In clinical practice, however, HRCT rarely is used to diagnose emphysema. Usually, some combination of a smoking history, a low diffusing capacity, airway obstruction on pulmonary function tests, and chest radiographs showing large lung volumes or lung destruction is sufficient to make the diagnosis. On the other hand, some patients with early emphysema present with clinical findings more typical of interstitial lung disease or pulmonary vascular disease, namely shortness of breath and low diffusing capacity, without evidence of airway obstruction on pulmonary function tests or emphysema on chest films. In such patients, HRCT can be valuable in making the diagnosis of emphysema, obviating lung biopsy.

HRCT also can be valuable in the preoperative assessment of patients before surgical treatment of emphysema (e.g., bullectomy, lung transplantation, volume reduction surgery). HRCT has become routine in the evaluation of such patients, both before and after operation. It is used to determine the type, severity, and distribution of emphysema (Fig. 24-14). Lung volume reduction surgery, in which areas of emphysematous lung are resected, works best when emphysema predominates in the upper lobes.

A

B

FIG. 24.12. Bullous emphysema in a young man. **A, B:** Large bullae are visible in the upper lobes, with displacement of normal lung to the bases. Bulla walls are visible (*arrows* in **B**).

A

B

FIG. 24.13. Bullous emphysema. **A:** Chest radiograph shows lucency in the lung apices. The right upper lobe is increased in volume with mediastinal shift to the left. Normal lung is compressed at the lung bases. **B:** HRCT shows large upper lobe bullae, right greater than left. Normal compressed lung is visible on the left. **C:** A large, right-sided bulla remains visible at the level of the carina. Normal right lung is compressed and atelectatic (*arrow*). The contour of this air collection indicates that it is a bulla instead of a pneumothorax; a pneumothorax would be concentric rather than rounded.

C

A

B

FIG. 24.14. Distribution of centrilobular emphysema shown using volumetric CT reformations. **A:** HRCT in a patient with centrilobular emphysema shows lucencies predominating in the right upper lobe. **B:** Minimum-intensity projection image at the same level shows the right upper lobe predominance of disease. **C:** Coronal minimum-intensity projection reformation shows the upper lobe predominance typical of centrilobular emphysema.

C

SELECTED READING

American Thoracic Society. Standards for the diagnosis and care of patients with chronic obstructive pulmonary disease (COPD) and asthma. Am Rev Respir Dis 1987; 136:225–243.

Arakawa H, Kurihara Y, Nakajima Y, et al. Computed tomography measurements of overinflation in chronic obstructive pulmonary disease: evaluation of various radiographic signs. J Thorac Imaging 1998; 13:188–192.

Burki NK. Roentgenologic diagnosis of emphysema: accurate or not? Chest 1989; 95:1178–1179.

Burki NL, Krumpelman JL. Correlation of pulmonary function with the chest roentgenogram in chronic airway obstruction. Am Rev Respir Dis 1980; 121:217–223.

Fishman A, Martinez F, Naunheim K, et al. A randomized trial comparing lung-volume-reduction surgery with medical therapy for severe emphysema. N Engl J Med 2003; 348:2059–2073.

Foster WL, Jr, Gimenez EI, Roubidoux MA, et al. The emphysemas: radiologic-pathologic correlations. Radiographics 1993; 13:311–328.

Gevenois PA, de Maertelaer V, De Vuyst P, et al. Comparison of computed density and macroscopic morphometry in pulmonary emphysema. Am J Respir Crit Care Med 1995; 152:653–657.

Gevenois PA, De Vuyst P, de Maertelaer V, et al. Comparison of computed density and microscopic morphometry in pulmonary emphysema. Am J Respir Crit Care Med 1996; 154:187–192.

Guest PJ, Hansell DM. High resolution computed tomography (HRCT) in emphysema associated with alpha-1-antitrypsin deficiency. Clin Radiol 1992; 45:260–266.

Janoff A. Elastases and emphysema. Current assessment of the protease-antiprotease hypothesis. Am Rev Respir Dis 1985; 132:417–433.

Lesur O, Delorme N, Fromaget JM, et al. Computed tomography in the etiologic assessment of idiopathic spontaneous pneumothorax. Chest 1990; 98:341–347.

Pratt PC. Role of conventional chest radiography in diagnosis and exclusion of emphysema. Am J Med 1987; 82:998–1006.

The National Emphysema Treatment Trial Research Group. Rationale and design of the National Emphysema Treatment Trial (NETT): a prospective randomized trial of lung volume reduction surgery. J Thorac Cardiovasc Surg 1999; 118:518–528.

Reich SB, Weinshelbaum A, Yee J. Correlation of radiographic measurements and pulmonary function tests in chronic obstructive pulmonary disease. AJR Am J Roentgenol 1985; 144:695–699.

Remy-Jardin M, Remy J, Gosselin B, et al. Sliding thin slab, minimum intensity projection technique in the diagnosis of emphysema: histopathologic-CT correlation. Radiology 1996; 200:665–671.

Sherman S, Skoney JA, Ravikrishnan KP. Routine chest radiographs in exacerbations of chronic obstructive pulmonary disease: diagnostic value. Arch Intern Med 1989; 149:2493–2496.

Slone RM, Gierada DS, Yusen RD. Preoperative and postoperative imaging in the surgical management of pulmonary emphysema. Radiol Clin North Am 1998; 36:57–89.

Stern EJ, Webb WR, Weinacker A, Müller NL. Idiopathic giant bullous emphysema (vanishing lung syndrome): imaging findings in nine patients. AJR Am J Roentgenol 1994; 162:279–282.

Sutinen S, Christoforidis AJ, Klugh GA, Pratt PC. Roentgenologic criteria for the recognition of nonsymptomatic pulmonary emphysema: correlation between roentgenologic findings and pulmonary pathology. Am Rev Respir Dis 1965; 91:69–76.

Thurlbeck WM, Müller NL. Emphysema: definition, imaging, and quantification. AJR Am J Roentgenol 1994; 163:1017–1025.

Thurlbeck WM, Simon G. Radiographic appearance of the chest in emphysema. AJR Am J Roentgenol 1978; 130:429–440.

Diffuse Cystic Lung Diseases

W. RICHARD WEBB

A *cyst* is a thin-walled, well-defined, air-containing lung lesion 1 cm or more in diameter. Cysts may be seen in patients with emphysema (i.e., bullae; see Figs. 24-3, 24-8, 24-12, and 24-13 in Chapter 24); honeycombing (i.e., large honeycomb cysts; see Fig. 10-17B in Chapter 10); pneumonia (i.e., pneumatoceles) (Fig. 25-1); cystic bronchiectasis (i.e., dilated bronchi) (Fig. 25-2; see also Fig. 9-28 in Chapter 9); subacute hypersensitivity pneumonitis; trauma with lung laceration (see Fig. 9-36 in Chapter 9); multiple healing cavities; and some parasitic infections (Table 25-1). The differential diagnosis (see Table 9-6 in Chapter 9) overlaps with that of multiple cavitary masses.

Several lung diseases are characterized by cysts as their primary abnormality. These are rare, and include Langerhans cell histiocytosis (LCH), lymphangiomyomatosis (LAM), tuberous sclerosis (TS), neurofibromatosis, lymphoid interstitial pneumonia (LIP), and Sjögren's syndrome. Another rare disease, tracheobronchial papillomatosis, is discussed in Chapter 3.

PULMONARY LANGERHANS CELL HISTIOCYTOSIS (PULMONARY HISTIOCYTOSIS X)

The term *Langerhans cell histiocytosis* refers to a group of diseases of unknown etiology, most often recognized in childhood, in which Langerhans cell accumulations involve one or more body systems, including bone, lung, pituitary gland, mucous membranes and skin, lymph nodes, and liver. This disease also is known as *histiocytosis X* or *eosinophilic granuloma* (Table 25-2). Lung involvement in LCH is common, seen in 40% of patients, and may be an isolated abnormality. In patients with multisystem disease, other commonly affected sites include bone and the pituitary gland.

In the early stage, pulmonary LCH is characterized by the presence of granulomas containing large numbers of Langerhans cells and eosinophils, resulting in destruction of lung tissue. LCH lesions typically are peribronchiolar in distribution. In the later stages of the disease, the cellular granulomas are replaced by fibrosis and lung cysts. Although LCH is characterized by a clonal proliferation of cells, it is likely that LCH in adults represents an abnormal immune response in response to an unidentified antigenic stimulus rather than a neoplasm.

Most patients with pulmonary LCH are young or middle-aged adults (average age, 32 years). Over 90% of adults with LCH are smokers, and this disease is considered to be related to smoking in most cases. Common presenting symptoms include cough and dyspnea. Up to 20% of patients present with pneumothorax.

Compared to patients with multisystem disease, the prognosis in patients with isolated pulmonary involvement is good; the disease regresses spontaneously in 25% and stabilizes clinically and radiographically in 50%. In the remaining 25% of cases, the disease follows a progressive downhill course, resulting in diffuse cystic lung destruction. In a small number of cases, death results from either respiratory insufficiency or pulmonary hypertension.

Radiographic Findings

The radiographic findings of LCH include reticular, nodular, and reticulonodular patterns, often in combination (Figs. 25-3, and 25-4A and B); a cystic appearance may

FIG. 25.1. Pneumocystis pneumonia with pneumatoceles. Ground-glass opacity representing acute pneumonia is associated with multiple clustered lung cysts. This appearance is common in pneumocystis pneumonia.

A

B

FIG. 25.2. Sarcoidosis with extensive upper lobe cystic bronchiectasis. **A:** Detail view of the right upper lobe from a chest radiograph shows a cystic appearance. **B:** HRCT shows cystic bronchiectasis, possibly associated with areas of emphysema. Abnormal bronchi and branching cysts (*arrows*) are a clue to the correct diagnosis.

mimic honeycombing. Abnormalities usually are bilateral, predominantly involving the middle and upper lung zones, with relative sparing of the costophrenic angles. Lung volumes are characteristically normal or increased (see Fig. 25-4A,B), an unusual appearance in the presence of reticular opacities or honeycombing.

TABLE 25.1 Multiple Lung Cysts

Bullae
Honeycombing
Pneumonia with pneumatoceles (e.g., pneumocystis)
Cystic bronchiectasis
Hypersensitivity pneumonitis (subacute)
Trauma with lung laceration
Healing cavities (e.g., abscesses, Wegener's, cavitary rheumatoid nodules)
Parasitic infections (e.g., Echinococcus, paragonimiasis)
Langerhans cell histiocytosis
Lymphangiomyomatosis
Tuberous sclerosis
Neurofibromatosis
Lymphoid interstitial pneumonia
Sjögren's syndrome

HRCT Findings

In almost all patients, HRCT demonstrates cystic air spaces, which are usually less than 10 mm in diameter (see Figs. 25-4 to 25-6). The lung cysts have walls, which range from being thin and barely perceptible to several millimeters thick. The presence of distinct walls makes it possible to differentiate these cysts from areas of emphysema. Although many cysts appear round, they can also have bizarre shapes, being bilobed or clover-leaf in appearance (see Figs. 25-4 to 25-6). An upper lobe predominance in the size and number of cysts is common (see Figs. 25-4 and 25-6). Large cysts or bullae (more than 10 mm in diameter) are seen in more than half of cases; some cysts are larger than 20 mm. True honeycombing, often suggested by the chest radiograph, does not occur.

In some patients, cysts are the only abnormality visible on HRCT, but in many cases, small nodules (usually less than 5 mm in diameter) are also present (see Figs. 25-3 and 25-5). Larger nodules, sometimes exceeding 1 cm, may be seen, but are less common (25%). Nodules can vary considerably in number in individual cases, probably depending on the activity of the disease; nodules can be few in number or myriad. The margins of nodules often are irregular, particularly when there is surrounding cystic or reticular disease. On HRCT, many nodules can be seen to be peribronchial or peribronchiolar, and, therefore, centrilobular in location. Some nodules, particularly those larger than 1 cm in diameter, may show lucent centers, presumably corresponding to small "cavities." These cavities, however,

TABLE 25.2 Langerhans Cell Histiocytosis

Lung involvement in 40%; may be an isolated abnormality
90% of adult patients are smokers
Granulomas in early stages
Lung cysts late in course
Cysts irregular in shape
Upper lobe predominance
Spare costophrenic angles
Nodules or cavitary nodules in some

FIG. 25.3. Langerhans cell histiocytosis in a 21-year-old smoker. **A:** Chest radiograph shows ill-defined nodules, predominating in the upper lobes. **B:** Detail view of the right upper lobe shows small nodules. **C:** HRCT through the upper lobes shows small nodules, cavitary nodules, and small irregular lung cysts. **D:** HRCT through the mid lungs shows a similar appearance. The lung bases were relatively normal.

sometimes represent a dilated bronchiolar lumen surrounded by peribronchiolar granulomas and thickened interstitium.

In nearly all cases, the lung bases and the costophrenic sulci are relatively spared (see Fig. 25-4). An upper lobe predominance in size and number of cysts is present in most patients (see Fig. 25-6), and a basal predominance is never observed.

Pulmonary lesions may evolve in a characteristic sequence, beginning with centrilobular nodules, followed by cavitation, the formation of thick-walled cysts, and, finally, thin-walled cysts. Nodular lesions may regress spontaneously or may be replaced by cysts, but cystic lesions, once formed, persist, eventually becoming indistinguishable from diffuse emphysema.

Associated hilar or mediastinal lymph node enlargement or lytic bone lesions also may be present (Fig. 25-7).

LYMPHANGIOMYOMATOSIS

Lymphangiomyomatosis or lymphangioleiomyomatosis is a rare disease characterized by progressive proliferation of immature-appearing smooth muscle cells (LAM cells) in relation to bronchioles, small pulmonary vessels, and lymphatics in the chest and abdomen (Table 25-3). Peribronchiolar infiltration eventually leads to bronchiolar obstruction and destruction of lung parenchyma with formation of isolated lung cysts. Very small nodules (1 to 3 mm) also may be present, representing focal proliferations of type II pneumocytes. Renal angiomyolipomas are present in 15% of cases.

Spindle cell proliferation also can involve the hilar, mediastinal, and extrathoracic lymph nodes, sometimes resulting in dilatation of intrapulmonary lymphatics and the thoracic

FIG. 25.4. Langerhans cell histiocytosis. PA (**A**) and lateral (**B**) chest radiographs show large lung volumes and a fine reticular pattern. **C:** HRCT through the upper lobes shows numerous thin-walled lung cysts, some irregular in shape. **D:** Near the level of the carina, a diffuse cystic abnormality persists. **E:** HRCT shows sparing of the costophrenic angles. **F:** This patient's lung removed at the time of lung transplantation shows cystic lesions with an upper lobe predominance.

FIG. 25.5. Langerhans cell histiocytosis. HRCT shows numerous irregularly shaped cysts in the upper lobes. Nodules (*arrows*) are visible as well.

FIG. 25.6. Langerhans cell histiocytosis. **A:** HRCT shows numerous irregularly shaped cysts in the upper lobes. The cysts are thick-walled. This is characteristic of early disease. Nodules (*arrows*) also are visible. **B:** HRCT at the right lung base shows smaller and less numerous cysts as well as nodules (*arrows*).

FIG. 25.7. Langerhans cell histiocytosis in a 2-year-old child. **A:** Chest CT shows hilar lymph node enlargement (*arrows*). **B:** A lytic lesion (*arrow*) in the skull also is visible.

duct. Involvement of the lymphatics can lead to chylous pleural effusions or ascites. Proliferation of cells in the walls of pulmonary veins may cause venous obstruction and lead to pulmonary venous hypertension with resultant hemoptysis.

LAM occurs almost exclusively in women of childbearing age, usually between 17 and 50 years. Occasional cases present in postmenopausal women probably as a result of slow progression. Although the etiology of LAM remains unclear, a chromosomal abnormality has been reported in some cases.

Most patients present with dyspnea, pneumothorax, or cough. The mean time interval from the onset of symptoms to diagnosis is typically 3 to 5 years. Sixty percent of patients have chylous pleural effusions; up to 80% have pneumothoraces; and 30% to 40% have blood-streaked sputum or frank hemoptysis. Nearly all patients have abnormal pulmonary function at presentation.

TABLE 25.3 Lymphangiomyomatosis

Proliferation of immature-appearing smooth muscle cells
Women of childbearing age
Identical to the lung disease seen in tuberous sclerosis
Cystic lung destruction
Chylous effusions
Renal angiomyolipomas are present in 15%
Lung cysts
Round in shape
Diffuse distribution
Involve the costophrenic angles
Nodules occasionally seen

Clinical improvement has been reported following treatment with progesterone, tamoxifen, or other antiestrogen agents; radiotherapy; or oophorectomy. Responses to such treatments are variable, however. Progression is typical, and most patients die within 5 to 10 years from the onset of symptoms. As a consequence, LAM is now considered an indication for lung transplantation. The abnormality may recur in the transplanted lung.

Radiographic Findings

On plain radiographs, 80% of patients with LAM show a fine reticular pattern. In patients with advanced disease, a cystic pattern mimicking that of honeycombing may be seen (Figs. 25-8 and 25-9). Lungs usually appear to be diffusely abnormal, with the lung bases involved to the same degree as the apices. As with Langerhans histiocytosis, lung volumes often appear increased despite the presence of reticulation.

FIG. 25.8. Lymphangiomyomatosis. Chest radiograph shows increased lung volume with reticular opacities at the lung bases. Blunting of the costophrenic angles results from chylous effusions.

Pleural abnormalities may precede, accompany, or be seen after the recognition of lung disease. About 50% of patients have radiographic evidence of pneumothorax at the time of presentation, and unilateral or bilateral pleural effusion is present in 10% to 20% of cases (see Fig. 25-8). About 10% to 25% of patients have normal-appearing radiographs at presentation despite the presence of lung cysts.

HRCT Findings

On HRCT, patients with LAM characteristically show numerous, isolated, thin-walled, rounded lung cysts (see Fig. 25-9). These cysts usually range from 2 to 5 mm in diameter, but may be larger. Their size tends to increase with progression of the disease. In patients with extensive disease in which 80% or more of the lung parenchyma is involved, most cysts are more than 1 cm in diameter. The walls of the lung cysts usually are thin and faintly perceptible. Irregularly shaped lung cysts, as are seen in patients with LCH, are uncommon.

The cysts are most often distributed diffusely throughout the lungs, from apex to base, and no lung zone is spared (see Fig. 25-9); diffuse lung involvement is seen even in patients with mild disease.

In most patients, the lung parenchyma between the cysts appears normal on HRCT. In some cases, however, a slight increase in linear interstitial markings, interlobular septal thickening, or patchy areas of ground-glass opacity also are seen. The latter probably represent areas of pulmonary hemorrhage. Small nodules occasionally are seen, but they are not a prominent feature of this disease as they are with LCH.

In many cases, a specific CT diagnosis may be made when characteristic diffuse, thin-walled, rounded lung cysts are identified in a woman of childbearing age.

On HRCT, as with chest radiography, pneumothorax may be seen to be associated with cysts in patients with LAM. Other features of LAM include pleural effusion and hilar, mediastinal, and retrocrural adenopathy. Renal angiomyolipomas may be visible on scans through the upper abdomen.

TUBEROUS SCLEROSIS

TS is an autosomal-dominant genetic disease of mesoderm associated with the classic triad of seizures, mental retardation, and adenoma sebaceum. It also is associated with abnormalities such as angiomyolipomas of the kidneys, cardiac rhabdomyomas, and retinal phacomas.

About 1% of patients with TS have lung disease virtually identical to that of LAM, although there may be subtle histologic differences between the two entities. It is not inappropriate to think of the lung disease of TS as a subtype of LAM.

Presenting symptoms are similar. Although TS affects both sexes equally, as with LAM, pulmonary abnormalities have been described almost exclusively in women. Radiographic findings are indistinguishable in individual cases (Figs. 25-10 and 25-11), although the presence of renal angiomyolipomas is more suggestive of TS. However, angiomyolipomas may be seen in LAM in the absence of TS.

FIG. 25.11. Tuberous sclerosis. **A:** CT through the lung bases shows cystic lesions and small nodules. Unenhanced (**B**) and enhanced (**C**) CTs show a low-attenuation angiomyolipoma (*arrow* in **B**) in the right kidney.

typically are increased, with flattening of the diaphragms. HRCT may show isolated cysts or bullae (Fig. 25-13).

LYMPHOID INTERSTITIAL PNEUMONIA AND SJÖGREN'S SYNDROME

LIP is a benign lymphoproliferative disorder characterized by a diffuse interstitial infiltrate of lymphocytes and plasma cells. LIP often occurs in association with collagen-vascular disease and Sjögren's syndrome.

Both LIP and Sjögren's syndrome may show a variety of radiographic and HRCT abnormalities, including a reticular or nodular pattern, patchy or diffuse ground-glass opacity (see Chapters 13 and 14), and multiple thin-walled lung cysts (see Figs. 13-32, 13-34, and 13-35 in Chapter 13). Cysts are most typical of LIP in Sjögren's syndrome. The cysts may be small or large, round or oval in shape, and thin-walled; they tend to be fewer in number than those seen in patients with LCH or LAM. Cysts may be an isolated abnormality or may be accompanied by other findings of LIP or Sjögren's syndrome.

A   B

FIG. 25.12. Neurofibromatosis. PA (**A**) and lateral (**B**) chest radiographs show large lung volumes with upper lobe lucency and a reticular pattern predominant at the lung bases.

FIG. 25.13. Neurofibromatosis. HRCT shows cysts and bullae indistinguishable from emphysema.

SELECTED READING

Aberle DR, Hansell DM, Brown K, Tashkin DP. Lymphangiomyomatosis: CT, chest radiographic, and functional correlations. Radiology 1990; 176:381–387.

Brauner MW, Grenier P, Mouelhi MM, et al. Pulmonary histiocytosis X: evaluation with high resolution CT. Radiology 1989; 172:255–258.

Chu SC, Horiba K, Usuki J, et al. Comprehensive evaluation of 35 patients with lymphangioleiomyomatosis. Chest 1999; 115:1041–1052.

Howarth DM, Gilchrist GS, Mullan BP, et al. Langerhans cell histiocytosis: diagnosis, natural history, management, and outcome. Cancer 1999; 85:2278–2290.

Johkoh T, Müller NL, Pickford HA, et al. Lymphocytic interstitial pneumonia: thin-section CT findings in 22 patients. Radiology 1999; 212: 567–572.

Kirchner J, Stein A, Viel K, et al. Pulmonary lymphangioleiomyomatosis: high-resolution CT findings. Eur Radiol 1999; 9:49–54.

Kitaichi M, Nishimura K, Itoh H, Izumi T. Pulmonary lymphangioleiomyomatosis: a report of 46 patients including a clinicopathologic study of prognostic factors. Am J Respir Crit Care Med 1995; 151:527–533.

Lenoir S, Grenier P, Brauner MW, et al. Pulmonary lymphangiomyomatosis and tuberous sclerosis: comparison of radiographic and thin-section CT findings. Radiology 1990; 175:329–334.

Moore AD, Godwin JD, Müller NL, et al. Pulmonary histiocytosis X: comparison of radiographic and CT findings. Radiology 1989; 172:249–254.

Müller NL, Chiles C, Kullnig P. Pulmonary lymphangiomyomatosis: correlation of CT with radiographic and functional findings. Radiology 1990; 175:335–339.

Templeton PA, McLoud TC, Müller NL, et al. Pulmonary lymphangioleiomyomatosis: CT and pathologic findings. J Comput Assist Tomogr 1989; 13:54–57.

The Pleura and Pleural Disease

W. RICHARD WEBB

INTERLOBAR FISSURES

The interlobar fissures represent invaginations of the visceral pleura that separate or partially separate the lobes of the lung. Recognizing the fissures is essential in the localization and diagnosis of both pleural and parenchymal abnormalities.

The Major (Oblique) Fissure

On the left, the major fissure separates the lower lobe from the upper lobe. On the right, it separates the lower lobe from the upper and middle lobes (see Figs. 2-29 and 2-30 in Chapter 2).

The major fissures originate posteriorly, above the level of the aortic arch, near the level of the fifth thoracic vertebra, and angle anteriorly and inferiorly, nearly parallel to the sixth rib. Posteriorly, the superior aspect of the left major fissure is cephalad to the right in 75%. They terminate along the anterior diaphragmatic pleural surface of each hemithorax, several centimeters posterior to the anterior chest wall.

Portions of one or both major fissures are almost always visible on the lateral radiograph. A thin triangular opacity representing fat is seen in 20% of cases at the point the major fissure contacts the hemidiaphragm. A similar opacity may be seen in the presence of a small amount of pleural fluid.

The major fissures can be distinguished on the lateral radiograph in several ways:

1. The surface of the right hemidiaphragm is visible in its entirety in most patients, while the anterior surface of the left hemidiaphragm is usually obscured by the heart; if a fissure is visible in continuity with the anterior part of a complete diaphragm, it is the right major fissure.
2. The left hemidiaphragm may be identified by its intimate relationship to the stomach bubble; this may in turn allow identification of the left posterior costophrenic angle, the left posterior ribs, and then the left major fissure in continuity with the posterior ribs.
3. The right posterior ribs are usually projected posterior to the left on a well-positioned left lateral radiograph and appear larger than the left ribs because they are farther from the film and more magnified. This is termed the

"big rib sign." A fissure in contiguity with "big ribs" is the right major fissure.
4. The right major fissure may be identified if it is seen contacting the minor fissure.

The major fissures are not clearly seen on frontal radiographs in normal subjects. In 5% to 10% of patients, however, a subtle arcuate opacity may be seen in the upper thorax, extending superiorly and medially from the lateral chest wall, representing contact of the superior part of the major fissure with the posterolateral thorax; this opacity is likely related to a small amount of fat or pleural fluid entering the edge of the fissure. Typically, it is sharply margined on its undersurface and ill defined superiorly. A similar but more pronounced opacity may be seen with pleural effusion (Fig. 26-1) extending into the posterior part of the major fissure.

On CT, the major fissures are oriented obliquely to the scan plane, and because of volume averaging, their appearance is variable and depends on slice thickness.

With thick slices, the fissures themselves are visible in only 40% of cases, although the location of each fissure can usually be inferred because of the presence of an avascular band, several centimeters thick, within the lung parenchyma. These bands appear "avascular" because of the small size of vessels located in the peripheral lung on either side of the fissure. In some cases, the major fissures are visible on thick slices as ill-defined bands of opacity, due to volume averaging of the fissure with adjacent lung, or hypoinflation of the dependent portions of the upper lobes, adjacent to the fissure. Occasionally, the fissure is visible as a linear opacity with thick slices.

On CT obtained using thin slices or high-resolution technique, the major fissures usually appear as thin, well-defined lines surrounded by a plane of relatively avascular lung measuring about 1 cm thick. The orientation of the major fissures varies at different levels. In the upper thorax, the major fissures angle posterolaterally from the mediastinum (see Fig. 2-30A in Chapter 2). Within the lower thorax, the major fissures angle anterolaterally from the mediastinum. In nearly 20% of cases, a focal thickening of the fissure is seen on CT just above its point of contact with the diaphragm; this represents fat extending into the fissure.

FIG. 26.1. Small pleural effusion outlining the posterior major fissure. The normal location of the major fissure where it contacts the posterolateral chest wall is well shown (*large arrows*). As in this case, it is sharply marginated on its undersurface and ill defined superiorly. The minor fissure is also visible (*small arrow*).

If a portion of the fissure is invisible on HRCT, it likely indicates that the fissure is incomplete with partial fusion of the lobes (Fig. 26-2). Incomplete fissures provide a pathway for collateral ventilation or spread of disease from one lobe to another. The right major fissure is incomplete in 70%, and some degree of fusion is present between the lower lobe and the upper lobe in 70% and between the lower lobe and middle lobe in 50%. On the left, the major fissure has been reported to be incomplete in 40% to 70% of patients.

In some cases, cardiac motion during the scan results in an artifact termed the *double-fissure sign*; when this artifact is present, the fissure is visible in two locations on the same scan separated by a few mm.

The Minor (Horizontal) Fissure

The minor or horizontal fissure separates the superior aspect of the right middle lobe from the right upper lobe. The minor

FIG. 26.2. Incomplete major fissures. **A, B:** HRCT shows normal-appearing major fissures laterally (*large arrows*). Medially, the fissures are incomplete and invisible on HRCT (*small arrows*).

fissure is incomplete in more than 80% of cases, most often laterally (see Figs. 2-29 and 2-30 in Chapter 2).

On a frontal radiograph, the minor fissure or a portion of the fissure is visible in 50% to 80% of cases, appearing as a roughly horizontal line, generally at or near the level of the anterior fourth rib. Its contour is variable, but its lateral part is often visible inferior to its medial part. Medially, the fissure usually appears to arise at the level of the right hilum and interlobar pulmonary artery.

On the lateral radiograph, the anterior part of the fissure often appears inferior to its posterior part. The posterior part of the fissure may be seen to end at the major fissure or may appear to extend posterior to it.

On CT obtained with thick slices, the minor fissure is rarely visible, as its position generally parallels the scan plane. Characteristically, however, the position of the minor fissure can be inferred because of a broad avascular region in the anterior portion of the right lung, anterior to the major fissure, at the level of the bronchus intermedius. This avascular region represents peripheral lung on each side of the fissure, lying in or near the plane of scan. The avascular region is often triangular, with the one corner of the triangle at the pulmonary hilum and the other two corners laterally. However, there is considerable variation in the appearance of the minor fissure due to variations in its orientation and curvature. In some cases, the avascular plane of the minor fissure appears rectangular, round, or elliptical.

The appearance of the minor fissure on HRCT scans is quite variable (Fig. 26-3). Depending on its orientation and contour, the fissure may appear as (1) a linear opacity, directed from anterior to posterior; (2) a linear opacity

FIG. 26.3. CT appearances of the minor fissure. **A:** HRCT through the lung bases shows the major fissures (*large arrows*) and the right minor fissure as a linear opacity extending from medial to lateral (*small white arrows*). The fissures delineate the upper (*UL*), middle (*ML*), and lower lobes (*LL*). A left minor fissure is also visible (*black arrows*), separating the lingula from the remainder of the upper lobe. **B:** At a higher level in the same patient, the minor fissure is visible as an arcuate or ringlike opacity (*arrows*). **C:** Slightly cephalad to (**B**), the fissure lies in the scan plane. The region of the fissure is visible as an avascular area (*arrows*).

extending from medial to lateral, paralleling and anterior to the major fissure (see Fig. 26-3A); (3) a circle or ring (see Fig. 26-3B); or (4) an ill-defined opacity or avascular regions resulting from the fissure lying in the plane of scan (see Fig. 26-3C).

Because the minor fissure often angles caudally, from posterior to anterior, the lower lobe, middle lobe, and upper lobe can all be seen on a single HRCT scan (see Fig. 26-3A). If this is the case, the major and minor fissures can have a similar appearance, with the major fissure being posterior and the minor fissure anterior; in this situation, the lower lobe is most posterior, the upper lobe is most anterior, and the middle lobe is in the middle. If the minor fissure is concave caudally, it can appear ring shaped, with the middle lobe in the center of the ring (see Fig. 26-3B).

Accessory Fissures

Accessory fissures separate a lung segment or a part of a lobe from the remainder of a lobe; numerous accessory fissures have been identified. As many as 50% of lungs show an accessory fissure, but these are less often visible radiographically.

An *azygos fissure* is present in 1 in 200 subjects, defining the presence of an *azygos lobe* (Fig. 26-4). An azygos lobe represents parts of the apical or posterior segments of the right upper lobe. An azygos fissure and azygos lobe are formed when the azygos vein invaginates the right upper lobe during gestation. The azygos fissure consists of four layers of pleura (two parietal and two visceral) and contains the arch of the azygos vein. On the frontal radiograph, the azygos fissure has a characteristic curvilinear appearance adjacent to

A

B

C

D

FIG. 26.4. Azygos fissure and azygos lobe. **A:** Chest radiograph shows the characteristic curvilinear appearance of the azygos fissure adjacent to the right mediastinum (*small arrows*). The azygos arch is visible within the right upper lobe (*large white arrow*) and has a teardrop appearance. The azygos arch is not visible in its normal location (*black arrow*). **B:** CT shows the typical curved appearance of the azygos fissure (*arrows*). **C:** At a lower level, the azygos arch (*small arrows*) extends from the right brachiocephalic vein anteriorly (*large arrow*) to a posterior and paravertebral location. **D:** Thickening of the azygos fissure (*arrows*) due to right pleural effusion in a different patient.

the right mediastinum, convex laterally; the azygos vein has a teardrop appearance at the inferior extent of the fissure. The azygos fissure is identifiable on CT as a thin, curved line. It extends from the right brachiocephalic vein, anteriorly, to a position adjacent to the right posterolateral aspect of the T4 or T5 vertebral body (see Fig. 26-4B and C). A left "azygos" fissure, associated with the left superior intercostal vein, is rarely seen.

The *inferior accessory fissure* separates the medial basal segment of either lower lobe from the remaining basal segments. It is present anatomically in 30% to 45% of lobes. On plain radiographs, this fissure is visible in 10%, extending superiorly and medially from the medial third of the hemidiaphragm. On CT, it is seen in 15% of cases, extending laterally and anteriorly from the region of the inferior pulmonary ligament to join the major fissure (Fig. 26-5).

The *superior accessory fissure* demarcates the superior segment from the remainder of the lower lobe; it is more common on the right. It is seen at about the same level as the minor fissure.

The *left minor fissure* is present anatomically in approximately 10% of normal lungs, separating the lingula from the remainder of the left upper lobe (Figs. 26-3A and 26-6). It is visible on plain radiographs in about 1%, appearing somewhat higher than the right minor fissure.

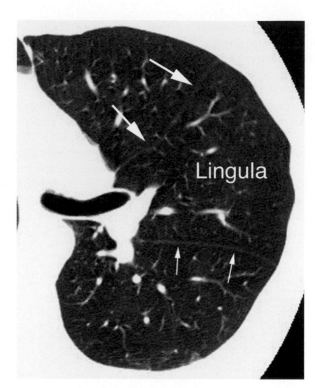

FIG. 26.6. Left minor fissure. The minor fissure (*large arrows*) separates the lingular segments from the remainder of the upper lobe. The major fissure (*small arrows*) is also seen.

INFERIOR PULMONARY LIGAMENTS AND PHRENIC NERVES

The right and left inferior pulmonary ligaments each represent a double layer of pleura that serves to anchor the lung to the mediastinum. They are formed as reflections of the visceral pleura lining the medial surfaces of the lower lobes onto the mediastinal pleural surface. They extend inferiorly and posteriorly from just below the pulmonary hila to the diaphragm. The ligaments can terminate before reaching the diaphragm or extend over the medial diaphragmatic surface. They may divide the medial pleural space below the hila into anterior and posterior compartments. The ligaments may also contain systemic vessels supplying the lung.

The inferior pulmonary ligaments are invisible on chest radiographs. On CT, they are visible as very short, thin, linear or triangular opacities below the level of the right and left inferior pulmonary veins, and often adjacent to the esophagus (Fig. 26-7). Although they do not extend into the lung parenchyma, they often appear contiguous with a connective tissue septum in the medial lung, termed the *intersublobar septum* (see Fig. 26-7B). On CT, the inferior pulmonary ligaments are visible in 40% to 70% of cases.

Similar thin lines may be seen on CT, anterior to the inferior pulmonary ligaments, representing pleural reflections

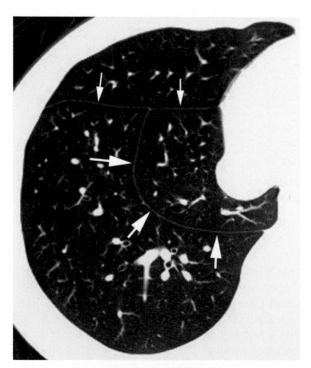

FIG. 26.5. Inferior accessory fissure. The fissure (*large arrows*) separates the medial basal segment of the lower lobe from the remainder of the basal segments. The major fissure (*small arrows*) is noted anteriorly.

A   **B**

FIG. 26.7. The inferior pulmonary ligaments and pleural reflections over the phrenic nerves. **A:** HRCT on the right shows the inferior pulmonary ligament as a thin triangular opacity (*large arrow*) arising in the region of the esophagus. The pleural reflection overlying the right phrenic nerve (*PN*) is seen lateral to the inferior vena cava (*IVC*). **B:** CT on the left shows the inferior pulmonary ligament as a triangular opacity (*large arrow*) lateral to the esophagus. A linear opacity extending from the inferior pulmonary ligament into the lung represents the intersublobar septum (*ISS*). The pleural reflection overlying the left phrenic nerve (*PN*) is seen more anteriorly.

over the right and left phrenic nerves (see Fig. 26-7). On the right, this opacity is usually seen lateral to the inferior vena cava (see Fig. 26-7A). The pleural reflections may be seen to extend over the surface of the diaphragm.

THE PLEURAL SURFACES AND ADJACENT CHEST WALL

A number of tissues, arranged in layers, surround the lung and line the inner aspect of the thoracic cavity. Knowledge of their anatomy is helpful in understanding normal radiographic and CT findings and the appearances of pleural diseases (Figs. 26-8 and 26-9).

The combined thickness of the layers of *visceral and parietal pleura* that surround the lung, and the fluid-containing pleural space, is less than 0.5 mm.

External to the parietal pleura is a layer of loose areolar tissue (*extrapleural fat*), which separates the parietal pleura from the endothoracic fascia. This fatty layer is very thin in most locations but can be markedly thickened over the

lateral or posterolateral ribs, resulting in extrapleural fat pads several millimeters thick.

The thoracic cavity is lined by the fibroelastic *endothoracic fascia* that covers the surface of the intercostal muscles and intervening ribs, blends with the perichondrium and periosteum of the costal cartilages and sternum anteriorly, and posteriorly is continuous with the prevertebral fascia that covers the vertebral bodies and intervertebral discs.

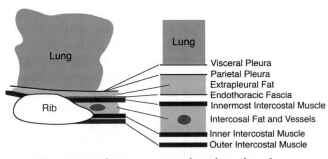

FIG. 26.8. Normal structures at the pleural surface.

FIG. 26.10. Parietal pleural thickening and calcification in asbestos exposure. **A:** Chest radiograph shows thickened pleura separating aerated lung from the adjacent ribs (*small arrows*). Pleural calcification (*large arrows*) is visible on the surface of the hemidiaphragms. **B:** CT shows thickened parietal pleura internal to the ribs (*large arrow*) and internal to the intercostal stripe (i.e., innermost intercostal muscle; *small arrows*). In both locations, a layer of thickened extrapleural fat separates the thickened pleura from the chest wall. Pleural calcification is also seen. **C:** Thickened parietal pleura (*small arrows*) is visible internal to the ribs and internal to the intercostal stripe (i.e., innermost intercostal muscle). A stripe of density in the paravertebral regions (*large arrows*) indicates pleural thickening. **D:** At the level of the diaphragm, thickened pleura is visible in the paravertebral regions and internal to the ribs (*small arrows*). Calcified pleura on the surface of the hemidiaphragms (*large arrows*) is typical of asbestos exposure.

Normal Fat Pads

Normal extrapleural fat is most abundant over the postero-lateral fourth to eighth ribs and can produce fat pads several millimeters thick that extend into the intercostal spaces.

On plain radiographs, the presence of a soft tissue stripe passing internal to the ribs, thus separating the lung from the chest wall, is generally taken to indicate the presence of a pleural thickening or effusion. However, in normal patients with extrapleural fat thickening or fat pads, a similar appearance may be seen.

Pleural disease and fat thickening can usually be distinguished; in contrast to pleural thickening or effusion, normal fat thickening is typically symmetrical and smooth in contour, appears low in attenuation, and is unassociated with costophrenic angle blunting.

Normal extrapleural fat can sometimes be seen on CT internal to the ribs. This appears very low in density and is easy to distinguish from thickened pleura.

The Subcostalis and Transversus Thoracis Muscles

These are invisible on chest radiographs. On CT, a 1- to 2-mm-thick line is sometimes seen internal to one or more ribs, along the posterior chest wall at the level of the heart, representing the subcostalis muscle (Fig. 26-11). This may closely mimic the appearance of focal pleural thickening. The subcostalis muscle is visible in a small percentage of patients.

Anteriorly, at the level of the heart and adjacent to the lower sternum or xiphoid process, the transversus thoracis muscles are nearly always visible on CT internal to the anterior ends of ribs or costal cartilages (see Fig. 26-11).

In contrast to pleural thickening, these muscles are smooth, uniform in thickness, and symmetric bilaterally.

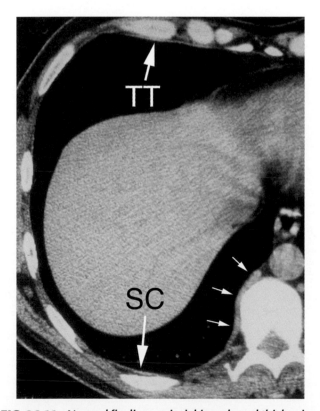

FIG. 26.11. Normal findings mimicking pleural thickening. CT shows the subcostalis muscle (*SC*), transversus thoracis muscle (*TT*), and intercostal veins (*small arrows*).

Paravertebral Intercostal Veins

These are invisible on chest radiographs. On CT, in some normal subjects, segments of intercostal veins seen in the paravertebral regions mimic pleural thickening. Continuity of these opacities with the azygos or hemiazygos veins is sometimes visible, allowing them to be correctly identified (see Fig. 26-11). Also, when viewed using lung window settings, these intercostal vein segments do not indent the lung surface; focal pleural thickening usually does.

DIAGNOSIS OF PLEURAL EFFUSION
Plain Radiographs

Pleural effusion cannot be distinguished from pleural thickening on chest radiographs unless high-density calcification or low-density fat is visible in relation to thick pleura, or air collections are visible within a pleural fluid collection.

The pleural space extends inferiorly, below the visible lung, in relation to the diaphragm and ribs. In upright subjects, pleural fluid first accumulates in the most inferior portions of the pleural space, including the costophrenic angles and subpulmonic regions. Costophrenic angle blunting is usually the first recognizable plain film finding of pleural fluid (Fig. 26-12A and B).

At least 175 mL of pleural fluid must be present to result in blunting of the lateral costophrenic angle on the frontal radiograph, and as much as 500 mL may be present without recognizable blunting. Blunting of the posterior costophrenic angle on the lateral view requires 75 mL (see Fig. 26-12B). Blunting of the posterior costophrenic angle may sometimes be diagnosed on the frontal view by looking through the shadow of the upper abdominal contents; posterior costophrenic angle blunting results in a sharper lower edge of the lung than normally seen. On a properly performed lateral decubitus film, as little as 10 mL of fluid may be seen. Very small pleural fluid collections, either unilateral or bilateral, are seen in a few normal individuals.

With increasing effusion, fluid may be seen lateral to the lower lobes, separating the lung from adjacent ribs. Because the lung is fixed medially by the hilum and inferior pulmonary ligament, medial pleural fluid collections are usually smaller (Fig. 26-13) and more difficult to recognize. Larger effusions result in a typical meniscus appearance with the level of the fluid and its density appearing greater in the lateral hemithorax. The edge separating the aerated lung from pleural fluid is often sharp and well defined.

Medial fluid collections may be seen when effusions are large. Most often, these accumulate in the posterior gutters, with thickening of the paravertebral stripes. The collections may be triangular, simulating lower lobe collapse.

Pleural fluid often accumulates in the subpulmonic pleural space (*subpulmonic effusion*), allowing the lung base to float superiorly. Subpulmonic fluid collections may be difficult to recognize on frontal radiographs, although some costophrenic angle blunting, a shallow costophrenic angle, or a hazy costophrenic angle is often present. However,

A

B

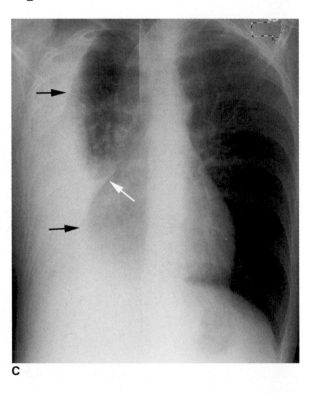

C

FIG. 26.12. Pleural effusion associated with cirrhosis. **A:** Posteroanterior chest radiograph shows blunting of the right costophrenic angle (*black arrow*). This usually indicates that 175 mL of pleural fluid is present. Fluid entering the minor fissure (*white arrow*) resembles a rose thorn. This is termed the "thorn" sign of pleural effusion. **B:** Lateral radiograph shows elevation of the lung base by a subpulmonic fluid collection and blunting of the posterior costophrenic angle (*arrow*). Posterior costophrenic angle blunting occurs with as little as 75 mL of fluid. **C:** Decubitus radiograph shows a large effusion (*black arrows*) separating the aerated lung from the chest wall. Fluid enters the major fissure (*white arrow*).

greater superior retraction of the lateral lung (likely because the medial lower lobe is fixed by the inferior pulmonary ligament) results in lateral displacement of what appears to the diaphragmatic dome or peak, with the lung lateral to the peak angling down sharply (Fig. 26-14). On the left side, 2 cm of separation of the lung base from the top of the stomach bubble is typically taken as evidence of a subpulmonic effusion, but this distance is variable in normal individuals.

On the lateral view (see Fig. 26-14B), a subpulmonic effusion often (1) elevates the posterior lung, flattening its undersurface; (2) insinuates itself into the major fissure, resulting in focal triangular thickening of the fissure; and (3) flattens the inferior contour of the lung anterior to the fissure, which then angles sharply downward.

Fluid may extend into the major or minor fissures. This is usually easy to recognize on the lateral radiographs as

A   **B**

FIG. 26.13. Pleural effusion with liver disease. **A:** Chest radiograph shows a large right pleural effusion with costophrenic angle blunting and a thorn sign (*arrow*). **B:** A large effusion is visible on CT. The lower lobe is collapsed. Because the lung is tethered medially by the hilar vasculature and inferior pulmonary ligament (*arrow*), most of the fluid accumulates laterally.

A   **B**

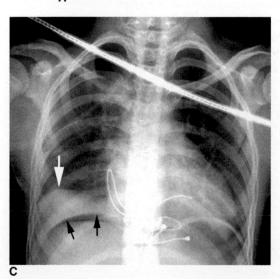

C

FIG. 26.14. Subpulmonic right pleural effusion. **A:** Posteroanterior chest radiograph shows no evidence of costophrenic angle blunting. There appears to be lateral displacement of the diaphragm dome (*arrow*). **B:** Lateral radiograph shows blunting of both costophrenic angles (*black arrows*), and fluid entering the right major fissure, resulting in a thorn sign (*white arrow*). Flattening of the undersurface of the lobes is also typical of subpulmonic effusion. **C:** Subpulmonic effusion in a patient with free abdominal air because of peritoneal dialysis. The free air outlines the undersurface of the right hemidiaphragm (*black arrows*). What appears to represent a laterally displaced dome of the right hemidiaphragm (*white arrow*) represents a subpulmonic effusion.

fissure thickening. On the frontal radiograph, fluid extending into the posterolateral major fissure typically results in an arcuate opacity, sharply defined medially and inferiorly (see Fig. 26-1). Fluid extending into the lateral aspect of the minor fissure and slightly separating the lobes often results in an opacity resembling a rose thorn (the "thorn sign"; see Figs. 26-12A, 26-13A, and 26-14B).

Large pleural effusions result in significant or complete lung atelectasis (see Fig. 26-13) and result in a mediastinal shift to the opposite side. Downward displacement or inversion of the hemidiaphragm may be recognized on the left because of downward displacement of the stomach bubble.

Supine and semierect radiographs are less sensitive in showing pleural effusion. Signs of effusion on supine radiographs include increased density of a hemithorax due to layering of the effusion posteriorly, blunting of the lateral costophrenic angle, obscuration or poor definition of the hemidiaphragm, and thickening of the paravertebral stripe, usually in the inferior hemithorax, due to accumulation of fluid in the posterior gutters. With large effusions, an apical cap may be seen.

On decubitus radiographs, an increase in separation of the lung from the chest wall indicates the presence of free pleural effusion (see Fig. 26-12C). Lack in change in thickness indicates pleural thickening or loculated pleural effusion.

CT Findings

Pleural effusion usually appears lower in attenuation than pleural thickening or consolidated or collapsed lung on unenhanced scans, and may be distinguished from them. On contrast-enhanced scans, both airless lung and thickened pleura enhance, and this difference is accentuated (see Fig. 26-13B). Small pleural effusions can be difficult to distinguish from pleural thickening.

In the supine position, free pleural effusion first accumulates in the most dependent part of the pleural space, posterior to the lower lobe. The thickness of a free pleural effusion usually decreases in less dependent parts of the thorax, anteriorly and superiorly. As the effusion increases in size, it becomes thicker and wraps around the lung, extending anteriorly and superiorly, and extending into the fissures.

When free pleural fluid accumulates, the lung decreases in volume but tends to maintain its normal shape. Thus, a free pleural effusion generally appears crescent-shaped on CT. Large effusions often extend into the major fissures, displacing the lower lobes medially and posteriorly. Atelectasis is common in patients with large effusions, and atelectatic lung may be seen floating within the fluid.

Pleural Effusion Versus Ascites

Subpulmonic effusion and pleural fluid in the costophrenic angles can be seen below the lung bases on CT and may mimic collections of fluid in the peritoneal cavity. The parallel curvilinear configuration of the pleural and peritoneal cavities at the level of the perihepatic and perisplenic recesses allows fluid in either cavity to appear as a crescentic collection displacing liver or spleen away from the adjacent chest wall.

However, pleural fluid collections and ascites may be distinguished in several ways.

Pleural fluid collections in the posterior costophrenic angle lie medial and posterior to the diaphragm and cause lateral displacement of the crus (the "displaced-crus sign"). Peritoneal fluid collections are anterior and lateral to the diaphragm; lateral displacement of the crus is not visible.

Pleural fluid can also be distinguished from ascites by the clarity of the interface of the fluid with the liver and spleen (the "interface sign"). With pleural fluid the interface is hazy, whereas with ascites it is sharp.

Fluid seen posterior to the liver is within the pleural space; the peritoneal space does not extend into this region, the so-called bare area of the liver (the "bare-area sign").

The most reliable method for localizing fluid is to identify its relationship to the diaphragm, if it is visible. In patients with both pleural and peritoneal fluid, the diaphragm often can be seen as a uniform, curvilinear structure of muscle density with relatively low-density fluid both anterior and posterior to it. Fluid posterior or lateral to the diaphragm is pleural (the "diaphragm sign").

A large pleural effusion will allow the lower lobe to float anteriorly and lose volume (Fig. 26-15). On CT, the posterior edge of the lower lobe, when surrounded by fluid both anteriorly and posteriorly, can appear to represent the diaphragm (i.e., a "pseudodiaphragm"), with pleural fluid posteriorly and ascites anteriorly. Sequential scans at more cephalad levels, however, generally will allow the correct interpretation to be made. Typically, the arcuate density of the atelectatic lower lobe becomes thicker superiorly, is contiguous with the remainder of the lower lobe, and often contains air bronchograms.

LOCULATED FLUID COLLECTIONS

Loculated pleural fluid collections are limited in extent by pleural adhesions. They often occur in association with exudative pleural effusions, high in protein, such as those that occur with empyema. Often they are elliptical or lenticular in shape.

Radiographic Findings

The appearance of loculated pleural fluid on chest radiographs varies with its location and the radiographic projection. Typically, a loculated collection appears sharply marginated when its surface is parallel to the x-ray beam and ill defined when viewed en face (Fig. 26-16A and B). Thus, a collection loculated in the lateral pleural space will appear sharply marginated on the frontal radiograph and ill defined on the lateral film. For a collection loculated anteriorly or posteriorly, the opposite is true.

FIG. 26.15. "Pseudodiaphragm" with pleural effusion and lower lobe collapse. **A:** Chest radiograph shows costophrenic angle blunting (*white arrow*) due to right pleural effusion. Air-fluid level represents a subphrenic abscess. **B:** CT shows the abscess cavity (*A*) in a subphrenic location. The liver (*L*) is also visible at this level. The collapsed lower lobe *(arrows)* surrounded by pleural fluid mimics the hemidiaphragm.

FIG. 26.16. Loculated pleural fluid collections in empyema. **A:** Posteroanterior chest radiograph shows evidence of a large right pleural effusion. **B:** Lateral radiograph shows a lenticular fluid collection anteriorly, with a sharply marginated edge (*arrows*). A large posterior fluid collection is also present. **C:** Contrast-enhanced CT shows multiple lenticular fluid collections (*arrows*), indicating the presence of loculation. Some fluid collections are nondependent, also a finding of loculation.

Localized fluid collections in the fissures may be loculated or may occur in the absence of pleural adhesions. They are most common in patients with congestive heart failure and often are transient. Since they mimic the presence of a focal lung lesion, they have been referred to as "phantom tumor" or "pseudotumor." Typically, fluid collections in a fissure are rounded or lenticular and may show a tapering triangular opacity or "beak" at the point they merge with the fissure itself (Figs. 26-17 and 26-18).

Fluid collections in the minor fissure often appear sharply marginated and lenticular on both posteroanterior and lateral radiographs. Collections in the major fissure may be ill defined on the frontal view.

CT Findings

CT findings of fluid loculation include (1) a localized collection, (2) an elliptical or lenticular shape (rather than crescentic), and (3) a nondependent location (i.e., anterior, lateral, or posterolateral; Figs. 26-16C and 26-18 to 26-20). If air is present within a loculated effusion, multiple septations may be seen, resulting in multiple air bubbles, localized air collections, or air-fluid levels (Fig. 26-21). Loculated effusions are often associated with pleural thickening, best seen with contrast enhancement (see Figs. 26-16C and 26-19). If both the visceral and parietal pleural surfaces are thickened, embracing the fluid collection, the *split-pleura sign* is said to be present (see Fig. 26-19).

A focal or loculated collection of pleural fluid in a major or minor fissure can have a confusing appearance on CT images and can be misinterpreted as a parenchymal mass. Careful analysis of sequential images usually will confirm the relationship of the "mass" to the plane of the fissure. If the abnormality is of fluid attenuation, the diagnosis is easier. The edges of the mass may taper to conform to the fissure, forming a "beak," especially if CT with thin collimation is used (see Fig. 26-18). Correlation of CT scans with the plain radiographs can help, particularly for fluid localized in the minor fissure.

TYPES OF EFFUSION: EXUDATES AND TRANSUDATES

Most pleural effusions are classified as exudates or transudates based on their composition. This distinction is usually made at thoracentesis. Other specific causes of pleura effusion are chylothorax and hemothorax.

Exudates

Exudative effusion reflects the presence of a pleural abnormality associated with increased permeability of pleural capillaries (Table 26-1). Exudative effusions have a high protein content. According to generally accepted criteria, an exudative effusion meets at least one of the following criteria:

1. A ratio of pleural fluid protein to serum protein higher than 0.5
2. A ratio of pleural fluid lactate dehydrogenase (LDH) to serum LDH that exceeds 0.6
3. A pleural fluid LDH level more than two thirds the upper limits of normal for serum

Less specific criteria used to diagnose an exudate include a pleural fluid specific gravity exceeding 1.016 and a pleural fluid protein level exceeding 3 g/dL.

A **B**

FIG. 26.17. Pseudotumor in congestive heart failure. **A:** Chest radiograph shows a rounded opacity (*arrows*) representing fluid localized to the major fissure. **B:** On the lateral view, the collection appears lenticular (*large arrows*). A beak (*small arrows*) is seen at its junction with the major fissure. This collection is resolved later.

FIG. 26.18. Fluid localized to the major fissure in a patient with cirrhosis and ascites. **A:** A lenticular collection of fluid (*white arrow*) is seen within the fissure. A loculated collection is also present peripherally (*black arrow*). **B:** At a lower level, a rounded collection is seen within the fissure. A beak (*arrow*) is visible medially. **C:** Sagittal reformation shows fluid thickening in the entire major fissure (*arrows*).

Common causes of exudative effusion include pneumonia with parapneumonic effusion, empyema, tuberculous pleuritis, neoplasm, pulmonary embolism, collagen diseases such as lupus or rheumatoid arthritis (RA), abdominal diseases (pancreatitis, abscess, surgery), Dressler's (postpericardiotomy) syndrome, asbestos exposure, Meigs syndrome, uremia, endometriosis, drug reactions, and therapeutic radiation.

Transudates

Transudative effusion is unassociated with pleural disease. It usually results from systemic abnormalities causing an imbalance in the hydrostatic and osmotic forces governing pleural fluid formation. A transudative effusion is low in protein and does not meet the criteria for an exudate listed above.

Common causes of a transudative effusion (Table 26-2) include congestive heart failure (CHF), pericardial disease, cirrhosis, pregnancy and delivery, hypoalbuminemia, overhydration, renal failure, nephrotic syndrome, peritoneal dialysis, and myxedema.

Distinguishing Exudate and Transudate

Distinguishing exudate from transudate is important in the differential diagnosis and clinical management of pleural effusion. CT numbers cannot be used to reliably predict the protein content or specific gravity of the fluid and whether it is a transudate or exudate. Most effusions appear to be near water in attenuation on CT, but range up to 20 to 30 HU regardless of their cause. Although the attenuation of exudates may be higher (average 7 to 17 HU) than transudates

FIG. 26.19. Streptococcal empyema. CT shows a loculated, lenticular fluid collection at the right base, associated with thickening of both the parietal (*large arrow*) and visceral (*small arrows*) pleural layers, the so-called split-pleura sign. The thickened pleura enhances following contrast infusion. The left pleural effusion is unassociated with pleural thickening and may be an exudate or transudate.

(average 10 to 12.5 HU), there is considerable overlap between the attenuation of exudates and transudates in the 10 to 20 HU range.

The appearance of the parietal pleura on contrast-enhanced CT is of value in predicting the nature of a pleural fluid collection. Visibility of the parietal pleura indicates that it is thickened (enhancing pleura is thickened pleura and thickened pleura enhances). The presence of thickened parietal pleura in association with a pleural effusion suggests that the fluid collection is an exudate (see Figs. 26-19 to 26-21). Parietal pleural thickening is present in about 60% of exudative effusions, and although the parietal pleural thickening can be seen in some patients with transudative effusion, the value of this finding in predicting the presence of an exudate is high (85% to 95%). Patients with transudative effusions who show pleural thickening on CT often have preexisting pleural disease. If pleural thickening is not visible on CT, an associated effusion may be an exudate or a transudate (see Fig. 26-19).

Using sonography, the presence of septation, complex nonseptation, or homogeneous echogenicity may be used to predict the presence of an exudate with a sensitivity and positive predictive value of 65% and 100%, respectively. Anechoic effusions may be either transudative or exudative.

If CT shows air within the fluid collection, for whatever reason (usually thoracentesis), and multiple air bubbles or multiple air-fluid levels are visible (rather than a single air-fluid level; see Fig. 26-21), the presence of proteinaceous and multiloculated effusion may be assumed. An exudate may be confidently diagnosed in this setting.

Causes of Pleural Effusion

Abdominal Abscess

Abdominal infections may be associated with ipsilateral pleural effusion. The effusion may be a transudate or exudate. Typical findings include small pleural effusion, elevation of the hemidiaphragm, and lower lobe atelectasis. Subphrenic abscess is associated with pleural effusion in 80% of cases;

A   B

FIG. 26.20. Empyema with multiple loculations. A, B: CTs at two levels show multiple loculated fluid collections with thickened parietal pleura (*arrows*).

FIG. 26.21. Empyema containing air due to thoracentesis. The parietal pleura is thickened (*arrows*). Multiple air bubbles indicate a multiloculated proteinaceous effusion. It may be concluded that this effusion is an exudate. The differential diagnosis of an air-containing fluid collection also included bronchopleural fistula and gas-forming organisms.

it may occur on either side. Hepatic abscess is associated with effusion in 20%, typically right-sided. Splenic abscess is associated with left-sided effusion in 30%.

Abdominal Surgery

Half of patients who undergo abdominal surgery have a small pleural effusion within the first 3 postoperative days. Effusions developing after this period likely have another cause.

TABLE 26.1   Causes of Exudative Effusion
Pneumonia (parapneumonic effusion)
Empyema
Tuberculous
Neoplasm
Pulmonary embolism
Collagen-vascular diseases
Abdominal diseases (pancreatitis, abscess, surgery)
Dressler's (postpericardiotomy) syndrome
Asbestos exposure
Meigs syndrome
Uremia
Endometriosis
Drug reactions
Radiation

TABLE 26.2   Causes of Transudative Effusion
Congestive heart failure
Pericardial disease
Cirrhosis
Pregnancy and delivery
Hypoalbuminemia
Overhydration
Renal failure
Nephrotic syndrome
Peritoneal dialysis
Myxedema

The incidence of pleural effusion is increased in association with upper abdominal surgery, peritoneal fluid, and atelectasis. Orthotopic liver transplantation is almost always associated with right-sided or bilateral effusions.

Asbestos Exposure

Asbestos-related pleural plaques are discussed in Chapter 18. Asbestos exposure can also result in benign exudative pleural effusion in a few percent of exposed individuals. The condition is likely inflammatory in nature and related to the presence of asbestos fibers at the pleural surface. It is dose-related and a relatively early manifestation of disease, usually occurring within 20 years of onset of exposure. Patients are often asymptomatic but may have chest pain. Effusions are usually unilateral and small to moderate in size. They are usually self-limited, lasting a few months, but may be recurrent. Diffuse pleural thickening results in about 20%. Rounded atelectasis may be associated.

Cirrhosis and Ascites

Cirrhosis is associated with pleural effusion, but the frequency of effusion is much higher if ascites is present. Effusions are typically right-sided or bilateral; isolated left-sided effusions are less common. Most important in the development of effusion is the passage of fluid into the chest through diaphragmatic defects. Reduction in plasma oncotic pressure due to hypoalbuminemia may also contribute to the formation of effusions. The effusions are transudates and may be large.

Collagen-Vascular Diseases

Exudative pleural effusion is common in patients with collagen-vascular disease, most commonly systemic lupus erythematosus (SLE) and RA.

SLE is associated with pleural effusion in as many as 70% of cases. Arthritis or arthralgia is commonly present. Effusions are usually small and bilateral and are exudates. Pericardial effusion may also be present. Symptoms include pleuritic pain, fever, and dyspnea.

About 5% to 20% of patients with RA have effusion. Effusions are exudates and have a low glucose, a high LDH, and a high rheumatoid factor. Eighty percent of patients with effusion are men, and 80% have subcutaneous nodules. Effusions in RA may be asymptomatic or associated with chest pain. They are usually small, unilateral, and right-sided. They may be transient, persistent, or recurrent. Pleural fibrosis may result. Empyema also has an increased incidence in patients with RA.

Congestive Heart Failure

Pleural effusion is present in about half of patients with CHF. CHF is the most common cause of transudative effusion, although exudative effusions may also occur. Pleura fluid accumulates in CHF primarily because pulmonary interstitial (edema) fluid crosses into the pleural space. Bilateral effusions are present in 70% of cases; when unilateral, pleural effusion is more common on the right (20%) than on the left (10%). Although unilateral effusion may be seen, a large unilateral pleural effusion suggests an alternative diagnosis. In a patient with CHF, thoracentesis may be performed for diagnosis if the patient has fever or pleuritic chest pain, the heart is normal in size, or if the effusion is unilateral or bilateral but asymmetrical.

Dressler's Syndrome

Dressler's syndrome (also known as postcardiotomy syndrome, postcardiac injury syndrome, and postmyocardial infarction syndrome) occurs in a few patients with myocardial infarction, pericardial or myocardial injury, or cardiac surgery. It typically occurs 2 or 3 weeks following the precipitating episode and is associated with chest pain, fever, dyspnea, and leukocytosis. Radiographs show pleural effusion (85%), lung consolidation (75%), and findings of pericardial effusion (50%). Pleural effusions are exudative and often bloody. They are usually bilateral and small; when unilateral, they are often left-sided. Dressler's syndrome may be self-limited or recurrent. It is thought to be immunologically mediated. Treatment includes aspirin, nonsteroidal antiinflammatory drugs, or steroids.

Drug Reactions

A number of drugs may result in pleural effusion, usually exudative. Effusion may be related to the development of drug-related SLE (see Chapter 14), may reflect an allergic reaction, or may be a primary drug effect. Allergic reactions with eosinophilia may be associated with pleural effusion in patients receiving methotrexate or other cytotoxic drugs, nitrofurantoin, propylthiouracil, and muscle relaxants (dantrolene); lung disease is commonly associated. The ergot-based drugs methysergide (migraine treatment) and bromocriptine (Parkinson's disease treatment) may cause pleural effusion and fibrosis.

Pleural Endometriosis

Catamenial pleural effusion or hemothorax can be associated with pleural endometrial implants. As with catamenial

pneumothorax described below, pleural endometriosis is right-sided in 90%, likely related to defects in the right hemidiaphragm that allow passage of endometrium into the thorax. Enhancing pleural nodules and masses, representing the endometrial implants, may be seen in addition to pleural effusion; they may be seen in the abdomen as well. The presence and size of the effusion and the size of masses wax and wane with hormonal changes.

Meigs Syndrome

Meigs syndrome was originally defined as ascites and pleural effusion associated with ovarian fibroma, but the definition has since extended to refer to other ovarian tumors. Pleural effusions are exudative or transudative and occur on the right side (65%), on the left side (10%), or bilaterally (25%); they may be large. Resection of the ovarian tumor results in resolution of the ascites and pleural effusion.

Myxedema

Pleural effusion occurs in as many as half of patients with myxedema, often associated with pericardial effusion. Associated heart failure or renal disease may be contributory. The effusion may be an exudate or transudate.

Neoplasm

Pleural effusion is common in patients with primary or metastatic pleural tumors. Effusions are usually exudative and may be bloody. Malignant effusions are always exudates, but not all exudative effusions in cancer patients are malignant. Exudative effusions in patients with malignancy may reflect pleural involvement by tumor, lymphatic obstruction, or pneumonia. Pleural effusion in patients with malignancy is described in detail below.

Pericardial Disease

Pleural effusion is common in patients with inflammatory pericardial disease. They are left-sided in 70%, bilateral in 20%, and right-sided in 10%. Left-sided effusion likely predominates because of local inflammation. In patients with constrictive pericarditis, effusions may result from elevated left- or right-sided venous pressures; in this setting, as in patients with CHF, effusions are most often bilateral or right-sided.

Pancreatitis

Acute pancreatitis results in effusion in 10% to 20%. Because of the relationship of the pancreatic tail to the left hemidiaphragm, these are usually left-sided (70%) or bilateral. They are exudative and often hemorrhagic and often contain high amylase levels.

Chronic pancreatitis may also be associated with a left-sided effusion, which contains high amylase. It is most often left-sided (70%) or bilateral. Pseudocyst is commonly present. Associated mediastinal pseudocyst with rupture into the pleural space may result in a pancreaticopleural fistula with a large pleural effusion.

Pancreatic abscess may be associated with pleural effusion containing high amylase levels. It is usually left-sided.

Parapneumonic Effusion and Empyema

Pleural effusion is common in patients with pneumonia; this is termed *parapneumonic effusion*. Parapneumonic effusions are typically exudates; they are small and sterile and have normal glucose and pH values. They usually resolve with appropriate antibiotic treatment but may progress to empyema. Empyema is an infected exudative effusion, often requiring tube drainage. These entities are described in detail below.

Pregnancy

Small bilateral transudative pleural effusions are seen in 10% of pregnant women. They are seen for a short time after delivery in up to 25% of women.

Pulmonary Embolism

Pleural effusion occurs in 30% of patients with pulmonary embolism, often associated with infarction. Effusion is more common in patients with the presenting complaint of hemoptysis or pleuritic chest pain (50%) than in those with dyspnea (25%). Exudate is more common (75%) than transudate (25%). They are often unilateral, but this depends on the distribution of emboli. Effusions are usually small and do not increase after 3 days. The majority resolve within a week. Consolidation is associated in half of cases.

Radiation (Therapeutic)

About 5% of patients having chest radiation develop a small exudative pleural effusion in association with radiation pneumonitis. The effusion occurs on the side of radiation and develops within 6 months of radiation. It resolves slowly with time.

Renal Disease

Several manifestations of renal disease may be associated with pleural effusion:

1. Renal failure with overhydration may result in transudative effusion. Acute glomerulonephritis may be responsible for this occurrence. Effusions are usually bilateral.
2. Nephrotic syndrome may result in transudative effusion because of increased hydrostatic pressure and hypoalbuminemia resulting in decreased plasma oncotic pressure. Effusions are often bilateral and subpulmonic in location.

3. Uremia may result in fibrinous pleuritis and a bloody exudative effusion that is often unilateral and large. Fever, chest pain, and dyspnea are often present. Pericardial effusion is often associated. Chronic fibrotic pleural thickening may result.
4. Hydronephrosis may result in retroperitoneal urinoma and ipsilateral pleural effusion. The effusion is a transudate but contains a high creatinine level.
5. Peritoneal dialysis may result in effusion, usually on the right side. Fluid likely enters the pleural space via diaphragmatic defects.

CHYLOTHORAX

Chylous effusion or *chylothorax* contains intestinal lymph (i.e., chyle), is high in protein and fatty acid, and is low in cholesterol. It typically appears milky. Chylothorax usually results from disruption of the thoracic duct (25%) or thoracic lymphatic obstruction by tumor (50% of cases). Simple obstruction of the thoracic duct does not result in chylothorax; it may be tied off without the development of chylothorax.

The thoracic duct originates at the cisterna chyli in the upper abdomen and enters the thorax along the right anterior aspect of the spine; it crosses to the left near the level of T6, lying along the left lateral wall of the esophagus, posterior to the descending aorta, and drains into the left brachiocephalic or subclavian vein. Approximately 2 L of chyle passes through the thoracic duct each day, although the volume varies with diet.

Chylous effusion is most common in patients with lymphoma, metastatic neoplasm, or other mediastinal masses (Table 26-3); following thoracic surgery (chylothorax is a complication in about 0.5% of cardiovascular and 4% of esophageal surgeries) or chest trauma (e.g., penetrating or nonpenetrating trauma, thoracic vertebral fracture); inflammatory mediastinal lymph node diseases; mediastinal fibrosis; central vein thrombosis; lymphangiomyomatosis; chylous ascites; and some congenital abnormalities.

Chylous effusions may be small or massive and unilateral or bilateral. They contain protein in addition to fat and appear to be near water in attenuation on CT (Fig. 26-22). Rarely, chylous effusion measures less than 0 HU in attenuation.

TABLE 26.3 Causes of Chylothorax

Cause	Prevalence (%)
Tumor	50
Lymphoma	35
Other tumor	15
Trauma	25
Surgery	20
Other trauma	5
Miscellaneous	25
Congenital	5
Other	20

FIG. 26.22. Chylous effusion in lymphoma. The effusion is unassociated with pleural thickening and has no distinguishing characteristics.

FIG. 26.23. Iatrogenic traumatic hemothorax related to thoracentesis. A large right pleural effusion shows a distinct fluid or hematocrit level (*arrows*). The dependent fluid measures in excess of 60 HU.

Following chest trauma and duct disruption, chyle typically accumulates in the mediastinum before leading to chylothorax. Mediastinal widening or a localized fluid collection may be seen days before development of the chylothorax. Because the location of the thoracic duct is to the right of midline in the lower thorax and to the left in the upper thorax, injury of the lower duct tends to cause right-sided effusion, while injury to the upper duct causes left-sided effusion. Postsurgical chylothorax is often left-sided. Closed trauma usually results in right-sided chylothorax.

Traumatic chylothorax will often resolve over time as the thoracic duct heals. Reduction in lymph flow may be helpful in achieving this result. A pleuroperitoneal shunt may be used. Tube drainage may lead to malnutrition. Ligation of the duct is curative. Chylothorax associated with lymphoma is usually treated with radiation.

Pseudochylous or *chyliform* effusion contains cholesterol but not chyle. It may be seen in patients with chronic inflammatory disease such as tuberculosis or RA or in patients with breakdown of cells present within a pleural effusion. Pseudochylous effusions are often chronic, being present for years.

HEMOTHORAX

The term "hemothorax" refers to a pleural fluid collection having a hematocrit over 50% of blood hematocrit. On CT, hemothorax results in fluid with high attenuation (usually higher than 50 HU), containing relatively dense clot or a fluid-fluid level, with the densest fluid being in the dependent portion of the pleural space (Fig. 26-23).

Most cases are traumatic, but a select list of entities can result in spontaneous hemothorax. These include rupture of an aneurysm or dissection, pulmonary or pleural neoplasm, pneumothorax, coagulopathy, rupture of a pulmonary arteriovenous malformation, and pulmonary or pleural endometriosis.

Treatment includes tube drainage or sometimes thoracotomy for control of bleeding. Empyema may complicate hemothorax. Organization of a hemothorax may result in pleural fibrosis and calcification.

PARAPNEUMONIC EFFUSION AND EMPYEMA

Pleural fluid accumulates in approximately 40% of patients with pneumonia. The term *parapneumonic effusion* is used to describe this occurrence. Parapneumonic effusions are usually classified into three stages. These are (1) the exudative stage (simple parapneumonia effusion), (2) the fibropurulent stage (empyema), and (3) the stage of organization (pleural peel). Progression from one stage to the next does not necessarily occur.

Stage 1 (Exudative Stage): Simple Parapneumonic Effusion

A simple parapneumonic effusion probably results from increased permeability of the visceral pleura occurring in association with pulmonary inflammation in patients with pneumonia (Table 26-4). Effusions in this stage are commonly exudates and are typically small and sterile and have a normal glucose level (more than 40 to 60 mg/dL) and pH (greater than 7.2).

Parapneumonic effusions usually (1) are small to moderate in size, (2) are dependent in location, (3) do not show evidence of loculation, (4) show a meniscus on plain radiographs, and (5) appear crescent-shaped on CT (Fig. 26-24).

TABLE 26.4 Simple Parapneumonic Effusion
Increased permeability of the visceral pleura
Commonly exudates
Sterile with normal glucose
Small to moderate in size
Dependent in location
No loculation
Meniscus on plain radiographs
Crescentic shape on CT
50% associated with pleural thickening
Resolve with appropriate antibiotic treatment

About 50% of parapneumonic effusions are associated with pleural thickening visible on CT. Visceral pleural thickening and the "split-pleura" sign also may be present.

Simple parapneumonic effusion will usually resolve with appropriate antibiotic treatment of the pneumonia and rarely needs tube drainage. A parapneumonic effusion that requires drainage is termed a *complicated parapneumonic effusion*. A complicated parapneumonic effusion is often an empyema.

Stage 2 (Fibropurulent Stage): Empyema

The term *empyema* is generally used when a pleural effusion is infected, although its true definition necessitates the presence of pus in the pleural space (Table 26-5). Although most empyemas occur in association with pneumonia, approximately 10% are unassociated with obvious lung disease.

Up to 75% of bacterial empyemas result from anaerobic infections or mixed anaerobic and aerobic infections. Common anaerobic organisms include *Bacteroides* species, Fusobacterium, anaerobic and microaerophilic cocci, and *Clostridium*. Common aerobic organisms are *Staphylococcus*

TABLE 26.5 Empyema
"Fibropurulent parapneumonic effusion"
Most empyemas occur with pneumonia
10% unassociated with lung disease
Anaerobic infections or mixed anaerobic and aerobic infections
Polymorphonuclear neutrophils in the fluid
Fibrin deposition along the pleural surfaces
Decreased glucose
Low pH values (<7.2)
Increased LDH (>1,000 IU/L)
Elliptical or lenticular shape on radiographs or CT
Nondependent location
Sharp demarcation from the adjacent lung
"Split-pleura" sign
Air = thoracentesis, bronchopleural fistula, gas-forming organism
Empyema necessitates—chest wall involvement, TB, actinomycosis, etc.

aureus, Streptococcus pneumoniae, Haemophilus influenzae, and Gram-negative enteric bacilli. Tuberculosis may result in empyema.

Empyema is characterized by the presence of infectious organisms in the pleural fluid, an increase in the size of the effusion, increased white blood cells and polymorphonuclear cells in the fluid, fibrin deposition along the pleural surfaces, a tendency for loculation, decreased glucose levels (less than 40 mg/dL) and pH (below 7.2), and increased LDH (over 1,000 IU/L).

In a patient who has pneumonia, the presence of a localized or loculated pleural effusion strongly suggests the presence of an empyema (see Figs. 26-16, 26-19, 26-20, and 26-21). On plain radiographs, empyemas often have a lenticular shape and tend to appear larger or better defined in one projection (e.g., as seen on the posteroanterior radiograph) than in the other (e.g., on the lateral radiograph; see Fig. 26-16). On radiographs, an empyema containing air may be difficult or impossible to differentiate from a peripheral lung abscess abutting the chest wall. This distinction can be an important one to make because empyemas are often treated by tube thoracostomy in addition to systemic antibiotics, whereas most lung abscesses require antibiotics only.

Classical CT findings of empyema (see Figs. 26-16 and 26-19 to 26-21) include an (1) elliptical or lenticular shape, (2) nondependent location, (3) sharp demarcation from the adjacent lung, (4) the split-pleura sign (the enhancing visceral and parietal pleural surfaces are split apart by the fluid collection), (5) smooth pleural thickening of uniform thickness (when enhanced by contrast or outlined by air), and (6) compression of lung and displacement of adjacent vessels.

In contrast to empyema, lung abscesses (see Figs. 9-39 and 9-40 in Chapter 9) tend to (1) be round, (2) be ill defined, (3) have shaggy walls of irregular thickness, and (4) destroy lung without displacing vessels.

FIG. 26.24. Simple parapneumonic effusion. The left pleural effusion is dependent, crescent-shaped, small, and unassociated with pleural thickening or findings of location. Bilateral pneumonia and a small right pleural effusion are present.

In patients with parapneumonic effusion or empyema, it is common (60% to 80% of cases) to see extrapleural fat thickening on CT when parietal pleural thickening is present. Increased attenuation of the thick extrapleural fat due to edema is less common (30% of cases).

Not all empyemas show classical findings. Many empyemas are crescent-shaped and dependent on location, without findings of loculation, and thus are indistinguishable from a simple parapneumonic effusion. Parietal pleural thickening or enhancement is always seen on CT, while visceral pleural thickening or enhancement is seen in half; thus, the split-pleura sign is absent in about half of cases.

Bronchopleural Fistula

Bronchopleural fistula (BPF) results from disruption of the visceral pleura, usually in association with lung abscess and empyema. Unless there has been a recent thoracentesis, gas within a pleural fluid collection is presumptive evidence of empyema and a BPF. The presence of a gas-forming organism is less often associated with gas in the pleural space. Rarely, in a patient with lung abscess, the site of BPF (i.e., the point of visceral pleural discontinuity) can be demonstrated on CT. BPF is an indication for chest tube drainage.

Empyema Necessitatis

Empyema can involve the chest wall by direct extension; this is termed *empyema necessitatis* or *empyema necessitans.* Tuberculosis accounts for about 70% of cases of empyema necessitatis, but other organisms such as *Actinomyces, Nocardia,* and other bacteria or fungi can be responsible. Extensive extrapleural fat thickening, edema or extrapleural fat, and subcutaneous collections of pus can be seen on CT.

Tube Drainage of Empyema

Indications for tube placement in patients with a parapneumonic effusion vary depending on the clinical setting, but one of the following criteria is usually sufficient: (1) thick pus on thoracentesis, (2) positive Gram stain from pleural fluid, (3) positive pleural fluid culture, (4) pleural fluid glucose below 60 mg/dL, (5) pleural fluid pH less than 7.2, and (6) LDH greater than 1,000 IU/L, or (6) a parapneumonic effusion that does not resolve with antibiotic treatment.

Stage 3 (Organization Stage): Pleural Peel or Fibrothorax

In patients with chronic empyema, ingrowth of fibroblasts and organization can result in extensive pleural fibrosis and the development of an inelastic fibrotic *pleural peel* or *fibrothorax* (Table 26-6). This can cause lung restriction and decreased lung volume ("trapped lung").

Smooth pleural thickening is typically visible on plain radiographs or CT (Fig. 26-25). Extrapleural fat thickening

TABLE 26.6 Pleural Peel
Chronic empyema
Pleural fibrosis
Restriction of lung function (i.e., trapped lung)
Smooth pleural thickening
Reduction in size of hemithorax
Pleural calcification

is frequently visible on CT, separating the thickened parietal pleura from the intercostal muscle or rib. Calcification, which usually is focal in its early stages, may become extensive. This is most common with tuberculosis. Chronic pleural effusion may occasionally be high in attenuation because of milk of calcium in the fluid (Fig 26-26).

A

B

FIG. 26.25. Pleural peel in two patients. **A:** In a patient with chronic empyema, smooth pleural thickening is visible (*arrows*) with reduction in volume of the affected hemithorax. **B:** Following tuberculous empyema, there is right pleural thickening and calcification (*white arrows*). Extrapleural fat is thickened (*black arrows*). The volume of the hemithorax is reduced.

FIG 26.26. Chronic pleural fluid collection in tuberculosis with milk of calcium. CT in a patient with a left upper lobe granuloma shows pleural thickening and high attenuation pleural fluid (*arrow*) in the right apex.

FIG. 26.27. Talc pleurodesis. Pleural thickening and dense talc (*arrows*) are visible.

A very important finding in diagnosing pleural peel on plain film or CT is reduction in volume of the affected hemithorax (see Fig. 26-25). Loculated fluid collections resulting from active infection may be seen on CT in association with the pleural peel.

In addition to chronic empyema, a pleural peel may result from chronic pleural effusion and inflammation in the absence of infection. This may be seen in patients with collagen-vascular diseases, asbestos exposure, uremia, and hemothorax.

Pleural Calcification

Pleural calcification may be associated with pleural fibrosis regardless of its cause. It is seen most commonly with pleural peel in patients with healed tuberculosis or bacterial empyema, hemothorax, or asbestos exposure. When present, it is commonly associated with increased thickness of extrapleural fat.

Talc Pleurodesis

Talc pleurodesis used to treat patients with chronic pleural effusion may mimic the appearance of pleural calcification. Dense accumulations of talc within the pleural space, in association with pleural thickening (Fig. 26-27), are typically seen. Talc is often visible in a clump posteriorly at the lung base.

PLEURAL NEOPLASMS

Neoplasm, either primary or metastatic, is a common cause of pleural mass, pleural effusion, or pleural thickening.

Pleural and Extrapleural Masses

Lesions located in the peripheral thorax, in contact with the chest wall, are generally classified as extrapleural, pleural, or parenchymal and are usually characterized radiographically by the angle (either acute or obtuse) formed by the interface between the lesion and the adjacent pleura.

Extrapleural masses usually displace the overlying parietal and visceral pleura, resulting in an obtuse angle between the lesion and the chest wall. Associated abnormalities including chest wall soft tissue mass or rib destruction may help to confirm the mass as extrapleural. Typically, extrapleural masses are sharply marginated at the point they contact the lung and displace pulmonary vessels away from them. Such masses may be related to rib lesions (tumor or fracture), soft tissue tumors, infection, or hematoma secondary to trauma.

Pleural masses, arising from the visceral or parietal pleura, usually remain confined to the pleural space and have an appearance similar to that of extrapleural lesions. The presence of an obtuse angle is common unless the lesion is large (Fig. 26-28). Large pleural lesions may have acute angles where they meet the chest wall, although some pleural thickening is often seen adjacent to them. As with extrapleural masses, pleural lesions are sharply marginated and displace pulmonary vessels away from them. Pleural masses or nodular pleural thickening suggests neoplasm, either primary to the pleura (e.g., mesothelioma, localized fibrous tumor (LFT), benign or malignant mesenchymal tumors) or metastatic, although the differential diagnosis includes organized and loculated fluid collections, pleural mesothelial cyst, fibrin ball or thoracolith (see below), splenosis (see below), and asbestos-related pleural plaques. (See Chapter 18).

Pulmonary parenchymal masses, when peripheral, may abut the pleura. A peripheral pulmonary lesion typically results in an acute angle with the pleural surface. Lung masses may result in obtuse angles at the chest wall in the presence

FIG. 26.28. Pleural metastases from chondrosarcoma. **A:** Chest radiograph shows a mass at the right apex. **B:** CT shows pleural masses with obtuse angles. No pleural effusion is associated; this is unusual with pleural metastases and implies a slow-growing lesion.

of pleural invasion. Pulmonary lesions are often ill defined along their inner aspect and may engulf rather than displace vessels. The differential diagnosis of pulmonary masses is long and described elsewhere.

Pleural Effusion with Neoplasm

Pleural effusion is common in patients with pleural malignancy, either primary or metastatic. Such effusions have a variety of causes but are usually exudates.

A *malignant effusion* is one secondary to pleural involvement by tumor and contains malignant cells. The most common causes of malignant effusion are lung cancer and breast cancer. Pleural fluid cytology is positive in 80% to 90% of patients with pleural malignancy, with the highest frequency in patients with adenocarcinoma. Malignant effusions are exudates.

Exudative effusions in patients with malignancy can also reflect the presence of obstructive pneumonia or lymphatic or pulmonary venous obstruction by tumor. This is particularly true of lung cancer; only patients with demonstration of tumor cells in the pleural fluid are considered to have unresectable disease.

Malignant effusions may be small or large and unilateral, bilateral, or asymmetrical. A large unilateral effusion suggests malignancy or infection (Figs. 26-29 to 26-31). Regardless of their cause, exudative effusions in cancer patients often require treatment by drainage.

Pleural Thickening with Neoplasm

The presence of pleural thickening on CT in a patient with malignancy and pleural effusion indicates the presence of an exudate (see Fig. 26-29), but is of little value in diagnosing malignant effusion. Pleural thickening is seen in 30% of cancer patients with a malignant effusion and 40% of those

with a benign effusion. Pleural effusion is usually the only abnormality visible on chest radiographs in patients with malignant effusion. In patients with gross pleural involvement by tumor, nodular pleural thickening may be seen (see Figs. 26-30 and 26-31). Metastatic tumor also may involve the pleural space in a concentric fashion.

The CT findings most specific in diagnosing malignant pleural disease are listed below. If one or more of these findings are considered to indicate malignancy, the overall diagnostic accuracy is about 75%.

1. Nodular pleural thickening (see Figs. 26-30 and 26-31)
2. Circumferential pleural thickening (pleural thickening surrounding the lung; Fig. 26-32)
3. Parietal pleural thickening greater than 1 cm
4. Mediastinal pleural thickening (see Fig. 26-32)

FIG. 26.29. Large unilateral malignant effusion. The effusion is large and the presence of pleural thickening (*arrows*) indicates that it is exudative.

A   B

FIG. 26.30. Pleural metastases. **A:** Chest radiograph shows a large right pleural effusion with mediastinal displacement to the left. **B:** CT shows nodular pleural thickening (*arrows*) with a large effusion and right lung collapse.

PLEURAL METASTASES

Pleural metastases typically result in pleural effusion. CT may show pleural effusion without pleural thickening, smooth pleural thickening (see Fig. 26-29), localized pleural masses (see Figs. 26-28, 26-30, and 26-31), or gross nodular pleural thickening (see Fig. 26-32). Localized pleural masses strongly suggest metastases. Nodular pleural thickening may be seen with metastatic tumor or mesothelioma. In patients with metastases, gross nodular pleural thickening is most typical of adenocarcinoma, but this is seen in a minority of cases.

On chest radiographs, pleural effusion is usually the only visible finding. However, in some patients with pleural metastases, particularly from invasive thymoma, pleural metastases may be unassociated with effusion and visible as rounded or lenticular pleural masses.

FIG. 26.31. Pleural metastasis in colon carcinoma with nodular pleural thickening. Gross nodular thickening of the parietal pleura is present (*arrows*). This appearance strongly suggests malignancy.

FIG. 26.32. Concentric pleural thickening with metastatic adenocarcinoma. Four findings of malignancy are visible: nodular pleural thickening, circumferential pleural thickening (*arrows*), parietal pleural thickening greater than 1 cm, and mediastinal pleural thickening.

LYMPHOMA

In patients with lymphoma, particularly those with Hodgkin's disease, exudative effusions commonly result from mediastinal lymphatic obstruction and resolve following mediastinal radiation; pleural thickening may or may not be present.

Marked thickening of extrapleural soft tissues may be seen with lymphoma or leukemia, often associated with posterior mediastinal lymph node enlargement. This may result in a rind of soft tissue mimicking the appearance of mesothelioma (see Figs. 5-25, 5-30, and 5-37 in Chapter 5). This appearance is associated with effusion.

MESOTHELIOMA

Mesothelioma (also known as malignant or diffuse mesothelioma) is a highly malignant, progressive neoplasm with an extremely poor prognosis (Table 26-7). In most patients, malignant mesothelioma is related to asbestos exposure. Although mesothelioma is rare in the general population, its incidence in heavily exposed asbestos workers is up to 5%. A latency period of 20 to 40 years between exposure and development of the tumor is typical. Mean age at diagnosis is 60. Symptoms include chest pain, dyspnea, and weight loss.

Mesothelioma arises in relation to the parietal pleura. It is classified pathologically as epithelial (50%), sarcomatous (25%), or mixed (25%). The epithelial type has a slightly better prognosis and tends to be associated with pleural effusion. Pleural effusion is small or absent with sarcomatous tumors. Histologic diagnosis of mesothelioma is difficult using pleural fluid cytology, and biopsy is usually required. Special histologic techniques may be needed to distinguish mesothelioma from adenocarcinoma.

TABLE 26.7   Mesothelioma
Commonly related to asbestos exposure
Incidence up to 5% in heavily exposed subjects
Latency period of 20–40 years
Arises in relation to the parietal pleura
Epithelial (50%), sarcomatous (25%), or mixed (25%) cell types
Pleural effusion
Concentric and lobulated pleural thickening
Frozen mediastinum sign
Involvement of fissure
Chest wall invasion or distant metastases
Poor prognosis

Mesothelioma is characterized morphologically by gross and nodular pleural thickening, which can involve the fissures. Hemorrhagic pleural effusion often occurs. Malignant mesothelioma spreads most commonly by local infiltration of the pleura. Hematogenous metastases are present in 50% of patients, although these are usually insignificant clinically.

Radiographic Findings

Plain radiographs may show pleural effusion as the initial abnormality (Fig. 26-33) or concentric and lobulated pleural thickening (Fig. 26-34). This may reflect tumor nodules, multiloculated pleural fluid collections, or both. Thickening of the major fissure is common due to tumor.

Because of pleural thickening and mediastinal infiltration, the involved hemithorax may be normal in volume, without mediastinal shift, despite the presence of a large effusion (the "frozen mediastinum sign"). The hemithorax may also be

A

B

FIG. 26.33. Asbestos exposure with mesothelioma. A: Chest radiograph shows pleural plaques and a large left pleural effusion. **B:** CT shows extensive pleural plaques and a left pleural effusion without obvious masses. This reflects left-sided mesothelioma.

FIG. 26.34. Asbestos exposure with mesothelioma. **A:** Chest radiograph shows lobulated right pleural thickening typical of this tumor. **B:** CT shows extensive nodular pleural thickening.

reduced in volume because of restriction of lung expansion. Asbestos-related pleural thickening or plaques may be seen (see Chapter 18).

CT Findings

Pleural fluid collections are visible on CT in 75% (see Fig. 26-33B). Pleural thickening is seen in 90%. Pleural effusion may be visible in the absence of visible pleural thickening in early disease, but this is uncommon.

Nodular concentric pleural thickening is highly suggestive of mesothelioma (Figs. 26-34B and 26-35). However, pleural thickening may also be thin and smooth (Fig. 26-36) or irregular in contour. Localized pleural masses are uncommon. In early disease, pleural thickening may appear discontinuous. As the disease progresses, pleural thickening becomes continuous, it increases in thickness and nodularity, and the amount of fluid may decrease as the pleural layers become fused.

Fluid can be difficult to distinguish from tumor on CT, since tumor nodules can sometimes appear low in attenuation (Fig. 26-37). However, decubitus scans or scans with the patient prone can help to distinguish underlying tumor from free fluid. Enhancement of the pleura after contrast infusion can also help differentiate tumor from adjacent fluid collections. Calcification usually reflects asbestos exposure, but calcification of tumor may be seen.

Although mesothelioma is most frequently visible along the lateral chest wall, mediastinal pleural thickening or

FIG. 26.35. Mesothelioma with concentric nodular pleural thickening. **A, B:** CTs at two levels show concentric nodular pleural thickening typical of mesothelioma. Note reduction in volume of the affected hemithorax because of lung restriction.

A

B

FIG. 26.36. Mesothelioma. CT shows mild pleural thickening (*arrows*) and pleural effusion. Extensive pleural plaques from asbestos exposure are also present.

concentric pleural thickening is seen with extensive disease. The abnormal hemithorax can appear contracted and fixed (40%), with little change in size during inspiration (see Fig. 26-35). Thickening of the fissures, particularly the lower part of the major fissures, can reflect tumor infiltration or associated pleural effusion; involvement of the fissures is seen on CT in 85% (see Fig. 26-35A).

Staging of Mesothelioma

Mesothelioma has a poor prognosis, with a mean survival of about 1 year and a 5-year survival rate of only a few percent. Extrapleural pneumonectomy may be used for treatment, often in combination with chemotherapy and radiation, and survival may be improved in patients with early disease. PET-CT is of value in determining the respectability of mesothelioma.

Staging systems have been proposed for mesothelioma similar to the TNM system used for lung cancer, but these have limited utility in clinical practice because of the poor prognosis associated with this tumor (Table 26-8; see Fig. 26-37).

LOCALIZED FIBROUS TUMOR OF THE PLEURA

LFT of the pleura was formerly known as benign mesothelioma, but it is not mesothelial in origin and is not necessarily benign. Approximately 30% of these tumors are malignant, although they have a good prognosis. It is unassociated with asbestos exposure (Table 26-9).

LFT is usually detected incidentally on chest radiographs. However, it can be associated with hypoglycemia (5% of cases) due to production of insulin-like growth factor type 2 (IGF-2), hypertrophic pulmonary osteoarthropathy (one third of cases), or chest pain. The symptoms resolve with resection.

FIG. 26.37. Mesothelioma with chest wall invasion. **A:** Chest radiograph shows a large effusion and a peripheral pleural nodule. **B:** The fluid and nodular areas of tumor are difficult to distinguish except for tumor invasion of the chest wall (*arrows*).

TABLE 26.8 Staging System for Mesothelioma

Stage[a]	Description
T1	Tumor limited to the ipsilateral parietal pleura or associated with scattered foci of visceral pleural involvement.
T2	Ipsilateral parietal pleural tumor with involvement of the diaphragm or confluent involvement of the visceral pleura
T3	Ipsilateral parietal pleural tumor with limited chest wall mediastinal, or pericardial invasion
T4	Extensive chest wall, subdiaphragmatic, mediastinal, or pericardial invasion

[a]T designations describe the extent of local invasion. N and M designations are identical to those used for lung cancer (see Chapter 3).

TABLE 26.9 Localized Fibrous Tumor

No relation to asbestos exposure
Associated with chest pain, hypoglycemia (5%),
   hypertrophic pulmonary osteoarthropathy (35%)
30% malignant; 70% benign
Arises in relation to the visceral pleura
Pleural effusion rare
Focal pleural mass
Good prognosis

LFT arises from the visceral pleura in 70%. It typically appears as a solitary, smooth, sharply defined, often large lesion, contacting a pleural surface (Figs. 26-38 and 26-39). When small, LFT tends to have obtuse angles at the pleural surface; when large, the angles are usually acute. LFT can be seen within a fissure, mimicking the appearance of loculated fluid. A "beak" or "thorn" sign is often visible on plain radiographs in patients with an LFT originating in or projecting into a fissure (see Fig. 26-38). They may also arise on a stalk and move with change in patient position. Pleural effusion is not usually present.

On CT, even if acute angles are visible, slight pleural thickening is usually visible adjacent to the mass (see Fig. 26-39). This thickening may reflect a small amount of fluid accumulating in the pleural space at the point where the visceral and parietal pleural surfaces are separated by the tumor. Masses may appear homogeneous. Necrosis can result in a multicystic appearance with or without contrast infusion. Large arteries supplying the mass may be seen. Calcification may be present (Fig. 26-40).

FIG. 26.39. Localized fibrous tumor appearing as a well-defined mass contacting the pleural surface. There is pleural thickening adjacent to the mass.

MESENCHYMAL TUMORS

Benign or malignant mesenchymal tumors (i.e., sarcomas) may arise from the pleura. These are rare. Pleural lipoma is a common benign tumor; they are typically 2 to 4 cm in diameter and of fat attenuation. Synovial sarcoma is a relatively common cell type of primary malignancy. Sarcomas tend to appear as large inhomogenous masses with areas of necrosis.

FIG. 26.38. Localized fibrous tumor in the right major fissure. The localized fibrous tumor (*LF*) lies in the plane of the major fissure and shows a small beak (*arrow*) at the point it contacts the fissure. The mass appears smooth and oval.

FIG. 26.40. Large localized fibrous tumor in the inferior pleural space. It appears somewhat inhomogeneous in attenuation, and focal calcification is visible (*arrow*).

FIBRIN BODY AND THORACOLITH

A resolving exudative effusion or hemothorax may deposit a clot of fibrin within the pleural space, termed a *fibrin body, fibrin ball,* or *pleural mouse.* A fibrin body appears as soft-tissue attenuation nodule, usually 1 to 2 cm in diameter. On radiographs or CT, a fibrin body contacts the pleural surface and is sometimes seen to move with change in patient position or on follow-up studies (Fig. 26-41). Fibrin bodies typically resolve over time but may remain stable or enlarge.

The presence of a calcified loose body in the pleural space has been termed *thoracolith.* Although various etiologies for thoracolith have been suggested, it most likely represents to fibrin body that has calcified. A thoracolith may range from a few millimeters to a few centimeters in diameter, and as with a fibrin body, it may show a change in location over time (Fig 26-42). They are most common on the left side.

FIG. 26.41. Fibrin ball. Coned-down lateral view shows a well-defined small nodular opacity at the pleural surface (*arrows*). This moved within the pleural space.

A

B

FIG. 26.42. Thoracolith. **A:** CT shows an oval calcification (*arrow*) in the medial left pleural space. **B:** CT 4 months later shows the calcification to have moved, being located posteriorly (*arrow*). **C:** Sagittal reconstruction at the time of (**B**). The calcification (*arrow*) is in contact with the pleura.

C

THORACIC SPLENOSIS

Thoracic splenosis is a rare condition resulting from simultaneous rupture of the spleen and left hemidiaphragm, with autotransplantation of splenic tissue into the left hemithorax. The splenic implants may be attached to the visceral or parietal pleura, may be located in a fissure, or may be found within the lung parenchyma, likely as a result of lung laceration occurring at the time of trauma.

Thoracic splenosis is usually an incidental finding on chest radiographs or CT, although it is rarely associated with hemoptysis. The interval between the initial trauma and detection of nodules ranges from 9 to more than 30 years. Radiographs and CT show sharply marginated, left-sided nodules in contact with the diaphragm or pleural surfaces (Fig 26-43). Findings of diaphragmatic rupture, splenic rupture, splenectomy, or peritoneal spenosis are usually associated. The radiologic diagnosis can be confirmed by using scintigraphy with ^{99m}Tc sulfur colloid, ^{99m}Tc-labeled heat-damaged erythrocytes, or ^{111}In-labeled platelets.

PNEUMOTHORAX

Pneumothorax is classified as spontaneous or traumatic.

A

B

C

FIG. 26.43. Thoracic spenosis. **A:** CT in a patient with a past history of trauma and splenectomy, shows multiple nodules in relation to the medial left pleural space (*arrows*). **B:** At a level just above the left hemidiaphragm, multiple nodules are visible (*arrows*). **C:** Sagittal reconstruction shows the relationship of one of the nodules to the diaphragm and pleural surface.

Spontaneous Pneumothorax

A spontaneous pneumothorax is one occurring without associated trauma. These are classified as primary or secondary.

Primary Spontaneous Pneumothorax

Primary spontaneous pneumothorax occurs without antecedent cause in an otherwise healthy patient. It often occurs at rest and is generally the result of rupture of an apical subpleural bulla (Fig. 26-44). There is an increased incidence of primary spontaneous pneumothorax in young patients (20 to 40 years), men (80% of affected patients are men), tall and thin patients, and smokers (90% are smokers). Pain is common, and a small pleural effusion is present in 10% to 20%, manifested as an air-fluid level. In half of patients, the pneumothorax recurs on the same side; recurrence on the opposite side occurs in 15%.

Secondary Spontaneous Pneumothorax

Secondary spontaneous pneumothorax occurs in patients with underlying lung disease. It is most commonly associated with chronic obstructive pulmonary disease. Other diseases include those associated with lung cysts (e.g., histiocytosis, lymphangiomyomatosis, pneumatocele), cavitation (e.g., tuberculosis, lung cancer, metastases, lung abscess, septic embolism; Fig. 26-45; see also Fig. 3-26 in Chapter 3), air trapping (e.g., asthma, cystic fibrosis), decreased lung compliance (e.g., any cause of fibrosis or honeycombing such as usual interstitial pneumonia, radiation, collagen-vascular disease, and sarcoidosis), or diseases of connective tissue (e.g., Ehlers-Danlos syndrome and Marfan's syndrome).

Because of underlying lung disease, patients with secondary spontaneous pneumothorax are often symptomatic. Such pneumothoraces have no specific characteristics, but underlying lung appears abnormal. Recurrence rates are higher than for primary spontaneous pneumothorax.

Pneumothorax Ex Vacuo

Pneumothorax ex vacuo is a rare cause of secondary spontaneous pneumothorax occurring in patients with acute lobar atelectasis, usually due to bronchial obstruction (see Fig. 3-27 in Chapter 3). Sudden collapse results in a rapid decrease in intrapleural pressure adjacent to the collapsed lobe. This in turn results in gas entering into the pleural space from tissue and blood. The resulting pneumothorax is seen adjacent to the collapsed lobe.

Catamenial Pneumothorax and Pleural Endometriosis

The development of pneumothorax coincident with menstruation, so-called catamenial pneumothorax, is rare. The onset of symptoms is within 48 hours of the onset of menses. It typically occurs in women over 30. Most cases (90%) occur on the right side. Recurrence is typical. Two primary mechanisms have been suggested:

1. Air may reach the peritoneum during menses via the vagina, uterus, and fallopian tubes. From there it may enter the pleural space through defects in the diaphragm, which are most common on the right side, or because of necrotic diaphragmatic implants of endometrium.
2. Endometrial implants may enter the pleural space by the same route, resulting in pleural endometriosis. If endometrial implants involve the visceral pleura and peripheral lung, their breakdown during menstruation may lead to pneumothorax and/or hemoptysis. This mechanism is more likely than the first.

Traumatic Pneumothorax

Traumatic pneumothorax refers to pneumothorax caused by chest trauma (penetrating or nonpenetrating, accidental

A   **B**

FIG. 26.44. Primary spontaneous pneumothorax in a smoker. **A:** Chest radiograph shows a large right pneumothorax (*white arrows*). An air-fluid level (*black arrows*) is visible at the right base. **B:** Follow-up CT shows apical bullae. Subcutaneous emphysema reflects chest tube drainage.

FIG. 26.45. Secondary spontaneous pneumothorax in a patient with cavitary metastatic giant cell tumor. Multiple lung nodules and a small left pneumothorax are visible.

or iatrogenic) or mechanical ventilation. Pneumothorax associated with mechanical ventilation is usually the result of high ventilator pressures; pneumothorax with mechanical ventilation usually occurs because of alveolar rupture, which

in turn causes interstitial emphysema, pneumomediastinum, and rupture of the pneumomediastinum into the pleural space. Pneumothorax does not cause pneumomediastinum; it is the other way around. Also, interstitial air may track to a subpleural location, form a subpleural bleb, and rupture directly into the pleural space. Traumatic pneumothorax usually requires chest tube drainage.

Radiographic Findings of Pneumothorax

Upright Patient

In an upright patient, air usually collects first above the lung apex. The visibility of pneumothorax is accentuated on expiration.

The presence of a visible *visceral pleural line* is key in making a definite diagnosis of pneumothorax in an erect patient (Fig. 26-46). In patients with pneumothorax, the visceral pleura is visible as a very thin line at the surface of the lung, with black air in the pleura space above or lateral to it, and air in lung below or medial to it. Air may enter the fissure, outlining its pleural surfaces.

FIG. 26.46. Pleural line in pneumothorax in three patients. **A–C:** A very thin line (*arrows*; thinnest in the patient in **A**) is visible at the edge of the lung. No lung markings are visible peripheral to it. A pleural line may also be seen medially (*large arrow* in **B**).

In the absence of underlying lung disease or pleural adhesions, the partially collapsed lung maintains its normal shape. Lung markings are not seen peripheral to the pleural line.

A skin fold may mimic pneumothorax, but a pleural line is not visible, and lung markings may be seen peripheral to it (Fig. 26-47). Pneumothorax increases in relative volume on expiration, although significant pneumothoraces are visible on inspiration (Fig. 26-48).

Distinction of a bulla from a pneumothorax is usually based on shape. Pneumothoraces are typically crescent-shaped and taper toward the lung base; bullae are rounded (see Fig. 24-13 in Chapter 24). However, this distinction may be difficult in some cases. Loculated pneumothorax may closely mimic a bulla.

Approximately half of the density of lung is blood, and when lung collapses in the presence of pneumothorax, a significant increase in lung density need not be visible. Reduction in lung volume also results in a reduction in lung perfusion. Until the lung becomes very small (Fig. 26-49), its density does not significantly increase.

Supine Patient

In supine patients, free pneumothorax usually collects within the anterior pleural space. A visceral pleural line may be

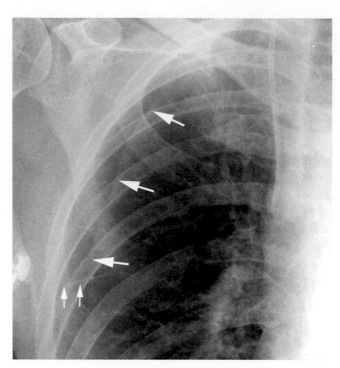

FIG. 26.47. Skin fold mimicking pneumothorax. A skin fold (*large arrows*) mimics pneumothorax, but a distinct pleural line is not visible, and lung markings (*small arrows*) may be seen peripheral to it.

A

B

FIG. 26.48. Inspiratory and expiratory radiographs in spontaneous pneumothorax. The relative volume of the pneumothorax (*arrows*) is smaller on inspiration (**A**) than on expiration (**B**).

FIG. 26.49. Total spontaneous pneumothorax. The left lung is reduced to the size of a fist (*arrows*). At this size, compressed lung tissue causes the lung to be dense. No mediastinal shift is present.

FIG. 26.50. The deep sulcus sign in pneumothorax. A supine radiograph in a patient with pulmonary edema shows a right pneumothorax manifested by a deep sulcus (*arrows*) on the right side. The right diaphragm and right heart borders appear sharp despite lung disease at the lung base.

seen medially in some patients (see Fig. 26-46B), mimicking pneumomediastinum. A subpulmonic pneumothorax with a visible visceral pleural line may be seen at the lung base. Less specific findings of pneumothorax in supine patients include the following:

1. The costophrenic angle may appear abnormally deep and lucent because of air in the anterolateral pleura space, the "deep-sulcus sign" (Fig. 26-50).
2. Increased lucency over the chest or upper abdomen
3. Visualization of the anterior costophrenic angle as an edge separate from the diaphragm but parallel to it (the "double-diaphragm sign")
4. Increased sharpness of the hemidiaphragm (because it is outlined by air), despite lung disease (see Fig. 26-50)
5. Increased sharpness of the cardiac border or mediastinum (because it is outlined by air; see Fig. 26-51)
6. Air in the minor fissure
7. A lumpy appearance at the cardiac apex due to alteration in the shape of the epicardial fat pad in the presence of pneumothorax (Fig. 26-51)

CT Findings of Pneumothorax

Upright expiratory radiographs and CT are equally sensitive in demonstrating a pneumothorax. CT is considerably more

FIG. 26.51. Tension pneumothorax with a deep sulcus sign. Left pneumothorax outlines fat at the cardiac apex, giving it a lumpy appearance (*arrows*). The left hemidiaphragm is displaced inferiorly and the mediastinum is shifted to the opposite side.

sensitive than supine radiographs in demonstrating pneumothorax.

On CT, a pneumothorax is imaged as air in the pleural space outside the lung and visceral pleura. Even a very small pneumothorax is visible in the anterior pleural space. Its diagnosis is usually straightforward, although differentiating a medial pneumothorax from pneumomediastinum may be difficult in some cases.

Tension Pneumothorax

Tension pneumothorax means that the pressure of intrapleural air exceeds atmospheric pressure, usually throughout the respiratory cycle; it may be life-threatening. True tension pneumothorax is uncommon. It is most often seen in mechanically ventilated patients or patients with chest trauma. Any pneumothorax in a patient on positive-pressure ventilation should be considered a tension pneumothorax.

Tension pneumothorax is difficult to diagnose on chest radiographs. Shift of the mediastinum away from the pneumothorax is not a reliable finding of tension and can be seen with any large pneumothorax. However, this finding in combination with clinical symptoms of circulatory compromise is usually considered diagnostic. Downward displacement or inversion of the hemidiaphragm also suggests tension (see Fig. 26-51).

In a patient with normal lungs, tension pneumothorax usually results in complete lung collapse. However, in the presence of underlying lung disease such as pulmonary edema, pneumonia, or chronic obstructive pulmonary disease, or in patients receiving positive-pressure ventilation, complete collapse need not occur. Also, complete lung collapse need not indicate tension (see Fig. 26-49).

Hydropneumothorax

Hydropneumothorax, the combination of fluid and air in the pleural space, is readily diagnosed in the upright position because of the presence of an air-fluid level (see Fig. 26-44). In supine or semierect patients, a visible pleural line or other findings of pneumothorax may be seen in combination with increased pleural density or findings of pleural fluid. A small amount of fluid is seen in 20% to 40% of patients with pneumothorax, regardless of its cause.

Estimating the Size of a Pneumothorax

There is no precise correlation between pneumothorax size and the need for treatment, although a 30% pneumothorax is generally considered to require treatment. Symptoms are more important in determining which patients require treatment, and this depends on both pneumothorax size and underlying lung disease. Nonetheless, an estimate of pneumothorax size is commonly requested.

The size of a pneumothorax may be estimated by using the average interpleural distance (Table 26-10). The distance

TABLE 26.10	Estimating the Size of a Pneumothorax	
Average Interpleural Distance (mm)	Percent Pneumothorax	
	Upright Film (%)	Supine Film (%)
10	14	19
20	23	29
30	32	39
40	40	49
50	49	59

separating the pleural surface of the lung from the adjacent chest wall (i.e., the depth or thickness of the pneumothorax) is measured in three locations (Fig. 26-52). To make these measurements, divide the hemithorax vertically into two halves, from the apex of the hemithorax to the costophrenic angle. Then measure the distance between the lung and the lateral chest at the midpoint of both the upper and lower halves; the third measurement is made vertically above the lung apex. The average of these measurements (i.e., the average interpleural distance) correlates with pneumothorax size in both upright and supine patients (see Table 26-10). Although the accuracy of this estimate is limited, so is the need to accurately determine the size of a pneumothorax. When reviewing Table 26-10, note that the average interpleural distance in millimeters is approximately equal to the pneumothorax percent in an upright patient; in a supine patient, add 9%.

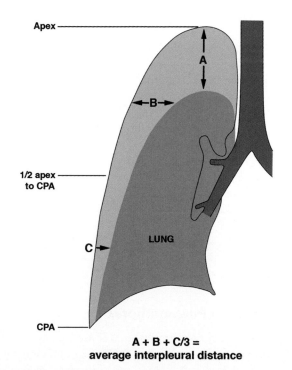

FIG. 26.52. Method of calculating average interpleural distance.

COMPRESSION ULTRASONOGRAPHY IN THE EVALUATION OF VENOUS THROMBOEMBOLISM

Compression ultrasonography is often used as an initial study in patients presenting with clinical suspicion of PE, particularly when patients present with unilateral DVT symptoms. Overall compression ultrasonography yields a diagnosis of DVT in 20% to 50% patients subsequently proven to have PE. In such instances, anticoagulation may be instituted without further testing. This approach is rapid and inexpensive, avoids the use of ionizing radiation, and is warranted for patients with lower extremity symptoms. However, compression ultrasonography is not recommended by either the American or British Thoracic Societies as a first-line examination for nonpregnant patients suspected of PE, in the absence of lower extremity symptoms, due to an unacceptably low positive predictive value. Although 90% of PEs originate in the lower extremity venous system (making it reasonable to begin the evaluation of VTE here), in one third of patients with proven PE, lower extremity CV is negative for DVT. Nonocclusive thrombus, unrecognized complete embolization of the thrombus without residua in the legs, and thrombus originating in nonimaged venous segments (e.g., deep pelvic veins), may account for this apparent discrepancy. So, it is clear that a negative lower extremity compression ultrasound examination is insufficiently sensitive to exclude PE in patients with clinical suspicion of PE.

For patients with nondiagnostic, (i.e., intermediate- or low-probability), $\dot{V}/\dot{P}$ scintigraphy results, compression ultrasonography may be obtained in an effort to avoid further diagnostic imaging. In this setting, if the compression ultrasound examination is positive, anticoagulation may be instituted without the need for further testing. Compression ultrasonography has been shown to be cost-effective when used in this fashion, because only those patients with normal lower extremity compression ultrasound examinations need further evaluation for suspected PE.

VENTILATION-PERFUSION SCINTIGRAPHY

Scintigraphy has occupied a central role in the evaluation of VTE for more than three decades. Although CT scanning has emerged as the initial diagnostic test at many institutions for patients suspected of PE, planar $\dot{V}/\dot{Q}$ lung scanning still is commonly used for the investigation of suspected PE.

Pulmonary Anatomy and Physiology

A basic understanding of normal pulmonary physiology is required to appreciate the alterations in lung function that occur in patients with PE. Reflex pneumoconstriction may occur in alveoli that are ventilated but not perfused (i.e., abnormally "high" $\dot{V}/\dot{Q}$); abnormally low carbon dioxide tension elicits this response. However, this reflex is not commonly observed and generally is transient, because patients inhale carbon dioxide from tracheal dead space into the poorly perfused alveoli, and bronchial circulation continues to deliver some carbon dioxide to ischemic alveoli, thus moderating this reflex bronchoconstriction. Abnormalities of ventilation may produce regional alveolar hypoxia, which, in turn, induces reflex pulmonary vasoconstriction. Thus, alveolar hypoxia (i.e., areas of abnormally low $\dot{V}/\dot{Q}$) causes redistribution of pulmonary blood flow away from hypoventilated alveoli. These pulmonary responses to alterations in regional ventilation and perfusion provide the basis for $\dot{V}/\dot{Q}$ scintigraphy.

Technique

Ventilation Scintigraphy

The agent most commonly used for ventilation scintigraphy is xenon-133 (^{133}Xe). ^{133}Xe is an inert gas with a principal photon energy of 81 keV and a physical half-life of 5.3 days. The advantages of ^{133}Xe are that it is relatively inexpensive, is widely available, and allows the acquisition of single-breath, equilibrium, and washout images. A disadvantage of ^{133}Xe is its low photon energy (81 keV), which generally requires that ventilation scans be obtained before perfusion scans. If technetium perfusion images are acquired prior to the ^{133}Xe ventilation study, the downscatter from the technetium-99m (^{99m}Tc) photons (140 keV principal photon energy) will be detected in the xenon window of the pulse height analyzer and will degrade the ventilation images. If the ventilation study must be performed or repeated after the perfusion study has been completed, ventilation images can be improved if a ^{99m}Tc background image is obtained using the ^{133}Xe window. This background image can then be subtracted from the subsequent ^{133}Xe ventilation images to improve image quality.

^{133}Xe images usually are obtained in the upright posterior projection to allow evaluation of the largest amount of lung volume. The single-breath image is obtained by having the patient exhale completely and then inhale approximately 5 to 20 mCi (200 to 740 MBq) ^{133}Xe gas, after which a 15- to 30-second breathhold is performed to obtain a static image. Then, the patient is instructed to breathe a mixture of the exhaled xenon and oxygen for 3 to 5 minutes, as tolerated, while static equilibrium images are obtained; images thus acquired represent the distribution of aerated lung volume. Finally, washout images are acquired by having the patient breathe fresh air, while serial 15- to 30-second images are obtained for a period of 3 minutes as xenon clears from the lungs. Normal xenon clearance is bilaterally symmetric and usually is complete in 2 to 3 minutes. Areas of delayed clearance may indicate regional air trapping and are commonly seen in patients with obstructive lung disease.

^{127}Xe has been used for ventilation scintigraphy and has the advantage of higher photon energies (172, 203, and 375 keV), societal recommendations favor the initial use of MSCTPA with dose reducing procedures. For example, the British Thoracic Society recommendations suggest that thoracic imaging for pregnant patients suspected of PE should begin with MSCTPA, whereas 69% of the PIOPED II investigators recommend initial investigation with V̇/Q̇ scanning. With attention to dose reduction, the fetal dose resulting from MSCTPA will usually be less than that of V̇/Q̇ scanning. While the maternal dose remains higher with MSCTPA, even with dose reducing techniques, the difference should be small when careful attention to technical factors is employed. Further innovations in dose reduction and noise reduction may eventually eliminate dose differences between MSCTPA and V̇/Q̇ scanning all together.

One of the main drivers for the recommendation of MSCTPA over V̇/Q̇ scanning for the evaluation of suspected PE in pregnant patients is the perception that MSCTPA is more likely to be diagnostic and also provides the ability to identify alternative causes of symptoms that prompted evaluation. The latter is important because the minority of patients who undergo imaging evaluation for suspected PE will actually be diagnosed with PE. Regarding the former, the "nondiagnostic" rate of MSCTPA is in the range of 5% to 10%, with limited data suggesting that this rate is increased in pregnant patients. The "nondiagnostic" rate of V̇/Q̇ scintigraphy in patients with suspected PE has been reported to range from 50% to 70% but has been suggested to be as low as 25% in pregnant patients suspected of PE. Therefore, in pregnant patients suspected of PE, V̇/Q̇ scintigraphy remains a useful test.

MAGNETIC RESONANCE IMAGING

MRI of the chest presents significant challenges, including the relative lack of signal due to the paucity of protons within the chest, susceptibility artifacts resulting from air and soft tissue interfaces within the thorax, and image degradation from respiratory and cardiac motion. The development of faster and stronger gradients and the evolution of contrast-enhanced magnetic resonance angiography (MRA) have made rapid high-resolution imaging of the thorax and pulmonary vascular system possible, and MRI of the pulmonary vascular system has evolved significantly. Additional techniques for cardiopulmonary imaging—pulmonary perfusion MRI and hyperpolarized 3-helium—also have been investigated and may provide unique diagnostic information. MRV of the pelvis and lower extremities has been shown to be an accurate technique for the diagnosis of DVT and may be combined with the thoracic examination to provide a comprehensive evaluation for patients with suspected VTE.

Techniques

Conventional MRA techniques, such as two- (2D) or three-dimensional (3D) time-of-flight, depend on blood flow to produce contrast between the vessels and the surrounding tissues. Early investigation with these methods yielded promising results for imaging of the pulmonary arteries, especially for evaluation of PE. However, time-of-flight methods suffer from several limitations, including insensitivity to slow flow, excessive respiratory and pulsation motion artifacts, and relatively poor spatial resolution. The introduction of 3D MRA techniques using intravenous gadolinium chelate contrast agents represents a major advance in MRI of PE. Because of the T1-shortening effect of gadolinium, contrast-enhanced 3D MRA does not rely on blood flow to produce images of vessels. Therefore, high-quality vascular imaging can be performed without artifacts due to flow phenomena. Single-breathhold monophasic protocols, with scan times of 20 seconds or less, or time-resolved multiphasic protocols, with scan times under 10 seconds, now are routinely possible and allow high-quality imaging, even in severely dyspneic patients.

The protocol for 3D MRA varies from institution to institution. Phased array coils are used to optimize the signal-to-noise ratio. A localizing sequence is obtained, typically in the transverse plane. The heavily T1-weighted 3D gradient echo MRA coronal acquisition may then be prescribed from the transverse images. Images are obtained using a slice thickness of 1 to 2 mm, repetition time (TR) of 3 to 5 milliseconds, and echo time (TE) of 1 to 2 milliseconds. Parallel imaging technique can be used for reduction of scan time by approximately 50%.

The angiographic sequence is completed during a breath-hold of approximately 20 seconds. To aid in breath holding, the patient can be provided with oxygen by nasal cannula, at a rate of 2 L/minute. Gadolinium contrast agent (0.1 mmol/mL) is administered via an antecubital vein with use of a power injector (2 to 5 mL/second) and is followed by a saline bolus. The scan begins approximately 5 to 10 seconds after the start of the injection of contrast medium when imaging the pulmonary arteries. Timing of the acquisition can be optimized with bolus-detection software or by performing a preliminary acquisition with use of a test bolus to estimate circulation time.

The complete sequence is performed in approximately 20 seconds, and the entire study can be completed in 30 to 45 minutes. Multiplanar maximum intensity projection reconstructions of the 3D MRA, performed on an off-line workstation, often are invaluable for interpretation of the study.

For optimal assessment of the vessels, 3D MRA can be supplemented in some cases by a sequence in the transverse plane, such as a steady-state free precession (SSFP) sequence (also referred to as balanced fast-field echo [bFFE], fast imaging with steady precession [True FISP], and fast imaging employing steady-state acquisition [FIESTA]). SSFP images are acquired using single-shot technique, typically with a TR and TE of approximately 3 and 1.5, respectively, and a flip angle of 60 degrees. Imaging may be performed in any desired plane. Images acquired in such a fashion have T2-weighting, with moving blood showing increased signal and stationary foci, such as emboli, showing decreased signal. An advantage of SSFP is the inherently high signal of moving blood relative to cardiac muscle and vascular walls. SSFP imaging in the coronal plane can be used as noncontrast MRA technique for evaluation of PE. This can be especially useful in patients with renal insufficiency. Moreover, SSFP can be performed in the short axis plane for the assessment of right ventricular function in patients with suspected PE.

Newer MR techniques that may play a role in PE imaging include MR pulmonary perfusion imaging. MR pulmonary perfusion imaging is a time-resolved technique performed with a fast, 3D low-angle shot (FLASH) gradient-echo sequence with typical sequence parameters including TR = 1.6, TE = 0.6, and a flip angle 25 degrees. Gadolinium contrast (0.5 mmol/mL solution with a dose of 0.125 mmol/kg) is injected at 4 mL/s followed by a 20 mL saline flush at the same rate. The number of phase-encoding steps depends on the size of the imaging volume, but imaging is very rapid, typically requiring 2 seconds or less. This sequence is repeated a number of times to image the first pass of contrast through the right ventricle and pulmonary arteries, over a period of about 35 to 55 seconds. Patients are asked to suspend respiration as long as possible to minimize diaphragmatic motion.

Both contrast enhanced MRA and pulmonary perfusion imaging may benefit from the recent introduction of parallel imaging techniques. Parallel imaging allows signal integration from multiple elements within a phased-array receiver coil to accelerate data sampling. This results in improved spatial resolution or volume of coverage, without requiring additional acquisition time. Alternatively, parallel imaging can be used to reduce imaging time (and breath holding time) by up to 50%. For pulmonary perfusion imaging, parallel imaging may allow for improvements in temporal resolution as well, as improvements in temporal resolution have more relevance for time-resolved imaging than improvements in volume of coverage or spatial resolution. Available parallel imaging techniques include sensitivity encoding (SENSE) and generalized autocalibrating parallel acquisition (GRAPPA).

Advantages and Disadvantages of MR for Diagnosis of Pulmonary Embolism

Gadolinium-enhanced 3D MRA has proved its utility for a number of thoracic applications, including diagnosis of PE. Advantages of MRA over MSCTPA and pulmonary angiography include the use of gadolinium-chelate contrast agent and the lack of ionizing radiation. Unlike iodinated contrast media, gadolinium chelates are not nephrotoxic (at the dose typically used for MR imaging), and the risk of contrast reaction is very low. Limitations of MRA include a relatively long breathhold time and the fact that MR is contraindicated in selected patients who may be at risk for PE, including those with pacemakers. Additionally, while contrast enhanced MRI was once considered a good option for vascular imaging in patients with renal insufficiency or failure, in whom iodinated contrast enhanced studies are contraindicated, the recent recognition of the association of nephrogenic systemic sclerosis with gadolinium administration in patients with renal insufficiency has tempered the utility of contrast enhanced MRI techniques in these patients.

Pulmonary Embolism Findings on MRI and MRA

MRI and MRA findings of PE depend on the imaging sequence employed. The short T1 signal of methemoglobin in pulmonary emboli produces high signal on T1-weighted imaging. On breathhold cine acquisition sequences, pulmonary emboli usually appear as very low signal intensity filling defects within high-signal blood pool, whereas on 3D contrast-enhanced MRA sequences, emboli appear as very low signal foci surrounded by high-signal intraluminal contrast.

Much like MSCTPA, acute PE is diagnosed when an intra-arterial filling defect is identified. Expanded, unenhanced pulmonary arteries also may suggest acute pulmonary embolization. Chronic thromboembolic disease may be suggested when eccentric filling defects (Fig. 27-20) or intravascular webs are identified, often in the presence of an enlarged main pulmonary arterial segment, reflecting pulmonary hypertension.

Accuracy of MRI and MRA for the Diagnosis of Pulmonary Embolism

Studies examining the utility and accuracy of MR techniques for the diagnosis of PE are smaller and far less numerous than studies detailing other imaging methods used to evaluate patients suspected of PE, including MSCTPA. Nevertheless, data are available from both experimental and clinical studies utilizing MR for the diagnosis of PE. Pooled analysis of the results of several studies shows that the sensitivity for MR techniques for the detection of PE ranges from 75% to 100%, with specificity usually exceeding 90%. Reports of the interobserver agreement of MR examinations for PE have shown good results, although the rate of technically inadequate studies has been slightly higher for MR than for MSCTPA. Predictably, MRI/MRA techniques show their highest sensitivity for central emboli, with diminishing sensitivity for smaller emboli, especially for subsegmental PE.

MR Perfusion and Ventilation Imaging of the Lung

Perfusion and ventilation imaging of the lung is now possible. Several methods for pulmonary perfusion imaging exist. Pulmonary perfusion may be performed in combination with 3D MRA, using gadolinium-based contrast agents and a sequence with short TR and TE, in a time-resolved fashion, by employing the first-pass effect as described above. As contrast enters the imaging volume, regions of diminished perfusion become increasingly apparent as first the vessels and then the pulmonary parenchyma enhance. This technique may allow the demonstration of pulmonary parenchymal perfusion defects as well as the intraluminal emboli producing the perfusion abnormalities. MR pulmonary perfusion may also be performed using blood pool agents. Because these agents circulate for a prolonged period of time,

A   **B**

FIG. 27.20. Chronic thromboembolic disease on MRA imaging. **A:** Coronal MRA image shows a peripheral, low-signal filling defect in the main pulmonary artery (*arrows*), representing chronic thromboembolic disease. **B:** Axial cine image shows low signal along the anterior wall of the right pulmonary artery (*arrow*).

perfusion imaging of the lung may be followed by lower extremity and pelvic imaging for potential DVT. Finally, MR pulmonary perfusion may be performed with noncontrast methods, such as arterial spin labeling; this technique is capable of distinguishing stationary from moving tissue, and thus may provide information on pulmonary blood flow.

Preliminary techniques for MR ventilation imaging have been studied in recent years. Using hyperpolarized noble gases or molecular oxygen, MR ventilation imaging is now possible. MR ventilation techniques may be combined with MR pulmonary perfusion methods to create a map of pulmonary ventilation and perfusion in a fashion similar to V̇/Q̇ scintigraphy. However, experience with these techniques currently is limited, and, although promising, further technical refinements will be required.

SELECTED READING

British Thoracic Society Standards of Care Committee Pulmonary Embolism Guideline Development Group. British Thoracic Society guidelines for the management of suspected acute pulmonary embolism. Thorax 2003; 58(6):470–83.

Chen M, Coakley FV, Kaimal A, et al. Guidelines for computed tomography and magnetic resonance imaging use during pregnancy and lactation. Obstet Gynecol 2008; 112(2 Pt 1):333–340.

Fink C, Ley S, Schoenberg SO, et al. Magnetic resonance imaging of acute pulmonary embolism. Eur Radiol 2007; 17:2546–2553.

Fraser RS, Müller NL, Colman N, Paré PD. Diagnosis of Diseases of the Chest. Philadelphia: WB Saunders, 1999: 1897–1945.

Frazier AA, Galvin JR, Franks TJ, Rosado-De-Christenson ML. From the archives of the AFIP: pulmonary vasculature: hypertension and infarction. Radiographics 2000; 20:491–524.

Ley S, Kauczor HU. MR imaging/magnetic resonance angiography of the pulmonary arteries and pulmonary thromboembolic disease. Magn Reson Imaging Clin N Am 2008; 16(2):263–273.

Marik PE, Plante LA. Venous thromboembolic disease and pregnancy. N Eng J Med 2008; 359:2025–2033.

Musset D, Parent F, Meyer G, et al. Diagnostic strategy for patients with suspected pulmonary embolism: a prospective multicentre outcome study. Lancet 2002; 360(9349):1914–1920.

Gotway MB, Patel RA, Webb WR. Helical CT for the evaluation of suspected acute pulmonary embolism: diagnostic pitfalls. J Comput Assist Tomogr 2000; 24:267–273.

Kubo T, Ohno Y, Gautam S, et al. Use of 3D adaptive raw-data filter in CT of the lung: effect on radiation dose reduction. AJR 2008; 191: W167–W174.

MacKenzie JD, Nazario-Larrieu J, Cai T, et al. Reduced-dose CT: effect on reader evaluation in detection of pulmonary embolism. AJR 2007; 189:1371–1379.

Stein PD, Woodard PK, Weg JG, et al. Diagnostic pathways in acute pulmonary embolism: recommendations of the PIOPED II investigators. Radiology 2007; 242(1):15–21.

Tapson VF, Carroll BA, Davidson BL, et al. The diagnostic approach to acute venous thromboembolism: clinical practice guideline. Am J Respir Crit Care Med 1999; 160:1043–1066.

van Beek EJR, Wild JM, Fink C, et al. MRI for the diagnosis of pulmonary embolism. J Magn Res Imaging 2003; 18:627–640.

28 Pulmonary Hypertension

MICHAEL B. GOTWAY

ANATOMY AND PHYSIOLOGY OF THE PULMONARY CIRCULATION

The pulmonary circulation consists of two parallel networks: the pulmonary arterial circulation and the bronchial arterial circulation. Pulmonary arteries course along the lobar, segmental, and subsegmental airways to the level of the terminal bronchioles. Small pulmonary arteries from the subsegmental level to the terminal bronchioles possess a thick muscular media, and range from 50 to 1,000 μm in size. These small pulmonary arteries progressively lose much of their muscle within the arteriolar media as well as their external elastic membrane. By the level of the respiratory bronchioles and alveolar ducts they are termed *pulmonary arterioles*, and range in size from 10 to 150 μm. These vessels ramify further within the alveolar walls to form a rich capillary network. Capillary blood collects in venules, which coalesce progressively to form veins, which course within the interlobular septa, eventually to empty into the left atrium.

The bronchial circulation, accounting for about 1% of the systemic cardiac output, originates from the thoracic aorta or intercostal arteries. Bronchial arteries, averaging two per lung, course within the pulmonary hila along the mainstem bronchi to the level of the terminal bronchiole and form a plexus that extends from the adventitia through to the submucosa of the associated airway. Bronchial arteries freely form anastomoses with pulmonary arteries, primarily at the capillary and postcapillary levels.

Unlike the tracheobronchial system, in which the major component to airflow resistance is located within the large airways, the major site of resistance to pulmonary arterial blood flow is located at the small muscular pulmonary arterial and arteriolar level. Caliber changes in the vessels at this level regulate pulmonary arterial pressure and are critical for optimizing ventilation and perfusion matching.

The pulmonary circulation is a low pressure system—the mean arterial pressure is approximately one sixth that of the systemic circulation. This low pressure is maintained at a relatively consistent level even with large increases in pulmonary blood flow such as may occur with exercise. This is possible because when the body is at rest, numerous pulmonary capillaries normally are not perfused; these capillaries are "recruited" when increased pulmonary blood flow must be accommodated.

PATHOGENESIS OF PULMONARY HYPERTENSION

Pulmonary hypertension (PH) is defined as a resting mean pulmonary arterial pressure (mPAP) ≥25 mm Hg at rest or 30 mm Hg with exercise. The subgroup of PH referred to as pulmonary arterial hypertension (PAH) adds the criterion that the pulmonary capillary wedge pressure is ≤15 mm Hg. Pulmonary venous hypertension is present when pulmonary venous pressure, usually approximated by measurement of the pulmonary capillary wedge pressure, is equal to or exceeds 18 mm Hg. Several mechanisms may produce a decrease in the total number of small pulmonary arteries, thereby increasing pulmonary vascular resistance and producing elevated pulmonary arterial pressure. These mechanisms include intraluminal arterial occlusion, muscular contraction of small pulmonary arteries, vascular remodeling with wall thickening, or conditions that produce pulmonary venous hypertension. Several of these mechanisms may be operative simultaneously in a patient with pulmonary hypertension.

The pulmonary vascular endothelium responds to changes in oxygen tension, transmural pressure, and pulmonary blood flow and participates actively in the regulation of pulmonary arterial pressure through the elaboration of various vasoactive substances, such as prostacyclin, nitrous oxide, and endothelin. The agents have a direct effect on pulmonary vascular smooth muscle tone (promoting relaxation and vasodilation) and also may directly affect platelet function. Abnormalities in endothelial cell function or injuries to these cells may be the fundamental derangement that ultimately produces the structural vascular changes observed in patients with pulmonary hypertension.

Various histopathological abnormalities may be observed in patients with pulmonary hypertension, varying somewhat depending on the cause of hypertension. In general, regardless of the specific cause of the pulmonary hypertension, the arteries are more commonly seen in patients with chronic thromboembolic pulmonary hypertension than patients with nonembolic causes of pulmonary hypertension, and the presence of these vessels tends to favor chronic PE over acute PE.

Right ventricular enlargement and hypertrophy are readily visible on MSCTPA studies in patients with chronic thromboembolic pulmonary hypertension. Leftward bowing of the interventricular septum may also be present. When the tricuspid annulus dilates, tricuspid regurgitation may develop and is associated with reflux of injected intravenous contrast into the inferior vena cava and hepatic veins; however, these findings can be seen as a result of increased right heart pressures in the absence of significant tricuspid valvular dysfunction also. Nonspecific MSCTPA findings in patients with chronic thromboembolic pulmonary hypertension include mild lymphadenopathy, pericardial effusion, and mild pericardial thickening.

$\dot{V}/\dot{Q}$ scanning often is interpreted as high-probability in patients with chronic thromboembolic pulmonary hypertension, although scintigraphy may underestimate the degree of hemodynamic derangement associated with chronic thromboembolic pulmonary hypertension. Furthermore, in the original Prospective Investigation of Pulmonary Embolism Diagnosis (PIOPED I) series, the positive predictive value of a high-probability $\dot{V}/\dot{Q}$ scan interpretation fell from 91% to 74% for patients with a prior history of thromboembolic disease, representing a loss of specificity in the high-probability scan interpretation. Other studies have shown that normal $\dot{V}/\dot{Q}$ scintigraphy results exclude chronic thromboembolic pulmonary hypertension with a high degree of certainty, whereas, as alluded to above, negative results on MSCTPA do not exclude this diagnosis, nor do they always establish or exclude the possibility of a favorable response to surgical intervention in patients with chronic thromboembolic pulmonary hypertension. For this reason, some investigators have recommended that $\dot{V}/\dot{Q}$ scintigraphy should remain the primary noninvasive imaging method for the investigation of suspected chronic thromboembolic pulmonary hypertension. It is likely, however, that combinations of $\dot{V}/\dot{Q}$ scintigraphy and MSCTPA examinations may provide the optimal ability to detect chronic thromboembolic pulmonary hypertension and guide management for these patients.

Findings of central chronic thromboembolic pulmonary hypertension on MRI and magnetic resonance angiography (MRA) are similar to those on CT. Chronic, organized thrombi appear as very low signal foci adjacent to the vascular wall on T1-weighted, gadolinium-enhanced MRA, and steady-state free precession images. Vascular webs and stenoses and hypertrophied bronchial arteries may be visible. MRI has the added utility of accurate assessment of right ventricular performance, and improvements in right ventricular ejection fraction and peak systolic pulmonary arterial flow velocity may be seen in patients with chronic thromboembolic pulmonary hypertension treated with endarterectomy. Additionally, velocity-encoded cine phase

contrast MRI has been used to assess the degree of bronchopulmonary shunt volume through hypertrophied bronchial arteries before and after surgical pulmonary endarterectomy—reduction of bronchopulmonary shunt volume represents a favorable response to surgical therapy in patients with chronic thromboembolic pulmonary hypertension.

Pulmonary angiography typically shows vascular tortuosity, webs, bands, stenoses, "pouching defects," and abrupt vascular cutoffs or occlusions in patients with chronic thromboembolic pulmonary hypertension.

NONTHROMBOTIC PULMONARY ARTERIAL EMBOLIZATION

Nonthrombotic emboli to the pulmonary arterial circulation may produce pulmonary hypertension. Potential etiologies include tumor emboli, particulates such as mercury and talc, and parasites.

Tumor Embolization
Etiology and Pathogenesis

Pulmonary hypertension resulting from microvascular obstruction caused by tumor emboli is classified in the 2008 Dana Point system as a Group 5.4 lesion, rather than with chronic thromboembolic pulmonary hypertension, but is considered here because tumor embolization shares a common theme with particulate and parasitic embolization: nonthrombotic pulmonary embolization.

As many as 25% of patients with a solid malignancy may have microemboli that lodge in the pulmonary circulation. The most common etiology of tumor microembolization is gastric cancer, but breast, lung, ovarian, renal, hepatocellular, and prostate cancers also may produce tumor emboli. Most emboli preferentially occlude small arteries and arterioles, with the exception of atrial myxomas and renal carcinomas, which may form larger, more centrally located, thromboemboli.

Histopathological specimens in patients with pulmonary tumor embolization show visible tumor within pulmonary arteries, often accompanied by lymphangitic tumor, organizing thrombi, pulmonary infarction, and intimal fibrosis (Fig. 28-10). Larger vessels may be affected, although small, peripherally located pulmonary arteries (at the centrilobular artery level) may be affected as well. Occasionally, myxoid intimal hyperplasia may be present and may induce arteriolar obliteration. This situation has been referred to as *thrombotic tumor microangiopathy*.

Clinical Presentation

Because tumor emboli are quite small, symptoms related to tumor embolization are uncommon. If the embolic load is

FIG. 28.10. Pulmonary arterial tumor embolism in a patient with carcinoma. This histopathological specimen shows tumor filling small pulmonary arterioles (*arrows*), producing a branching configuration. Hemorrhagic infarction also is present (*arrowheads*).

great enough, patients may present with dyspnea on exertion, hypoxemia, chest pain, cough, syncope, and even right-sided heart failure.

Imaging Manifestations

Chest radiographs in patients with intravascular tumor embolization often are normal, but sometimes they may resemble pulmonary lymphangitic carcinomatosis.

In addition to the characteristic findings of pulmonary hypertension and thromboembolism described previously, thoracic CT of patients with tumor emboli may reveal lymphadenopathy, lymphangitic carcinomatosis, and peripheral, wedge-shaped opacities representing infarction. When emboli affect larger vessels, such as subsegmental arteries, CT may reveal a "beaded" appearance of these vessels. When smaller vessels are affected (at the centrilobular level), beading and nodularity may be observed, and the affected vessels may assume a branching configuration, resembling "tree-in-bud."

Lung scintigraphy may reveal subsegmental unmatched perfusion defects, indistinguishable from thromboembolic disease. Pulmonary angiography may show a delayed arterial phase, intravascular filling defects with a beaded appearance, and peripheral pruning.

Particulate Embolization

Etiology and Pathogenesis

Intravascular mercury embolization may produce pulmonary hypertension. After injection, mercury embolizes small vessels and eventually migrates from the vessel into the surrounding pulmonary interstitium, where the metal

elicits an inflammatory, granulomatous response that produces vascular obstruction and, eventually, pulmonary hypertension.

Pulmonary talcosis results from the intravascular injection of talc. Talc is an insoluble filler used as a binding agent in several medications. When intravenous drug users abuse medications containing talc, they intravenously inject a suspension containing crushed tablets intended for oral use, thereby embolizing small pulmonary arterioles with talc. The talc may migrate from the vessels into the surrounding pulmonary interstitium, where its presence elicits a foreign body granulomatous response. Vascular thrombosis with recanalization, medial arterial hypertrophy, fibrosis, and refractile talc particles are present in histopathological specimens.

Clinical Presentation

Mercury may be injected into the vascular system accidentally or intentionally. Intentional mercury injection most often represents a suicide attempt.

Pulmonary talcosis usually produces few symptoms, but patients may present with chronic, progressive shortness of breath, dyspnea on exertion, and cough. Symptoms may progress even after cessation of drug abuse.

Imaging Manifestations

On chest radiography, mercury embolization appears as fine, branching, symmetric, very dense nodules representing intra-arterial mercury deposits. Metal deposits also may collect within the heart, particularly at the apex of the right ventricle.

Chest radiographs in patients with talc embolization show diffuse, bilateral, small nodular opacities about 1 to 2 mm in diameter throughout the lung parenchyma. Perihilar conglomerate masses associated with fibrosis, producing retraction of lung parenchyma and relative hyperlucency in the lower lung, may be seen in some patients.

CT may demonstrate numerous, small micronodules with or without patchy ground-glass opacity. Upper lobe fibrotic opacities, resembling progressive massive fibrosis, may be present. These fibrotic opacities may show high attenuation due to the presence of talc.

Parasitic Embolization

Etiology and Pathogenesis

Pulmonary hypertension resulting from schistosomiasis is considered a Group 1 lesion (PAH) in the 2008 Dana Point classification (see Table 28-2), but is considered here since parasitic embolization shares similar pathophysiological mechanisms to other nonthrombotic pulmonary emboli. Cardiopulmonary schistosomiasis most often is the result of infection with *Schistosoma mansoni*, which is endemic in the Middle East, Africa, and South America. There usually is a latency period of 5 years or more after the onset of infection before cardiopulmonary disease develops. Secreted ova migrate to the lungs via portal-systemic collaterals and lodge within medium-sized muscular arteries and arterioles. Within the pulmonary circulation, the eggs elicit an inflammatory reaction that results in medial hypertrophy, granuloma formation, intimal hyperplasia, collagen deposition and fibrosis, and obliterative arteritis. An associated eosinophilic alveolitis may be present.

Clinical Presentation

Presenting symptoms of parasitic embolization include hepatosplenomegaly, symptoms of right heart failure, dyspnea, and cough. Patients with cardiopulmonary schistosomiasis always have cirrhosis and portal hypertension.

Imaging Manifestations

Chest radiography in patients with parasitic embolization shows findings consistent with pulmonary hypertension. Small nodules, representing parasitic granulomas, may be evident. Pulmonary infarction rarely is seen with parasitic embolization.

HRCT may demonstrate nodules, interstitial prominence and thickening, and ground-glass opacity associated with the classic findings of pulmonary hypertension.

PULMONARY HYPERTENSION WITH UNCLEAR OR MULTIFACTORIAL MECHANISMS

Various, seemingly disparate, conditions may produce pulmonary hypertension and are classified under Group 5 in the 2008 Dana Point classification system as "pulmonary hypertension with unclear multifactorial mechanisms." Pulmonary hypertension in these conditions shares the same imaging characteristics as other causes of pulmonary hypertension, although some of the diseases in this category may show thoracic imaging findings suggestive of a particular disorder. The specific imaging features of such disorders have been reviewed elsewhere.

The first subcategory of the Group 5 2008 Dana Point classification of disorders producing pulmonary hypertension includes hematological disorders, such as myeloproliferative diseases, polycythemia vera, essential thrombocytosis, chronic myeloid leukemia, and splenectomy. A number of mechanisms may result in pulmonary hypertension in patients with these conditions, including high cardiac output, congestive heart failure, asplenia, or mechanical pulmonary arterial obstruction due to circulating megakaryocytes. Other systemic conditions included in Group 5 include sarcoidosis, Langerhans cell histiocytosis,

lymphangioleiomyomatosis, pulmonary vasculitis, and neurofibromatosis. In patients with sarcoidosis, postulated mechanisms producing pulmonary hypertension include capillary bed destruction due to fibrosis, pulmonary artery and venous compression by lymphadenopathy, and granulomatous inflammation directly involving the pulmonary vessels, particularly the veins. Elevated pulmonary arterial pressure in patients with end-stage Langerhans cell histiocytosis is not uncommon and may be related to a combination of pulmonary parenchymal destruction with associated hypoxemia and vasculopathy. Pulmonary hypertension is relatively uncommon in patients with lymphangioleiomyomatosis, but, when present, has been thought to be the result of hypoxemia due to capillary destruction caused by the cystic lesions that characterize this condition.

Also in Group 5 of the 2008 Dana Point classification of pulmonary hypertension are a number of metabolic disorders, such as Gaucher disease, glycogen storage disease, and thyroid conditions. Various mechanisms for the development of pulmonary hypertension in these conditions include hypoxemia, pulmonary parenchymal disease, portocaval shunts (in the case of type Ia glycogen storage disease), and capillary blockade by Gaucher cells. The mechanisms by which thyroid disorders may produce pulmonary hypertension are unclear, but an association between autoimmune thyroid disease and PAH raises the possibility of a linked genetic pathogenesis.

The final subcategory of Group 5 in the 2008 Dana Point classification includes several disorders that produce mechanical obstruction of the pulmonary arteries and/or veins, including central obstructing tumors, metastatic microvascular obstruction, and fibrosing mediastinitis. Also included in this category is pulmonary hypertension associated with end-stage renal disease on long-term hemodialysis. Among these disorders, fibrosing mediastinitis may present with suggestive thoracic imaging findings and is discussed in detail.

Fibrosing Mediastinitis

Fibrosing mediastinitis represents a progressive proliferation of collagenous and fibrous tissue throughout the mediastinum, producing encasement and compression of mediastinal structures. Granulomatous infections, particularly *Histoplasma capsulatum* and *Mycobacterium tuberculosis*, are among the most common causes of fibrosing mediastinitis.

The deposition of fibrous tissue in fibrosing mediastinitis commonly affects relatively deformable structures, such as the superior vena cava, the trachea and central airways, the pulmonary arteries, the pulmonary veins, and the esophagus. Pulmonary hypertension may be produced by fibrous encasement of either the pulmonary arteries or draining pulmonary veins. The former produces precapillary pulmonary hypertension, which often is mistaken for chronic thromboembolic disease, and the latter produces postcapillary

FIG. 28.11. Pulmonary hypertension secondary to fibrosing mediastinitis. CT scan shows abnormal soft tissue within the anterior mediastinum and compression of the main pulmonary artery (*arrows*). Note the presence of an intensely enhanced hemiazygos vein (*arrowhead*). Multiple biopsies revealed fibrous tissue, consistent with fibrosing mediastinitis.

pulmonary hypertension. Pulmonary venous obstruction is patchy in distribution, producing wide variations in pulmonary capillary wedge pressure measurements, although the wedge pressure usually is elevated. Cardiac catheterization reveals normal left heart size and pressures.

Fibrosing mediastinitis produces histopathological changes characteristic of venous hypertension, including medial hypertrophy, septal thickening secondary to edema, hemosiderin-laden macrophages, venous infarction, and the typical vascular changes of pulmonary hypertension. Thrombi may be found within affected veins.

The predominant symptoms of fibrosing mediastinitis depend on the structures most severely involved. Patients often present with nonspecific symptoms of pulmonary venous hypertension such as dyspnea and hemoptysis. The treatment for the disorder is limited; if focal fibrosis of a pulmonary vein is diagnosed, surgical treatment may be effective. Corticosteroids have shown limited efficacy in reversing the disease.

Chest radiographs often show a widened mediastinum with hilar prominence and calcified lymph nodes. Findings of pulmonary venous hypertension, including interlobular septal thickening and alveolar edema, may be present. Fibrosing mediastinitis may result in airway stenoses which may cause lobar volume loss.

CT reveals extensive infiltration of the mediastinum with abnormal soft tissue. Fibrosing mediastinitis due to *H. capsulatum* usually produces extensive lymph node calcification, which is readily identified with CT. Contrast-enhanced CT may show extensive collateral vein formation due to fibrotic involvement of systemic thoracic veins such as the superior vena cava or azygos vein. Pulmonary artery compression may be visualized directly (Fig. 28-11). Pulmonary venous infarcts, appearing as subpleural, wedge-shaped consolidations, may be seen in patients with pulmonary venous involvement. V̇/Q̇ scintigraphy may show focal unmatched perfusion defects. Unilateral lack of perfusion of one lung has been reported in patients with fibrosing mediastinitis.

Pulmonary angiography findings vary depending on the location of obstruction. If the arterial circulation is affected primarily, asymmetric narrowing of the pulmonary arteries will be present. When pulmonary veins are affected primarily, venous phase angiography will show stenoses, dilation, or obstruction, often near the junction of the affected vein and the left atrium.

SELECTED READING

Castañer E, Gallardo X, Ballesteros E, et al. CT diagnosis of chronic pulmonary thromboembolism. Radiographics 2009; 29(1):31–50; discussion 50–53.

Fraser RS, Müller NL, Colman N, Paré PD. Diagnosis of Diseases of the Chest. Philadelphia: WB Saunders, 1999: 1897–1945.

Frazier AA, Galvin JR, Franks TJ, Rosado-DeChristenson ML. From the archives of the AFIP: pulmonary vasculature: hypertension and infarction. Radiographics 2000; 20:491–524.

Hoeper MM, Barberà JA, Channick RN, et al. Diagnosis, assessment, and treatment of non-pulmonary arterial hypertension pulmonary hypertension. J Am Coll Cardiol 2009; 54(1 Suppl):S85–S96.

McLaughlin VV, Archer SL, Badesch DB, et al. ACCF/AHA 2009 expert consensus document on pulmonary hypertension: a report of the American College of Cardiology Foundation Task Force on Expert Consensus Documents and the American Heart Association developed in collaboration with the American College of Chest Physicians; American Thoracic Society, Inc.; and the Pulmonary Hypertension Association. J Am Coll Cardiol 2009; 53(17):1573–1619.

Simonneau G, Robbins IM, Beghetti M, et al. Updated clinical classification of pulmonary hypertension. J Am Coll Cardiol 2009; 54(1 Suppl):S43–S54.

Multislice CT and MRI of the Thoracic Aorta

GAUTHAM P. REDDY, MARTIN GUNN, LEE M. MITSUMORI, MICHAEL B. GOTWAY, AND CHARLES B. HIGGINS

INTRODUCTION

The aorta can be imaged with a number of modalities: x-ray angiography, transesophageal echocardiography (TEE), multislice computed tomography (MSCT), and magnetic resonance imaging (MRI). Because some diseases of the thoracic aorta are life threatening, the aorta must be fully evaluated when pathology is suspected. For comprehensive diagnostic assessment of the thoracic aorta, the lumen, aortic wall, and periaortic region must be depicted to assess intraluminal, mural, and extramural disease. Aortic pathology can involve any or all of these three locations. Imaging techniques must have the capability of evaluating the entire thoracic aorta as well as the origins of the arch vessels to define the extent of involvement. In some patients the status of the aortic valve and annulus must also be delineated. Imaging studies are used both for the initial diagnosis and for the surveillance of disease progression over time.

MSCT and MRI are the mainstays of evaluation of the thoracic aorta. The use of MSCT or MRI is dependent upon the information required, the clinical status of the patient, history of contrast reaction, and institutional practice.

The advantages of MSCT are its speed, ease of use, and lack of operator dependence. At many institutions, MSCT is the examination of choice for evaluation of acute aortic pathology, including dissection, intramural hematoma, aneurysm rupture, penetrating ulcer, and acute traumatic injury. MSCT can be used to evaluate the lungs and pleura in patients with suspected aortic disease, a capability that can be especially important in the acute setting because vascular and nonvascular diseases can have similar clinical presentations and may be difficult to differentiate on the basis of signs and symptoms. At many centers, MSCT is preferred for acutely ill patients and MRI for patients who are stable.

MRI is a valuable technique for comprehensive non-invasive morphologic and functional evaluation of the thoracic aorta. MRI has several advantages, including high intrinsic contrast between the blood pool and vessel wall, a wide range of soft tissue contrast that allows the delineation of the vascular and perivascular structures, the ability to evaluate both morphology and function of the vascular system, multiplanar imaging, avoidance of iodinated contrast agent, and absence of ionizing radiation. Because of its robustness, MRI remains the optimal method of evaluating aortic disease in patients who are not acutely ill. MRI can serve as a complementary imaging modality in acute aortic syndromes when CT is contraindicated (such as in patients with renal failure) or when CT does not provide complete evaluation of the disease process.

TECHNIQUES

MSCT

MSCT techniques have evolved rapidly, as scanners with additional detector rows have become available. Nonetheless, certain variables must be optimized to yield the highest image quality: collimation, pitch, field-of-view, reconstruction increment, amount, rate and timing of contrast administration, distance to be scanned, mA, and tube rotation time. Occasionally, a compromise among these parameters is necessary to optimize the scan.

MSCT of the thoracic aorta usually begins with a noncontrast series. Slice thickness of 5 mm is sufficient for the unenhanced scan, which is followed by the contrast-enhanced scan.

Optimal postcontrast imaging requires a slice thickness of 0.6 to 2.5 mm, which provides excellent spatial resolution and allows for high quality reconstructed images. A pitch of 1.375 to 2 allows a large volume of coverage to be obtained rapidly. The field of view should include at least the outer rib to outer rib at the widest portion of the thorax.

There is no consensus regarding the iodine concentration that should be used for MSCT. Undiluted (300 or 360 mg I/mL) contrast agent is usually appropriate. Approximately 80 to 140 mL of contrast agent is injected at a rate of 3 to 5 mL/s. These rates can be achieved using a 20-gauge intravenous catheter. A standard scan delay of 25 seconds after start of injection will usually suffice for MSCT. However, patients with diminished cardiac function or an unsuspected stenosis of the injected vein may require longer delays to achieve optimal opacification of the vessel. Therefore, either a test bolus to determine contrast transit time, or bolus triggering software allow for synchronization of CT acquisition with optimal contrast opacification in nearly all patients.

The contrast-enhanced MSCT should extend from the thoracic inlet to below the aortic bifurcation in the pelvis, to assess the possibility of pathology extending into the arch vessels and iliac arteries.

The mA used is critical for obtaining high quality studies. Values of 120 to 150 mA per tube rotation will usually suffice for most patients, but heavier individuals may need an upward adjustment in the mA. Automated exposure algorithms that permit axial and longitudinal (XYZ) dose modulation exist for most scanners with nonelectrocardiographic (ECG) synchronized helical acquisitions. The use of prospective ECG gating will reduce motion artifact and should be used when available. MSCT of the aorta is best achieved with the shortest available tube rotation time, as low as 330 to 350 ms with currently available machines.

MRI

Several MRI techniques are useful for imaging the thoracic aorta. The most important sequences are ECG-gated black blood double inversion recovery and white blood steady-state free precession (SSFP) cine sequences as well as contrast-enhanced three-dimensional (3D) MR angiography (MRA). With respect to the long axis of the aorta, images can be acquired parallel (sagittal oblique or sagittal) or perpendicular (transverse). Use of orthogonal planes helps to distinguish among intraluminal, mural, and extramural pathologies and reduces partial volume averaging. ECG gating is used for black blood and SSFP cine acquisitions but not for MRA.

A typical protocol for imaging of the thoracic aorta consists of black blood, SSFP cine, and MRA sequences. Transverse images are acquired from a level several centimeters above the aortic arch to the level of the diaphragm, using a slice thickness of approximately 5 mm. Transverse breath hold SSFP cine MRI is performed in the same anatomic region. A slice thickness of 4 to 6 mm is used for the cine sequence. A black blood inversion recovery sequence is acquired in the oblique sagittal or sagittal plane (slice thickness 3 to 5 mm) to display the entire length of the aortic arch, along with the ascending aorta and proximal descending aorta, on the same image. This sequence may be useful to visualize the origins of the arch vessels, which is important when aortic dissection is suspected. The oblique sagittal imaging sequence is prescribed from the transverse image at the level of the aortic arch. Contrast-enhanced 3D MRA is performed in the sagittal or oblique sagittal plane to reduce the number of phase encodes required, resulting in shorter acquisition times and/or better spatial resolution.

For black blood imaging, double inversion recovery technique is used to suppress the signal of the intraluminal blood. The aortic lumen is therefore homogeneously black. Although this technique can be valuable, the luminal signal is not completely black when flow is inordinately slow.

SSFP sequences render the blood pool homogeneously bright. These sequences are especially useful for aortic evaluation because they demonstrate intraluminal pathology as a "filling defect" in the bright blood pool. The bright signal of the blood on SSFP images is secondary to "flow-related" enhancement. With SSFP imaging radiofrequency (RF) pulses are applied to saturate a volume of tissue. Because the TR is short, there is little time for signal recovery from stationary tissue. Therefore the maximum signal is emitted by blood flowing into the volume of tissue, because this blood contains the only protons that have not been saturated by the RF pulses. Slow blood flow, which results in decreased flow enhancement, is the primary factor that causes signal depression on these images. Signal loss also can occur as a consequence of disturbed flow caused by intravoxel phase dispersion, such as occurs with turbulence from a flow jet.

In the thorax, SSFP sequences are frequently performed as breath hold cine acquisitions. SSFP cine images are acquired at multiple contiguous slice locations. An ECG signal is acquired along with the imaging data so that images can be reconstructed at multiple phases (frames) of the cardiac cycle. Generally at least 16 to 32 frames are acquired at each anatomic level.

Three-dimensional MRA with intravenous gadolinium chelate contrast agent relies on the T1-shortening effect of gadolinium to produce high-signal intensity in blood vessels, thereby avoiding flow-related artifacts. The protocol for 3D MRA varies from institution to institution. One of the most effective prescribes MRA in the sagittal or oblique sagittal planes. ECG gating is not required to perform this sequence. Thirty to sixty images are typically obtained using a slice thickness of 1 to 2 mm.

The MRA sequence is performed during a breath hold of approximately 15 to 25 seconds. The patient can be provided with oxygen by nasal cannula, at a rate of 2 L/min, to aid in breath holding. The contrast agent is administered via an antecubital vein with use of a power injector (2 mL/s, 0.1 mmol/kg total). Timing of the acquisition can be optimized by using real-time imaging for bolus detection or by performing a preliminary acquisition employing a test bolus to estimate circulation time.

Image postprocessing of the CT and MRI data sets can include:

- maximum intensity projection; uses include calcifications and small vessels (such as collaterals)
- multiplanar reformations and curved planar reformation; uses include measurement of perpendicular aortic dimensions and centerline lengths for graft planning
- volume rendering; uses include 3D display of aortic course, and extent of disease involvement

NORMAL RANGE OF THORACIC AORTIC DIMENSIONS

The sizes of the thoracic aorta (mean and standard deviation) as measured on axial MRI or CT images are:

- Sinus of Valsalva 3.3 ± 0.4 cm
- Mid-ascending aorta 3.0 ± 0.4 cm
- Proximal descending aorta 2.4 ± 0.4 cm

These normal measurements were determined in a population of young adults.

THORACIC AORTIC ANEURYSM

Aortic diameter exceeding 4 cm is called dilatation, and a diameter over 5 cm is termed an aneurysm. The maximum diameter of the aorta is an important determinant of the risk of rupture. When the aortic diameter is more than 6 cm, the risk of rupture in the next 5 years is greater than 30%.

Thoracic aortic aneurysms vary in shape and size. Saccular aneurysms are localized and do not involve the entire circumference of the aorta (Fig. 29-1). Fusiform aneurysms involve the entire aortic circumference and may extend over a great length of the vessel (Fig. 29-2). Annuloaortic ectasia results from cystic medial necrosis, which is associated with Marfan syndrome; although it can be idiopathic. In annuloaortic ectasia the aortic root, and often the entire ascending aorta, is enlarged (Figs. 29-3 and 29-4). Many aneurysms involving the thoracic aorta also involve the abdominal aorta.

In a true aneurysm, all three layers of the aortic wall are intact, whereas a false aneurysm results from a focal disruption of the aortic wall contained by the adventitia and surrounding fibrous tissue. Common causes of false aneurysm are trauma (Fig. 29-5), infection, and surgery (Fig. 29-6). True aneurysms most frequently are secondary to atherosclerosis. Other etiologies of true aneurysms include connective tissue disorders such as Marfan syndrome, arteritis (Takayasu or giant cell arteritis), idiopathic cystic medial necrosis, relapsing polychondritis, complications of aortic valve disease, and aneurysm of the ductal remnant.

Mycotic aneurysms result from infection of the aortic wall and occlusion of the vasa vasorum by septic emboli; this causes weakening of the wall resulting in aneurysm formation. Etiologies of mycotic aneurysm include septic emboli from intravenous drug use and indwelling catheters, infection of prosthetic valves, or infection of atherosclerotic plaque. Common infectious agents include *Salmonella*, *Staphylococcus aureus*, streptococci, tuberculosis, and fungi, such as Candida and *Aspergillus*. Mycotic aneurysms are usually saccular, and they may grow quickly. Mycotic aneurysms can be associated with periaortic fat infiltration and inflammation or gas formation. Mycotic aneurysms are at high risk for rupture.

Imaging Evaluation of Aneurysm

In the imaging evaluation of thoracic aortic aneurysm, the primary goals are measurement of the maximum diameter of the aorta, demonstration of the extent of the aneurysm, identification of branch vessel involvement, compression of adjacent structures, and detection of periaortic hematoma. The demonstration of mural thrombus is important in patients who present with peripheral embolization.

MSCT findings of aortic aneurysm rupture include high-density fluid in the wall of the aorta, pleural space, or pericardium

A   **B**

FIG. 29.1. Saccular aneurysm of the aortic arch. A: Contrast-enhanced CT of the thoracic aorta demonstrates a large eccentric saccular aneurysm arising in a patient with atherosclerosis. **B:** The aneurysm (∗) is more proximal than the location of the aortic isthmus (*black arrow*), and there was no history to suggest major trauma.

A

B

FIG. 29.2. Fusiform aneurysm. **A:** There is dilation of the sinuses of Valsalva and ascending aorta with **(B)** complete effacement of the sinotubular junction of the aorta (between *arrows*), consistent with annuloaortic ectasia.

(Fig. 29-7). Mediastinal hematoma also suggests the possibility of aneurysm rupture. The "draped aorta" sign may indicate an early, contained rupture. This sign manifests as indistinctness of the posterior wall or close alignment of the posterior wall with the contour of the adjacent vertebral bodies.

MRI also readily depicts the size and extent of an aneurysm of the ascending or descending thoracic aorta. The outer dimension of the aneurysm and the size of the patent lumen can be seen. Because it can demonstrate the outer wall of the aorta, unlike angiography, MRI allows accurate measurement of the aneurysm diameter even when there is wall thickening or mural thrombus. Mural thrombus and atherosclerotic plaque are depicted as eccentric or concentric thickening of the aortic wall. The patent lumen can usually be determined

FIG. 29.3. Focal dissection in a patient with annuloaortic ectasia. Oblique sagittal maximum intensity projection of a gadolinium-enhanced MR angiogram demonstrates an intimal flap (*arrow*) in the aortic arch. Note the aneurysm of the aortic root and ascending aorta (A), consistent with annuloaortic ectasia.

FIG. 29.4. Annuloaortic ectasia in a patient with Marfan syndrome. Note the marked, diffuse enlargement of the aortic root and ascending aorta (A).

FIG. 29.5. Chronic pseudoaneurysm secondary to deceleration injury. Oblique sagittal maximum intensity projection of an MR angiogram demonstrates a pseudoaneurysm (*arrow*) in the ductal region, a classic location for a traumatic pseudoaneurysm. The patient had been involved in a high-speed motor vehicle accident several years before.

by the flow void on black blood MRI. However, slow flow can produce intraluminal signal on black blood images. Slow flow can be differentiated from thrombus with SSFP cine MRI or contrast-enhanced MRA. MRA is especially effective for demonstrating the extent of thoracic aortic aneurysm, the relationship to the aortic branches, and the precise dimensions—especially in the aortic arch.

Identification of periaortic or mediastinal hematoma is vital in the evaluation of aneurysm rupture. On black blood images hematoma appears as an area of high-signal intensity, although this appearance may not be seen early. It may produce intermediate signal intensity during the first few hours after bleeding. MRI can delineate the extent of the hemorrhage, which may spread through the mediastinum or be localized to the periaortic region, pleural space, subpleural space, or pericardium.

MRI is an effective noninvasive means of monitoring the progression of thoracic aortic aneurysms. If the aortic diameter is greater than 6.0 cm or if there is a rapid increase in diameter, surgical repair is generally necessary. Because it is noninvasive and accurate, MRI is also the optimal method for sequential follow-up of the aorta in patients with a high risk for developing dissection, such as those with Marfan or Ehlers-Danlos syndromes (see Fig. 29-3).

False aneurysms can be revealed by MSCT, contrast-enhanced MRA, or a combination of transverse and sagittal or sagittal oblique MR images. MRI is useful for depiction of

A

B

FIG. 29.6. False aneurysms following an ascending aortic interposition graft. **A:** 3D-volume rendered projection shows a large false aneurysm at the lower anastomosis (*arrows*) of the graft (g). **B:** A smaller false aneurysm is present at the superior anastomosis. Hematoma (∗) is present adjacent to the false aneurysms, indicating blood loss.

FIG. 29.7. Acute rupture of a thoracic aortic aneurysm. **A:** Noncontrast CT demonstrates a large right pleural effusion containing hyperdense blood clot (*) and a calcified aortic valve (*white arrow*). The aneurysm (a) is better seen with the contrast enhanced CT **(B)**, in addition to a small area of active vascular extravasation (*black arrow*). **C:** 3D volume rendered reconstruction shows that the aneurysm contains both fusiform and saccular (*arrows*) components.

the longitudinal extent of the false aneurysm. Post-traumatic false aneurysms seen on MSCT and MRI are most frequently located at the site of ligamentum arteriosum and involve either the entire aortic circumference or only the anterior wall (see Fig. 29-5).

ACUTE AORTIC SYNDROMES

Aortic Dissection and Intramural Hematoma

Aortic dissection is a separation of the aortic wall that results from a tear in the intima. Blood can enter the aortic wall through an intimal disruption and extend proximally and distally in the media, displacing the intima inward. The dissection may reenter the lumen at one or more sites of fenestration. Typically blood flows in both the true and false channels, although the false channel is sometimes thrombosed. The dissection may disrupt the adventitia and cause pericardial tamponade, exsanguination, pleural hemorrhage, or periaortic hematoma. If the dissection involves or occludes branches of the aorta, cerebral ischemia, myocardial infarction, renal insufficiency, or mesenteric infarction can ensue.

Aortic dissection can result from an intramural hematoma, which is caused by rupture of the vasa vasorum, the arteries that supply the aortic wall. The ruptured vasa vasorum bleed into the aortic wall, which can result in an intimal tear and separation of the wall. If the intima does not rupture, causing a frank dissection, then an intramural hematoma remains. The intramural hematoma may be localized, or it can extend along the wall in antegrade or retrograde direction or sometimes rupture through the adventitia. An intramural hematoma can be considered to be a form of dissection, and management is similar to that of a frank dissection.

The most common predisposing factor for aortic dissection is hypertension. Other etiologies include connective tissue disorders such as Marfan syndrome or Ehlers-Danlos syndrome, bicuspid aortic valve, aortic aneurysm, and arteritis.

The longitudinal extent of the dissection or intramural hematoma is an important factor in determining management. A dissection can begin at any location in the aorta; the most common sites of origin are just above the sinuses of Valsalva or just beyond the origin of the left subclavian artery. Dissections typically progress in the direction of blood flow (antegrade dissection), although on occasion they can proceed opposite to the blood flow (retrograde dissection). Depending on the site and extent of aortic involvement, aortic dissection can be classified as Stanford type A (involving the ascending aorta) or type B (involving the descending aorta only, beyond the left subclavian artery origin). Another classification, the DeBakey system divides dissections into three types: Type I involves the ascending aorta and extends into the descending aorta; type II involves the ascending aorta only; and type III involves the descending aorta only, distal to the origin of the left subclavian artery.

There are four life-threatening complications of type A (I and II) dissection: pericardial hemorrhage and tamponade; aortic valve rupture and acute aortic insufficiency; coronary artery dissection and myocardial infarction; and carotid artery dissection and stroke. Therefore, patients with type A dissection usually undergo immediate surgery. Type B usually can be managed medically. Intramural hematoma can also be classified as type A and B. The natural history of type A and B intramural hematoma is similar to that of other type A and B dissections. However, the prognosis of type A intramural hematoma with medical therapy is better than that of type A dissection. With either surgical or medical management the dissection is not completely eradicated. Close monitoring is therefore necessary to assess progression or complications.

Approach to the Evaluation of Aortic Dissection

Because it is life-threatening, aortic dissection must be diagnosed rapidly and definitively. The primary goals of imaging examinations are: to establish the diagnosis by demonstrating the intramural hematoma or the intimal flap and false channel; and to identify the extent of dissection. Involvement of the arch vessels and coronary arteries must be assessed. It is also vital to identify pericardial hematoma, which can result in tamponade and is an indication for immediate surgery. Other findings that should be identified are peri-aortic or mediastinal hematoma, as well as pleural hemorrhage.

Because of the noninvasive nature of MSCT and MRI, they are ideal techniques for the initial evaluation of aortic dissection and for surveillance of patients treated for dissection.

Imaging of Aortic Dissection

The MSCT diagnosis of aortic dissection is based on evaluation of both unenhanced and enhanced images. Unenhanced scans are useful for demonstrating high attenuation intramural hematoma or thrombosis of the false lumen (Fig. 29-8). Unenhanced images may also show inward displacement of intimal calcification. The most reliable finding for the diagnosis of dissection on MSCT is the presence of an intimal flap separating the true and false channels (Figs. 29-9 and 29-10). Contrast enhanced scans can also reveal the patency of branch vessels and can demonstrate differential flow rates between the true and false channels.

Intramural hematoma appears as crescentic or circumferential area of high-density thickening of the aortic wall on noncontrast MSCT. Although the hyperattenuation may be appreciated on postcontrast images, this finding is usually more easily seen on noncontrast images (see Fig. 29-8).

On MRI examinations, the definitive diagnosis of dissection requires the identification of the intimal flap or an intramural hematoma. The intimal flap frequently appears as a linear structure within the aorta (Fig. 29-3). When there is rapid flow in the true and false channels, the intimal flap is discerned between the flow void in both channels on black blood images. The dissection usually extends over a long region of the aorta; however, focal dissection can occur (see Fig. 29-3). Blood flow is often slower in the false channel, resulting in partial or complete filling of this lumen with signal of variable intensity, thereby allowing differentiation between the true and the false channels. SSFP cine MRI or MRA may be used to distinguish between slow flow and thrombus in the false lumen.

MRI can be used to determine whether aortic branches (such as the arch arteries, celiac, superior mesenteric, and renal arteries) arise from the true or false channel (Fig. 29-11). MRI can also identify extension of the intimal flap into the aortic arch branches. Intramural hematoma is diagnosed on black blood images by the presence of intermediate- or high-signal intensity material within the wall of the aorta (Fig. 29-12). The wall is thickened eccentrically or circumferentially.

MSCT and MRI can assess the most critical complication of dissection: blood leaking from the aorta into the pericardium, mediastinum, or pleura (Fig. 29-13). The signal intensity of blood within the first few hours after hemorrhage usually has high-signal intensity on black blood images.

Occasionally, it can be difficult to differentiate between the true and false channels. The true lumen is usually located

(text continues on page 709)

FIG. 29.8. Acute intramural hematoma. **A:** Gated MRI double inversion black blood sequence demonstrates a hyperintense crescent of intramural met-hemoglobin (*white arrow*), which is faintly visible as a hyperdense crescent on noncontrast CT **(B)**, and as diffuse mural thickening (*black arrowheads*) on an oblique sagittal maximal intensity projection (MIP) of a postcontrast CT **(C)**.

FIG. 29.9. Two patients with a type A dissection. **A:** Electrocardiogram gated CTA of the aorta clearly shows the relationship of the intimo-medial flap (*black arrow*) and the origin of the right coronary artery (*white arrow*). **B:** Nongated CTA of the aorta shows the intimo-medial flap (*black arrow*) but in addition a simulated second flap is present (*white arrowheads*) from pulsation artifact and the status and location of the right coronary artery origin (white arrow) are difficult to evaluate.

A   B

FIG. 29.10. Acute type B aortic dissection with signs to differentiate the true and false lumens. **A:** Contrast axial CT reconstruction demonstrates a small cobweb (*arrowhead*) and an acutely angled "beak sign" (*arrow*) in the crescent shaped false lumen (f). Both of these signs are specific for the false lumen (f). The smaller and more ovoid true lumen (t) is contracted anteriorly. **B:** Oblique sagittal MIP demonstrates extension of the intimo-medial flap (*white arrows*) into the superior mesenteric artery (*black arrow*).

FIG. 29.11. Type B dissection sparing the arch vessels. Sagittal source image of a contrast-enhanced MR angiogram demonstrates an intimal flap (*black arrowhead*) beginning just distal to the origin of the left subclavian artery (*white arrow*). The dissection does not extend into the left subclavian artery.

FIG. 29.12. Type A intramural hematoma. ECG-gated sagittal black blood double inversion recovery MR images shows intermediate-to-high signal thickening (*arrows*) of the wall of the ascending aorta (A), consistent with an intramural hematoma.

FIG. 29.13. Hemopericardium as a complication of type A aortic dissection. Contrast-enhanced CT reveals a high-density pericardial effusion (h) indicating hemopericardium. The intimo-medial flap (*white arrows*) extends to the sinuses of Valsalva and down the descending aorta.

along the left posterolateral aspect of the descending thoracic aorta and abdominal aorta. Frequently the true lumen is compressed by the false lumen. When the dissection flap appears as a circular or oval structure within the center of the

aorta, the center of the circular, or oval structure represents the true lumen.

For assessment of dissection, the diagnostic accuracy of MRI and helical CT are high. Sensitivity and specificity are over 95%. The diagnostic accuracy of MRI and CT has been compared to that of TEE. Whereas the sensitivities of the three techniques are almost 100%, some studies have shown that the specificity of MRI and CT may be significantly better. Gadolinium-enhanced MRA has similar accuracy to black blood and SSFP MRI. However, MRA is less sensitive for intramural hematoma and periaortic pathology. Because the diagnostic accuracies of MRI and CT are similar, they can be used interchangeably for evaluation of aortic dissection. At some institutions, MSCT may be preferred in the acute setting and MRI when the situation is not acute.

Follow-up of Patients with Aortic Dissection

Type A dissections are treated by surgery, whereas type B dissections are usually managed medically. In both groups of patients, MSCT and MRI can be used to monitor the progression of disease and to identify complications such as aneurysm formation of the false lumen (Fig. 29-14), compression and occlusion of branch vessels, and recurrent progressive dissection. MRI has shown aneurysmal dilatation of the false channel in type A and B dissections and persistent patency of the false lumen in the majority of patients after repair of the ascending aorta. Thrombosis of the false

A   **B**

FIG. 29.14. Aneurysm of the false lumen. **A:** Sagittal maximum intensity projection (MIP) of a contrast-enhanced MR angiogram approximately 1 month after repair of a type A dissection with a graft in the ascending aorta. Note the artifact at the anastomotic site (*arrowhead*), giving the misleading appearance of slight narrowing. The false lumen (f) is largely thrombosed and therefore poorly opacified. t, true lumen. **B:** Sagittal MIP of a contrast-enhanced MR angiogram 9 months later shows an aneurysm (*arrow*) of the false lumen (f), as well as outpouching (∗) of the true lumen (t) in the aortic arch.

channel and remodeling of the thoracic aorta can occur in some patients.

ATHEROSCLEROSIS AND PENETRATING AORTIC ULCER

Aortic thrombus is frequently present in the wall of aneurysms and sometimes in regions of atherosclerosis. Aortic thrombus may lead to peripheral embolization. In a patient with peripheral embolization, the left atrium, left ventricle, and the aorta are evaluated for the source of the embolus. The most common sources are the left atrium in patients with atrial fibrillation or the left ventricle in patients with dilated cardiomyopathy or recent myocardial infarction. Embolization from aortic thrombus occurs less frequently.

SSFP cine MR images are useful because they depict the motion of the clot within the aortic lumen and can distinguish the thrombus from signal due to slow blood flow. MRA is also effective for differentiating thrombus from slow flow (Fig. 29-15). Black blood double inversion recovery images are also useful, but may be difficult to interpret if slow flow produces intraluminal signal. By evaluating the heart and aorta in a single examination, MRI can be used to provide comprehensive investigation of the possible sources of peripheral embolization.

MSCT readily depicts the location and morphology of aortic thrombus and atherosclerotic plaque. Thrombus and plaque typically appear as low-density material adjacent to the aortic wall, on the luminal side of intimal calcifications. Although TEE is more frequently used for the specific investigation of aortic thrombus, disease in the cranial aspect of the ascending aorta and arch may be more effectively identified with MSCT.

Penetrating Aortic Ulcer

Penetrating aortic ulcer occurs when atherosclerotic plaque ulcerates, disrupts the intima, and extends into the media. This can result in mural hemorrhage (intramural hematoma) and extension along the media, or rarely frank dissection or rupture through the adventitia. The most common location is the mid descending thoracic aorta. The clinical presentation of aortic ulcer is similar to that of dissection, usually with sudden onset of chest or back pain. Penetrating ulcer involving the ascending aorta is treated surgically, whereas those in the descending aorta can usually be managed medically.

Penetrating aortic ulcer appears on unenhanced MSCT as an intramural hematoma. Contrast-enhanced MSCT shows a focus of contrast agent projecting beyond the confines of the lumen (Fig. 29-16). Aortic mural enhancement and, rarely, active contrast extravasation may be seen. Complications, such as dissection, pseudoaneurysm, or aortic rupture may be present (see Fig. 29-7B).

MRA may be especially effective for demonstration of a penetrating ulcer. Black blood or SSFP sequences are valuable for showing an intramural hematoma associated with an ulcer, as well as pseudoaneurysm caused by extension through the adventitia.

ACUTE TRAUMATIC AORTIC INJURY

Acute traumatic aortic injury (ATAI) is usually the result of severe deceleration, such as a high speed motor vehicle collision or a fall from a great height. ATAI results in exsanguination and immediate death in 80% to 90% of patients. Among patients with ATAI who survive the initial trauma, the mortality of untreated ATAI may be as high as

A   B

FIG. 29.15. Aortic thrombus. **A:** ECG-gated axial black blood MR image and **(B)** sagittal source image from a gadolinium-enhanced MR angiogram demonstrate multiple areas of aortic thrombus (*arrows*), felt to be the source of peripheral emboli.

FIG. 29.16. Penetrating aortic ulcer. Contrast enhanced CT of the chest at baseline **(A)**, 10 days **(B)** after baseline, and 19 days **(C)** after baseline show an eccentric ulcer (*arrow*) arising from the lumen of the descending thoracic aorta (a) that deforms the contour of the aorta. Subsequent examinations demonstrate increasing size of the ulcer, with progressive dilation of the aorta in the region of the ulcer.

1% per hour for the first 48 hours. Chronic pseudoaneurysm may occur in untreated long-term survivors.

The most common sites of injury are the aortic isthmus (90%), the great vessel origins (5% to 10%), the aorto-cardiac junction (1%), and the descending aorta near the diaphragmatic hiatus (1% to 3%). A nearly circumferential laceration is frequently present. Minimal aortic injuries or isolated intimal injuries have been more recently recognized with MSCT. Arch vessel injuries may coexist.

MSCT Evaluation

MSCT has largely replaced diagnostic catheter angiography in the assessment of ATAI.

For the diagnosis of ATAI, the sensitivity of helical CT approaches 100%, and the specificity is more than 80% to 96%. MSCT findings of ATAI can be classified as direct or indirect. The most common direct finding of ATAI is a pseudoaneurysm (Fig. 29-17). Other direct signs include an abnormal aortic contour or abrupt change in caliber, kinking of the aorta (pseudocoarctation), occlusion of a segment of aorta, and an intimal flap. Extravasation of contrast agent is rarely depicted on imaging examinations. Patients with direct findings of ATAI are usually treated by endovascular repair or surgery.

Indirect signs of ATAI include mediastinal and retrocrural hematoma. Although mediastinal or retrocrural hematoma raises the possibility of ATAI, it is not specific because it may result from bleeding of small mediastinal veins or arteries or adjacent fractures. When a mediastinal hematoma is noted, its relationship to the aorta should be determined. If the hematoma is in direct contact with the aorta, the aorta and branch vessels should be carefully evaluated with thin section reconstructions and MPRs for direct signs of injury. Recent evidence with MSCT suggests that when there is no direct evidence of aortic injury, catheter angiography may be unnecessary. Occasionally, aortic injuries can occur without periaortic hematoma.

The high quality of modern MSCT scans allows the identification of subtle aortic injuries such as small intimal

FIG. 29.17. Acute traumatic aortic injury. Contrast enhanced CT with and axial reconstruction **(A)** demonstrates a large pseudoaneurysm (∗) arising from the lumen of the descending thoracic aorta (L). This appearance has been termed the "Beret" sign. There is periaortic hematoma (h) surrounding the aorta. Multiplanar reformation **(B)** and volume rendered image **(C)** shows the pseudoaneurysm (between *arrowhead* and *arrows*) in the typical location of the aortic isthmus, by far the most common site of blunt aortic injury.

injuries (Fig. 29-18) and intramural hematoma; these were less likely to have been recognized by single-slice CT scanning and catheter angiography.

PERIAORTIC ABSCESS

In patients with bacterial endocarditis, MRI can be used to identify complications such as a periaortic abscess. The abscess cavities may be similar to a false aneurysm, with a cavity communicating with the aorta. MRI may show a flow void in the cavity, which implies communication with the aortic lumen (Fig. 29-19). MRI can be used to monitor progression of these abscess cavities.

AORTITIS

Aortitis is defined as inflammation of the aortic wall that can be in an active or healing phase. The aortic inflammation results from tissue proliferation and wall thickening that can cause progressive luminal stenosis, and structural weakening of the aortic wall that can lead to aneurysm formation, dissection, and rupture.

Noninfectious aortitis comprises several disorders that include giant cell arteritis, Takayasu arteritis, aortic inflammation associated with other miscellaneous systemic diseases, and an isolated type with aortic inflammation not associated with a known co-existing systemic autoimmune disorder.

FIG. 29.18. Minimal aortic injury following major trauma. **A:** Axial contrast enhanced CT showing a small intraluminal filling defect in the aorta at the level of the aortic hiatus of the diaphragm (*black arrow*). **B:** There are small infarcts in the right kidney (*black arrowheads*) indicating emboli. Follow up CT 48 hours later showed resolution of the aortic intimal injury.

The clinical features of aortitis can be divided into an early and late phase. Signs and symptoms of the early phase include nonspecific complaints of malaise, low-grade fevers, weight loss, arthralgias, myalgias, fatigability, sweating, and weakness. The presence of active aortic inflammation can be indicated by laboratory abnormalities such as an elevated erythrocyte sedimentation rate, leukocytosis, and elevated C-reactive protein. Unfortunately, in many cases of pathologically documented aortitis, a history of acute phase symptoms was not elicited, and up to 40% of asymptomatic patients with normal laboratory tests have progressive aortic disease.

The late phase occurs weeks to months after the acute phase. In contrast to the early phase, the symptoms of this phase are related to arterial stenosis and occlusion. Because of the lack of specific symptoms in the early phase, the diagnosis of noninfectious aortitis in the majority of patients is most commonly made in the late stage.

Medical treatment is primarily based on corticosteroids, which are administered to suppress active inflammation, stabilize the arterial abnormalities, and prevent further vascular damage. The magnitude of therapy depends on the degree of disease activity and the complications that may develop.

FIG. 29.19. Periaortic abscess and pseudoaneurysm. **A:** ECG-gated axial black blood MR image shows a pseudoaneurysm (*arrowhead*) of the ascending aorta (A) secondary to a periaortic abscess. **B:** Gadolinium-enhanced ECG-gated axial black blood MR image demonstrates periaortic enhancement (*arrow*) at the site of the abscess.

Symptomatic vascular lesions and critical stenoses are treated with angioplasty/stenting or surgical revision, with procedures timed during periods of disease remission to reduce the incidence of complications due to the weakened inflamed tissue.

Giant Cell Aortitis

Giant cell arteritis is a systemic panarteritis that is currently the most common autoimmune condition associated with aortitis. While originally believed to be a disease solely of the temporal and cranial arteries, aortic inflammation is found in 10% to 15% of these patients. The disease mainly involves the thoracic aorta and is emerging as an important cause of ascending thoracic aortic aneurysm in the elderly. Since patients with giant cell arteritis are 17 times more likely to develop a thoracic aortic aneurysm than the general population, the detection of aortic involvement is important due to the risk of rupture. Giant cell arteritis can be difficult to recognize because of the indolent course of the disease and the low specificity of the clinical manifestations.

Noninvasive imaging is used to confirm and characterize the severity of large vessel involvement, monitor the course of disease, and disclose the presence of subclinical active inflammation. The detection of active vascular inflammation (vessel wall thickening, mural enhancement and edema) is helpful to indicate the presence of early stages of the disease before luminal changes are present, and to indicate when therapy may need to modified.

Takayasu Arteritis

Takayasu arteritis is a large vessel vasculitis that affects the aorta, the main arterial branches, and the coronary and pulmonary circulation. Pathologically the disease is characterized by multi-focal vascular stenoses and/or aneurysms with intervening unaffected segments. There can be diffuse involvement of the aorta with or without isolated disease of individual branch arteries. The branch vessels most frequently affected are the subclavian (90%), carotid (45%), vertebral (25%), and renal (20%) arteries. As with giant cell arteritis, Takayasu disease can be difficult to diagnose due to nonspecific signs, symptoms, and laboratory abnormalities.

One classification scheme has been described that divides Takayasu disease into six types, based on the anatomic distribution of disease (Fig. 29-20). Imaging findings consist of arterial narrowing, wall thickening, dilation or aneurysm formation, luminal irregularity, or any combination of these features in the aorta or its main branches (Fig. 29-21). Active aortic inflammation can be indicated by enhancement of a thickened aortic wall on contrast enhanced CT and MRI (Fig. 29-22). The ability to identify active disease allows earlier diagnosis before luminal changes occur, assessment of disease activity to modify treatment, and confirmation of response to therapy.

THORACIC AORTIC NEOPLASM

Secondary involvement of the aorta by a mediastinal tumor or bronchogenic carcinoma can occur. Staging CT and MRI can show involvement of the aorta, which renders the tumor inoperable. Primary aortic neoplasms are rare and include angiosarcoma or spindle cell sarcoma.

Aortic neoplasm can manifest as an irregular mass projecting into the vessel lumen. MSCT and MRI can define the intraluminal and perivascular extent of the neoplasm. Findings that suggest secondary tumor involvement are irregular thickening of the aortic wall, intraluminal mass, and tumor extending around more than 180 degrees of the aortic circumference.

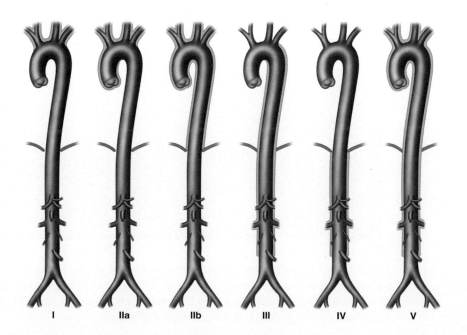

FIG. 29.20. Classification of Takayasu arteritis.

Type I: the branches of the aortic arch only

Type IIa: ascending aorta and/or arch, and possibly arch vessels

Type IIb: descending thoracic aorta and possibly the ascending aorta, arch, or arch vessels

Type III: descending thoracic aorta, abdominal aorta, and/or renal arteries; no involvement of ascending aorta, arch, or arch vessels

Type IV: abdominal aorta and/or renal arteries only

Type V: generalized

FIG. 29.21. Takayasu arteritis, late stage. **A:** Axial thin slab maximum-intensity-projection (MIP) of a contrast enhanced MR angiogram. High grade stenosis of the right pulmonary artery (*arrow*). **B:** Volume MIP showing pseudoaneurysm in the right subclavian artery (*white arrow*), and long areas of narrowing in the bilateral common carotid arteries (*white arrowheads*) and right subclavian artery (*gray arrowhead*).

THORACIC ENDOVASCULAR AORTIC REPAIR

Thoracic endovascular aortic repair (TEVAR) of thoracic aortic aneurysm, aortic dissection, penetrating aortic ulcer, and traumatic aortic injury (Fig. 29-23) is associated with low early morbidity and mortality rates and reduces aneurysm-related deaths.

Commercially available thoracic stent grafts have a stainless steel or nitinol skeleton with a polyester fabric covering. The proximal or distal ends of most stents have an uncovered skeletal section, for better fixation without occlusion of side branches.

Preprocedure Planning

Preprocedural imaging is necessary in order to determine location and configuration of the aortic pathology, determine whether the patient is a stent graft candidate, choose the appropriate type and size of stent and best location for placement, and plan the interventional approach.

FIG. 29.22. Takayasu arteritis, active phase (early stage). **A:** Noncontrast and **B:** Contrast-enhanced ECG-gated axial black blood MR images show thickening (**A**, *arrow*) and enhancement (**B**, *arrow*) of the wall of the brachiocephalic artery.

A   B

FIG. 29.23. Type I endoleak with aortic rupture weeks following endovascular repair of acute traumatic aortic injury. Axial reconstruction **(A)** and oblique sagittal MIP **(B)** of a contrast enhanced CT of the chest demonstrate a type Ia endoleak (*white arrow*) with contrast agent leaking between the stent (*black arrow*) and the aorta, arising from the proximal attachment site. Hyperdense peri-aortic material (∗) is consistent with blood. Apparent collapse of the stent-graft (*black arrowhead*) is due to partial volume artifact.

Ideally, a landing zone of normal aorta about 15 mm above and below the abnormal section of aorta is desired for optimal stent-graft fixation and seal, usually measured along the greater curvature of the aorta. However, the left subclavian artery origin can be covered in many patients if there is a short proximal landing zone. This may be accompanied with a subclavian artery bypass procedure if compromise to the vertebrobasilar or left upper extremity arterial supply is envisaged. MSCT may also be useful in identifying the location of the artery of Adamkiewicz, and the contour of the distal landing zone.

Usually a stent device is selected which has a diameter 10% to 15% greater than the diameters at the proximal or distal landing zones.

A   B

FIG. 29.24. Small type II endoleak best seen on the delayed phase. Arterial phase CTA of the aorta **(A)** demonstrates a very subtle area of enhancement (*white arrow*) within the native lumen but outside the aortic stent graft. On the 120 second delayed phase image **(B)** the endoleak is clearly visible (*white arrow*) outside of the stent graft (*black arrowhead*).

TABLE 29.1	**Classification of Endoleaks**
I	Attachment site leak
	A. Proximal
	B. Distal
II	Collateral vessel leak(s)
	A. Single vessel
	B. Two or more vessels
III	Graft failure, junctional leak, or disconnection fabric disruption.
	A. Junctional separation (modular devices)
	B. Endograft defect
IV	Graft-wall porosity (rare)
V	Endotension

Generally, imaging of the abdominal aorta, iliac arteries, and proximal femoral arteries is also necessary to detect significant kinking or stenosis that could limit access by the large deployment devices.

Surveillance

Life-long surveillance following TEVAR is currently recommended. MSCT is the mainstay of imaging surveillance, although MRI can be performed in patients with nitinol stents, and may be more sensitive for minor endoleaks. Although imaging protocols vary, surveillance is typically performed after 1, 6, 12 months, and then annually. During surveillance, the addition of a delayed phase scan 90 to 120 seconds following contrast administration increases the detection of small endoleaks (Fig. 29-24).

Complications of TEVAR include endoleaks, kinking, migration, and collapse.

Endoleaks

Endoleaks are blood flow within the aortic sac, but outside the stent graft lumen following TEVAR (Table 29.1).

Type I endoleaks (see Fig. 29-23) usually do not resolve spontaneously, and should be considered significant, because of the acute curvature of the aortic arch, particularly in younger patients; there may be inadequate apposition between the stent graft and the inner aortic surface. Type II endoleaks (Fig. 29-25) occur uncommonly, and are usually caused by retrograde flow through bronchial or intercostal arteries. Incomplete coverage of the left subclavian artery is associated with a high risk of endoleak.

Migration

Stent graft fixation depends on outward radial force on the aortic wall, supplemented by barbs in some devices. Inadequate early fixation or subsequent aortic remodeling may lead to loss of this fixation, and migration of the stent, sometimes leading to endoleaks.

A

B

FIG. 29.25. Type II endoleak. Axial MIP of a contrast CT of the chest **(A)** demonstrates a small posterior intercostal vessel (*white arrow*) that feeds into an endoleak (*arrowhead*) between the aortic lumen (a) that is surrounded by a stent and outer wall of the aorta. **(B)** 3D volume rendered reconstruction demonstrates the endoleak (*arrowhead*) passing caudally between the native aortic sac and the stent.

SELECTED READING

Agarwal PP, Chughtai A, Matzinger FR, et al. Multidetector CT of thoracic aortic aneurysms. Radiographics 2009; 29:537.

Chao CP, Walker TG, Kalva SP. Natural history and CT appearances of aortic intramural hematoma. Radiographics 2009; 29:791.

Chughtai A, Kazerooni EA. CT and MRI of acute thoracic cardiovascular emergencies. Crit Care Clin 2007; 23:835.

Gotway MB, Araoz PA, Macedo TA, et al. Imaging findings in Takayasu's arteritis. AJR Am J Roentgenol 2005; 184:1945.

Pua U, Tay KH, Tan BS, et al. CT appearance of complications related to thoracic endovascular aortic repair (TEVAR): a pictorial essay. Eur Radiol 2009; 19:1062.

Shiga T, Wajima Z, Apfel CC, et al. Diagnostic accuracy of transesophageal echocardiography, helical computed tomography, and magnetic resonance imaging for suspected thoracic aortic dissection: systematic review and meta-analysis. Arch Intern Med 2006; 166:1350.

Singhal P, Lin Z. Penetrating atheromatous ulcer of ascending aorta: a case report and review of literature. Heart Lung Circ 2008; 17:380.

Steenburg SD, Ravenel JG, Ikonomidis JS, et al. Acute traumatic aortic injury: imaging evaluation and management. Radiology 2008; 248:748.

Ueda T, Fleischmann D, Rubin GD, et al. Imaging of the thoracic aorta before and after stent-graft repair of aneurysms and dissections. Semin Thorac Cardiovasc Surg 2008; 20:348

Radiography of Acquired Heart Disease

CHARLES B. HIGGINS

T he thoracic radiograph is one of the earliest points of departure in the evaluation of heart disease. It may provide the first indication that cardiac disease is present, but more frequently it is used to determine the severity of known or suspected disease. The severity of some cardiac diseases is readily reflected on the thoracic radiograph, while other significant diseases cause little or no alterations in the pulmonary vessels or cardiac silhouette. Consequently, the thoracic radiograph may have only limited value in the assessment of some diseases, while in others it may serve as one of the most sensitive and reliable gauges of the course of the disease. The propensity of various cardiac diseases to cause substantial cardiomegaly serves as the major dividing line in our system for cataloging acquired heart disease.

APPROACH TO THE CHEST X-RAY IN ACQUIRED HEART DISEASE

A systematic approach is directed toward discerning the pertinent findings from the radiograph and, for each finding, narrowing the array of diagnostic considerations. A free-floating approach places one into the unnecessary jeopardy of failing to examine salient features of the cardiovascular anatomy.

A five-step systematic approach permits the orderly examination of the thoracic radiograph, and at each step it is possible to narrow the diagnostic possibilities (Figs. 30-1 and 30-2). A radiographic classification of acquired heart disease is used in association with this five-step examination (see Fig. 30-2; Table 30-1).

The five steps in the examination of the thoracic radiograph in patients with suspected cardiac disease are (1) thoracic musculoskeletal structures, (2) pulmonary vascularity, (3) overall heart size, (4) specific chamber enlargement, and (5) great arteries (ascending aorta, aortic knob, main pulmonary arterial segment).

Thoracic Musculoskeletal Structures

Examination of the thoracic wall discloses evidence of prior operations, such as rib or sternal deformities or sternal wire sutures. Sternal deformities such as pectus may serve as a

clue to cardiac lesions associated with it, such as Marfan's syndrome and mitral valve prolapse; or perhaps the deformity is responsible for a cardiac murmur or even symptoms caused by cardiac compression. Narrow anteroposterior diameter of the thorax can be caused by a straight thoracic spine (straight-back syndrome) or pectus excavatum. A narrow anteroposterior diameter is defined as a distance between the sternum and the anterior border of the vertebral body that measures less than 8 cm and a ratio of the transverse diameter (determined by frontal view) to the anteroposterior diameter (determined by lateral view) exceeding 2.75. The anteroposterior diameter is the maximum diameter from the undersurface of the sternum to the anterior border of the vertebral body.

Pulmonary Vascularity (Pulmonary Edema)

There are three steps in assessing pulmonary vascularity: the type of abnormality (pulmonary arterial overcirculation vs. pulmonary venous hypertension [PVH]); the severity of the pulmonary vascular abnormality; and determination of the symmetry, asymmetry, or even focal nature of the abnormality. In patients with acquired heart disease, the type

FIG. 30.1. Five-step approach to analysis of the thoracic radiograph in cardiac disease.

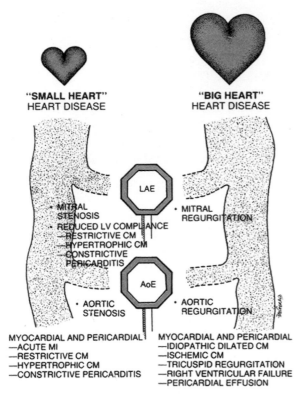

FIG. 30.2. Diagnostic pathway for the identification of the hemodynamically predominant cardiac lesion. Signposts gleaned from the thoracic radiograph guide the analysis.

of abnormality is usually PVH. The major signs of PVH are equalization or larger diameter of the upper compared to the lower lobe vessels; loss of prominence or clear visualization of the right lower lobe pulmonary artery; prominence of the interstitial markings, especially the appearance of Kerley A and B lines; indistinctness of the pulmonary vascular margins and/or hilar vessels; loss of the right hilar angle; and alveolar filling (Figs. 30-3 to 30-6). After repeated episodes of pulmonary edema in longstanding cases of mitral valve disease, permanent interstitial lines or ossific nodules may appear. Ossific nodules are small foci of bony metaplasia that appear in the lungs only after multiple episodes of edema and chronic PVH. Foci of hemosiderin may form fibrotic

TABLE 30.1 Radiographic Classification of Acquired Heart Disease

Small Heart (C/T < 0.55)	Large Heart (C/T > 0.55)
Aortic stenosis	Aortic regurgitation
Arterial hypertension	Mitral regurgitation
Mitral stenosis	Tricuspid regurgitation
Acute myocardial infarction	High-output states
Hypertrophic cardiomyopathy	Congestive cardiomyopathy
Restrictive cardiomyopathy	Ischemic cardiomyopathy
Constrictive pericarditis	Pericardial effusion
	Paracardiac mass

FIG. 30.3. Pulmonary venous hypertension in mitral valve disease. Radiograph demonstrates redistribution of pulmonary blood flow (upper lobe vessels larger than lower lobe vessels) indicating grade I pulmonary venous hypertension. There is cardiomegaly and straightening of the upper left cardiac border indicative of left atrial enlargement.

nodules in patients with multiple episodes of edema as well as after multiple episodes of pulmonary hemorrhage.

The severity of PVH can be gauged by the signs observed. The radiographic severity of PVH can be divided into three grades: grade I (redistribution of pulmonary blood volume); grade II (interstitial pulmonary edema); and grade III (alveolar

FIG. 30.4. Interstitial pulmonary edema after acute myocardial infarction. Radiograph demonstrates interstitial pulmonary edema with Kerley B lines, indistinct vascular margins, and peribronchial cuffing.

FIG. 30.5. Noncardiac pulmonary edema. Alveolar pulmonary edema with normal heart size in a child after drowning.

pulmonary edema; Table 30-2). The pulmonary venous pressure (or mean left atrial wedge pressure) associated with edema varies depending on whether the cardiac dysfunction is acute or chronic (Table 30-3). The venous pressure in chronic disease is approximately 5 mm Hg greater for each grade of PVH compared to that in acute disease.

Asymmetric PVH

Asymmetric distribution of PVH or pulmonary edema raises a number of diagnostic possibilities (Table 30-4,

FIG. 30.6. Alveolar pulmonary edema with normal heart size in a patient with left atrial myxoma obstructing the mitral valve.

TABLE 30.2	**Signs of Pulmonary Ventricular Hypertension by Grade of Severity**

Grade I: vascular redistribution
Equal upper and lower lobe vessels
Larger upper lobe vessels

Grade II: interstitial edema
Kerley A or B lines
Increased prominence of "interstitial markings"
Peribronchial cuffing
Loss of the hilar angle
Enlargement and indistinctness of hila
Subpleural edema (increased thickness of pleura)
Loss of visibility of much of the descending branch of the right pulmonary artery

Grade III
Confluent acinar shadows (pulmonary alveolar edema)
Perihilar alveolar filling
Lower lobe or more generalized alveolar filling

Fig. 30-7). The most frequent cause of such asymmetry is probably gravitational; patients with heart disease frequently sleep lying on their right side because of consciousness of the prominent left-sided pulsation (prominent point of maximum impulse in the presence of cardiomegaly). The next most frequent cause is underlying lung disease such as chronic obstructive pulmonary disease, which obliterates portions of the pulmonary vascular bed. Edema or pulmonary venous distention appears in the normal or less severely abnormal portions of the lungs. Unilateral pulmonary edema may occur contralateral to an occluded or severely stenotic pulmonary artery. Such unilateral edema might appear contralateral to a pulmonary embolism, or a pulmonary artery stenosis caused by congenital anomalies (branch pulmonary arterial stenosis, proximal interruption or agenesis of a pulmonary artery) or acquired diseases (bronchogenic carcinoma, Takayasu's arteritis, fibrosing mediastinitis, mediastinal tumors). Unilateral edema is infrequently used by unilateral obstruction of pulmonary veins caused by mediastinal or lung tumors, primary and

TABLE 30.3	**Correlates of Left Atrial Pressure (Mean)[a] and Pulmonary Vascular Hypertension Grade**

	Left Atrial Pressure	
	Acute Disease (Myocardial Infarction)	Chronic Disease (Mitral Stenosis)
Grade I	12–19 mm Hg	15–25 mm Hg
Grade II	20–25 mm Hg	25–30 mm Hg
Grade III	25 mm Hg	30 mm Hg

[a]Left atrial mean pressure is usually inferred from the mean pulmonary wedge pressure. Correlation between left atrial pressure and radiographic signs of pulmonary edema is only fair because of phase lag between rapid pressure changes and slower changes inradiographic alterations.

TABLE 30.4 Unilateral Pulmonary Edema

Gravitational
Chronic lung disease (emphysema)
Unilateral pulmonary arterial obstruction
    Thromboembolic disease
    Extrinsic obstruction of pulmonary artery
    Lung cancer, thoracic aortic aneurysm, mediastinal fibrosis
Unilateral pulmonary venous obstruction
    Left atrial tumor
    Mediastinal tumor encasing pulmonary veins
    Mediastinal fibrosis
Reexpansion pulmonary edema
    Postpneumothorax, postthoracentesis

TABLE 30.5 Noncardiogenic Pulmonary Edema

Drowning
Asphyxia
Upper airway obstruction
High altitude
Increased intracranial pressure
Reexpansion pulmonary edema
Noxious gases
    Smoke inhalation
    Nitrous dioxide (silo filler's disease)
    Sulfur dioxide
    Others
Drugs
    Aspirin
    Valium, librium, barbiturates, heroin, cocaine, methadone
Poisons—parathion
Blood transfusion reaction
Contrast media reaction
Adult respiratory distress syndrome

secondary tumors of the heart and pericardium, mediastinal fibrosis, and complications of the Mustard procedure and other procedures used in congenital heart disease. Finally, pulmonary edema induced by reinflation of a collapsed lung or after thoracentesis must be considered.

Pulmonary edema may occur in the absence of underlying cardiac disease. Such noncardiogenic edema is usually due to damage to the alveolar-capillary membrane, causing a leak of fluid into the lung at normal or near-normal pulmonary venous pressure and capillary oncotic pressure. A partial list of the many settings in which this occurs is shown in Table 30-5.

Overall Heart Size

Acquired heart disease can be divided into two groups, depending on the presence or absence of substantial

cardiomegaly. "Small heart" heart disease is associated with a normal heart size or only mild cardiomegaly. For the sake of our discussion, we will set a cardiothoracic (CT) ratio of less than 0.55 as consistent with this group of lesions. The choice of 0.55 is obviously somewhat arbitrary. The CT ratio is calculated using the convention of measuring the thoracic diameter as the distance from the inner margin of the ribs at the level of the dome of the right hemidiaphragm and the cardiac diameter as the horizontal distance between the most rightward and most leftward margins of the cardiac shadow. The second group, called "big heart" heart disease, is characterized by substantial cardiomegaly (CT ratio greater than 0.55).

The pathophysiologic factors associated with "small heart" heart disease are pressure overload and reduced ventricular compliance. The pathophysiologic factors associated with "big heart" heart disease are volume overload and myocardial failure. Pericardial effusion also is included in this group.

The cardiac lesions included in the two groups are listed in Table 30-1. The major pressure overload types of acquired lesions are aortic and mitral stenosis and hypertension. The major volume overload types of acquired lesions are aortic, mitral, and tricuspid regurgitation and high output states. Cardiac diseases that cause reduced left ventricular (LV) compliance or resistance to full expansion of the ventricles are acute myocardial infarction (MI), hypertrophic cardio-myopathy, restrictive cardiomyopathy, and constrictive pericardial disease.

Specific Chamber Enlargement

It is not until the fourth step in the examination of the chest x-ray that attention should be directed to determining specific chamber enlargement. A critical observation is the identification of left atrial enlargement. It is also useful to determine which ventricle is enlarged or if both

FIG. 30.7. Asymmetric pulmonary edema. Unilateral pulmonary edema in a patient with a metastatic tumor selectively obstructing the right pulmonary veins. Note the increased density of the right lower lung field.

ventricles are enlarged. It is sometimes not possible to clearly determine the type of ventricular enlargement on the thoracic radiograph. The radiographic signs observed with enlargement of each of the cardiac chambers are given below.

Left Atrial Enlargement

1. Right retrocardiac double density. Distance from the middle of the double density (lateral border of left atrium) to the middle of the left bronchus is less than 7 cm in greater than 90% of normal subjects and greater than 7 cm in 90% of patients with left atrial enlargement, proven by echocardiography (Figs. 30-8 and 30-9). In cases of severe left atrial enlargement, the right atrial border may extend further to the right than the right atrial border (Fig. 30-10).
2. Enlargement of the left atrial appendage. This is seen as a bulge along the left cardiac border just beneath the main pulmonary artery segment (see Figs. 30-8 to 30-10). Using the left bronchus as an orientation point, the bulge above it is the main pulmonary artery segment, while the bulge at the level of and/or just below the left bronchus is the left atrial appendage.
3. Splaying of the carina and/or elevation of the left bronchus (see Figs. 30-10 and 30-11)
4. Horizontal orientation of the distal portion of the left bronchus
5. Posterior displacement of the left upper lobe bronchus (see Fig. 30-11). On the lateral radiograph, the circular

FIG. 30.9. Left atrial double intensity in mitral regurgitation. The left atrial dimension is the length of a line from the middle of the double density to the medial border of the left bronchus. A value greater than 7 cm indicates left atrial enlargement. Note also enlargement of the left atrial appendage (*arrowheads*).

shadow of the right upper lobe and left bronchi is located within the tracheal air column. Left atrial enlargement causes displacement of the left bronchus posterior to this level and beyond the plane of the trachea.

FIG. 30.8. Mitral stenosis causing left atrial enlargement. Subtle convexity along the upper left cardiac border is caused by enlargement of the left atrial appendage (*arrowhead*). Note right retrocardiac double density (*arrow*) caused by enlargement of the left atrial chamber.

FIG. 30.10. Mitral regurgitation. There is cardiomegaly and marked left atrial enlargement with pulmonary ventricular hypertension. The left atrium is enlarged to the extent that it forms the right heart border on the frontal view (*arrows*).

FIG. 30.11. Mitral and tricuspid regurgitation. Frontal (**left**) and lateral (**right**) radiographs show prominent double densities on both sides of the spine due to marked left atrial enlargement. Right atrial enlargement is shown by the elongation of the right-sided convexity on the front view. Prominent upper left cardiac border on frontal view is caused by dilatation of the right ventricular outflow region. Lateral view shows posterior displacement of the left bronchus (*arrow*) by the enlarged left atrium and obliteration of the retrocardiac space by right ventricular enlargement.

Right Atrial Enlargement

1. Lateral bulging of the right heart border on the posteroanterior radiograph (see Fig. 30-11)
2. Elongation of the right heart border on the posteroanterior view. A rough rule is that a right atrial border exceeding 60% in length of the mediastinal cardiovascular shadow is a sign of substantial right atrial enlargement (Fig. 30-12).

FIG. 30.12. Tricuspid regurgitation. Severe right atrial enlargement is evident by the elongation of the right atrial shadow. The length of the right atrial border exceeds 60% of the height of the mediastinal cardiovascular structures.

Left Ventricular Enlargement

1. On the posteroanterior view, leftward and downward displacement of the cardiac apex. The vector of enlargement of the LV is leftward and downward compared with the vector of right ventricular enlargement, which is leftward only or perhaps leftward plus upward (Figs. 30-13 and 30-14).
2. On the lateral view, the posterior border of the heart is displaced posteriorly. The Hoffman-Rigler sign is measured 2.0 cm above the intersection of the diaphragm and the inferior vena cava. A positive measurement for LV enlargement is a posterior border of the heart extending more than 1.8 cm behind the inferior vena caval shadow at this level.

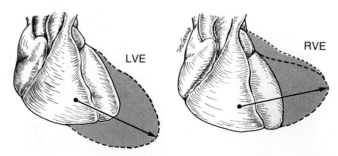

FIG. 30.13. "Vectors of enlargement" for the left and right ventricles. For left ventricular enlargement (*LVE*), the vector is directed leftward and caudal. For right ventricular enlargement (*RVE*), the vector is directed leftward or leftward and slightly cranial.

FIG. 30.14. Aortic regurgitation. The ventricular contour is enlarged along a left inferolateral vector, causing the apex to droop over the left hemidiaphragm. Concavity along the upper left cardiac border indicates that the right ventricle is not enlarged. There is enlargement of the thoracic aorta.

Right Ventricular Enlargement

1. On the posteroanterior view, the left border of the heart is enlarged directly laterally or laterally and slightly superiorly (see Fig. 30-13). In some instances, this causes the apex to be displaced superiorly ("upward tipped apex"; Fig. 30-15); in the extreme form this causes a "boot shape" (Fig. 30-16).
2. On the lateral view, the retrosternal space is encroached upon by the enlarged right ventricle. Right ventricular enlargement is inferred by contact of the right heart border over greater than one third of the sternal length. A prominent convexity to the anterior border rather than the usual straight surface is an early sign of right ventricular enlargement.

Signposts for Cardiac Valvular Lesions

There are three signposts on the thoracic radiograph that direct attention to a certain cardiac valve:

1. Left atrial enlargement
2. Ascending aortic enlargement
3. Right atrial enlargement

These signs point specifically to the following:

1. Mitral valve (left atrium)
2. Aortic valve (ascending aorta)
3. Tricuspid valve (right atrium)

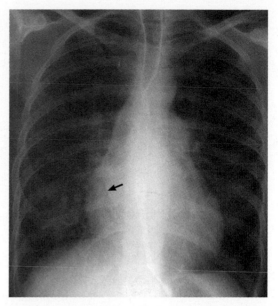

FIG. 30.15. Mitral stenosis with pulmonary arterial hypertension and interstitial pulmonary edema. Cardiomegaly is caused by right ventricular enlargement. The vector of enlargement of the ventricle is directly lateral, indicating right ventricular enlargement. The most lateral portion of the apex is located above the diaphragm. Left atrial enlargement is indicated by double density (*arrow*). Pulmonary arterial hypertension is indicated by pulmonary arterial enlargement.

Using our classification system ("big heart" vs. "small heart" heart disease) and applying the signpost, we can analyze the thoracic radiograph in accordance with the flow diagram shown in Figure 30-2. This schema obviously works well

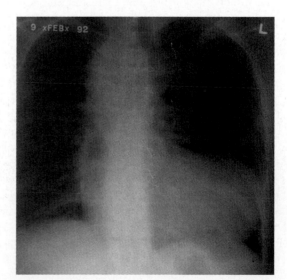

FIG. 30.16. Tetralogy of Fallot after total correction with severe pulmonary regurgitation. Substantial right ventricular enlargement is evident. The vector of enlargement of the ventricle is leftward and cranial, causing uplifting of the apex in relation to the diaphragm. Note the right aortic arch.

FIG. 30.17. Aortic stenosis with calcification in 43-year-old man. Frontal radiograph (**left**) shows a nearly normal appearance except for enlargement of the ascending aorta. Lateral view (**right**) demonstrates heavy calcification (*arrow*) of the aortic valve.

for diseases causing typical alterations in the chest x-ray. Of course, a specific cardiac lesion does not always cause typical features because of other associated abnormalities or because the lesion is very mild or has been present for insufficient time to alter the cardiac morphology to a degree discernible on the thoracic radiograph.

The schema can be briefly described by considering the chest x-ray that shows a normal heart size or mild cardiomegaly in a patient with significant heart disease. This means that the lesion likely causes pressure overload (hypertension, aortic stenosis, or mitral stenosis) or reduced LV compliance. If the left atrial signpost is present, then attention is directed to the mitral valve (see Fig. 30-8). The diagnosis should be either mitral valvular stenosis or resistance to left atrial emptying. Diseases that significantly reduce LV compliance (and increase LV diastolic pressure) cause resistance to left atrial emptying and thereby induce left atrial enlargement. Diseases that may reduce LV compliance are hypertrophic cardiomyopathy, restrictive cardiomyopathy, and constrictive pericardial disease. Acute MI may also reduce LV compliance, but usually this has not been present for a sufficient time to cause left atrial enlargement. LV hypertrophy from any cause can reduce LV compliance if it is sufficiently severe.

If the ascending aorta is enlarged, then this signpost points to the aortic valve, indicating aortic stenosis (Fig. 30-17). Systemic hypertension can produce a similar appearance, although it usually causes enlargement of the entire thoracic aorta rather than the ascending aorta alone. If no signposts are present, then the diagnosis is unlikely to be a valvular lesion. The absence of signposts should direct attention to a disease directly afflicting the myocardium or pericardium, such as acute MI, hypertrophic cardiomyopathy, restrictive cardiomyopathy, and constrictive pericardial disease. However, even these latter diseases sometimes induce left atrial enlargement, as stated above.

The schema for a patient with substantial cardiomegaly proceeds along the following path. The big heart suggests that there is either a volume overload lesion (valvular regurgitation) or myocardial failure or pericardial effusion. High output states are certainly a volume overload and can cause substantial cardiomegaly, but sometimes they cause only mild cardiomegaly. If left atrial enlargement is noted, then the signpost points to mitral regurgitation (Figs. 30-18 and 30-19). If the ascending aorta is enlarged in "big heart" heart

FIG. 30.18. Mitral regurgitation with pulmonary arterial hypertension. There is cardiomegaly and left ventricular and left atrial enlargement. The pulmonary arterial enlargement indicates pulmonary arterial hypertension. There is also right lower lobe pneumonia.

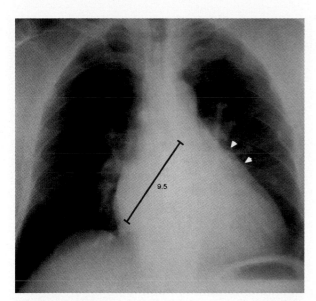

FIG. 30.19. Mitral regurgitation causing cardiomegaly and left ventricular and left atrial enlargement. Note the enlarged left atrial appendage (*arrowheads*). Left atrial dimension is 9.5 cm.

FIG. 30.20. Aortic stenosis. Frontal radiograph shows normal cardiac size and normal pulmonary vascularity. The sole abnormality in this 40-year-old subject is enlargement of the ascending aorta (*arrows*). The posterior aortic arch is normal in size.

disease, then this signpost points to aortic regurgitation (see Fig. 30-14). If the right atrium is enlarged, then this signpost points to tricuspid regurgitation (see Fig. 30-11). Acquired pulmonic regurgitation is rare, except as a consequence of operation for right ventricular outflow obstruction, and is not considered in this schema. If no signposts are present, then the favored diagnostic considerations are congestive (dilated) cardiomyopathy or pericardial effusion.

RADIOGRAPHIC FEATURES OF SPECIFIC CARDIAC LESIONS

Aortic Stenosis

Aortic stenosis is a pressure overload lesion for which the compensatory mechanism is concentric LV hypertrophy (Table 30-6). Concentric LV hypertrophy causes a slight reduction in the volume of the LV but little increase in the

overall cardiac size. Consequently, aortic stenosis, for much of its natural history, is a disease that is clearly "small heart" heart disease. There is little or no cardiac enlargement. The characteristic radiographic feature is enlargement of the ascending aorta (see Figs. 30-17, 30-20, and 30-21). The pulmonary vascularity is also generally normal for much of the course of aortic stenosis. However, in the decompensated phase of aortic stenosis, there may be evidence of PVH due to LV failure. Occasionally, when LV hypertrophy has reduced LV compliance considerably, there may also be signs of PVH even in the absence of LV enlargement.

TABLE 30.6 Salient Radiographic Features of Aortic Stenosis

Enlargement of the ascending aorta due to poststenotic dilatation (see Figs. 30-17 and 30-20)
Mild or no cardiomegaly in compensated stage
Substantial cardiomegaly occurs only after myocardial failure has ensued
No pulmonary venous hypertension or pulmonary edema is seen during most of the course of this disease
Calcification of aortic valve may be discernible on radiograph but is more readily shown on CT (see Fig. 30-21)

FIG. 30.21. CT scan shows calcification of the aortic valve (*arrow*) in a patient with valvular aortic stenosis.

TABLE 30.7 Salient Radiographic Features of Arterial Hypertension

Enlargement of the thoracic aorta—ascending, arch, and descending aorta (see Fig. 30-22)
Mild or no cardiomegaly until the onset of myocardial failure
No pulmonary edema or pulmonary venous hypertension until the occurrence of diastolic dysfunction due to severe left ventricular hypertrophy or myocardial failure

Hypertension

Hypertensive heart disease is a pressure overload lesion and consequently is associated with a normal heart size for much of the compensated phase of this disease (Table 30-7; Fig. 30-22). The severity or even the presence of LV hypertrophy cannot be reliably determined from the thoracic radiograph.

Mitral Stenosis

The features of a thoracic radiograph are frequently diagnostic for mitral stenosis (see Figs. 30-8, 30-15, 30-23, and 30-24). Likewise, the radiograph provides considerable insight into the severity of mitral stenosis. While mitral stenosis is a pressure overload lesion that causes little increase in overall heart size during the early phase of the disease, it does produce characteristic enlargement of the left atrium and the left atrial appendage and produces signs of PVH (Table 30-8).

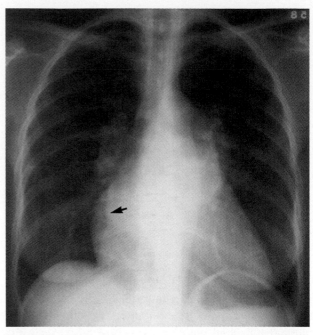

FIG. 30.23. Mitral stenosis. Frontal thoracic radiograph demonstrates left atrial and right ventricular enlargement. Left atrial enlargement is indicated by right retrocardiac double density (*arrow*) on the frontal view. There is pulmonary arterial hypertension as shown by enlargement of the main and central pulmonary arteries. The thoracic aorta is inconspicuous. Right ventricular enlargement is indicated by lateral displacement of the ventricular margin (apex uplifted) on the frontal view.

Hypertrophic Cardiomyopathy

The chest radiograph is neither specific nor sensitive for the diagnosis of hypertrophic cardiomyopathy. More than 50% of patients with hypertrophic cardiomyopathy have a normal chest x-ray. In a few patients there is some abnormality of the chest x-ray, which is usually relatively vague and not particularly indicative of this disease. Since some patients with hypertrophic cardiomyopathy have a reduction in LV compliance, the radiograph sometimes demonstrates PVH. The PVH is usually relatively mild. The overall heart size is generally normal. In patients with reduced LV compliance, left atrial size may be increased. Approximately 30% of patients with symptomatic hypertrophic cardiomyopathy have associated mitral regurgitation. Because of the mitral regurgitation, there again is a proclivity to left atrial enlargement. A few patients have a squared appearance of the left cardiac border. This is caused by a prominent evagination on the upper left cardiac border. This focal enlargement is a consequence of extreme enlargement of the upper or outflow portion of the ventricular septum (Table 30-9).

FIG. 30.22. Systemic hypertension. Frontal view shows borderline cardiomegaly and prominence of the entire thoracic aorta.

FIG. 30.24. Mitral stenosis causing moderate enlargement of the left atrium and appendage. The wall of the appendage is calcified (*arrow*).

Restrictive Cardiomyopathy

Restrictive cardiomyopathy is a relatively rare disease that may occur in an idiopathic form or may be the form of cardiomyopathy that is a consequence of various infiltrative

TABLE 30.8 Salient Radiographic Features of Mitral Stenoses

Pulmonary venous hypertension or edema is present (see Fig. 30-15).
Pulmonary edema may be observed intermittently.
Mild cardiomegaly is seen in isolated mitral stenosis (see Figs. 30-8, 30-15, and 30-24).
Enlargement of the left atrium is characteristic (see Figs. 30-8, 30-15, 30-23, and 30-24).
Enlargement of the left atrial appendage is frequent and suggests a rheumatic etiology (see Figs. 30-8 and 30-24).
Right ventricular enlargement indicates some degree of pulmonary arterial hypertension or associated tricuspid regurgitation.
Enlargement of the pulmonary arterial segment is indicative of associated pulmonary arterial hypertension (see Fig. 30-23).
Right ventricular enlargement in the absence of prominence of the main pulmonary artery suggests associated tricuspid regurgitation. The right atrium is also enlarged with tricuspid regurgitation (see Fig. 30-11).
The ascending aorta and aortic arch are usually inconspicuous in isolated mitral stenosis. Even slight enlargement of the thoracic aorta raises the question of associated aortic valve disease.

TABLE 30.9 Salient Radiographic Features of Hypertrophic Cardiomyopathy

Normal in most patients
Mild cardiomegaly and pulmonary venous hypertension in a minority of patients
Left atrial enlargement can be caused by associated mitral insufficiency or reduced left ventricular compliance.
In the obstructive form (subaortic stenosis), ascending aortic enlargement is infrequent.
Left ventricular enlargement may occur in end-stage disease.

diseases of the LV. Types of infiltrative processes of the LV that may produce restrictive cardiomyopathy include sarcoidosis, hemochromatosis, and amyloidosis.

During the early stage of restrictive cardiomyopathy the cardiac size is within normal limits. Restrictive cardiomyopathy has as its main physiologic deficit a reduction of LV compliance. Because of the reduced compliance, there is frequently an elevation in pulmonary venous pressure, which of course is reflected on the chest radiograph as various degrees of PVH (Figs. 30-25 and 30-26). Likewise, because of the reduced LV compliance, there is a rise in left atrial pressure, which may cause a left atrial enlargement to be visible on the radiograph. Because the major radiographic features of this disease are PVH and left atrial enlargement, the plain radiograph may mimic the appearance of mitral stenosis. In advanced disease there is frequently some degree of LV enlargement, which along with the left atrial enlargement usually results in a mild to moderate cardiomegaly (see Fig. 30-26). However, in some patients the restrictive cardiomyopathy may progress to congestive cardiomyopathy, which is associated with considerable cardiomegaly and LV enlargement (Table 30-10).

FIG. 30.25. Restrictive cardiomyopathy. Normal cardiac size with left atrial enlargement.

FIG. 30.26. Restrictive cardiomyopathy. Frontal (**left**) and lateral (**right**) radiographs show interstitial pulmonary edema and left atrial and right ventricular enlargement.

Acute Myocardial Infarction

The plain radiograph is obtained in the emergency room in most patients with an acute MI. The initial chest x-ray or a chest x-ray within the first 24 hours after the onset of acute MI is normal in approximately 50% of patients with initial acute MI. In the other 50% of patients, the most frequent finding is some degree of PVH or pulmonary edema, along with a normal heart size (Fig. 30-27). The major physiologic deficit in the early phase of acute MI is an abrupt decrease in LV compliance, which results in an increase in pulmonary venous pressure. The increase in pulmonary venous pressure is reflected on the chest x-ray by varying degrees of PVH or pulmonary edema. It is unusual for the patient with a first acute MI, even when the infarction is severe and eventually lethal, to have cardiomegaly or perceptible LV enlargement.

The plain chest x-ray does provide some insight into the severity of the acute MI. The gauge of severity is the degree of PVH. Indeed, a relationship has been shown between the degree of PVH on the plain radiograph within the first 24 hours and the early and late survival rates after the initial MI (Fig. 30-28). The plain radiograph may also be useful in

demonstrating complications of acute MI, such as cardiac rupture; pericardial effusion; LV aneurysm, both true and false; papillary muscle rupture; and intractable congestive heart failure.

Some patients with a true LV aneurysm demonstrate a normal chest x-ray. However, in many patients there is evidence of an abnormal cardiac configuration, especially an abnormal evagination along the midportion of the left cardiac border or in the region of the cardiac apex (Fig. 30-29). The abnormal contour generally occurs in these sites because the most frequent location of a true LV aneurysm is the anterolateral wall or the apical wall of the

TABLE 30.10 Salient Radiographic Features of Restrictive Cardiomyopathy

Pulmonary venous hypertension is typical.
Pulmonary edema may occur intermittently.
Normal heart size or mild cardiomegaly in most patients (see Figs. 30-25 and 30-26)
Left atrial enlargement (see Fig. 30-26)
Left atrial appendage is typically not enlarged.
Moderate to severe cardiomegaly can ensue in end-stage disease.

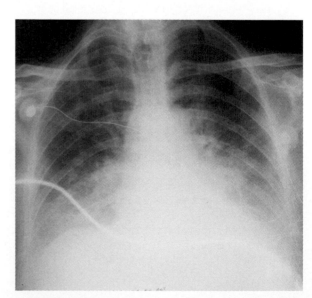

FIG. 30.27. Acute MI with alveolar pulmonary edema. Note alveolar filling in perihilar regions and lower lobes with normal heart size.

FIG. 30.28. Thirty-day, 6-month, and 12-month survival rates in relation to the severity of pulmonary ventricular hypertension (PVH) on the initial chest x-ray of patients after acute MI. With any degree of PVH, survival is decreased compared to patients with no PVH. (From Battler A, Karliner JS, Higgins CB, et al. The initial chest x-ray film in acute myocardial infarction: prediction of early and late mortality and survival. Circulation 1980; 61:1004.)

LV. Calcification of the anterolateral region of the LV is suggestive of LV aneurysm (Fig. 30-30). Calcification of an infarct is more readily displayed on CT (Fig. 30-31).

An abnormal evagination that is localized to the posterior wall or the diaphragmatic wall of the LV should raise the possibility of a false LV aneurysm (Fig. 30-32). While only approximately 5% of true LV aneurysms involve the upper diaphragmatic and posterior wall, these sites are the most frequent ones for false LV aneurysm. Consequently, an abnormal contour or a double density localized to these sites should raise the consideration of this diagnosis. The differentiation of a false aneurysm from a true aneurysm becomes important because of the known propensity of false aneurysms to be complicated by late rupture. Other plain radiographic signs of a false aneurysm are an aneurysm that is extremely large with a prominent projection off the posterior or diaphragmatic surface of the heart (see Fig. 30-32), and an increase in the size of the aneurysm on sequential studies. A false aneurysm is more frequently associated with occlusion of either the circumflex or right coronary artery, while a true aneurysm is most frequently associated with occlusion of the left anterior descending coronary artery.

Papillary muscle rupture is a dramatic event that usually induces severe and many times intractable pulmonary edema. Partial rupture of the papillary muscle, resulting in less severe mitral regurgitation, may produce a moderate degree of mitral regurgitation and less severe or even no evidence of pulmonary edema. The dramatic radiographic findings in acute papillary muscle rupture are pulmonary edema with little increase in left atrial size or cardiomegaly. If the patient survives beyond several weeks or months, then varying degrees of left atrial enlargement and cardiomegaly may be present.

Postinfarction rupture of the ventricular septum may produce a radiographic appearance very similar to that of acute mitral regurgitation. The radiographic signs of acute ventricular septal defect include an increase in the prominence of the pulmonary arteries (i.e., pulmonary arterial overcirculation), usually pulmonary edema, and mild degrees of cardiomegaly. Again, if the patient tolerates

FIG. 30.29. True left ventricular aneurysm complicating myocardial infarction. Frontal (**left**) and lateral (**right**) views. Abnormal evagination of left cardiac border (*arrowheads*) is typical for an aneurysm involving the anterolateral and/or apical segment of the left ventricle. Lateral view demonstrates an anterior double density (*arrows*), characteristic of an anterolateral aneurysm.

FIG. 30.30. Calcified apical left ventricular aneurysm. Lateral thoracic radiograph shows calcification (*arrows*) on the anteroapical region of the left ventricle.

FIG. 30.31. CT scan shows mural calcification at the site of an old apical myocardial infarction.

the episode and survives for several weeks to months, then the degree of cardiomegaly may be more considerable, and there may even be signs of left atrial enlargement.

Dressler's syndrome, another complication of acute MI, occurs within the first weeks to months after an acute MI. This is an autoimmune response to various antigens that are released during the acute MI. This autoimmune response involves the pericardial and pleural surfaces, eventuating in pericardial and pleural effusions. Chest radiographs in this syndrome demonstrate an increase in cardiac size as a consequence of the pericardial effusion, along with evidence of unilateral or bilateral pleural effusions (Table 30-11).

Constrictive Pericarditis

Constrictive pericarditis is a disease that is being encountered with increasing frequency. Currently, the major causes are iatrogenic. The most frequent inciting factor is postoperative bleeding associated with cardiac surgery, especially coronary revascularization procedures. The second most frequent inciting factor is mediastinal irradiation; the third most common cause

FIG. 30.32. False left ventricular aneurysm complicating myocardial infarction. Frontal (**left**) and lateral (**right**) radiographs show left retrocardiac density (*arrow*) on the frontal view and large posterior evagination (*arrowheads*) of left ventricular contour on the lateral view. Large size and posterior location are characteristics of false aneurysm.

TABLE 30.11 **Salient Radiographic Features of Acute Myocardial Infarction**

Normal chest x-ray in about 50% of first acute infarctions.
Normal heart size with pulmonary venous hypertension or pulmonary edema in about 50% of first acute infarctions (see Fig. 30-27).
Cardiomegaly is usually indicative of acute infarction in a patient with history of previous infarctions.
Cardiomegaly may be indicative of ischemic cardiomyopathy.

Signs of complication of acute myocardial infarction
Intractable pulmonary edema may occur with papillary muscle rupture (mitral regurgitation) or ventricular septal rupture (left to right shunt).
Enlarged cardiac silhouette may be caused by pericardial effusion.
Abnormal cardiac contour may be a sign of true (bulge of the anterolateral or apical regions; see Fig. 30-29) or false (bulge of the posterior or diaphragmatic regions) aneurysms (see Fig. 30-32).

is repeated episodes of viral pericarditis. Uremic pericardial disease may also eventuate in constrictive pericarditis, but usually this disease produces an effusive/constrictive type of pericardial disease. In Third World countries, tuberculosis continues to be a major cause of constrictive pericarditis.

The plain radiograph is frequently but not always abnormal in patients with hemodynamically significant constrictive pericarditis. Because of pericardial constriction there is restriction to left atrial emptying during diastole, with a subsequent rise in left atrial and pulmonary venous pressures. The rise in pulmonary venous pressure is reflected on the chest radiograph by signs of PVH, such as redistribution and interstitial or alveolar pulmonary edema. The overall cardiac size is usually normal or there is only mild cardiomegaly (Fig. 30-33). There is frequently left atrial enlargement but normal ventricular size. Recognition of pericardial calcification supports or may initially suggest the diagnosis of constrictive pericarditis (Fig. 30-34; Table 30-12).

"BIG HEART" HEART DISEASE

Aortic Regurgitation

Aortic regurgitation is characterized on the plain radiograph by a substantial degree of cardiomegaly, which is due predominantly to LV enlargement (see Figs. 30-14 and 30-35). A signpost pointing to the aortic valve is present in this disease, consisting of enlargement of the ascending aorta, aortic knob, and usually the descending thoracic aorta. As opposed to aortic stenosis, the enlargement of the thoracic aorta involves the aortic knob as well as the ascending aorta. Consequently, "big heart" heart disease with the aortic signpost is indicative of aortic regurgitation.

The severity of aortic regurgitation is reflected on the plain radiograph. Since this is a volume overload lesion, the extent of the increase in volume of the heart is related to the severity and the duration of aortic regurgitation. For most of the course of aortic regurgitation, the pulmonary vascularity is normal. Consequently, the presence of PVH in a patient with aortic regurgitation is indicative of LV failure and is frequently associated with end-stage aortic valve disease (Table 30-13).

FIG. 30.33. Constrictive pericarditis. Frontal (**left**) and lateral (**right**) radiographs show grade I pulmonary ventricular hypertension and flattened right cardiac contour (*arrows*), which are characteristics of constrictive pericarditis. Lateral view demonstrates calcification (*arrowhead*) in the posterior interventricular groove.

FIG. 30.37. Congestive dilated cardiomyopathy. Frontal radiograph shows biventricular enlargement and mild pulmonary ventricular hypertension (grade I). Enlargement of the left ventricle is indicated by a vector of ventricular enlargement directed laterally and caudally on the frontal view. Right ventricle enlargement is indicated by the prominent convexity of the upper left cardiac border on the frontal view.

Myocardial Disease as a dilated cardiomyopathy without known etiologic identification (Table 30-16).

Pericardial Effusion

The cardiac configuration in pericardial effusion is relatively nonspecific. It has been assumed that the presence

FIG. 30.38. Congestive dilated cardiomyopathy. Frontal radiograph shows moderate cardiomegaly with biventricular but no discernible left atrial enlargement.

TABLE 30.16 Salient Radiographic Features of Congestive (Dilated) Cardiomyopathy

Pulmonary venous hypertension or pulmonary edema may be but is not invariably present.
Moderate to severe cardiomegaly (see Figs. 30-37 and 30-38)
Left ventricular enlargement
Left atrial enlargement is infrequently evident but can be caused by mitral regurgitation caused by left ventricular enlargement.

of substantial cardiomegaly in the absence of signs of PVH should be a clue to the presence of pericardial effusion (Figs. 30-39 and 30-40). This radiographic appearance is actually quite nonspecific. Similar to the appearance of congestive cardiomyopathy, the cardiac configuration is that of cardiomegaly without a radiographic signpost. A specific appearance providing a diagnosis of pericardial effusion is relatively infrequent in this entity. The so-called water-bottle appearance of the heart is nonspecific and difficult to recognize. The "fat pad" sign seen on the lateral radiograph does permit identification but occurs in only a few patients (see Fig. 30-39). The varying density sign is also sometimes present on the frontal radiograph (see Fig. 30-40). This consists of a lesser density at the periphery of the cardiac contour compared to the central portion of the cardiac contour. The cause of this varying density is that the x-ray beam encounters only fluid toward the periphery of the pericardial effusion, while in the center of the pericardial effusion the radiographic beam must pass through both water anteriorly and the cardiac substance more centrally.

With the frequent use of echocardiography, large pericardial effusions are being encountered less frequently. The presence of any degree of pericardial effusion can be easily recognized by echocardiography (Table 30-17).

Paracardiac Masses

Enlargement of the cardiac contour may not always be indicative of cardiac enlargement itself or pericardial effusion. One must also consider the infrequent possibility that the enlargement represents a cardiac or paracardiac mass (Figs. 30-41 and 30-42). Such consideration should be prompted by recognition of an unusual cardiac contour. The various causes of paracardiac masses are legion, but considerations are pericardial cysts, paracardiac tumors such as lymphoma and germinal cell tumor, cardiac tumors such as rhabdomyoma or various sarcomas, metastasis to lymph nodes within the pericardiophrenic angle, eventration or hernia of the diaphragm, neural tumors of the phrenic nerve, and various types of skeletal muscle tumors arising from the diaphragm. The diagnosis of the paracardiac mass can be readily made by CT and even more precisely with gated MRI.

FIG. 30.39. Pericardial perfusion. "Fat pad" sign is shown on lateral view (**right**). A stripe of water density (*arrow*) separates two fat layers on the outer surface of the parietal pericardium and beneath the visceral pericardium.

ABNORMAL CARDIAC CONTOURS

Enlargement of the Main Pulmonary Arterial Segment

Enlargement of the main pulmonary arterial segment is usually due to enlargement of the main pulmonary artery itself (Fig. 30-43). There are a number of causes of enlargement of the main pulmonary artery (Table 30-18).

Enlargement of the main pulmonary artery segment is the main indicator of pulmonary arterial hypertension (see Fig. 30-43). Severe pulmonary hypertension may cause calcification of the central pulmonary arteries (Fig. 30-44). Whenever one recognizes enlargement of the main pulmonary artery segment in a patient with no known pulmonary valvular disease, the differential diagnosis of pulmonary arterial hypertension must be considered. The differential diagnosis of pulmonary hypertension should lead to a systematic organization of the diagnostic possibilities. There are five diagnostic categories for pulmonary arterial hypertension: (1) pulmonary arterial hypertension resulting from PVH; (2) pulmonary arterial hypertension resulting from left-to-right shunts resulting in pulmonary arteriolar disease (arteriolopathy); (3) pulmonary arterial hypertension resulting from obliteration of the pulmonary vascular bed from chronic lung disease; (4) pulmonary arterial hypertension resulting from obliteration of the pulmonary vascular bed as a consequence of pulmonary embolic disease or schistosomiasis; and (5) primary pulmonary hypertension. Radiographic signs that permit the differential diagnosis of the various causes include recognition of the following:

1. Signs of PVH would indicate the likelihood that the pulmonary arterial hypertension is secondary to PVH.
2. Signs of chronic lung disease such as chronic obstructive pulmonary disease or interstitial lung disease would indicate this as the etiology.

FIG. 30.40. Pericardial perfusion. Varying cardiac density sign caused by transition of density near the margin of the cardiac silhouette (*arrows*).

TABLE 30.17 Salient Radiographic Features of Pericardial Effusion

No pulmonary venous hypertension or pulmonary edema
Moderate to severe enlargement of cardiac silhouette
Associated pleural effusion is not uncommon
Specific features, such as "fat pad" and/or "variable density" signs, are infrequently evident (see Figs. 30-39 and 30-40)

FIG. 30.41. Right paracardiac mass caused by loculated pericardial hematoma after cardiac surgery.

FIG. 30.42. Pericardial cyst. Frontal radiograph shows a mass (*arrow*) adjacent to the cardiac apex.

3. Asymmetric pulmonary vascularity or signs of pulmonary scarring might indicate the presence of chronic thromboembolic disease.
4. Marked enlargement of the central pulmonary arteries or signs of enlargement of the specific cardiac chambers may indicate the presence of a previous left-to-right shunt that has resulted in Eisenmenger's syndrome.

FIG. 30.43. Marked dilatation of the pulmonary artery (*arrow*) due to Eisenmenger's syndrome caused by patent ductus arteriosus. The main pulmonary artery and aortic arch are moderately enlarged.

Enlargement of Left Atrial Appendage Region or Middle Segment of Left Heart Border

An evagination ("mogul") in the region of the left atrial appendage on the frontal view should lead to a series of differential diagnostic considerations. The left atrial appendage region is considered to be the region immediately adjacent to and below the left bronchus (see Figs. 30-8, 30-10, 30-18, and 30-19). This is in contradistinction to the region of the main pulmonary artery segment, which is above the left bronchus. The two normal structures that reside within this area are the left atrial appendage and the right ventricular outflow tract; the left atrium is situated posterior to the right ventricular outflow region. The outflow portion of the ventricular septum is also located within this region. The pericardium covers the left atrial appendage and the right ventricular outflow tract in this region as in other parts of the heart. Other

TABLE 30.18 Enlargement of Main Pulmonary Artery: Etiology

Pulmonary arterial hypertension
Excess pulmonary blood flow (left to right shunts, chronic high output states)
Valvular pulmonic stenosis
Pulmonary regurgitation
Congenital absent pulmonary valve (aneurysmal pulmonary artery)
Absence of left pericardium
Aneurysm of pulmonary artery
Idiopathic dilatation of pulmonary artery

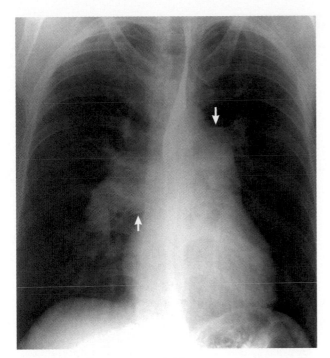

FIG. 30.44. Pulmonary arterial hypertension due to Eisenmenger's complex; the underlying lesion was an atrial septal defect. Frontal view shows the markedly enlarged main (*arrow*) and right pulmonary arterial segments. There is calcification (*arrow*) in the pulmonary arteries consistent with a systemic arterial pressure level in the pulmonary circulation.

structures are occasionally abnormally positioned at this site. The abnormally positioned structures that can lie within this site are a juxtaposed right atrial appendage and a transposed ascending aorta with the associated inverted right ventricular outflow region.

TABLE 30.19 Enlargement Of The Middle Segment of Left Heart Border: Etiology
Dilated left atrial appendage (rheumatic mitral valve disease)
Partial absence of left pericardium (see Fig. 30-45)
Enlargement of right ventricular outlet region such as occurs with left-to-right shunts
Asymmetric form of hypertrophic cardiomyopathy (occurs in small minority of cases)
Levo transposition of the great arteries
Juxtaposition of atrial appendages (rare anomaly usually associated with tricuspid atresia)
Left ventricular aneurysm
Cardiac tumor
Aneurysm or pseudoaneurysm of left circumflex coronary artery
Pericardial cyst or tumor
Mediastinal tumor

The differential diagnoses of an enlargement or evagination of the middle segment of the left heart border are multiple (Table 30-19; Fig. 30-45).

Enlargement of the Left Lower Cardiac Border—Ventricular Region

Enlargement along the lower left cardiac border in the region of the ventricles is most frequently caused by enlargement of either the right or the left ventricle (see Fig. 30-13). An abnormal convexity evagination within this region has a limited differential diagnosis (Table 30-20).

Enlargement of the Right Heart Border

Enlargement of the right heart contour in the frontal view is generally ascribed to right atrial enlargement. There are a few

FIG. 30.45. Complete (**left**) and partial (**right**) absence of left pericardium. Complete absence causes a shift of the heart to the left without a shift of the mediastinum (note the central position of the trachea) and a prominent convexity of the upper left cardiac margin. Lung (*arrow*) is insinuated between the aorta and pulmonary artery, indicating an absence of the pericardium at this site. Partial absence causes a prominent convexity (*arrowhead*) of the mid-left cardiac margin, especially in the region of the left atrial appendage segment.

TABLE 30.20	Evagination of Left Lower Heart Border: Etiology
Ventricular aneurysm	
Ventricular tumor	
Pericardial cyst, diverticulum or tumor	
Left ventricular diverticulum	
Mediastinal or lung tumor	
Pericardial fat pad	

TABLE 30.21	Enlargement of Right Heart And Border
Right atrial enlargement	
Pericardial fat pad	
Eventration or hernia of diaphragm	
Pericardial cyst or diverticulum	
Pericardial tumor	
Cardiac tumor	
Diaphragmatic tumor	
Mediastinal tumor	

other abnormalities that can also enlarge this contour and produce an abnormality in the contour (Table 30-21).

Cardiac Calcification

Calcification in the central cardiovascular structures is frequent and is an important diagnostic sign. In a few instances, calcification of a specific shape and location is pathognomonic for a disease. The various cardiovascular calcifications include the following:

1. Ascending aortic calcification. This is most frequently observed on the right anterolateral margin of the ascending aorta in elderly individuals, especially in the presence of aortic valve disease. In the past, it was considered to be a characteristic of luetic aortitis.
2. Mitral annular calcification (Fig. 30-46). This is a dense C-shaped calcification in the region of the mitral valve. It may be a causative factor of mitral regurgitation. It

is frequently observed in apparently normal elderly patients.
3. Aortic annular calcification, a circular calcification in the region of the aortic valve. Extension of this calcification into the region of the conducting system can produce complete heart failure.
4. Valvular calcification (aortic and mitral). Calcification of the aortic valve of sufficient density and extent to be visualized on the radiograph (see Fig. 30-17) is nearly always associated with hemodynamically important aortic stenosis (gradient more than 50 mm Hg).
5. Coronary arterial calcification. Coronary arterial calcification is frequently observed by fluoroscopy or CT. It must be both dense and extensive to be recognized on the thoracic radiograph (Fig. 30-47).
6. LV mural calcification. This is most frequently located in the anterolateral or apical regions of the LV and marks the site of a transmural MI or aneurysm (see Figs. 30-30 and 30-31).

FIG. 30.46. Mitral annular calcification. Frontal (**left**) and lateral (**middle**) views and CT scan (**right**) show a C-shaped calcification (*arrows*) in the mitral annulus.

FIG. 30.47. Calcification in the left anterior descending coronary artery (*arrow*). This is the most frequent site where coronary arterial calcification is observed on the frontal radiograph.

7. Pericardial calcification is indicative of constrictive pericarditis. It is located usually in the interventricular or atrioventricular grooves of the heart (see Figs. 30-33 and 30-34).

8. Unusual sites of calcification may represent intracardiac tumor (left atrial myxoma), pericardial tumor (dermoid), or healed granulomas (myocardial tuberculoma). An extremely rare process of the LV, Loeffler's eosinophilic fibroplasia, can cause calcification of the LV wall.

SELECTED READING

Higgins CB. Essentials of Cardiac Radiology and Imaging. Philadelphia: JB Lippincott, 1992.

Miller SW. Cardiac Radiology: The Requisites. Boston: Mosby-Year Book, 1996.

Skorton DJ, Shelbert HR, Wolf GL, et al. Cardiac Imaging. Philadelphia, PA: WB Saunders, 1996.

Steiner RM. Radiology of the heart and great vessels. In: Braunwald E, Zipes DP, Libby P (eds). Heart Disease, 16th ed. Philadelphia: WB Saunders, 2001.

FIG. 31-4. Truncus arteriosus, type I. Note pulmonary arterial overcirculation in the presence of cyanosis and cardiomegaly. There is an enlarged aorta with right arch (*arrow*).

FIG. 31-5. Atrial septal defect. Frontal (**left**) and lateral (**right**) views. Pulmonary arterial overcirculation is shown by large hilar and segmental pulmonary arteries. The absence of left atrial enlargement, indicated by no impression on the barium-filled esophagus, is characteristic for an atrial-level shunt.

It is frequently difficult to distinguish between normal and diminished pulmonary vascularity. This observation can be greatly simplified, however, when one remembers that normal pulmonary vascularity, as gleaned from the radiograph in a patient with cyanosis, can be equated with decreased pulmonary vascularity. Consequently, the major observation on the radiograph in terms of pulmonary vascularity in the cyanotic patient is to determine whether the pulmonary vascularity is increased. Normal or diminished pulmonary vascularity in a patient with cyanosis indicates that the lesion produces a right-to-left shunt. Increased pulmonary vascularity in a cyanotic patient indicates that there is an admixture lesion; the cyanosis is indicative of right-to-left shunting, and increased pulmonary vascularity is a sign of left-to-right shunting.

GROUPS OF CONGENITAL HEART LESIONS

Group I

Group I contains all of the left-to-right shunts; consequently, this is the group into which most patients with congenital heart disease are classified. The criteria that place a patient within this category are for the most part dependent on the clinical recognition of the absence of cyanosis with the subsequent demonstration on the chest radiograph of increased pulmonary arterial vascularity (see Figs. 31-1 and 31-5 to 31-9). The degree of cardiomegaly is usually in proportion to the increase in pulmonary vascularity. The left-to-right shunts are volume overload lesions. Consequently, there is frequently cardiomegaly, and this cardiomegaly should in general be in proportion to the prominence of the pulmonary vascularity.

FIG. 31-6. Ventricular septal defect. Frontal (**left**) and lateral (**right**) views. Pulmonary arterial overcirculation is evidenced by shunt vessels and prominent hilar vessels. Heart size is increased in proportion to overcirculation. Left atrial enlargement produces impression on and displacement of the barium-filled esophagus, as shown on the lateral view.

FIG. 31-7. Patent ductus arteriosus. Frontal (**left**) and lateral (**right**) views. Note pulmonary arterial overcirculation and cardiomegaly. The prominent aortic arch (*arrow*) and descending aorta are diagnostic signs of patent ductus arteriosus. On the lateral view, the enlarged left atrium causes posterior displacement of the left bronchus (*arrowhead*).

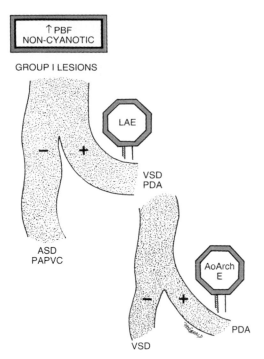

FIG. 31-8. Signposts on the diagnostic pathway of left-to-right shunts.

When cardiomegaly exists out of proportion to the pulmonary arterial vascularity, then one must consider a number of possibilities. One of the possibilities is that the left-to-right shunt is diminishing in size because of a decrease in the size of the ventricular septal defect (VSD). Another consideration is the coexistence of additional cardiac lesions, such as primary myocardial disease or coarctation of the aorta.

Two signposts can be used to help distinguish among the various types of left-to-right shunts (see Fig. 31-8). The

first of these is the left atrium. Left atrial enlargement indicates that the predominant lesion is not an atrial level shunt but rather a VSD or a patent ductus arteriosus (PDA). The atrial septal defect and partial anomalous pulmonary venous connection lack both of these signposts (see Fig. 31-5). The next signpost is the aortic arch. A prominent aortic arch distinguishes between the PDA and the VSD. The aortic arch usually has a normal dimension or is small in VSD (see Fig. 31-6). PDA is associated with left atrial enlargement and a prominent aortic arch (see Figs. 31-1 and 31-7). In infants, prominence of the aortic arch may be difficult to recognize, so this signpost may not always be available. Consequently, since a VSD is a more frequent lesion, this should be the diagnosis when there is left atrial enlargement and no clearly discernible enlargement of the aortic arch. An exception to this rule is in the premature infant, where a PDA is statistically by far the most frequent congenital heart lesion. The radiograph of the premature infant with PDA usually does not disclose signs of left atrial and aortic arch enlargement.

The plain radiograph may be useful in determining the severity and progression of left-to-right shunts. The severe volume overload with large left-to-right shunts causes pulmonary venous congestion or pulmonary edema in addition to pulmonary arterial overcirculation (see Fig. 31-9). In individuals with large left-to-right shunts, there should also be substantial cardiomegaly.

Group II

A lesion is included in group II when there is cyanosis and the plain radiograph demonstrates diminished or normal pulmonary vascularity and the absence of substantial cardiomegaly (see Figs. 31-2, 31-10, and 31-11). The pathophysiology that produces this constellation of findings

FIG. 31-9. Ventricular septal defects. Large-volume left-to-right shunt causing pulmonary edema, severe pulmonary arterial overcirculation, and cardiomegaly. Indistinct hilar and segmental arteries on the right side are caused by interstitial edema.

FIG. 31-10. Tetralogy of Fallot. Note pulmonary oligemia with more diminished vascularity on the left, especially the left upper lobe. Normal heart size and concave pulmonary artery segment are characteristic features in the infant.

FIG. 31-27. Atrioventricular septal defect/primum atrial septal defect. Radiography shows pulmonary arterial overcirculation and cardiomegaly due to right atrial and ventricular enlargement. The vector of ventricular enlargement is laterally and superiorly, causing the apex to be located high above the diaphragm. Prominent bulging of the upper right atrial border is a feature of primum atrial septal defects.

by malposition of the outlet septum, resulting in a small right ventricular outflow region and an aorta overriding the septal defect (tetralogy of Fallot). VSDs are not uncommonly multiple. Multiple defects in the trabecular septum may produce a "Swiss cheese septum."

A small VSD is one in which the diameter or cross-sectional area is less than that of the aortic annulus. A large or nonre-

FIG. 31-28. Atrioventricular septal defect (atrioventricular canal). Pulmonary arterial overcirculation and cardiomegaly due to right atrial and ventricular enlargement are present. There is elongation of the right atrial border, indicating substantial right atrial enlargement.

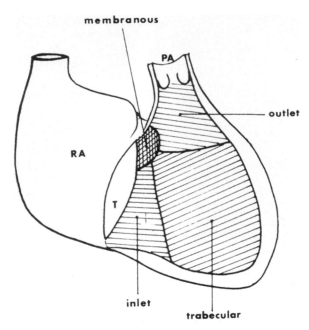

FIG. 31-29. The regions of the ventricular septum. The types of defect are named according to the region of the septum that is completely or partially defective. *PA*, pulmonary artery; *RA*, right atrium; *T*, tricuspid valve. (From **Higgins CB, et al**. Congenital Heart Disease: Echocardiography and Magnetic Resonance Imaging. New York: Raven Press, 1990.)

strictive defect has a diameter or cross-sectional area exceeding the aortic annulus. A nonrestrictive defect permits equalization of pressures in the two ventricles. Isolated VSD causes a left-to-right shunt in which the volume is determined by the cross-sectional area of the defect and pulmonary vascular resistance. With large defects, shunting is not restricted by the defect but is controlled only by pulmonary vascular resistance. With low pulmonary vascular resistance the volume of the shunt is great, causing severe pulmonary overcirculation and eventually pulmonary edema and elevated left ventricular end-diastole pressure. With higher resistance the flow is less severe and there is pulmonary arterial hypertension. Increased pulmonary vascular resistance and pulmonary arterial hypertension may be due to pulmonary arteriolar constriction (reversible) or arteriolopathy (irreversible).

Most isolated VSDs close spontaneously. The process of closure is frequently marked by a ventricular septal aneurysm. The aneurysm usually consists of portions of the septal leaflet of the tricuspid valve adherent to the rim of the defect; a hole may develop in the adhesed leaflet. Although the supracristal defect may be obstructed by the prolapsed sinus of Valsalva, it does not actually close. The inlet VSD (part of the AVSD) rarely closes spontaneously.

In the early postpartum period, pulmonary vascular resistance has not declined completely to adult levels, and the elevated resistance limits the left-to-right shunting through large defects. Pulmonary arteriolar resistance tends to reach a nadir 4 to 6 weeks postnatally and pulmonary overcircu-

TABLE 31.8 Salient Radiographic Features of Hemodynamically Significant Ventricular Septal Defect

Pulmonary arterial overcirculation (see Figs. 31-6 and 31-9): With large shunts pulmonary edema is frequent during infancy.

Enlargement of the left atrium (see Figs. 31-6 and 31-30): This may not be easy to identify during infancy.

Enlargement of either or both ventricles

Enlargement of main and central pulmonary arterial segments (see Fig. 31-9)

Disproportionate enlargement of central pulmonary arteries compared with peripheral vasculature suggests the Eisenmenger's complex but can also be observed with very large shunts. Pulmonary arterial calcification can occur in Eisenmenger's complex.

Small thoracic aorta: Right aortic arch is alleged to occur in about 2% of ventricular septal defects.

TABLE 31.9 Salient Radiographic Features of Hemodynamically Significant PDAS

Pulmonary arterial overcirculation (see Figs. 31-1 and 31-7)

Enlargement of left atrium (see Fig. 31-7)

Enlargement of left ventricle (see Figs. 31-1 and 31-7)

Enlargement of aortic arch (see Figs. 31-1 and 31-7): While this may not be evident with infants, it is an invariable feature in the older child and adult. It may also be possible to identify prominence of the ascending aorta and lateral displacement of the descending aorta.

Enlargement of the main and central pulmonary arterial segments: This tends to be less prominent than in atrial septal defect.

Abnormal contour of the posterior aortic arch and proximal descending aorta: In many normal subjects, there is a localized dilatation of the aorta at the site of attachment of the ligamentum arteriosus, the aortic spindle (also called infundibulum). This aortic spindle is enlarged in patients with patent ductus arteriosus. The combined shadows of the posterior arch and aortic spindle cause apparent elongation, prominence or atypical contour of the aortic knob. The aorticopulmonary window may be obliterated or convex due to the patent ductus arteriosus.

Calcification in the aorticopulmonary window due to calcification of the walls of the ductus in older individuals (see Fig. 31-32)

lation peaks. Because of the process of gradual closure and a relative decrease in the defect due to cardiac growth, the defect is physiologically maximal during the first year of life. Since VSD is a volume overload lesion and the volume overload is directly related to the excess pulmonary blood flow, cardiac enlargement is proportional to the degree of overcirculation (Table 31-8; see Figs. 31-6, 31-9, and 31-30).

Patent Ductus Arteriosus

The ductus arteriosus connects the proximal descending aorta to the proximal left pulmonary artery just beyond

the pulmonary arterial bifurcation. With mirror-image right aortic arch, the ductus usually connects the distal left innominate artery to the left pulmonary artery. With non–mirror-image right arch (retroesophageal left subclavian artery), the ductus connects the proximal right descending aorta to the proximal left pulmonary artery and causes a vascular ring.

PDA closes within the first day of life in full-term neonates, but persistent PDA is frequent in the premature infant. Significant left-to-right shunting in a premature infant during the early neonatal period is nearly always due to PDA. The shunt is predominantly left to right and causes pulmonary overcirculation and, if severe, pulmonary edema. However,

FIG. 31-30. Ventricular septal defect. Radiograph shows increased pulmonary blood flow and cardiomegaly. A right retrocardiac double density (*arrowheads*) indicates left atrial enlargement. Aortic arch is normal in size.

TABLE 31.10 Salient Radiographic Features of Patent Ductus Arteriosus with Pulmonary Arterial Hypertension

Enlarged main and central pulmonary arteries (see Fig. 31-31)

Disparity in enlargement of central and lobar arteries compared with peripheral arteries

Calcification of main or central pulmonary arteries

Calcification of the ductus (track-like calcification in the aorticopulmonary window (see Figs. 31-31 and 31-32).

Onset of pulmonary arterial hypertension is usually accompanied by a decrease in cardiomegaly or normal heart size (see Fig. 31-31).

Enlargement of the aortic arch and proximal descending aorta (see Fig. 31-31)

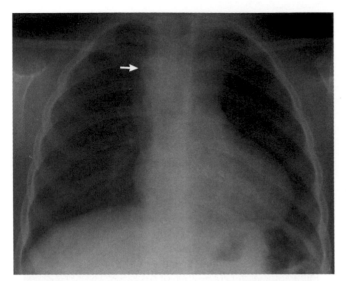

FIG. 31-33. Tetralogy of Fallot. Radiograph shows reduced pulmonary vascularity, normal heart size, right ventricular prominence, concave main pulmonary arterial segment, and right aortic arch (*arrow*).

After surgical repair of tetralogy, a number of radiographic findings may be identified, such as aneurysm of a right ventricular outflow patch; asymmetry of pulmonary vascularity due to persistent branch pulmonary arterial stenosis; and progressive right ventricular enlargement due to pulmonary regurgitation complicating a transannular patch (Fig. 31-35). Pulmonary arterial overcirculation can develop when a hemodynamically significant residual VSD exists after successful repair of outflow stenosis.

Transposition of Great Arteries

TGA is one of several abnormalities of arterioventricular connection. The others are double-outlet right ventricle, double-outlet left ventricle, and truncus arteriosus. All of these anomalies are admixture lesions, all produce cyanosis, and in the absence of obstruction to blood flow, all are associated with pulmonary arterial overcirculation.

In TGA, the aorta arises from the right ventricle and the pulmonary artery arises from the left ventricle. The base of the aorta is positioned anterior to pulmonary artery. If the aorta lies to the right of the pulmonary artery, the name d-TGA (dextro-TGA) applies, while if the aorta lies to the left of the pulmonary artery, the name l-TGA (levo-TGA) applies. If the aorta is directly anterior to the pulmonary artery, the term a-TGA (antero-TGA) is sometimes used.

The physiologic consequence of TGA is pulmonary arterial overcirculation and cyanosis due to the combination of left-to-right and right-to-left shunts (admixture lesion). Because the pulmonary and systemic circulations are parallel, most of the blood ejected by the left ventricle into the pulmonary artery is recirculated. The severity of overcirculation is usually greater in the presence of VSD and reduced in the presence of pulmonic stenosis. Cardiac size increases in rela-

A

B

FIG. 31-34. Tetralogy of Fallot with absent pulmonary valve in an adult (**A**) and an infant (**B**). Aneurysmal dilatation of main and right pulmonary arterial segments is diagnostic of this anomaly. Note the disparity in size of the right hilar arterial region and the peripheral segments of the pulmonary arteries.

tion to the pulmonary overcirculation. Pulmonary arterial hypertension and arteriolopathy tend to ensue early in life in children with TGA. Pulmonary arteriolopathy and fixed hypertension not uncommonly develop at 6 to 12 months of age in children with TGA with VSD.

TGA is the most frequent cyanotic heart lesion. Without surgical intervention, most of the infants would die in the first year of life.

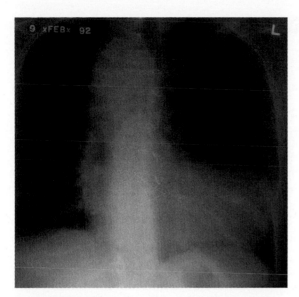

FIG. 31-35. Tetralogy of Fallot with severe pulmonary regurgitation several years after repair. The cardiomegaly is caused by marked right ventricular enlargement, as indicated by the uplifted apex.

The radiographic appearance is influenced a great deal by the associated lesions. TGA is the most frequent anomaly causing pulmonary overcirculation in a cyanotic infant (see Fig. 31-16). The presence of significant pulmonic stenosis

produces a radiographic appearance similar to tetralogy of Fallot (i.e., decreased pulmonary vascularity and normal heart size in a cyanotic infant). The radiographic appearance during the first day or first few days of life may not be characteristic, since a prominent thymus conceals the narrow great vessel region and pulmonary blood flow is still limited by high pulmonary vascular resistance persisting from intrauterine life. After thymic involution in the stressed newborn, the narrow base of the heart becomes evident (Table 31-14; see Fig. 31-16).

Corrected Transposition (l-TGA)

Corrected transposition consists of arterioventricular transposition and atrioventricular discordance. The aorta originates from the right ventricle and the right ventricle is inverted with connection to the left atrium. There is an L-ventricular loop with the morphologic right ventricle to the left of the morphologic left ventricle. Thus, blood flow in the central circulation is corrected; pulmonary venous blood flows to the left atrium, to the right ventricle, and into the aorta. Most patients with corrected transposition have significant additional cardiac anomalies. The most frequent ones are pulmonic stenosis, VSD, Ebstein's anomaly (tricuspid regurgitation into the left atrium), and complete heart block (Table 31-15; Fig. 31-36).

Double-Outlet Right Ventricle

Double-outlet right ventricle is an anomaly in which more than 50% of both great vessels originate from the right ventricle. The aorta is positioned further to the right of the pulmonary artery and originates completely from the right ventricle, while the pulmonary artery may originate entirely from the right ventricle or have a biventricular origin (Taussig-Bing malformation). A VSD is always present, and other associated anomalies are frequent. The physiology of double-outlet right ventricle is determined to a great

TABLE 31.14 Salient Radiographic Features of Transposition
Pulmonary arterial overcirculation: Asymmetry of pulmonary flow, greater on the right side, is sometimes apparent.
Pulmonary edema is frequent, especially in the presence of a VSD or PDA.
Cardiomegaly: A cardiothoracic ratio exceeding 0.58 constitutes cardiomegaly in the neonatal period.
In newborns, specific chamber enlargement is difficult to identify. In older children, there is left atrial and right ventricular enlargement.
Narrow vascular pedicle: The great vessels are usually but not invariably inconspicuous (see Fig. 31-16). The ascending aorta occupies a more medial position than normal and is hidden in the mediastinum. Likewise, the pulmonary artery lies medially within the mediastinum, so a typical main pulmonary arterial segment is not present. Thus, there is the incongruity of pulmonary arterial overcirculation with a small or absent main pulmonary arterial segment. Infrequently, even in complete TGA, the aorta lies to the right or left of the pulmonary artery, causing a normal or even increased width of the pedicle.
Right aortic arch occurs in about 5% of patients with TGA, usually in association with pulmonic stenosis and VSD.
In the presence of pulmonic stenosis and VSD, there is decreased pulmonary vascular size and normal heart size, producing an appearance similar to tetralogy of Fallot.

ASD, atrial septal defect; TGA, transposition of the great arteries; VSD, ventricular septal defect.

TABLE 31.15 Salient Radiographic Features of Corrected Transposition
Prominent convexity of upper left cardiac border (see Fig. 31-36): The convexity may extend nearly to the arch or merely involve the base of the heart.
Ascending aortic shadow on the right is not visible (see Fig. 31-36).
Crossing of the edge of the ascending aorta and the lateral edge of the proximal descending aorta
Conspicuous absence of a convex main pulmonary arterial segment even in the presence of pulmonary arterial overcirculation: Sometimes there is upward tilt of the right and downward tilt of the left pulmonary artery.
Left atrial enlargement can be caused by pulmonary overcirculation caused by the ventricular septal defect or by tricuspid regurgitation caused by Ebstein's anomaly.

FIG. 31-36. Corrected transposition of great arteries (L-ventricular loop with l-TGA). There is a prominent elongated convexity (*arrow*) of the upper left cardiac border.

degree by the position of the VSD. A VSD oriented to the aortic valve (subaortic VSD) causes preferential flow from the left ventricle into the aorta and is frequently associated with significant pulmonic stenosis, resulting in physiology and radiographic appearance similar to tetralogy of Fallot. In the absence of pulmonic stenosis, preferential left ventricular to aortic flow may make cyanosis minimal. A VSD located beneath the pulmonic valve (Taussig-Bing malformation) causes preferential flow from the left ventricle into the pulmonary artery and consequently severe pulmonary arterial overcirculation. The right ventricular outflow is preferentially into the aorta; consequently, there is also cyanosis. Coarctation or interruption of the aortic arch is sometimes associated with the subpulmonic VSD. A large VSD may be situated beneath the origin of both great vessels (doubly committed VSD) or may be displaced away

TABLE 31.16 Salient Features of DORV Without Significant Pulmonic Stenosis

Pulmonary arterial overcirculation: It is one of the causes of cyanosis and pulmonary arterial overcirculation (see Fig. 31-37).
Cardiomegaly
Enlargement of left atrium, left ventricle, and right ventricle: Distinction between left and right ventricle enlargement during infancy is usually inconclusive.
Widened great artery pedicle due to side-by-side position of aorta and pulmonary artery (see Fig. 31-37): This is not always evident. It can be a distinguishing feature when compared to the appearance of d-TGA.
Prominent main pulmonary arterial segment: This can also be a distinguishing feature for DORV in comparison with d-TGA.
Signs of coarctation or interruption of the aortic arch

DORV, double-outlet right ventricle; TGA, transposition of the great arteries.

TABLE 31.17 Salient Radiographic Features of DORV with Pulmonic Stenosis

Decreased pulmonary vascularity
Normal or nearly normal cardiac size
Right ventricular prominence
Inconspicuous main pulmonary arterial segment
Right aortic arch in about 10%–15% of patients

from both origins (noncommitted VSD). The great arteries tend to be side by side at the base of the heart, but either vessel can be located more anteriorly.

This is an admixture lesion that causes the combination of cyanosis (right-to-left shunt) and pulmonary arterial overcirculation (left-to-right shunt). The severity of pulmonic stenosis and the position of the VSD initially determine the relative severity of the two shunts.

Double-outlet left ventricle is an exceedingly rare anomaly in which both arteries originate from a morphologic left ventricle. The presentation and radiologic appearance are similar to double-outlet right ventricle (Tables 31-16 and 31-17; Fig. 31-37).

Tricuspid Atresia

Tricuspid atresia is the absence of a direct connection of the right atrium to the right ventricle. The atresia can be due to a membrane or a ridge of muscle between the chambers. An atrial septal defect or patent foramen ovale is always present. Other associated lesions are frequent and are usually important in determining the physiology and clinical presentation. The most frequently associated lesions are TGA, VSD, and pulmonic stenosis. A classification of tricuspid atresia is based on the presence or absence of these associated lesions. Tricuspid atresia without TGA can be (1) with pulmonary

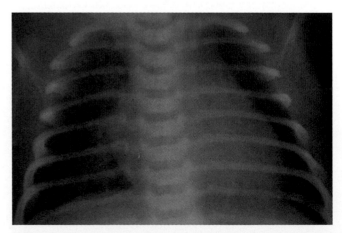

FIG. 31-37. Double-outlet right ventricle. Note pulmonary arterial overcirculation and cardiomegaly. Prominent great vessel region is shown in contradistinction to narrow great vessel region as seen in d-TGA.

TABLE 31.18 Salient Radiographic Features of Tricuspid Atresia

With normally related great vessels, VSD, and pulmonic stenosis, the appearance is similar to tetralogy of Fallot (see Fig. 31-12). There is decreased pulmonary vascularity, small central pulmonary arteries, and normal or nearly normal heart size. A distinguishing feature from tetralogy, if discernible, is prominence of the left atrium and left ventricle and flat right atrial border (see Fig. 31-12).

With TGA, VSD without pulmonic stenosis, the typical feature of d-TGA, is present. There is pulmonary overcirculation, cardiomegaly, and a narrow vascular pedicle. A distinguishing feature may be the right atrial border. The right atrial border (right atrial enlargement) is frequently prominent in d-TGA, but it is not prominent or even flat in tricuspid atresia when the interatrial communication is large (see Figs. 31-12, 31-38, and 31-40).

With a small (restrictive) interatrial communication, the right atrium may enlarge considerably. The right atrium enlarges to the extent of causing considerable cardiomegaly as depicted on the frontal radiograph (see Fig. 31-39).

Tricuspid atresia with TGA is sometimes associated with left juxtaposition of the atrial appendages: the right atrial appendage extends posteriorly behind the great arteries and lies above the left atrial appendage. This causes a prominent upper left cardiac border and flattening of the right cardiac border (see Fig. 31-40).

VSD, ventricular septal defect; TGA, transposition of the great arteries.

FIG. 31-39. Tricuspid atresia with small (restrictive) atrial septal defect and large ventricular septal defect. Small atrial septal defect is responsible for right atrial enlargement (*arrow*) and thus cardiomegaly. Large ventricular septal defect results in pulmonary arterial overcirculation.

atresia and no VSD; (2) with pulmonary stenosis and a small restrictive VSD; or (3) with no pulmonary stenosis and a large nonrestrictive VSD. Tricuspid atresia with TGA can be (1) with pulmonary atresia and a large VSD; (2) with pulmonary stenosis and a large VSD; or (3) with no pulmonary stenosis and a large VSD.

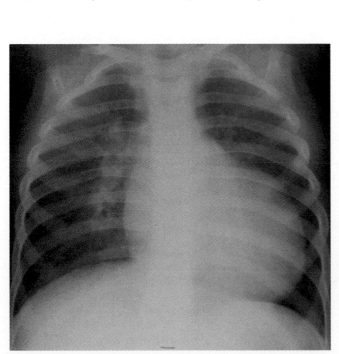

FIG. 31-38. Tricuspid atresia with transposition of great arteries. Radiograph shows the narrow base of the heart that is characteristic for transposition. Flat right atrial border is a feature of tricuspid atresia with nonrestrictive atrial septal defect.

FIG. 31-40. Tricuspid atresia, transposition, and juxtaposition of atrial appendages. Prominent upper left cardiac border (*arrows*) is due to the abnormal position of the right atrial appendage on the left, above the left atrial appendage. The flat contour of the right atrium is also characteristic of this anomaly.

TABLE 31.19 Salient Radiographic Appearance of Single Ventricle

With normally related arteries and no pulmonic stenosis, the appearance is like a VSD or d-TGA, depending on the preferential streaming in the ventricle. There is pulmonary overcirculation and cardiomegaly.

With significant pulmonic stenosis and normally related great arteries, the appearance is reduced pulmonary vascularity and normal or nearly normal heart size. The appearance is similar to tetralogy of Fallot.

With d-TGA, the appearance can be typical of d-TGA. Pulmonary blood flow may be increased or decreased.

With l-TGA, the appearance can be typical of l-TGA. Pulmonary blood flow may be increased or decreased. A notch along the upper left cardiac border may be due to the intersection of the contour of an inverted right ventricular outlet chamber with the dominant ventricle (see Fig. 31-41).

VSD, ventricular septal defect; TGA, transposition of the great arteries.

The most common form is tricuspid atresia with pulmonic stenosis and normally related great arteries and restrictive VSD. TGA is present in about 30% of patients with tricuspid atresia. It is usually associated with VSD and no pulmonic stenosis.

When the VSD is large and the pulmonary stenosis mild or nonexistent, there is pulmonary overcirculation. This is the situation both for normally related arteries and TGA. Restriction of pulmonary blood flow usually exists at pulmonic valvular and subvalvular levels or at a restrictive VSD. A small atrial septal communication also limits pulmonary flow and additionally causes the right atrium to enlarge. Despite obstruction to the right atrial outlet, the right atrium usually does not dilate since a large interatrial communication causes the right atrium to function as a venous conduit similar to the vena cavae (Table 31-18; Figs. 31-12 and 31-38 to 31-40).

FIG. 31-41. Single ventricle with inverted outlet chamber (L-loop) and l-TGA. Prominent convexity of upper left cardiac border represents the inverted right ventricle outlet chamber (*arrows*) and the l-transposed ascending aorta.

Single Ventricle

Single ventricle consists of a predominant ventricle that receives both atrioventricular valves (double-inlet ventricle) and a tiny remnant portion of the other ventricle. A more specific term for most of the anomalies grouped under this title is *univentricular atrioventricular connections.* The great arteries can both originate from the dominant ventricle, or one may originate from the small ventricle. The dominant ventricle can be either the left or right.

TABLE 31.20 Two Classification Systems for Truncus Arteriosus

Type	Description
Grouped according to the site of origin of the pulmonary arteries from the truncus	
I	A main pulmonary artery originates from the proxima portion of the truncus, usually from the left posterolateral aspect
II	Right and left pulmonary arteries have individual origins from the posterior aspect of the truncus
III	One of both pulmonary arteries arises from the lateral aspect of the truncus
IV	No pulmonary arteries arise from the ascending truncus (aorta) but rather from the descending aorta. This type is not really a truncus arteriosus but rather pulmonary atresia with VSD and major pulmonary blood flow from bronchial and other systemic arteries originating from the descending aorta.
Classification of Van Pragh and Van Pragh	
I	Common pulmonary artery arises from truncus
II	Right and left pulmonary arteries arise separately from truncus
III	Absence of one pulmonary artery, other pulmonary artery arises from ductus
IV	Common pulmonary artery arises from truncus with arch interruption

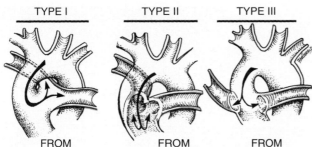

FIG. 31-42. The types of truncus arteriosus: type I, single origin of main pulmonary artery; type II, separate origins of left and right pulmonary arteries from dorsal aspect of the truncus; type III, separate origins of left and right pulmonary arteries from the left and right side of the truncus.

Single ventricle is frequently associated with an abnormality of arterioventricular connection, such as TGA or double-outlet right ventricle. Normally related great vessels are uncommon with single ventricle. The left ventricular type of single ventricle is frequently associated with an inverted right ventricular outlet chamber and l-TGA. The dominant ventricle communicates with the outlet chamber through a "bulboventricular foramen."

The physiology is determined to a substantial degree by associated obstruction of the outflow to the pulmonary artery or aorta. There is an admixture of systemic and pulmonary venous blood in the dominant ventricle, so both cyanosis and

TABLE 31.21 Salient Radiographic Features of Truncus Arteriosus

Pulmonary arterial overcirculation (see Fig. 31-4 and 31-17): Asymmetry of flow is not uncommon, even to the extent of plethora on one side and oligemia on the other.
Pulmonary venous hypertension or edema is frequent, especially in type I.
Cardiomegaly: The heart size is frequently, but not always, proportionate to the pulmonary overcirculation. Cardiomegaly may also be related to truncal insufficiency. Four-chamber enlargement may be present. Enlargement of left atrium and left ventricle is generally identified.
Prominent main pulmonary arterial segment (type I; see Fig. 31-4) or reduced main pulmonary arterial segment (type II or III): In type I, the left pulmonary artery has a higher position than usual, and a comma-shaped configuration ("hilar comma") as it curves upward and leftward (see Fig. 31-4).
Right aortic arch in about 35% of patients (see Figs. 31-4 and 31-17).
Dilated ascending aorta: There are two cyanotic lesions that are frequently associated with a large ascending aortic shadow: one causes decreased pulmonary vascularity (tetralogy of Fallot) and the other causes increased pulmonary vascularity (truncus arteriosus).

TABLE 31.22 Frequency of Right Aortic Arch in Congenital Heart Disease

Abnormality	Frequency (%)
Tetralogy of Fallot	20
Pulmonary atresia with ventricular septal defect	25
Truncus arteriosus	35
Double outlet right ventricle	12
Tricuspid atresia	10–15
Transposition of great arteries	5–8
Ventricular septal defect	2

pulmonary overcirculation occur. The presence and severity of the pulmonary overcirculation are regulated by pulmonary stenosis. If pulmonary stenosis is severe, the physiology and clinical presentation are similar to tetralogy of Fallot. If obstruction to pulmonary blood flow is not present, then the physiology and clinical presentation are similar to transposition. The physiology of the common ventricle is identical to a large VSD, which is really the proper designation for this lesion (Table 31-19; Fig. 31-41).

Truncus Arteriosus

Truncus arteriosus is a single trunk originating from the heart and supplying the pulmonary, systemic, and coronary arteries. The truncus straddles a large VSD. It is an admixture lesion, with both left-to-right and right-to-left shunts. Two classification systems for truncus arteriosus are extant currently. The older and more familiar one was proposed by Collett and Edward in 1949. The types are grouped according to the site of origin of the pulmonary arteries from the truncus (Table 31-20; Fig. 31-42).

The truncal valve can have two to five cusps. The valves with numbers of cusps more or less than three are frequently incompetent, and truncal insufficiency can be severe. Hemitruncus is not infrequent; one pulmonary artery originates from the ascending aorta and the other arises directly from the right ventricle. Stenosis at the origin of the right and/or left pulmonary arteries is common, especially in types II and III of Collett and Edwards. Consequently, asymmetry of blood flow occurs with this anomaly. A right aortic arch is common (Tables 31-21 and 31-22).

The physiology is characterized by excess pulmonary blood flow and frequent volume overload of especially left-sided chambers. This is one of the lesions causing pulmonary arterial overcirculation in a cyanotic patient. Congestive heart failure and pulmonary edema are common.

Total Anomalous Pulmonary Venous Connection

All pulmonary veins connect to a systemic venous structure or the right atrium directly in this anomaly. This is another admixture lesion. Generally, the pulmonary veins form a central confluence before entering the systemic venous site.

TABLE 31.23 Salient Radiographic Features of TAPVC without Venous Obstruction

Pulmonary arterial overcirculation (see Figs. 31-18 and 31-43). Pulmonary venous hypertension and edema may be present with extreme volume overload.

Cardiomegaly. This is usually proportionate to the pulmonary arterial overcirculation.

Enlargement of right atrium and right ventricle

The enlarged systemic vein into which drainage occurs or the anomalous connecting vein may be visible as the "snowman appearance" (see Figs. 31-18 and 31-43), dilated right superior vena cava, or dilated azygous vein or coronary sinus.

TAPVC, total anamalous pulmonary venous connections.

FIG. 31-43. Total anomalous pulmonary venous connection, supracardiac type (type I). Note pulmonary arterial overcirculation, cardiomegaly, and enlargement of superior mediastinum ("snowman" appearance). The snowman is caused by the dilated vertical vein connecting to the left innominate vein (left-sided enlargement) and the dilated superior vena cava (right-sided enlargement).

Infrequently, they do not all join together and may drain to different sites. This anomaly is divided into three types based on the site of pulmonary venous drainage.

In the supracardiac type, connections are to the left innominate vein, right superior vena cava, or azygos vein. A left-sided vertical vein connects the pulmonary venous confluence to the left innominate vein. The cardiac type has connections to the right atrium or coronary sinus. In the infracardiac type, connection is below the diaphragm to the portal vein or one of its branches, ductus venosus, or hepatic vein. In this type, a long vein courses from the pulmonary venous confluence and through the esophageal hiatus to its site of infradiaphragmatic connection. Pulmonary venous drainage is always obstructed with this type because of a variety of mechanisms, including narrowing or stenosis of the connecting vein at its site of connection with the systemic vein, or the systemic vein itself. The need for pulmonary venous blood to pass through the hepatic sinusoids has also been held to be an additional site of obstruction. However, portal venous pressure is not higher than pulmonary venous pressure in normal individuals. Infrequently, total anomalous pulmonary venous connection above the diaphragm is associated with pulmonary venous obstruction.

The physiology of total anomalous pulmonary venous connection depends on whether pulmonary venous obstruction exists. Mixing systemic and pulmonary venous blood occurs in the right atrium, and there is an obligatory right-

to-left shunt of mixed venous blood through an interatrial connection. The size of the communication determines the volume of the flow to the left heart. Preferential flow from the right atrium is usually to the right ventricle and pulmonary artery, causing a large volume of recirculated blood. In total anomalous pulmonary venous connection above the diaphragm, the volume of pulmonary blood flow is very high and is the major feature, while cyanosis may be mild. The volume overload of the lungs may be so great that pulmonary edema occurs.

In total anomalous pulmonary venous connection with obstruction, the major feature is pulmonary venous hypertension and edema. The flow to the lungs is not very great.

TABLE 31.24 Salient Radiographic Features of TAPVC with Venous Obstruction

Pulmonary edema (see Fig. 31-21)

Normal heart size

Prominence of right atrium and less frequently, right ventricle

Infrequently the connecting vein can be identified on the lateral view in a position behind the heart. A barium swallow may show an anterior impression on the esophagus.

TAPVC, total anamalous pulmonary venous connections.

TABLE 31.25 Salient Radiographic Features of Ebstein's Anomaly

Decreased pulmonary vascularity (see Figs. 31-3 and 31-14)

Cardiomegaly (see Figs. 31-3 and 31-14)

Enlarged right atrium: The right heart border is elongated, with a prominent convexity.

Enlargement of right ventricle. The right ventricle is less conspicuous than the atrium.

Main pulmonary arterial segment and hilar segments are small. However, the right ventricular outflow tract may produce a prominent bulge just caudal to the pulmonary arterial segment on the frontal view.

Small thoracic aorta

TABLE 31.26 Salient Radiographic Features of Type I Pulmonary Atresia

Decreased pulmonary vascularity
Normal cardiac size or only slight cardiomegaly
Concave main pulmonary arterial segment and small hilar pulmonary arteries
Uplifted apex: This appearance may be due to left ventricular enlargement in the presence of a diminutive right ventricle.
Thoracic aorta can be enlarged.

TABLE 31.28 Salient Features of Compensated Valvular Pulmonic Stenosis

Normal pulmonary vascularity
Normal cardiac size
Right ventricular enlargement or prominence: This is usually detected initially on the lateral view as a prominent convexity of the anterior cardiac border or filling of the retrosternal space.
Poststenotic dilatation of main pulmonary arterial segment (see Fig. 31-44)
Dilated and usually laterally displaced left pulmonary artery (see Fig. 31-44)

Because there is less pulmonary venous blood to mix with the desaturated systemic venous blood, cyanosis is conspicuous. Total anomalous pulmonary venous connection can occur in association with a number of other cardiac anomalies. It is a frequent lesion in patients with the asplenia syndrome (Tables 31-23 and 31-24; Fig. 31-43).

Ebstein's Anomaly

Ebstein's anomaly is a deformity of the tricuspid valve in which one or more leaflets are displaced into the inflow portion of the right ventricle. The leaflets have lines of attachment to the right ventricle of varying length. The displacement into the right ventricle and the deformity of the valve cause tricuspid regurgitation, and the mural attachments in the right ventricle may cause obstruction to pulmonary blood flow. The septal and posterior leaflets are involved, while the anterior leaflet usually has a normal attachment to the atrioventricular ring. A small to substantial portion of the inflow region of the right ventricle has a thin wall and lacks ventricular myocardium (atrialization of the right ventricle). A patent foramen ovale or secundum atrial septal defect is present in about 80% of cases.

The physiologic consequence of the lesion is nearly always tricuspid regurgitation and usually a small-volume right-to-left shunt. Cyanosis may be absent or very mild. Occasionally the major effect is tricuspid obstruction, due to limitation of the atrioventricular inlet to only narrow slits in the displaced leaflets of the valve. In this circumstance the right-to-left shunt is more severe. In the 20% or so of patients without an interatrial communication, cyanosis is not present (Table 31-25).

Pulmonary Atresia with Intact Ventricular Septum

Pulmonary atresia with intact ventricular septum exists in two forms: hypoplasia of the right ventricle and tricuspid valve with little or no tricuspid regurgitation (type I) or a normal or enlarged right ventricle with significant tricuspid regurgitation (type II). This entity is distinct from pulmonary atresia with VSD (extreme form of tetralogy of Fallot).

The physiology of this lesion is reduced pulmonary blood flow, so that the volume of fully oxygenated blood entering the left atrium is small. The shunting of nearly all systemic venous blood occurs through the interatrial communication. There is admixture of desaturated and oxygenated blood in the left atrium. Because the volume of pulmonary venous blood is reduced, cyanosis is severe. Blood reaches the lung by a PDA and/or bronchial arteries (Tables 31-26 and 31-27).

Pulmonic Stenosis

Pulmonary valvular stenosis exists in two distinct syndromes. The most frequent type presents in an innocuous manner with mild symptoms, a systolic murmur, and a slightly abnormal thoracic radiograph. Infrequently, infants present with severe symptoms and marked cardiomegaly. The severity of the valvular stenosis is so great that the right ventricle dilates markedly and right ventricular failure ensues. Because of the elevated right-sided diastolic pressure, there is considerable right-to-left shunting across a secundum atrial septal defect or stretched foramen ovale. When the stenosis

TABLE 31.27 Salient Radiographic Features of Type II Pulmonary Atresia

Decreased pulmonary vascularity (see Fig. 31-13)
Cardiomegaly (see Fig. 31-13)
Right atrial and right ventricular enlargement
Small pulmonary arterial segment
Thoracic aorta may be enlarged.

TABLE 31.29 Salient Radiographic Features of Critical Pulmonic Stenosis

Decreased pulmonary vascularity
Cardiomegaly
Enlargement of right atrium and ventricle
Enlarged main pulmonary arterial segment

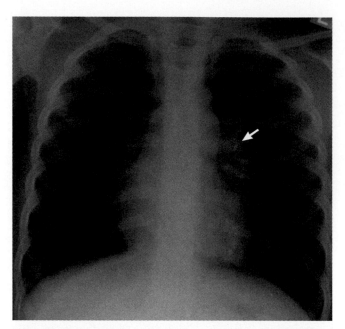

FIG. 31-44. Valvular pulmonic stenosis. Radiograph shows enlargement of the main and left pulmonary arterial (*arrow*) segments. The descending branch of the left pulmonary artery is frequently very prominent.

is so severe that right ventricular failure occurs, the entity is called critical pulmonary stenosis (Tables 31-28 and 31-29; Fig. 31-44).

Hypoplastic Left Heart

This lesion consists of several or all of the following features: hypoplastic ascending aorta, severe aortic stenosis or atresia, hypoplastic left ventricle (thick wall and diminutive cavity), and mitral atresia. The coronary arteries are perfused by right-to-left flow across a PDA and retrograde into the ascending aorta. An atrial septal communication is present so that admixture of pulmonary and systemic venous blood occurs in the right atrium. Consequently, there is volume overload of the right-sided chambers and excess pulmonary blood flow. The usual clinical presentation is severe congestive heart failure in the first few days of life (Table 31-30; see Fig. 31-22).

TABLE 31.30 Salient Radiographic Features of Hypoplastic Left Heart

Pulmonary arterial overcirculation and/or pulmonary edema (see Fig. 31-22)
Cardiomegaly (see Fig. 31-22)
Prominent right-sided chambers, especially the right atrium (see Fig. 31-22)
Because of the patent ductus, the aortic arch may be prominent (see Fig. 31-22).

TABLE 31.31 Cause of Rib Notching

Aortic obstruction
  Coarctation of the aorta
  Interruption of the aorta
  Acquired obstruction of the aorta: Takayasu's aortitis, atherosclerotic obstruction, etc.
  Unusual causes of coarctation: neurofibromatosis, Williams' syndrome, rubella syndrome
Subclavian arterial obstruction
  Blalock-Taussig shunt (upper 2 ribs)
  Takayasu's arteritis (usually unilateral)
  Atherosclerosis
Severely reduced pulmonary blood flow
  Tetralogy of Fallot
  Pulmonary atresia
  Tricuspid atresia
  Unilateral absence or atresia of a pulmonary artery
  Pulmonary emphysema
  Chronic pulmonary thromboembolic disease
  Superior vena canal obstruction
Vascular shunts
  Pulmonary arteriovenous shunt
  Intercostal arteriovenous shunt
  Intercostal to pulmonary arterial shunt
  Intercostal neuroma
  Poliomyelitis (upper margin)
  Hyperparathyroidism

(Modified from Felson B. *Chest Roentgenology*. Philadelphia: WB Saunders; 1973.)

Coarctation of the Aorta

Coarctation of the aorta is a narrowing of the distal aortic arch and/or proximal descending aorta due to a discrete fibromuscular ring or a long- or short-segment tunnel narrowing of the aortic isthmus. There may also be hypoplasia of the posterior portion of the aortic arch. The coarctation usually occurs adjacent to the site of attachment of the ligamentum arteriosus and distal to the left subclavian artery.

TABLE 31.32 Salient Radiographic Features in Compensated Coarctation

Rib notching (see Fig. 31-45)
Retrosternal undulating soft tissue due to dilated tortuous internal mammary arteries (site of collateral flow)
Abnormal appearance of the aortic arch (see Fig. 31-45)
A notch on the proximal descending aorta followed by poststenotic dilatation causes a figure-3 sign on the aorta (see Fig. 31-45) and a reverse figure-3 sign on the barium-filled esophagus.
Left ventricular prominence
Prominent ascending aorta
A duplicated aortic "knob" may be caused by tortuosity of the posterior arch and proximal descending aorta causing kinking of the aorta: This is called pseudocoarctation of the aorta when no pressure gradient exists.

TABLE 31.33 Salient Radiographic Features in Decompensated Coarctation

Pulmonary venous hypertension or edema
Cardiomegaly (see Fig. 31-46)
Left ventricular enlargement
Pulmonary arterial overcirculation is present, with associated ventricular septal defect and patent ductus arteriosus.
Rib notching is not present during infancy.
The aortic knob is usually not characteristic during infancy. The only sign may be lateral displacement of the descending aortic stripe.

The coarctation is infrequently proximal to the origin of the left subclavian artery. The coarctation can extend into the origin of the left subclavian artery, causing stenosis of this artery. Both of these situations cause lower arterial pressure in the left compared to the right pulmonary artery. Anomalous origin of the right subclavian artery (retroesophageal right subclavian artery) from a site distal to the coarctation causes lower arterial pressure in the right arm.

Coarctation may be associated with a wide variety of congenital lesions, but two occur with noticeable frequency: PDA and VSD. The triad of coarctation, VSD, and PDA has been called the coarctation syndrome and is especially

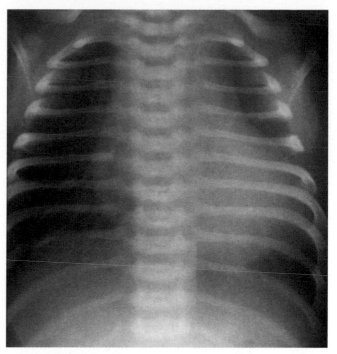

FIG. 31-46. Coarctation of the aorta in a newborn. Radiograph shows severe cardiomegaly without pulmonary arterial overcirculation. This is characteristic of a group V lesion, of which coarctation is the most frequent cause after 1 week of age.

frequent when the lesion presents in early infancy. A bicuspid aortic valve occurs in a high percentage of patients.

The physiology is hypertension in arteries originating proximal to the site of coarctation and reduced blood flow to arteries arising below the coarctation. If the coarctation occurs proximal to the site of origin of one of the subclavian arteries, then there is hypertension in only one arm and rib notching on only the side with hypertension. The numerous causes of rib notching are listed in Table 31-31. The 4th to 8th ribs are the ones usually notched; the 3rd and 9th ribs are less frequently notched. The notching consists of scalloped

FIG. 31-45. Coarctation of the aorta. Abnormal contour of arch and proximal descending aorta. The duplicated aortic knob is due to poststenotic dilatation (*arrow*) in the proximal descending aorta. There is outward displacement of the lateral margin of the descending aorta. A figure-3 configuration is caused by the notch at the site of the coarctation with poststenotic dilatation. Rib notching is present (*arrowheads*).

TABLE 31.34 Salient Radiographic Features of Interruption of Aortic Arch

Isolated variety has the appearance as described for coarctation.
Interruption with ventricular septal defect and patent ductus arteriosus causes pulmonary arterial overcirculation and usually severe pulmonary edema with cardiomegaly (see Fig. 31-47).
The trachea is sometimes identified to lie exactly in the midline, and there is no indentation on the trachea (see Figs. 31-47 and 31-48).
If a patent ductus arteriosus is present, the posterior arch may be prominent yet the trachea, not indented, lies exactly in the midline (see Fig. 31-47).

FIG. 31-47. Interruption of aortic arch with ventricular septal defect and patent ductus arteriosus. Radiograph shows pulmonary arterial overcirculation, cardiomegaly due to left ventricular enlargement, and enlargement of main pulmonary arterial and aortic arch segments. Despite the enlarged aortic arch segment (*arrow*), the trachea (*T*) is situated directly in the midline.

regions on the undersurface of the posterior portion of the ribs. The posterior upper surface is infrequently involved. Sclerosis may outline the scalloped sites. Rib notching is unusual in patients younger than 5 years of age. Rib notching depends on the origin of the ipsilateral subclavian artery

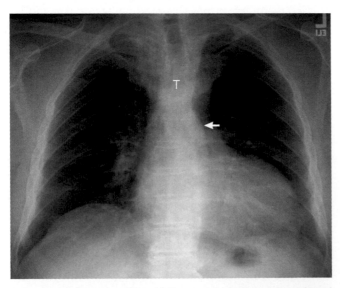

FIG. 31-48. Interruption of the aortic arch as an isolated anomaly. Radiographs show midline trachea and dilated proximal descending aorta (*arrow*) below the narrow site of interruption.

TABLE 31.35 Salient Radiographic Features in Uncomplicated Aortic Stenosis
Normal heart size
Enlargement of ascending aorta: This occurs in valvular stenosis and about half of patients with discrete membranous subvalvular stenosis.
Ascending aorta is small in supravalvular form (see Fig. 31-49).

proximal to the site of the coarctation. Coarctation proximal to the left subclavian arterial origin causes right-sided rib notching only, while an anomalous origin of the right subclavian artery from a site below the coarctation produces unilateral left-sided notching.

Hypertension usually causes left ventricular hypertrophy but may induce left ventricular dilatation and failure if extremely severe. Left ventricular dilatation, myocardial failure, and pulmonary edema are most likely to occur in early infancy (Tables 31-32 and 31-33; Figs. 31-45 and 31-46).

Interruption of Aortic Arch

The arch can be interrupted at any of three sites: beyond the left subclavian artery (type A); between the left subclavian and left common carotid arteries (type B); and between the innominate artery and left carotid artery (type C). Types A and B occur with approximately equal frequency; type C is rare. The right subclavian artery sometimes originates ectopically as a fourth aortic branch in this anomaly, which is called a type B2 interruption. In this circumstance, hypertension is confined to the carotid arteries.

This lesion can exist in an isolated form but usually is associated with VSD and PDA. There is an association with double-outlet right ventricle with subpulmonic VSD (Taussig-Bing malformation; Table 31-34; Figs. 31-47 and 31-48).

Aortic Stenosis

Congenital aortic stenosis is caused by a bicuspid aortic valve, unicuspid and unicommissural, or dysplastic valves. It may be so severe as to induce intractable left ventricular failure in the neonate (critical aortic stenosis). Stenosis also occurs at the subvalvular (discrete membranous or tunnel forms) and supravalvular sites (Tables 31-35 and 31-36; Figs. 31-49 and 31-50; see also Table 32-1 in Chapter 32).

TABLE 31.36 Salient Radiographic Features of Critical Aortic Stenosis
Pulmonary venous hypertension or edema (see Fig. 31-50)
Cardiomegaly (see Fig. 31-50)
Left ventricular enlargement

FIG. 31-50. Critical aortic stenosis. Radiograph in an infant shows pulmonary edema and cardiomegaly.

FIG. 31-49. Supravalvular aortic stenosis. Concavity is seen in the region occupied by the ascending aorta.

SELECTED READING

Elliott LB. Cardiac Imaging in Infants, Children, and Adults. Philadelphia: JB Lippincott, 1991.
Higgins CB. Radiography of congenital heart disease. In: Essentials of Cardiac Radiology and Imaging. Philadelphia: JB Lippincott, 1992:49.

CHAPTER

32

Valvular Heart Disease

CHARLES B. HIGGINS AND KAREN ORDOVAS

The goals of imaging in valvular heart disease are as follows:

1. Identification of stenosis or insufficiency of one or more valves.
2. Estimation of the pressure gradient (or valve orifice area) and severity of regurgitation (regurgitant fraction).
3. Quantification of ventricular volumes, mass, and function.
4. Sequential monitoring of ventricular volumes, mass, and function. Determination of response to therapy.
5. Exclusion of significant coronary artery disease, especially prior to surgery.

Echocardiography is the most commonly used technique for the evaluation of valvular disease. For the most part, it has replaced cardiac catheterization for definitive diagnoses and assessment of severity of valvular dysfunction. The echocardiographic aspects of valvular heart disease are the topic of a number of chapters in other textbooks. The current role of angiography is the exclusion of significant coronary artery disease before surgery or as a contributing factor for heart failure in these patients. In the future, noninvasive imaging of coronary arteries by multidetector CT may suffice for these purposes.

All valvular lesions exert a stress on the supporting ventricle. Valvular stenosis exerts a pressure overload, which involves the compensatory mechanism of myocardial hypertrophy. Regurgitation exerts a volume overload, which involves chamber dilatation. Eventually, these compensatory mechanisms are dissipated, and in the end stage of valvular heart disease, myocardial failure and low cardiac output state ensue.

AORTIC STENOSIS

Aortic stenosis usually is described at three anatomic levels: supravalvular, valvular, and subvalvular. The classification of the types of aortic stenoses is presented in Table 32-1.

Supravalvular stenosis nearly always is a congenital anomaly, either as an isolated lesion or as part of the Williams' syndrome. The supravalvular narrowing has roughly three configurations: focal constriction at the sinotubular junction (hourglass configuration) with post-stenotic dilation

of the mid and distal ascending aorta, focal membrane at the sinotubular junction, and tubular narrowing from the sinotubular junction to just below the origin of the innominate artery. The Williams' syndrome is characterized by hypercalcemia, elfin facies, variable mental retardation and characteristic personality ("cocktail party personality"), hypertension, and additional peripheral arterial stenoses.

Concomitant cardiovascular lesions variably associated with supravalvular aortic stenosis include (1) aortic and pulmonary valvular stenoses, (2) peripheral pulmonary arterial stenoses, (3) diffuse hypoplasia of the aorta, (4) discrete stenoses of branches of the aortic arch and abdominal aorta, and (5) stenoses at origin of the coronary arteries. However, the coronary arteries usually are ectatic because they originate below the obstruction at the sinotubular junction and are thereby subjected to elevated pressure.

Rarely, supravalvular stenosis is acquired. This can be a sequelae of aortitis. Another possible cause is exaggerated scarring at the site of aortotomy performed for aortic valve replacement.

Valvular aortic stenosis may have either a congenital or acquired etiology. The congenital cause most often is a bicuspid aortic valve. A less common cause is a unicuspid valve; this type of valve causes more severe stenosis, usually presenting in the first year of life. A rare pathology is the primitive valve, usually consisting of a hypoplastic annulus containing a ring of gelatinous tissue. This lesion also presents most often during infancy. Rheumatic valvular aortic stenosis commonly occurs in association with mitral stenosis or regurgitation. Degenerative aortic stenosis is now the most frequent cause of calcific aortic stenosis in the adult. Although degenerative aortic stenosis once was considered to be a result of premature fibrosis and calcification of a bicuspid aortic valve, it is now recognized as degeneration of tricuspid aortic valves in elderly patients. The bicuspid aortic valve degenerates into hemodynamically significant aortic stenosis in the fourth and fifth decade; the tricuspid aortic valve degenerates into hemodynamically significant stenosis usually after the sixth decade. With the aging of the population, this type of aortic stenosis is becoming the most commonly encountered type. All types of acquired aortic stenosis are characterized by heavy calcification (calcific aortic stenosis).

Subvalvular aortic stenosis: Congenital subvalvular stenosis is caused most commonly by a thin membrane situated within 1 cm beneath the aortic cusps. Other

TABLE 32.1 Classification of Aortic Stenosis

Supravalvular
Congenital
  Hourglass shape
  Membranes or fibrous diaphragm
  Diffuse
  Acquired (aortitis; operative scarring)

Valvular
Congenital
  Bicuspid
  Unicuspid
  Primitive (dysplastic)
  Annular hypoplasia
Acquired
  Rheumatic
  Degenerative

Subvalvular
Congenital
  Discrete
  Membranous
  Fibromuscular tunnel
  Extra mitral valve tissue
  Idiopathic hypertrophic subaortic stenosis (hypertrophic cardiomyopathy-asymmetric type)

types consist of a discrete fibromuscular ring or tunnellike narrowing of the left ventricular (LV) outlet region. Redundant gelatinous tissue attached to the anterior mitral valve leaflet also may rarely cause subvalvular stenoses, either alone or as part of an endocardial cushion anomaly. Muscular subaortic stenosis is caused by the asymmetric form of hypertrophic cardiomyopathy. It is due to the combination of asymmetric hypertrophy of the upper septum and systolic anterior motion of the anterior leaflet of the mitral valve.

Radiography

The findings on chest x-ray in **valvular aortic stenosis** depend on the severity and level of the obstruction and the age at presentation (see Table 30-6 in Chapter 30). The x-ray image in infants presenting with symptoms of heart failure is characterized by pulmonary edema and cardiomegaly. Cardiomegaly without pulmonary edema also may occur. On the other hand, x-rays in older children and adults may display only enlargement of the ascending aorta. In the presence of severe LV hypertrophy (reduced ventricular compliance) or with the onset of myocardial failure, pulmonary venous hypertension or edema may become evident. This usually occurs late in the natural history of uncomplicated valvular aortic stenosis. The extent and density of aortic valvular calcification roughly parallel the severity of the stenosis in adults before the seventh decade. On the other hand, ascending aortic dilation does not correlate with severity of stenosis and may be substantial with a nonobstructive bicuspid valve.

Supravalvular aortic stenosis may cause a narrow base of the heart with inconspicuous ascending aortic region (right superior mediastinum; see Chapter 31). With **subvalvular aortic stenosis**, enlargement of the ascending aorta often is not evident on the chest x-ray. Ascending aortic enlargement is discernible in about 50% of patients with the membranous type of subvalvular stenosis.

Magnetic Resonance Imaging

Magnetic resonance imaging (MRI) can be used to identify valvular dysfunction and to assess the effect of the lesion on ventricular volumes, mass, and function (Table 32-2). In addition to identifying stenosis and regurgitation, the gradient across stenotic valves and volume of valvular regurgitation can be quantified. Sequential MRI studies can be used for monitoring the severity of the valvular lesion and ventricular function over time and in response to therapy.

Identification of Aortic Stenosis

Aortic stenosis is identified using cine MR images. Cine MR imaging consists of multiple gradient echo (GRE) or balanced steady-state free precession (b-SSFP) images in which the blood under normal flow conditions has bright (white) signal intensity. High-velocity jet flow, such as occurs with the flow across a valvular stenosis or the retrograde flow across a regurgitant orifice, produces a signal void (low-signal region within the bright signal of the blood pool) on GRE cine. Identification of valvular stenosis on GRE images is based on the typical appearance of the downstream chamber or great artery. The signal void of a dysfunctional valve appears as an area of diminished or absent signal persisting for most of systole or diastole. Aortic stenosis is detected readily on images in coronal, axial, and vertical long-axis planes, which display an area of signal loss distal to the valve during ventricular systole (Fig. 32-1).

Recognition of the signal void on cine MR images is critically dependent on the TE value employed. The signal void diminishes in area with decreasing TE value. Indeed, the signal void may not be discernible with TE values of less than 6 ms. For depiction of the signal void, a TE value of 12 or greater is generally used.

In recent years, the SSFP cine sequence has replaced GRE cine. With the former sequence, the high-velocity signal void is minimized and more complex. At moderately increased

TABLE 32.2 MR Features of Valvular Aortic Stenosis

1. Thickening and limitation of systolic excursion of cusps
2. +/− Bicuspid aortic valve
3. High-velocity jet (central increased signal and peripheral signal void) on cine—SSFP
4. Dilatation of proximal ascending aorta
5. Symmetric increase in LV wall thickness (≥12 mm)
6. Increase in LV mass—measured at end diastole on cine—SSFP in short-axis plane
7. Hyperdynamic LV contraction in compensated state

FIG. 32.1. Cine (gradient echo) MR image in the coronal plane during systole demonstrates a signal void emanating from the aortic valve in a patient with valvular aortic stenosis.

FIG. 32.3. Cine MR image on the left ventricular outflow tract view in systole shows a flow jet starting at the level of the aortic valve and extending to the ascending aorta (Ao). Periphery of the flow jet shows low signal intensity (*arrows*) and center of the flow jet (*arrowhead*) shows increased signal intensity (vena contracta). Note the post-stenotic dilatation of the ascending aorta.

velocities, the flow jet has increased signal (Fig. 32-2), but at very high velocities, the center of the jet shows high signal while the periphery may show a signal void (Fig. 32-3).

Estimation of the Valve Gradient

The valve gradient is estimated using velocity-encoded cine (VEC; phase contrast) MRI. VEC MRI measures the phase

FIG. 32.2. Cine MR image parallel to the aortic valve orifice shows a high-intensity flow jet (*arrow*) and thickened aortic valve leaflets in a patient with aortic stenosis.

shifts that accumulate as hydrogen nuclei move through a magnetic field gradient. The net phase shifts of protons within various voxels are displayed in gray levels, in proportion to the degree of phase shift. Because phase shift is basically proportional to motion over time, VEC MRI can be used to measure flow velocity. Reconstruction of VEC data provides a magnitude image (anatomic information) and a phase image (velocity information in selected direction; Fig. 32-4A). The velocity-encoding direction can be selected in any orientation or in all three dimensions. The cross-sectional area of the vessel can be measured by drawing a region of interest on the magnitude (amplitude) image. The same region of interest is then applied on the corresponding phase image, where spatial mean velocity is measured. The product of area and spatial mean velocity provides the instantaneous flow volume for a specific time frame of the cardiac cycle. Integration of all instantaneous flow volumes throughout the cardiac cycle (usually 16 or higher) gives volume flow per heartbeat (see Fig. 32-4B). This technique has been validated in vitro with flow phantoms and in vivo by comparing flow measurements in the pulmonary artery and the aorta with left and right stroke volumes measured by cine MRI in healthy volunteers.

The signal void on cine GRE caused by turbulence allows identification of stenosis or regurgitation. The currently employed SSFP cine sequence mitigates the signal

A   B

FIG. 32.4. A: Four magnitude (**top**) and phase (**bottom**) images acquired during the cardiac cycle to measure blood flow in the aorta. Regions of interest are drawn around the aorta on magnitude images to measure cross-sectional area and around phase images to measure spatial average velocity. Volumetric flow is the product of cross-sectional area and spatial average velocity. **B:** Schematic diagram of aortic blood flow versus time curve during an average cardiac cycle. Each point on the curve is derived from a pair of images acquired at 16 time points during a cardiac cycle.

void of high-velocity flow. The high-velocity jet of aortic stenosis may cause a central hyperintense jet with low signal or signal void at the edges of the jet (Fig. 32-3). The central hyperintensity corresponds to the vena contracta. Peak systolic jet velocities over 5.0 m/s have been measured with

this technique in patients with aortic stenosis. These values determined by phase-shift GRE have correlated with Doppler flow and catheter measurements. The peak velocity is determined by identifying the voxel with highest velocity on the phase contrast image in peak systole (Fig. 32-5). Using

A   B

FIG. 32.5. Magnitude **(A)** and phase **(B)** images from velocity-encoded cine MR sequence on the left ventricular outflow tract plane in systole show a flow jet in the ascending aorta starting at the level of the aortic valve, consistent with aortic stenosis. A manual region of interest outlines the area containing the peak velocity.

the measurement of peak velocity by VEC MR imaging, the pressure gradient can be estimated by the modified Bernoulli equation as $\Delta P = 4V^2$, where ΔP = pressure drop across the stenosis (mm Hg) and V = peak velocity (m/s). An example of the use of VEC to estimate the gradient across valvular aortic stenosis as derived from VEC measurement of a peak velocity of 4 m/s looks like this:

$$\Delta P = 4V^2$$
$$\Delta P = 4(4)^2$$
$$\Delta P = 64 \text{ mm Hg}$$

However, it should be noted that this measurement by VEC has limitations. The number of images reconstructed for a cardiac cycle may lack temporal resolution for capturing the exact instant when peak velocity occurs. The direction of flow encoding may differ from the flow direction of the jet. These limitations can be minimized by using three-dimensional flow encoding, but this further reduces temporal resolution.

Calculation of the Aortic Valve Orifice Area

The estimated gradient is dependent on the stroke volume, ejection time, and aortic pressure. It provides an incomplete assessment of severity of aortic stenosis. Indeed, depression of LV myocardial contractile state may cause the gradient to decline when heart failure ensues in end stage decompensated aortic stenosis. Consequently, it is important to determine the aortic valve area. Severe AS is defined as an aortic valve area less than 1.0 cm^2 (less than 0.60 cm^2/m^2). Perpendicular cine views through the aortic valve can show the number of valve leaflets, excursion of leaflets, and the aortic valve orifice. These images can be used to measure

the aortic valve area. For this measurement, the area of flow through-plane at the level of the origin of the flow jet is used (Fig. 32-6). As an alternative, application of the continuity equation on VEC MRI profiles in the LV outflow tract (LVOT) (velocity measured below the valve) and aorta (Ao) (just above the valve in the aorta) can also be used (Fig. 32-7). The velocity time integral (VTI) is measured for systolic forward flow in both planes (planes perpendicular to LVOT and Ao, Fig. 32-7). The aortic valve area A (centimeters squared) is given by

$$A_{AO} = A_{LVOT} \, (VTI_{LVOT}/VTI_{AO})$$

where A_{LVOT} = LVOT area in cm^2, VTI_{LVOT} is LVOT VTI, and VTI_{Ao} is A_O VTI.

Quantification of LV Volumes, Mass, and Function

Ventricular mass and function can be measured precisely from a three-dimensional set of cine MR images that can be acquired in any plane. In contrast to echocardiography and cineangiocardiography, MR imaging does not rely on geometric assumptions or calculations based on partial sampling of the cardiac volume. Typically, a set of contiguous tomograms encompassing the entire heart from the apex to the bifurcation of the pulmonary artery is acquired. Cine MR images typically are acquired at 16 phases of the cardiac cycle. These images can be laced together and displayed in a cinematic format. When viewed in the cinematic format, it is possible to assess global right ventricular (RV) and LV function and to assess wall thickening and motion to define regional myocardial function. In recent years, hybrid echo planar and b-SSFP sequences have been

A   **B**

FIG. 32.6. Magnitude **(A)** and phase **(B)** images from velocity-encoded MR sequence parallel to the aortic valve orifice show the blood flow (*arrows*) across the maximum opening of the valve at peak systole. The valve area was measured as 0.9 cm^2 (0.45 cm^2/m^2).

FIG. 32.7. Velocity time integrals are calculated at two different positions before and after the aortic valve to calculate functional aortic valve area by means of the continuity equation. Velocity time integral is the summation of the area bounded by the peak velocity versus time curve during systole (shaded area). Reproduced from **Caruthers SD, et al**. Practical value of CMR Imaging for clinical evaluation of aortic valve stenosis. Circulation 2003; 108:2236–2243, with permission.

developed that provide more images (frames) per cardiac cycle and substantially reduce image acquisition time. The optimal technique for maximizing contrast between blood and myocardium is the use of b-SSFP sequences—true fast imaging with steady precession, balanced fast-field echo, and FIESTA (Figs. 32-8 and 32-9). This sequence has replaced the cine GRE.

Ventricular cavity volumes are simply calculated as the sum of the cavity area times the slice thickness (Fig. 32-9). Interobserver variabilities for LV end-diastolic volume and LV end-systolic volume have been shown to be less than 5% and 10%, respectively. Mass measurements are highly accurate, with excellent interstudy and interobserver variabilities for LV mass of less than 5%. Because interstudy variabilities of ventricular volumetric and mass measurements by cine MR imaging are small, this technique is ideal for monitoring the effectiveness of therapy in patients with aortic stenosis.

EVALUATION OF ASCENDING AORTA

In patients with aortic stenosis, there is usually post-stenotic enlargement of the proximal ascending aorta. (greater than 4.0 cm or 2.2 cm/m²) (Figs. 32-1 and 32-3). This is especially so for some types of bicuspid aortic valves. The dimensions of the ascending aorta can be initially made and monitored with cine MR imaging in the axial plane or a plane perpendicular to the long axis of the ascending aorta.

AORTIC REGURGITATION

Aortic regurgitation imposes a volume overload on the left ventricle as a consequence of retrograde flow across the aortic valve during diastole. Because of the excessive diastolic volume, the left ventricle becomes dilated. Regurgitation may be caused by lack of coaptation of the valvular cusps, annular dilatation, or ascending aortic dilatation. Aortic regurgitation has a number of possible causes (Table 32-3); moreover, it may be a component of several systemic diseases and inherited syndromes (Table 32-4). With some causes, there may be abnormalities at more than one site (e.g., Marfan's syndrome, aortoannular ectasia, and relapsing polychondritis).

Radiography

Findings on the chest x-ray are governed by the severity and chronicity of aortic regurgitation and whether there is associated pathology of the ascending aorta (see Table 30-13 in Chapter 30). The typical features of chronic regurgitation are (1) absence of pulmonary venous hypertension or edema, (2) cardiomegaly due to LV enlargement, and (3) ascending aortic and arch enlargement. Pulmonary venous hypertension and edema usually occur late in the natural history of chronic aortic regurgitation and signify the onset of myocardial failure. On the other hand, acute regurgitation such as occurs with infective endocarditis may produce severe pulmonary edema even with normal cardiac size. Severe

FIG. 32.8. Magnified views of cine MR images (balanced steady-state free precession) in the left ventricular outflow plane depict opening and closing of aortic and mitral valves. Images show three time points: diastole (**left**), near end diastole (**center**), and systole (**right**).

A   B

FIG. 32.9. Cine MR images in the short-axis plane demonstrate left ventricular circumferential wall thickening at end diastole **(A)** and nearly complete cavity obliteration at end systole **(B)** in a patient with severe aortic stenosis and left ventricular hypertrophy. *LV*, left ventricle; *RV*, right ventricle.

enlargement of the ascending aorta may reflect specific pathologies such as aortoannular ectasia, Marfan's syndrome, or ascending aortic aneurysm.

Magnetic Resonance Imaging

MRI is used to identify the presence and quantify the volume of aortic regurgitation. It also is used to monitor the effect of regurgitation on LV volumes, mass, and function (Table 32-5).

TABLE 32.3   Etiology of Aortic Regurgitation

Aortic cusps abnormality
    Bicuspid aortic valve
    Rheumatic disease
    Infective endocarditis
    Supracristal ventricular septal defect
    Syphilis
Aortic annulus abnormality
    Aortoannular ectasia
    Systemic hypertension
    Marfan's syndrome
    Aortic dissection (type A)
    Ankylosing spondylitis
    Relapsing polychondritis
Ascending aorta abnormality
    Aortoannular ectasia
    Marfan's syndrome
    Ehlers-Danlos syndrome
    Aortic dissection (type A)
    Relapsing polychondritis
    Ascending aortic aneurysm

Identification of Aortic Regurgitation

Cine MR imaging demonstrates the regurgitant jet as a signal void. This signal void emanates from the closed aortic valve and projects into the left ventricle during most or all of the diastolic period (Figs. 32-10 to 32-12). The area and volume of the signal void correspond roughly to the severity of regurgitation and thus serve as a semiquantitative estimate of aortic regurgitation. However, the size of the signal void depends on the TE value used and may not be evident with reduction of the TE below 6 ms. Additionally, the size of the signal void can be influenced by regurgitant orifice, LV diastolic pressure and function, aortic pressure, and orientation

TABLE 32.4   Systematic Diseases or Inherited Syndromes Associated with Aortic Regurgitation

Inherited syndromes
Marfan's syndrome
Ehler-Danlos syndrome
Osteogenesis imperfecta
Pseudoxanthoma elasticum

Systemic diseases
Rheumatoid arthritis
Rheumatoid variants
    Ankylosing spondylitis
    Psoriatic arthritis
    Reiter's syndrome
Relapsing polychondritis
Giant cell aortitis
Syphilis (luetic aortitis)

TABLE 32.5 MR Features of Aortic Regurgitation

1. Diastolic signal void starting at closed aortic valve on cine MRI
2. Increased LV stroke volume (effective stroke volume + regurgitant volume)
3. Increased LV end-diastolic and end-systolic volumes
4. Forward (stroke volume) and retrograde (regurgitant volume) on VEC (phase contrast) MRI

of the imaging plane to the direction of the regurgitant jet. The flow void is attenuated on the currently used cine MR images (cine SSFP) (Fig. 32-12).

Acceleration of flow proximal to the regurgitant orifice (proximal convergence zone) produces a second flow void in the aorta just above the valve. The area of this signal void also provides an estimate of the severity of regurgitation. However, this measurement is not employed in clinical practice.

Quantification of Regurgitant Volume

Cine MR imaging also can be used for assessment of regurgitant volume by determining RV and LV stroke volumes. In the normal subject, RV stroke volume is nearly equivalent to LV stroke volume. Stroke volumes are calculated from a stack of MR images as the difference between end-diastolic and end-systolic volumes of each ventricle. The regurgitant volume can be calculated by the difference between RV and LV stroke volumes. These calculations are valid only for patients

FIG. 32.11. Axial cine MR images starting at end systole (**top left**) and in early, mid, and late diastole (**bottom right**). A signal void emanates from the aorta valve in diastole, indicating aortic regurgitation.

with a single regurgitant valve. In patients with combined aortic and mitral regurgitation, this method assesses the total regurgitant volume of the left side of the heart.

Another method for quantification of regurgitation is VEC (phase contrast) MRI. With this technique, regurgitant

FIG. 32.10. Coronal cine MR images in systole (**top**) and diastole (**bottom**). The signal void emanating from the closed aortic valve in diastole indicates aortic regurgitation.

FIG. 32.12. Cine MR image on the left ventricular outflow tract view in diastole shows a flow jet (*arrow*) starting at the level of the aortic valve and extending to the left ventricle (LV), consistent with aortic regurgitation. *Ao,* Ascending aorta.

volume can be calculated in two different ways. First, the regurgitant volume can be assessed by the difference between the systolic flow in the ascending aorta (LV stroke volume) and the systolic flow in the main pulmonary artery (RV stroke volume). The two stroke volumes are calculated from time-integrated measurements of flow volumes during systole on imaging perpendicular to the proximal ascending and another perpendicular to the main pulmonary.

VEC MRI can discriminate between antegrade and retrograde flow during the cardiac cycle, enabling retrograde flow to be measured directly to quantify regurgitation. For example, bright voxels in the ascending aorta during systole indicate antegrade flow, whereas dark voxels in diastole represent retrograde flow caused by aortic regurgitation (Fig. 32-13). High accuracy and interstudy reproducibility ($r = 0.97$) of VEC MRI measurement of retrograde diastolic flow in the ascending aorta have been found in patients with chronic aortic regurgitation. Diastolic retrograde aortic flow equals aortic regurgitant volume (see Fig. 32-13). The measurements of regurgitant volume and fraction by this method correlate closely with volumetric cine MRI measurements ($r > 0.97$). Measurement of regurgitant volume by this method in a group of patients evaluated at two separate occasions demonstrated high interstudy reproducibility ($r > 0.97$). This suggests that this approach is useful for follow-up and monitoring response to therapy in patients with aortic regurgitation.

Quantification of LV Volumes, Mass, and Function

As discussed earlier in the section on aortic stenosis, cine MRI provides a highly accurate and reproducible measurement of ventricular volumes, mass, and function. The high

interstudy reproducibility of these measurements makes it attractive for monitoring these parameters over time in patients with aortic regurgitation in order to document response to pharmacologic therapy and to recognize the appropriate time for valve replacement.

Cine MRI has disclosed the typical effect of aortic regurgitation on the left ventricle. According to the severity of regurgitation, there is an increase in LV end-diastolic and end-systolic volumes. Although LV wall thickness may be within the normal range (less than 12 mm at end diastole), the total LV mass may be increased substantially because of the increase in end-diastolic volume (mass = mean wall thickness × end-diastolic volume). Cine MRI demonstrates elevated LV stroke volume. The total stroke volume consists of the effective stroke volume and regurgitant volume. During the compensated phase of aortic regurgitation, the effective stroke volume remains in the normal range.

The following formulas are relevant for aortic regurgitation:

Total LV stroke volume = effective stroke volume
+ regurgitant volume

Regurgitant volume = LV stroke volume − RV stroke
volume

Regurgitant fraction = regurgitant volume/total LV
stroke volume

MITRAL STENOSIS

Mitral stenosis usually is acquired and nearly always is caused by rheumatic fever. It is the salient lesion of rheumatic heart disease. Other etiologies are rare; these include

FIG. 32.13. A: Velocity-encoded cine MR images in the axial plane in aortic regurgitation. Magnitude (**top**) and phase (**bottom**) images in systole (**left**) and diastole (**right**). Note that on the phase images antegrade flow in systole is represented by bright voxels, whereas retrograde flow (aortic regurgitation) in diastole is represented by dark voxels in the ascending aorta. **B:** A flow versus time curve derived from image pairs at 16 phases of the cardiac cycle shows negative values (retrograde flow) in diastole. The area under the curve with negative values is the volume of aortic regurgitation.

congenital valvular, subvalvular (parachute mitral valve), or supravalvular stenoses; left atrial myxoma; and exuberant mitral annular calcification. Mitral stenosis often is accompanied by a variable degree of mitral regurgitation.

Mitral stenosis causes elevated left atrial pressure throughout diastole, and pulmonary venous hypertension produces pulmonary arterial hypertension. In long-standing mitral stenosis, pulmonary arterial hypertension may be severe, and pulmonary regurgitation eventually ensues across a dilated pulmonary annulus. The right ventricle eventually dilates, causing tricuspid regurgitation from a dilated annulus.

Radiography

The chest x-ray provides good insight into the severity of mitral stenosis by showing the relative severity of pulmonary venous hypertension (see Table 30-8 in Chapter 30). In mild disease, there may be only equalization or reversal of the diameter of upper and lower lobe pulmonary vessels (cephalization). In more severe disease or with an imposed hypervolemic state, interstitial pulmonary edema or alveolar pulmonary edema becomes evident. Interlobular septal thickening (Kerley B lines) usually is a sign of interstitial edema but may become permanent as a consequence of fibrosis or deposition of hemosiderin after multiple episodes of pulmonary edema. Rarely, high-density nodules (ossific nodules) in the lower lobes may be a consequence of multiple episodes of alveolar pulmonary edema and hemorrhage.

In compensated mitral stenosis, only mild cardiomegaly or normal heart size is seen. The left atrium invariably is enlarged, causing a right retrocardiac double density. A convexity on the upper left cardiac border in the frontal view indicates enlargement of the left atrial appendage. This finding nearly always is evident in rheumatic mitral stenosis. Enlargement of the pulmonary arterial segment and right heart indicates pulmonary arterial hypertension. Enlargement of the right heart in the absence of pulmonary arterial enlargement usually indicates concomitant rheumatic tricuspid regurgitation.

The ascending aorta and aortic arch are characteristically small in isolated mitral valve disease. Even slight prominence of the thoracic aorta should raise suspicion of associated rheumatic aortic valve disease.

Magnetic Resonance Imaging

MRI can be used to identify mitral valvular stenosis and any associated mitral regurgitation; estimate the gradient across the valve; and quantify ventricular volumes, mass, and function (Table 32-6).

Identification of Mitral Stenosis

Cine MR images demonstrate a signal void emanating from the opened mitral valve in diastole and projecting into the left ventricle (Fig. 32-14). This signal void is depicted well on

TABLE 32.6 MR Features of Mitral Stenosis

1. Diastolic signal void (or hyperintensity) emanating from mitral valve in diastole on cine MRI
2. Thickened and limited excursion of leaflet on cine MRI
3. Left atrial enlargement
4. Normal LV end-diastolic and end-systolic volumes
5. High-velocity flow on VEC (phase contrast) cine MRI

images acquired in the axial or horizontal long-axis planes. Associated mitral regurgitation appears as a signal void projected into the left atrium during systole. Likewise, signal voids may be recognized in right-sided cardiac chambers if there is any associated pulmonary or tricuspid regurgitation.

Estimation of the Valve Gradient

VEC (phase contrast) MRI is acquired in planes perpendicular or parallel to the stenotic jet (flow void) to sample the peak velocity of the jet (as discussed earlier in the section on aortic stenosis). The diastolic phase image containing the highest velocities can be selected. Then, the voxels with peak velocity on that phase image can be sought (Fig. 32-15). Using the measurement of peak velocity, the pressure gradient can be estimated by the modified Bernoulli equation as $\Delta P = 4V^2$, where ΔP = peak pressure gradient of mitral stenosis and V = peak diastolic velocity across the mitral valve. In general, the MR method is expected to underestimate the pressure gradient compared with Doppler echocardiography because it has a lesser sampling rate. Comparative studies have shown a good correlation between the two techniques, but the MR method has tended to underestimate the gradient.

FIG. 32.14. Axial cine MR image acquired in diastole shows a signal void arising at the opened mitral valve leaflets. This is caused by mitral stenosis.

FIG. 32.15. A: Phase (velocity) image acquired in a plane perpendicular to the direction of flow across a stenotic mitral valve. The high-intensity elliptically shaped area is the flow channel of the stenotic mitral valve (*MV*). This area is interrogated for the peak velocity during diastole to estimate the pressure gradient using the modified Bernoulli equation (peak gradient = 4 × peak velocity²). **B:** Velocity versus time curve in mitral stenosis. The peak velocity in early diastole is slightly lower than the peak velocity measured by Doppler echocardiography.

Quantification of LV Volumes, Mass, and Function

Some version of cine MR images is performed for quantification of LV volumes, mass, and function. As discussed earlier, cine MR imaging is a highly accurate and reproducible method of monitoring LV function. Isolated mitral stenosis usually is associated with smaller than average LV volumes and normal ejection fraction.

MITRAL REGURGITATION

Mitral regurgitation may be caused by an abnormality of any portion of the mitral apparatus or by LV dilatation. The dysfunction may involve one or more of several components: leaflets, chordae, anterior and posterior papillary muscles, or annulus. The etiologies of mitral regurgitation are presented in Table 32-7.

Chronic mitral regurgitation produces left atrial and LV enlargement. Pulmonary venous hypertension or edema usually is less severe than with mitral stenosis. Pulmonary arterial hypertension is less common and less severe than with stenosis.

Acute onset of mitral regurgitation such as might occur with chordal or papillary muscle rupture imposes sudden onset of pulmonary venous hypertension with no time for compensating mechanisms to become operative. Severe pulmonary edema may ensue as a result. In this event, the left atrium and ventricle are normal in size. It has been noted that rupture of the posterior papillary muscle or chordae supported by it may cause pulmonary edema confined to or more severe in the right upper lobe.

Mitral annular calcification occasionally is the sole cause of regurgitation. The cause of the calcification usually is unknown, but such calcification occurs more often in

hypertension, aortic stenosis, hypertrophic cardiomyopathy, hyperlipidemia, and hypercalcemia. It is easy to distinguish mitral valve prolapse from flail. **Prolapse** is ballooning of the middle of the valve beyond the annulus during systole; the tips of the leaflets to which the chordae attach do not pass beyond the annulus. **Flail** is indicated by passage of the tips of the mitral leaflets beyond the annulus and into the left atrium during systole.

Radiography

The radiographic features of mitral regurgitation are regulated by the duration and severity of the lesion and

TABLE 32.7   Etiology of Mitral Regurgitation

Leaflet distortion or perforation
  Rheumatic carditis
  Myxomatous degeneration (mitral valve prolapse)
  Bacterial endocarditis
  Asymmetric form of hypertrophic cardiomyopathy
  Left atrial tumor (myxoma)
  Congenital (parachute mitral valve; cleft mitral valve)
  Systemic lupus erythematosus
Chordae
  Myxomatous degeneration (spontaneous chordal rupture)
  Traumatic (weight lifting, etc.)
  Bacterial endocarditis
Papillary muscle
  Rupture from acute infarction
  Dysfunction during myocardial ischemia
  Congenital (parachute mitral valve)
Annulus
  Annular dilation with left ventricular enlargement
  Annular (periannular) calcification
  Myxomatous degeneration

associated lesions of the mitral and other valves (see Table 30-14 in Chapter 30). Isolated chronic mitral regurgitation is a volume overload lesion that causes left atrial and LV enlargement. In the absence of myocardial failure, the degree of cardiomegaly bears a rough relation to the severity of regurgitation. Signs of pulmonary venous and arterial hypertension are less prominent than with mitral stenosis. Nonrheumatic causes of mitral regurgitation usually do not cause radiographically discernible enlargement of the left atrial appendage.

Acute onset of mitral regurgitation is characterized by pulmonary edema with a normal heart size. Rupture of the posterior papillary muscle or associated chordae may cause focal or more severe pulmonary edema of the right upper lobe.

Mitral Valve Prolapse

Mitral valve prolapse is observed on about 5% of left ventriculograms. Pathologically, it is caused by myxomatous degeneration of the mitral valve leaflets and chordae tendineae. Some patients with prolapse have mitral regurgitation, which often is mild. However, one complication that may occur—rupture of a chordae tendineae—can induce severe regurgitation. Other complications include supraventricular and ventricular arrhythmias, bacterial endocarditis, and cerebral emboli. Abnormal contraction of segments of the left ventricle and abnormal shape of the left ventricle have been observed in some patients with mitral valve prolapse.

Magnetic Resonance Imaging

MRI can be used to identify mitral regurgitation, quantify the regurgitant volume, and measure LV volumes, mass, and function (Table 32-8).

Identification of Mitral Regurgitation

Cine MR images in the axial, horizontal long axis (four-chamber), or vertical long axis can be employed to demonstrate the signal void caused by the jet flow of mitral regurgitation. The signal void originates at the closed valve in systole and is directed into the left atrium (Figs. 32-16 and 32-17). The signal void prominence and size increase with increasing TE. The signal void appears through most or all of systole. The signal void is attenuated on SSFP cine MR images.

TABLE 32.8 MR Features of Mitral Regurgitation

1. Systolic signal void (or hyperintensity) into the left atrium during systole
2. Left atrial enlargement
3. Increased LV end-diastolic and end-systolic volumes
4. Mitral inflow greater than aortic outflow on VEC (phase contrast) MRI

FIG. 32.16. Axial cine MR image in systole shows a flow void emanating from the closed mitral valve and projecting into the left atrium. This is caused by mitral regurgitation.

Quantification of Mitral Regurgitation

Mitral regurgitation is quantified using VEC MRI acquired in a plane parallel to and near the mitral annulus. One approach is to measure the retrograde flow across the valve (into the left atrium) during the systolic phase. This has proved to be complicated, however, because the flow jets occur in multiple orientations in any individual. Another and more robust approach has involved measuring LV diastolic inflow across the mitral annulus and systolic outflow in the proximal ascending aorta (Fig. 32-18). In normal

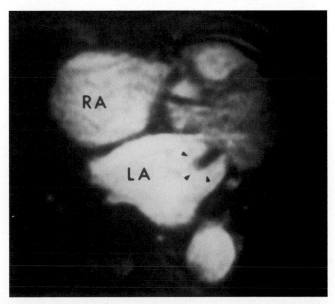

FIG. 32.17. Axial cine MR image in systole shows a flow void (*arrows*) projected into the left atrium (*LA*), indicating mitral regurgitation. *RA*, right atrium.

FIG. 32.18. Magnitude (**left**) and phase (**right**) images at the mitral annulus (**top**) and at the proximal ascending aorta (**bottom**). These are used to measure inflow and outflow of the left ventricle. Inflow exceeds outflow volume by the mitral regurgitant volumes (see Fig. 32-13).

subjects, these values are equivalent, and each represents a measurement of stroke volume (Fig. 32-19). In mitral regurgitation, the diastolic mitral inflow exceeds the systolic aortic outflow; the difference represents the regurgitant volume (see Fig. 32-19). Any concomitant aortic regurgitation invalidates this approach.

As discussed earlier, a volumetric method also may be used to estimate the volume of mitral regurgitation. Using cine MR images (short-axis plane) encompassing the length of the ventricles, the area of the left and right ventricles is

measured on end-diastolic and end-systolic images at each anatomic level to provide end-diastolic and end-systolic volumes. The stroke volume of the left ventricle exceeds the stroke volume of the right ventricle by a volume equal to the mitral regurgitant volume. This method is valid only for isolated mitral regurgitation; it does not apply in the presence of a regurgitant lesion of the right ventricle or aortic regurgitation.

The following formulae are relevant to calculations in mitral regurgitation:

Stroke volume = end-diastolic volume − end-systolic volume (volumetric method)

Mitral regurgitant volume = LV stoke volume − RV stroke volume (volumetric method)

Mitral regurgitant fraction = regurgitant volume/LV stroke volume (volumetric method)

Mitral regurgitant volume = mitral inflow − aortic outflow (VEC method)

Mitral regurgitant fraction = regurgitant volume/mitral inflow (VEC method)

Quantification of LV Volumes, Mass, and Function

Cine MR images encompassing the left ventricle are used for assessing the LV volumes, mass, and function. Because of the precision and reproducibility of LV volumetry using cine MR images, this technique is optimal for monitoring LV volumes and function to assess therapy or to define criteria for surgical intervention.

PULMONARY STENOSIS

Pulmonary stenosis results when egress of blood from the right ventricle is obstructed. It can be divided into four types, depending on the level of obstruction: valvular, supravalvular, subvalvular, and midventricular. Pulmonary stenosis usually is a congenital anomaly.

FIG. 32.19. Flow versus time curve for proximal aorta (left ventricular outflow) and mitral valve (left ventricular inflow) in a normal subject and a patient with mitral regurgitation. The area under the inflow curve is considerably greater than the area under the outflow curve in the patient with mitral regurgitation.

Pulmonary stenosis rarely is caused by rheumatic disease. The etiology of pulmonary stenosis is given in Table 32-9.

Radiography

The typical feature of valvular pulmonic stenosis is enlargement of the main and left pulmonary arterial segments. In the absence of an associated intracardiac defect, there is no oligemia. Obstruction at any level may cause RV enlargement. The radiographic features of congenital pulmonic stenosis are discussed in Chapter 31 (Table 31-28).

Magnetic Resonance Imaging

Cine MRI demonstrates the signal void caused by the jet flow of pulmonic stenosis (Fig. 32-20). The site of origin of the signal void indicates the level of obstruction. A signal void originating at the valve and projecting into the pulmonary artery indicates valvular pulmonic stenosis. MRI can be used to exclude rare causes of stenosis such as tumors or hypertrophic cardiomyopathy.

VEC MRI can be used to estimate the gradient across the stenotic valve. Cine MR imaging is the most accurate technique for quantifying RV volumes and mass. Mass is calculated as the mass of the RV free wall (the septum is assigned to the left ventricle by convention).

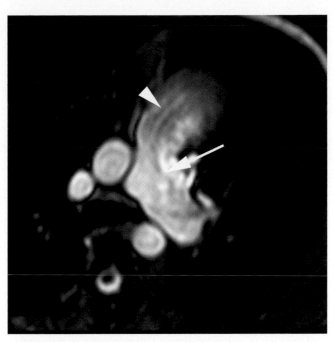

FIG. 32.20. Axial cine MR image at the level of the pulmonary arteries shows large main and left pulmonary arteries. Note the flow jet emanating from the pulmonary valve level (*arrowhead*) and directed toward the left pulmonary artery (*arrow*).

TABLE 32.9 Etiology of Pulmonary Stenosis

Valvular Stenosis
Congenital
  Central perforated diaphragm
  Biscupid valve
  Dysplastic valve
  Hypoplastic annulus
  Tetralogy of Fallot
Acquired
  Rheumatic carditis
  Carcinoid syndrome

Supravalvular
Congenital
  William's syndrome
  Tetralogy of Fallot
Acquired
  Surgical (banding, etc.)
  Carcinoid syndrome
  Rubella syndrome
  Behcet's disease
  Takayasu's arteritis

Subvalvular
Congenital
  Isolated infundibular narrowing
  Tetralogy of Fallot
Acquired
  Infundibular hypertrophy (hypertrophic cardiomyopathy)
  Tumor
Midventricular
Anomalous muscle bundles (double-chamber right ventricle)

PULMONARY REGURGITATION

Pulmonary regurgitation most often is caused by pulmonary arterial hypertension. It can occur in a congenital anomaly in which the pulmonary valve is absent. It nearly always occurs after pulmonary valvuloplasty and surgical correction of tetralogy of Fallot. Pulmonary regurgitation can be severe after repair of tetralogy and over many years can cause severe RV dilatation and failure. Many patients with pulmonary regurgitation also have tricuspid regurgitation as a result of RV dilatation.

Radiography

The major feature of pulmonary regurgitation is enlargement of the main pulmonary arterial segment, central pulmonary arteries, and right ventricle.

Magnetic Resonance Imaging

Cine MRI demonstrates a diastolic signal void emanating from the pulmonary valve and projecting into the right ventricle (see Chapter 36). VEC MRI can be used to quantify the volume of regurgitation. Currently, it is used to monitor the regurgitant volume of patients after the repair of tetralogy of Fallot. The total regurgitant volume of valvular regurgitation on the right side of the heart (pulmonary and tricuspid regurgitation) can be measured as the difference between RV and LV stroke volumes employing volumetric measurements of a stack of short-axis cine MR images that encompass the length of the heart. Pulmonary regurgitation is usually assessed using VEC (PC) MRI (see Chapter 36). If the volume of pulmonary regurgitation is measured directly by VEC MRI in a plane perpendicular to the main pulmonary artery, tricuspid regurgitant volume can be assigned as the difference between the regurgitant volume measured by the two techniques. The volumetric technique gives the total right-sided regurgitant volume; VEC MRI measurement in the pulmonary artery gives pulmonary regurgitant volume only.

Cine MRI can be used to quantify RV volumes, mass, and function. It has demonstrated substantial increases in RV volumes and mass and generalized hypokinesis in patients with severe pulmonary regurgitation after repair of tetralogy of Fallot.

TRICUSPID STENOSIS

Acquired **tricuspid stenosis** is uncommon in comparison with stenosis of left-sided valves. Congenital tricuspid stenosis is rare in comparison with congenital pulmonary stenosis. Other causes of tricuspid stenosis are rare (Table 32-10).

Radiography

The major feature of radiography is isolated right atrial enlargement. Enlargement of the right atrium may be difficult to discern on the chest x-ray. The superior vena cava and azygos vein may be dilated.

Magnetic Resonance Imaging

Cine MRI demonstrates the signal void across the stenotic tricuspid valve in diastole. VEC (phase contrast) MRI may be used to measure the peak velocity and thereby estimate the peak pressure gradient.

TRICUSPID REGURGITATION
Radiography

Tricuspid regurgitation produces cardiomegaly with right atrial and RV enlargement (see Table 30-15 in Chapter 30).

TABLE 32.10 Etiology of Tricuspid Stenosis
Congenital
Rheumatic carditis
Carcinoid syndrome
Right ventricular or atrial tumors
Pericardial and paracardiac tumors (compression of tricuspid annulus)
Focal constrictive pericarditis (constriction of the tricuspid annulus)
Tricuspid annular (periannular) calcification

The most remarkable degree of cardiomegaly may occur with chronic severe tricuspid regurgitation. A cardiac silhouette extending from one lateral chest wall to the other ("wall to wall") usually is due to severe tricuspid regurgitation. This lesion does not produce pulmonary venous hypertension or edema. In severe cases, the pulmonary vascularity may appear attenuated.

Magnetic Resonance Imaging

Cine MRI demonstrates a systolic signal void into the right atrium emanating from the tricuspid valve. Cine MRI also is used to quantify RV volumes, mass, and function. With isolated tricuspid regurgitation, the stroke volume of the right ventricle exceeds that of the left ventricle by a volume equal to that of the tricuspid regurgitant volume.

SELECTED READING

Braunwald E. Valvular heart disease. In: Braunwald E, Zipes DP, Libby P (eds). Heart Disease, 6th ed. Philadelphia: Saunders Publishing Co., 2001: 1643.

Boegaert J, Dymorkowski S, Herregods MC, Taylor, AM, et al. Valvular heart disease. In: Higgins CB, de Roos A (eds). MRI and CT of Cardiovascular System, 2nd ed. Philadelphia: Lippincott Williams & Wilkins, 2006: 183.

Caruthers SD, Jiuanlin S, Brown P, et al. Practical value of CMR imaging for clinical evaluation of aortic valve stenosis. Circulation 2003; 108:2236.

Didier D. Detection and qualifications of valvular heart disease with dynamic CMR imaging. Radiographics 2000; 20:1279.

Dulce MC, Mostbeck GH, Higgins CB. Severity of arortic regurgitation: interstudy reproducibility of measurement with VEC cine MRI. Radiology 1992; 185:235.

Fujita N, Hartiala JJ, Higgins CB. Qualifications of mitral regurgitation by velocity encoded cine MR. J Am Cardiol 1994; 23:951.

33 Myocardial Diseases

CHARLES B. HIGGINS AND KAREN ORDOVAS

Magnetic resonance imaging (MRI) is highly effective for the morphologic and functional evaluation of myocardial diseases. It is used much less frequently than echocardiography, however, for the diagnosis and monitoring of cardiomyopathies. In comparison with echocardiography, the three-dimensional (3D) data set available with MRI provides a more precise and reproducible method for qualifying ventricular volumes, mass, and function. ECG-referenced multidetector CT (MDCT) and electron-beam CT also provide 3D data and consequently should have similar capabilities. CT is not used much in the evaluation of nonischemic myocardial diseases.

Considerable new information has been produced in the past few years showing the value of MRI in various myocardial diseases. It has become clear that this technique provides insight into ventricular morphology and function and myocardial tissue characterization. Indeed tissue characterization with delayed contrast enhancement provides insight into the etiology of a number of myocardial diseases.

TECHNIQUES

The ECG-gated spin-echo (SE) acquisitions in the axial and coronal planes are customarily used to demonstrate the morphology of the ventricles and pericardium. Sharp demarcation of the endocardium is achieved on single- or multiple-slice breath-hold turbo SE images with preparatory double-inversion recovery pulses applied to vitiate the signal of the blood pool (Fig. 33-1). Contrast-enhanced T1-weighted gradient-echo (GRE) inversion recovery images may be applied to demonstrate regional or focal differential (hyper-) enhancement at sites of inflammation, ischemic injury, or fibrosis associated with some myocardial diseases (Fig. 33-2). New T2-weighted sequences can demonstrate myocardial edema.

Cine MR images are acquired for the purpose of quantifying ventricular volumes, mass, and global function. Cine MR images are now usually done with some form of balanced steady state free precession sequence. A set of these images at multiple levels encompassing the heart provides a volumetric data set for the direct measurement of the end-diastolic, end-systolic, and stroke volumes, mass, and ejection fraction of both the left ventricle and right ventricles. The blood pool is bright on cine MRI. The balanced steady-state free precession techniques represented by true fast imaging with steady precession (FISP), fast imaging employing steady-state acquisition (FIESTA), and balanced fast field echo (bFFE) sequences provide a homogeneous bright signal of the blood pool throughout the cardiac cycle and relatively high temporal resolution in a short acquisition period (Fig. 33-3). Cine MRI sequences are usually acquired in the cardiac short axis plane encompassing both ventricles from base to apex and in one or more long-axis planes for the quantification of ventricular volumes and function (Fig. 33-4). On cine MR images, valvular regurgitation associated with cardiomyopathies or subvalvular stenosis accompanying some forms of hypertrophy cardiomyopathy may be recognized by a signal void (high-velocity jet flow; Fig. 33-5). High velocity flow can also cause a circumscribed jet of high signal when the velocity is below a certain threshold.

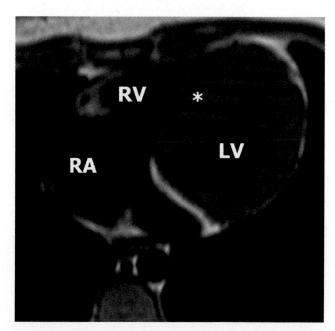

FIG. 33.1. Asymmetric hypertrophic cardiomyopathy. T1-weighted spin-echo image in the axial plane shows thickening of the ventricular septum (*asterisk*) with a normal thickness of the left ventricular (*LV*) lateral wall. *RV*, right ventricle; *RA*, right atrium.

FIG. 33.2. Delayed-enhancement image in the horizontal long axis plane demonstrates patchy areas of delayed enhancement within the hypertrophied ventricular septum (*arrows*).

Velocity-encoded (VEC; phase contrast) cine MRI can be used to measure blood flow into the aorta or pulmonary artery to quantify the left ventricular (LV) or right ventricular (RV) stroke volume, respectively. It has also been used for direct measurement of the volume of valvular regurgitation, which may accompany some cardiomyopathies. Velocity encoded (phase contrast) cine MR in LV outflow tract (LVOT) plane can be used to estimate gradient across LVOT in obstructive hypertrophic cardiomyopathy (Fig. 33-6).

Delayed contrast-enhanced MR (DE-MR) involves the application of an inversion recovery GRE sequence at a delay time after administration of a gadolinium chelate (0.1 to 0.2 mmol/kg). The delay time is 10 to 15 minutes after injection and the inversion time is set to null the signal of normal myocardium. The usual inversion time is in the range of 225 to 300 ms. Abnormal myocardium appears bright in contrast to normal myocardium (Fig. 33-2). The abnormal bright region can be due to edema, necrosis, fibrosis, or various infiltrates which expand the extracellular space of the myocardium.

A

B

FIG. 33.3. End-diastolic cine MR images in the short axis plane at the left ventricular basilar (**A**), midventricular (**B**), and apical levels (**C**) demonstrate severe hypertrophy of the ventricular septum (*VS*). *LV*, left ventricle.

C

FIG. 33.4. Top and center: Series of cine MR (balanced FFE) images in the cardiac short axis plane from apex (**top left**) to base (**bottom right**). **Bottom:** Images in the horizontal long axis (**left**), vertical long axis (**middle**), and left ventricular outflow planes (**right**).

FIG. 33.5. Systolic cine MR image in the left ventricular outflow tract plane shows subaortic stenosis due to a thick ventricular septum (*asterisk*) in a patient with hypertrophic cardiomyopathy. Note the flow jet (*arrow*) starting at the level of the subaortic stenosis and extending to the ascending aorta (*Ao*). There is also a flow jet (*arrowhead*) consistent with associated mitral regurgitation. *LV*, left ventricle; *LA*, left atrium.

CLASSIFICATION OF CARDIOMYOPATHIES

According to the consensus of the World Health Organization and the International Society and Federation for Cardiology, cardiomyopathies are defined as diseases of the myocardium associated with cardiac dysfunction. Based on pathophysiologic features, they have been divided into four main categories: dilated, hypertrophic, restrictive, and arrhythmogenic RV cardiomyopathy (Table 33-1). In addition, diseases of the myocardium that are associated with specific systemic disorders are termed specific cardiomyopathies. Cardiomyopathies caused by pathologic

substances or cells infiltrating the myocardium are called infiltrative cardiomyopathies such as amyloid and sarcoid myocardial disease (cardiomyopathy). Infiltration and fibrosis of the endocardium and subendocardium is very rare in temperate climates and is called endomyocardial infiltrative cardiomyopathy. These rare forms are now classified as restrictive cardiomyopathies.

A

B

FIG. 33.6. Magnitude (**A**) and phase (**B**) images of velocity encoded cine sequence in the left ventricular outflow tract. Note the flow jet (*arrow*) starting at the subaortic region, consistent with subaortic stenosis. *LV*, left ventricle; *LA*, left atrium; *Ao*, aorta.

TABLE 33.1 Classification of Cardiomyopathies
Clinico-anatomical Classification
Dilated cardiomyopathy
Hypertrophic cardiomyopathy
Restrictive cardiomyopathy
Arrhythmogenic right ventricular vardiomyopathy
(dysplasia)
Pathological Classification
Infiltrative

TABLE 33.3 Phenotypes of Hypertrophic Cardiomyopathy
1. Asymmetric septal
obstructive
nonobstructive
2. Concentric
3. Apical
4. Midventricular
5. Right ventricular
6. Restrictive without hypertrophy

Dilated Cardiomyopathy

This entity is characterized by dilation and diminished contraction of the left or both ventricles. End-systolic and end-diastolic volumes are increased, whereas stroke volume and ejection fraction are decreased. Mild to moderate mitral regurgitation and tricuspid regurgitation are frequently associated with the ventricular enlargement. The wall thickness of the left ventricle is usually within the normal range, so that an overall increases in LV mass results. There are many causes of dilated cardiomyopathy (Table 33-2). However, most cases have no identifiable cause (idiopathic). The most common cause of dilated cardiomyopathy is myocardial ischemia secondary to coronary artery disease in which the degree of myocardial dysfunction is frequently not explained by the obvious extent of myocardial infraction. Hypertension, viral diseases, alcoholism, diabetes, obesity, several toxins, and hereditary factors also lead to dilated cardiomyopathy. The most common clinical feature of dilated cardiomyopathy is LV failure. Mural thrombus may form in the dilated left ventricle.

Hypertrophic Cardiomyopathy

A variety of distribution patterns of inappropriate myocardial hypertrophy develop in the absence of an obvious hemodynamic stress (increased afterload), such as aortic stenosis or systemic hypertension (Table 33-3). The disease is genetically transmitted in about half of the cases and follows an autosomal dominant inheritance pattern with

TABLE 33.2 Some Etiologies of Dilated Cardiomyopathy
Ischemic
Familial
Alcohol
Cocaine
Postmyocarditis
Drug toxicity (doxorubicin)
Cobalt (beer drinkers cardiomyopathy)
Obesity
Metabolic (e.g., carnitine deficiency, thiamine deficiency, scurvy)
Endocrine (e.g., acromegaly, myxedema, thyrotoxicosis, etc.)
Postpartum (peripartum)
Tachyarrhythmia
Idiopathic

variable penetrance. Possible manifestations are symmetric involvement of the entire left ventricle or both ventricles or asymmetric hypertrophy of the upper septum, midportion of the ventricular septum, or apex. Nonobstructive and obstructive hypertrophic cardiomyopathy can be distinguished by the associated hemodynamic alterations. Asymmetric septal hypertrophic cardiomyopathy can cause obstruction of the LV outflow tract. The hallmark is dynamic subvalvular aortic stenosis. During diastole, the LV outflow tract appears normal or slightly narrowed because of the presence of upper septal hypertrophy. Increasing stenosis develops during systole as the anterior leaflet of the mitral valve moves in an anterior direction toward the septum, thereby narrowing the outflow tract. Although uncommon in the Western world, apical hypertrophy is prevalent in Japan. This type of hypertrophic cardiomyopathy does not cause obstruction of the outflow tract. Midventricular type involves hypertrophy of the middle of the LV with mid cavity obliteration in systolic causing high wall tension in the isolated LV apex. LV apical dyskinesis or aneurysm is frequent. Symmetric hypertrophic cardiomyopathy is also recognized and may be a particularly severe form. Involvement of the right ventricle is a feature of the disease in infants and children.

Restrictive Cardiomyopathy

This entity is characterized by hampered ventricular filling secondary to myocardial diastolic stiffness. Flow into the ventricles is rapid during early diastole; it then plateaus, and little filling takes place in late diastole. End-diastolic pressure is elevated in both ventricles, whereas systolic function is normal or only slightly reduced. Endomyocardial fibrosis and Loeffler endocarditis are now classified as types of restrictive cardiomyopathy. Loeffler endocarditis is associated with hypereosinophilia. Degranulation of endomyocardial eosinophils is suspected to be responsible for focal necrosis and subsequent fibrosis and for the formation of mural thrombus. Increased stiffness of the ventricular walls and reduction of the cavity by organized thrombus contribute to the restrictive filling pattern. Endomyocardial fibrosis, a different entity with a peak geographic distribution in equatorial Africa, is not associated with hypereosinophilia. In this disease, fibrosis of the apex and subvalvular regions leads to restrictive cardiomyopathy. Glycogen storage diseases, radiation fibrosis,

TABLE 33.4 Types of Infiltrative Diseases of Myocardium and Endocardium

1. Amyloidosis
2. Sarcoidosis
3. Loeffler's eosinophilic endocardial fibroplasia
4. Endomyocardial fibrosis
5. Hemochromatosis
6. Glycogen storage diseases
7. Mucopolysaccharidoses
8. Anderson-Fabry's disease
9. Whipple's disease
10. Gaucher's disease
11. Sphingolipidoses

and certain infiltrative diseases, such as amyloidosis and sarcoidosis, can also cause restrictive cardiomyopathy. Many cases of restrictive cardiomyopathy are idiopathic.

Specific cardiomyopathies are myocardial diseases that are associated with a specific cardiac or systemic disease. Hemochromatosis, sarcoidosis, amyloidosis, and hypertensive or metabolic cardiomyopathy are examples of specific cardiomyopathies. Dilated cardiomyopathy may be the result of inflammation (myocarditis).

Several classifications also consider infiltrative cardiomyopathy as an additional category (Table 33-4). The definition of infiltrative cardiomyopathy refers solely to the histopathologic mechanism of infiltration of myocardial tissue, and the diseases in this group may cause either restrictive or dilated cardiomyopathy. Hemochromatosis is an example of an infiltrative cardiomyopathy in which the cardiomyopathy is of the dilated type, whereas amyloidosis usually causes a restrictive pattern.

FIG. 33.7. Cine MR images at two levels at end diastole (**left**) and end systole (**right**) in a patient with dilated cardiomyopathy.

IMAGING FEATURES

Dilated Cardiomyopathy

The morphologic characteristics of dilated cardiomyopathy are clearly depicted on ECG-gated SE MRI or cine MRI (Figs. 33-7 and 33-8) (Table 33.5). Morphologic changes include enlargement of the left ventricle and sometimes the right ventricle and atria. The thickness of the LV wall usually remains normal. The MRI features in dilated cardiomyopathy are frequently nonspecific, so that the

FIG. 33.8. Short axis cine MR images in the end-diastolic (**A**) and end-systolic (**B**) frames demonstrate a severely enlarged left ventricle (*LV*) with poor systolic function. *RV*, right ventricle.

TABLE 33.5 Imaging Features of Dilated Cardiomyopathy

1. Increased LV end diastolic volume
2. Increase LV end systolic volume
3. Decreased LV stroke volume
4. Decreased LVEF
5. Normal LV wall thickness
6. ± Decreased RVEF

various underlying causes cannot be distinguished. However, it is usually possible to distinguish between ischemic and nonischemic forms of dilated cardiomyopathy. In most cases of nonischemic dilated cardiomyopathy, the wall thickness of the left ventricle is uniform; no regional wall thinning is recognized. If the cardiac dilation is caused by prior myocardial infarction and ischemia, usually one or more regional areas of severe wall thinning with or without ventricular aneurysm are seen. MRI may demonstrate localized ventricular dilation after occlusion of a major coronary artery rather than global dilation; the latter is characteristic of dilated cardiomyopathy. Delayed contrast-enhanced MRI may be used to demonstrate regional hyperenhancement in a subendocardial or transmural distribution at the site of prior myocardial infarction to distinguish patients with ischemic cardiomyopathy (Fig. 33-9). Regional delayed hyperenhancement is not a usual feature of idiopathic dilated cardiomyopathy (Fig. 33-9).

A minority of patients (almost 30%) with idiopathic dilated cardiomyopathy show delayed contrast enhancement. The hyperenhancement is not subendocardial but rather in a midwall distribution especially in the septum. These may be cases of myocarditis presenting in the chronic phase as dilated cardiomyopathy.

Ventricular mass, ventricular thickness, and ventricular volumes can be quantified with cine MRI to determine the severity of dilated cardiomyopathy. Cine MRI measurements of LV volumes, mass, and ejection fraction in dilated cardiomyopathy have been shown to be highly reproducible between studies. The 3D data set with MRI is especially useful for monitoring LV dimension and function over time. Because of its high degree of accuracy and reproducibility, MRI can be used to monitor the effect of treatment in individual patients and in clinical studies to assess the efficacy of new therapeutic interventions. For example, significant decreases in LV systolic volume, wall stress, and mass and increase in ejection fraction have been shown in dilated cardiomyopathy after angiotensin-converting enzyme inhibitor treatment and other therapies.

Although the right ventricle is usually less dilated and its systolic function is less severely depressed, RV diastolic abnormalities, such as an increased time to peak filling rate, have been detected using cine MRI and VEC (phase contrast) cine MRI. The profile of diastolic inflow velocity measured in the region of the tricuspid valve is flattened in comparison with that in healthy volunteers. It is suspected

A   B

FIG. 33.9. Delayed-enhancement image in two different patients. **(A)** shows no delayed-enhancement in an axial plane image of a patient with idiopathic dilated cardiomyopathy (same patients as in Fig. 33.8). **(B)** shows short-axis image with transmural delayed-enhancement in the inferolateral wall, consistent with prior myocardial infarction in a patient with ischemic dilated cardiomyopathy. *LV*, left ventricle; *RV*, right ventricle.

FIG. 33.10. Cine MR image in a patient with hemochromatosis. Note the low signal of the myocardium caused by iron deposition.

that the altered morphology and function of the left ventricle causes functional changes in RV filling.

The signal intensity on SE and GRE images has not been found to be consistently altered in dilated cardiomyopathy, except in cardiomyopathy associated with hemochromatosis (Fig. 33-10). Shortening of relaxation rates has been shown on SE, T2*, and GRE images of myocardium overloaded with iron.

Mural LV thrombus can be readily identified on cine MR images and on DE-MR (delayed gadolinium-enhanced inversion recovery GRE) images. The most frequent site of thrombus is the LV apex (Fig. 33-11).

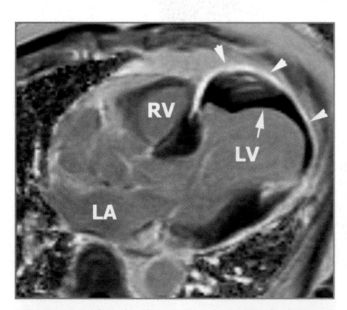

FIG. 33.11. Delayed enhancement image in the horizontal long axis plane shows transmural hyperenhancement (*arrowheads*) and left ventricular thrombus (*arrow*) in a patient with ischemic cardiomyopathy consistent with prior myocardial infarction. *LA*, left atrium; *LA*, left ventricle; *RV*, right ventricle.

TABLE 33.6	Imaging Features of Hypertrophic Cardiomyopathy

1. Normal LV end diastolic volume
2. Normal or reduced LV end systolic volume
3. Normal or increased LVEF
4. Increased LV wall thickness (>12 mm)
5. Asymmetric or symmetric increased LV wall thickness
6. Septal to posterolateral wall thickness ratio >1.5
7. Increased RV wall thickness (especially children)
8. Delayed gadolinium hyperenhancement in septum or junction of septum-anterior wall
9. Mimics restrictive cardiomyopathy rarely
10. Myocardial crypts—genotypes without hypertrophy

Hypertrophic Cardiomyopathy

The initial diagnosis of hypertrophic cardiomyopathy is nearly always established by echocardiography (Table 33.6). The typical diagnostic feature on any imaging modality is a ratio of the end-diastolic thickness of the septum to the posterolateral wall greater than 1.5. Because not all patients have asymmetric hypertrophy, an additional criterion is concentric hypertrophy (end-diastolic wall thickness greater than 1.2 cm) in the absence of a cause for hypertrophy, such as hypertension, aortic stenosis, or extreme isometric exercise. MRI enables a precise delineation of the location and extent of hypertrophic myocardium in persons with hypertrophic cardiomyopathy (see Figs. 33-1 to 33-3, 33-5, and 33-12 to 33-16). One of the major clinical roles of MRI is to evaluate unusual forms of hypertrophy that are difficult to assess with echocardiography (Figs. 33-17 and 33-18). Another indication for MRI is sequential monitoring of the LV mass and assessment of prognosis using delayed MRI, the extent of delayed enhancement is related to morbidity and mortality.

FIG. 33.12. ECG-gated spin-echo transaxial image of patient with the asymmetric form of hypertrophic cardiomyopathy. Note asymmetric thickening of ventricular septum (*VS*).

disease. Secondary hemochromatosis develops mainly when repeated blood transfusions are required to treat thalassemia and hemolytic anemias. It may also occur in hepatic failure due to chronic elevated levels of serum ferritin. Other common causes are chronic alcohol abuse and long-term hemodialysis. In primary hemochromatosis, iron is deposited in the liver and pancreas but the spleen remains normal. This characteristic distinguishes primary from secondary hemochromatosis, in which iron is also deposited in the spleen. Increased iron deposition in the cardiac myocytes in hemochromatosis causes diastolic and systolic cardiac dysfunction. After an initial asymptomatic period, cardiopathy caused by iron overload initially presents as diastolic dysfunction with a restrictive filling pattern. When the iron overload reaches a critical level, systolic functional abnormalities occur, and the disease take the form of a dilated cardiomyopathy.

Iron reduces the T1 and T2 relaxation rates by introducing local magnetic field inhomogeneities, causing myocardial signal intensity to be reduced, especially on cine MR images (see Fig. 33-10). The amount of signal decrease on T2-weighted images correlates with the iron level in tissue but not with serum iron levels. MRI is a valuable tool for noninvasively estimating the iron concentration in the heart and for monitoring therapy.

Assessment for myocardial dysfunction caused by myocardial iron deposition is most effectively done using a cine MR acquisition in the short axis plane in order to calculate the LVEF. A specialized T2* (star) sequence is done which produces an array of images at varying T2 delays. From this acquisition a T2* value can be calculated. A value below 20 milliseconds is considered indicative of some amount of iron deposition in the myocardium. Myocardial dysfunction with depressed LVEF is associated with a value of less than 10 milliseconds.

Myocardial Vasculitis

Myocardial vasculitis such as Churg-Strauss syndrome (eosinophilia, skin rash, asthma, pulmonary infiltrates) can produce regional LV dysfunction and delayed gadolinium hyperenhancement. Similar to myocardial infarction, hyperenhancement is subendocardial.

Rare Myocardial Disease Associated with Delayed Hyperenhancement

Delayed gadolinium hyperenhancement of regional myocardium has been reported in numerous unusual or rare myocardial and systemic diseases (Table 33-10). The delayed enhancement is usually not subendocardial so nonischemic etiology is suggested. The site in the LV may be so specific as to suggest the etiology such as the inferobasal segment as occurs in Anderson-Fabry's disease. The delayed hyperenhancement may be diffuse subendocardial in Loeffler's eosinophilic fibroplasia (Fig. 33-22).

TABLE 33.10 Myocardial Abnormalities Associated with Delayed Gadolinium Hyperenhancement

1. Acute and chronic myocardial infarction
2. Acute myocarditis
3. Hypertrophic cardiomyopathy
4. Dilated cardiomyopathy (minority of cases)
5. Restrictive cardiomyopathy (some cases—usually infiltrative type)
6. Amyloidosis
7. Sarcoidosis
8. Anderson Fabry's disease
9. Endomyocardial Fibrosis
10. Postoperative and adult congenital heart disease (some cases especially postoperative tetralogy of Fallot)
11. Ebsteins anomaly (fibrotic atrialized portion of RV)
12. Myocardial vasculitis (Churg-Strauss syndrome)
13. Lyme carditis
14. Fibroma

Arrhythmogenic Right Ventricular Cardiomyopathy

Arrhythmogenic right ventricular cardiomyopathy (ARVC) may have characteristic features on SE and cine MRI (Table 33.11). Typical findings are transmural fatty deposition in the RV free wall as displayed on T1-weighted SE images (Figs. 33-25 and 33-26). T1-weighted SE images may also demonstrate the focal deposition of fat in the myocardial wall as bright spots surrounded by the medium signal intensity of myocardium. Another feature is regional bulging or thinning of the RV free wall (Fig. 33-27). Thinning of the RV free wall is difficult to interpret because the thickness of the free wall varies among normal persons. Additional morphologic features include

FIG. 33.25. ECG-gated spin-echo image shows transmural fat in the right ventricular (*RV*) free wall in a patient with arrhythmogenic RV dysplasia.

FIG. 33.26. ECG-gated T1-weighted spin-echo image displays transmural fat in the right ventricular (*RV*) wall in a patient with arrhythmogenic RV dysplasia.

FIG. 33.27. Cine MR image shows regional dyskinesis (*arrow*) of the right ventricle in a patient with arrhythmogenic right ventricular dysplasia. *LA*, left atrium; *RA*, right atrium; *RV*, right ventricle.

FIG. 33.28. Severe arrhythmogenic right ventricular dysplasia. Axial T1-weighted spin-echo image (**A**) shows prominent trabeculation (*arrows*) in the right ventricular (*RV*) free wall. Delayed enhancement image in the same plane (**B**) shows transmural hyperenhancement (*arrowheads*) of the RV free wall. Short-axis cine MR images at end-diastole (**C**) and end-systole (**D**) demonstrate RV dilatation and global hypokinesis. *LV*, left ventricle; *RA*, right atrium.

SELECTED READING

Buser PT, Keller DI, Bremerich J. Arrhythmogenic right ventricular cardiomyopathy. In: Higgins CB, de Roos A (eds). MRI and CT of the Cardiovascular System, 2nd ed. Philadelphia: Lippincott Williams & Wilkins, 2006:154.

Friedrich MG, Sechtem U, Schulz-Menger J, et al. Cardiovascular MR in Myocardites: a JACC White Paper. J Am Coll Cardiol 2009; 53:1475.

Friedrich MG, Wassmuth R. Magnestic resonance of cardiomyopathy and myocarditis. In: Higgins CB, de Roos A (eds). MRI and CT of the Cardiovascular System, 2nd ed. Philadelphia: Lippincott Williams & Wilkins, 2006:121.

Kirk P, Roughton M, Porter JB, et al. Cardiac T2* magnetic resonance for prediction of complications in thalassemia major. Circulation 2009; 120:1961.

Maceira AM, Joshi J, Prasad SK, et al. Cardiovascular Magnetic Resonance in Cardiac Amyloidosis. Circulation 2005; 111:186.

Patel MR, Cawley PJ, Heitner JF, et al. Detection of myocardial damage in patients with sarcoidosis. Circulation 2009; 120:1969.

Richardson P, McKenna W, Bristow M, et al. Report of the 1995 World Health Organization/International Society and Federation of Cardiology Task Force on the Definition and Classification of Cardiomyopathies. Circulation 1996; 93:841.

Tandri H, Bluemke DA, Ferrari VA, et al. Findings on MRI of idiopathic right ventricular dysplasia. Am J Cardoil 2004; 94:1441.

Pericardial Diseases

CHARLES B. HIGGINS AND KAREN ORDOVAS

Pericardial disease may be primary and involve the pericardium alone. It is also frequently a manifestation of a wide variety of systemic diseases or secondary to cardiovascular disease.

There are several imaging techniques that are effective for the diagnosis of pericardial diseases. The imaging modality initially and most frequently utilized is transthoracic echocardiography. Asymptomatic abnormalities of the pericardium are occasionally identified on computed tomography (CT) of the thorax.

The imaging modality of choice for initial evaluation of patients with suspected pericardial effusion is transthoracic echocardiography. This widely available and relatively low-cost method has a high accuracy for detection of pericardial effusion and signs of tamponade. It is also a good method for guiding diagnostic or therapeutic pericardiocenteses. The main limitation of echocardiography in pericardial diseases is its inability to assess the entire pericardial extension. It is also not very accurate for depiction of pericardial thickening, because echogenicity of the pericardium is similar to adjacent tissues.

Major indications for further investigation with CT or magnetic resonance imaging (MRI) are the visualization of loculated pericardial effusion; evaluation of complicated pericardial effusion (hemorrhagic vs. nonhemorrhagic); measurement of pericardial thickness; assessment of enhancement of the pericardium and characterization of pericardial masses.

CT and MRI provide excellent delineation of the mediastinal anatomy, with high soft-tissue contrast and spatial resolution. The visualization of the entire chest can also give important information for differential diagnosis and extent of pericardial diseases. Both methods provide some information on tissue characterization, which is useful for the diagnosis of pericardial masses and pericardial inflammation.

CT is the best method for depiction of pericardial calcification, a finding suggestive of constrictive pericarditis in the appropriate clinical setting. CT-guided pericardiocenteses is a well-established technique for management of loculated pericardial effusions. Electrocardiogram-gated CT can eliminate the artifacts related to cardiac motion and is superior to nongated studies for the evaluation for pericardial abnormalities.

MRI has the advantage of avoiding iodinated contrast media and ionizing radiation as well as providing imaging in multiple planes. The major indication for MRI is the measurement of pericardial thickness, which is useful for diagnosis of constrictive pericarditis in patients with constrictive/restrictive physiology. Cine MRI can usually differentiate a small pericardial effusion from pericardial thickening, which can be misinterpreted by CT.

TECHNIQUES

Multidetector CT imaging with cardiac gating is ideally used to assess pericardial anatomy and cardiac function with adequate temporal and high spatial resolution. However nongated multidetector CT is usually adequate for diagnosis of pericardial disease.

Electrocardiogram-gated MRI studies with morphologic and functional sequences allow a complete evaluation of the pericardium with high soft-tissue contrast and spatial resolution. Images of the entire heart can be acquired with a few breath holds or during free-breathing. New techniques with a phased-arrayed coil can image the heart with a high temporal resolution.

Turbo spin-echo (SE) T1-weighted images are usually acquired at least in the axial and coronal planes for morphologic assessment of the pericardium. SE or inversion recovery gradient-echo (GRE) images after administration of gadolinium chelates may be used to detect enhancement caused by inflammatory processes of the pericardium. Cine MR images using GRE or steady-state free precession sequences are acquired to evaluate ventricular function, ventricular sliding motion over the pericardium, and diastolic ventricular septal motion.

NORMAL PERICARDIUM AND PERICARDIAL RECESSES

The pericardium is a compliant sac that envelops the heart and the origin of the great vessels. It is attached to the sternum anteriorly and to the diaphragm inferiorly. The left atrium is only partially covered by the pericardium. Parietal pericardium consists of fibrous tissue with an inner layer of mesothelial cells that reflect in the regions of pericardial attachment and cover the surface of the heart, forming the visceral pericardium. On MRI and CT studies, the normal pericardium is usually less than 2 mm thick (Figs. 34-1 and 34-2). A thickness greater than 4 mm is considered abnormal. CT can overestimate pericardial

A   **B**

FIG. 34.10. Pericardial hematoma on CT. Contrast-enhanced CT at the level of the right pulmonary artery (**A**) shows a type A aortic dissection (*arrows*) associated with a high-density pericardial effusion (*asterisk*) consistent with acute hemopericardium. CT image at the level of the base of the heart (**B**) in another patient after cardiac surgery shows a large heterogeneous collection on the anterior aspect of the pericardium (*arrows*). Note the compression of the right ventricle by the hematoma.

A   **B**

C   **D**

FIG. 34.11. MR appearance of pericardial hematoma. Axial SE MR images at the midventricular level show different ages of pericardial blood. The homogeneous high-intensity collection adjacent to the right atrium (*arrow*) is an acute hematoma (**A**). Note the low intensity of simple pericardial effusion at the left side of the cavity (*asterisk*). Subacute pericardial hemorrhage with areas of low and high signal intensity is shown in loculated (**B,C**) pericardial hematomas (*arrows*). The homogeneous low-intensity collection compressing the left ventricle (**D**) is a typical presentation of an old chronic hematoma (*arrow*).

TABLE 34.2 Hemorrhagic Versus Nonhemorrhagic Pericardial Effusion

Hemorrhagic effusion
1. High density on CT (higher than 40–45 density units)
2. High intensity on T1-weighted spin echo MR
3. Heterogeneous (high, medium, low) on T1-weighted spin echo MR
4. Heterogeneous or low signal on gradient echo (cine MR) and balanced steady state free precession (cine MR) images
5. Low signal on all types of MR sequences (old loculated pericardial hematoma)

Nonhemorrhagic effusions
1. Low (water density) on CT (usually <20 density units)
2. Low signal (less than myocardium) on T1-weighted spin echo images
3. Homogeneous high signal on T2-weighted spin echo images
4. Homogeneous high signal on gradient echo (cine MR) and balanced steady state free precession (cine MR) images

TABLE 34.3 Etiologies of Acute Pericarditis

1. Infection
   a. Viral (Coxsackie A, Coxsackie B, echovirus, adenovirus, hepatitis B, herpes virus, parvovirus, AIDs, etc.)
   b. Bacterial (staphylococcal, streptococcal, pneumococcal, etc.)
   c. Fungal (histoplasmosis, coccidioidomycosis, Candidosis, aspergillosis, cryptococcosis, etc.)
   d. Tuberculosis
2. Acute myocardial infarction
3. Acute myocarditis (myopericarditis)
4. Neoplastic (especially lymphoma, melanoma, lung cancer, breast cancer, leukemia)
5. Radiation
6. Collagen-vascular diseases (especially systemic lupus erythematosus, rheumatoid arthritis, scleroderma, mixed connective tissue disease)
7. Sarcoidosis
8. Systemic diseases (amyloidosis, Behcet's disease, inflammatory bowel disease)
9. Drug reaction (adriamycin, hydralyzine, procainamide, diphenylhydantoin, methysergide)
10. Post-myocardial infarction (Dressler's syndrome)
11. Postpericardiotomy syndrome
12. Thoracic trauma
13. Idiopathic

a small simple effusion and the adjacent low signal of normal parietal pericardium. However, small volume of fluid and pericardium may be indistinguishable on spin echo MR and thereby simulate pericardial thickening. Pericardial effusion shows no increase in signal on T1-weighted images after administration of gadolinium chelate. This feature aids in distinguishing between pericardial fluid and pericardial or myocardial tumor on T1-weighted SE images. CT and MRI are very sensitive for the detection of generalized or loculated pericardial effusions. CT and MRI can detect pericardial effusion as small as 30 mL. Both provide information on the location of pericardial effusion and are especially effective for demonstrating loculated effusions (Fig. 34-11A). Because of uneven distribution, the total fluid volume cannot be calculated from the width of the pericardial space by applying a simple formula. However, a semiquantitative estimation can be obtained by measuring the width of the pericardial space in front of the right ventricle. A moderate effusion is associated with a width of more than 5 mm. Loculated effusion occurs when fluid is trapped by adhesions between the parietal and visceral pericardium. MRI is more sensitive than echocardiography in detecting loculated effusion because of its wide field of view.

ACUTE PERICARDITIS

Acute pericarditis is an inflammation of the pericardium due to a multiple etiologies (Table 34-3) of which the most frequent is viral. The diagnostic features are effusion and thickened pericardium. The thickening of the pericardium is due to fibrinous exudates and edema.

The thickened pericardium and effusion can be identified on CT and MR (Fig. 34-12). After contrast media administration, the pericardium shows various levels of enhancement (Fig. 34-12). Enhancement of the pericardium is more reliably demonstrated on spin echo MR, especially using fat saturation technique (Fig. 34-13). The diagnostic features of acute pericarditis are summarized in Table 34-4.

CONSTRICTIVE PERICARDITIS

Constrictive pericarditis is due to progressive pericardial fibrosis, which impedes diastolic ventricular expansion. It is a nonspecific reaction to various conditions, such as infectious pericarditis, connective tissue disease, neoplasm, trauma, long-term renal dialysis, cardiac surgery, and radiation therapy (Table 34-5). Currently, constrictive pericarditis is most often a sequela of cardiac surgery in Europe and North America. However, tuberculous pericarditis remains a leading cause of constrictive pericarditis in Third World countries.

As a result of inflammatory processes, fibrosis of the pericardium and/or pericardial adhesions may occur, sometimes with concomitant calcifications. The less compliant pericardium impedes ventricular and/or atrial filling, depending on the extent of the disease. Another consequence of the rigid pericardium is ventricular interdependence. Because the free walls of ventricular chambers have restricted expansion during diastole, the volumetric capacity of one ventricle is strictly related to the filling of the opposite-sided ventricle. Therefore, minimal and instantaneous differences in ventricular filling result in diastolic ventricular septal motion toward the left ventricle.

FIG. 34.23. Pericardial cyst. CT image (**A**), axial T1-weighted (**B**) and T2-weighted (c) SE images. Cystic mass (**C**) conforms to the contour of the heart and main pulmonary artery. The cyst has water density on CT, homogeneous low to intermediate signal intensity on the T1-weighted images, and homogeneous high signal intensity on the T2-weighted images.

FIG. 34.24. Pericardial cyst. CT images before (**A**) and after (**B**) the administration of contrast media show a homogeneous mass at the right cardiophrenic angle with water attenuation (*arrow*). No enhancement is observed in the postcontrast image.

FIG. 34.25. ECG-gated spin-echo coronal images at the level of the right pulmonary artery (**left**) and 1 cm further ventral (**right**) show an extensive pericardial sarcoma. The tumor infiltrates throughout the left side of the pericardial cavity and the superior recesses (*arrow*). The tumor is located between the left ventricle and the pericardium (*arrowhead*), with an additional component that extends outside the pericardium.

cine MR images and do not enhance on spin echo images after gadolinium.

PERICARDIAL TUMORS

Primary pericardial tumors are rare, with mesothelioma being the most frequent. Sarcoma, lipoma, hemangioma, dermoid, and teratoma can also occur in the pericardium (Fig. 34-25).

Secondary tumors of the pericardium are far more common. These occur from local invasion of lung and mediastinal malignancies and from distant metastases. Lymphomas, melanomas, lung, and breast carcinomas are the most common primary tumors that involve the pericardium (Fig. 34-26).

Most neoplasms have medium signal intensity on T1-weighted SE images and high signal intensity on T2-weighted SE images. Melanoma is an exception with characteristic high intensity on T1-weighted images.

Pericardial hemorrhagic effusion caused by a malignant primary or secondary tumor of the heart pericardium can be

A

B

C

FIG. 34.26. Pericardial neoplastic invasion in three patients. Contrast-enhanced CT at the level of the great vessels (**A**) shows invasion of the pericardium by a bronchogenic carcinoma (*BC*). Note obliteration of the pericardial line (*arrow*) and pericardial effusion (*asterisk*). Contrast-enhanced CT at the level of the right pulmonary artery (**B**) in another patient shows a mediastinal lymphoma (*L*) involving the pericardial cavity. Contrast-enhanced CT at the midventricular level (**C**) in a third patient demonstrates another invasive lymphoma (*L*) obliterating the adjacent pericardial line, with an associated pericardial effusion (*asterisk*).

A **B**

FIG. 34.27. Pericardial metastases. CT images before (**A**) and after (**B**) administration of contrast media show a loculated pericardial effusion (*asterisks*). There are enhancing pericardial nodules on the visceral pericardium (*arrows*).

recognized by MRI and CT. A hemorrhagic effusion should raise suspicion for tumor involvement of the pericardium. Pericardial metastases can also be recognized as enhancing nodules or masses on the visceral or parietal pericardium after administration of contrast media (Fig. 34-27).

The characteristic signal intensity of masses such as cyst, lipoma, hemangioma, and melanoma metastases allows a high probability of a histologic diagnosis based on MRI. However, detection, evaluation of the tumor extension, and differentiation between benign and malignant appearance are the most important roles of cross-sectional imaging in this setting. Nevertheless, definitive differentiation between benign and malignant tumors is frequently not possible.

SELECTED READING

Axel L. Assessment of pericardial disease by MRI and CT. J Magn Reson Imaging 2004; 19:816.

Giorgi B, Mollet NRA, Dymarkowski S, et al. Clinically suspected constrictive pericarditis: MRI assessment of ventricular septal motion and configuration in patients and healthy subjects. Radiology 2003; 228:417–424.

Maui T, Frick S, Higgins CB. Constrictive pericarditis and restrictive cardiomyopathy: evaluation with MRI. Radiology 1992; 182:369–373.

Reinmüller R, Gröll R, Lipton MJ. CT and MRI of pericardial disease. Radiol Clinics N. Am. 2004; 42:587–601.

Spodick DH. Pericardial diseases. In Braunwald, E, Zipes, D, Libby, P. eds. Heart Disease. 6th Ed. Philadelphia: WB Saunders, 2001:1823–1876.

35 Cardiac and Paracardiac Masses

CHARLES B. HIGGINS AND KAREN ORDOVAS

he goals of tomographic imaging in evaluation of cardiac masses are the following:

1. Identify an intracardiac or extracardiac mass.
2. Demonstrate the extent and invasiveness of the mass (staging of tumor).
3. Distinguish between benign and malignant tumor if possible.
4. Distinguish between primary and secondary tumor.
5. Distinguish between tumor and thrombus.

The term *mass* is used rather than *tumor* in this chapter because the most frequent mass within a cardiac chamber is thrombus rather than tumor. Primary tumors are rare. Secondary tumors, either metastatic or representing direct extension of primary tumors of another organ, are about 40 times more frequent than primary cardiac tumors.

Computed tomography (CT) and magnetic resonance imaging (MRI) can help determine the presence and extent of cardiac and paracardiac tumors. These modalities, especially MRI, can also sometimes characterize the mass. Although CT may be adequate for the evaluation of cardiac and paracardiac mass, MRI is usually employed for this purpose. Consequently, this chapter focuses on the findings on MRI.

Because of a wide field of view that encompasses the cardiovascular structures, mediastinum, and adjacent lung simultaneously, CT and MRI can display the intracardiac and extracardiac extent of tumors. In addition, the ability to image in multiple planes makes MRI especially suited for the demarcation of the spatial relationship of a mass to the various cardiac and mediastinal structures. Multiplanar images or reconstructions overcome the volume-averaging problem at the diaphragmatic interface encountered with a solely transaxial imaging plane. These features permit a clear delineation of the possible infiltration of a mass lesion into cardiac and adjacent mediastinal structures. MRI allows the assessment of functional parameters such as ventricular wall thickening, ejection fraction, or flow velocity in adjacent vessels. Therefore, the impact of a tumor on cardiac function can be evaluated.

In clinical practice, MRI and CT are most often used to verify or exclude a possible mass suggested initially by echocardiography. Echocardiography clearly depicts cardiac morphology and provides an assessment of functional parameters. The effectiveness of transthoracic echocardiography is limited by the acoustic window, however, which varies considerably with patient habitus. Image quality of echocardiography may be severely decreased by obesity or chronic obstructive pulmonary disease. Transesophageal echocardiography overcomes this problem but adds invasiveness. The soft tissue contrast achieved with echocardiography remains limited in comparison with that obtained with MRI and CT. Usually, pericardial involvement and infiltration of the myocardium can be better visualized with MRI and CT.

Tissue characterization based on specific T1 and T2 relaxation times is possible to a limited degree. Nevertheless, definitive differentiation between benign and malignant tumors is sometimes not possible. Most cardiac tumors have low to intermediate signal intensity on T1-weighted images and high signal intensity on T2-weighted images. However, the combination of imaging characteristics of a cardiac mass, such as location, signal intensity on T1- and T2-weighted images, possible hyperenhancement after the administration of paramagnetic contrast agents, and possible suppression of signal with the application of a fat-saturation technique, may render a specific tissue diagnosis highly probable in some cases.

TECHNIQUES

Computed Tomography

Multislice or spiral single-slice CT scans in the axial plane after contrast enhancement are used to identify and determine the extent of masses (Fig. 35-1). For this evaluation, ECG-gated multislice CT acquisitions are not necessary. However, ECG-gated multislice CT is now sometimes used especially for evaluation of an intracardiac mass. Collimation is usually 1.25 to 2.5 mm. Retrospective reconstruction of volumetric data in the sagittal or coronal plane may be useful. Reconstructions in the sagittal and coronal planes are done routinely using the multislice axial data usually with slice thickness of 1.25 mm or less. Positron emission tomography/CT can also be used to indicate the likely malignant nature of intracardiac and paracardiac tumors (Fig. 35-2).

FIG. 35.1. Contrast-enhanced CT in the axial plane shows a low-density left ventricular mass involving the apex (*arrows*). Coronal reconstruction from the CT better demonstrates the relationship of the mass (*arrowheads*) with the left ventricular apex. Note the peripheral rim of high density with some calcifications surrounding the lower density central mass (fibroma). *LV*, left ventricle; *LA*, left atrium; *RV*, right ventricle; *Ao*, aorta.

Magnetic Resonance Imaging

ECG-gated transaxial T1-weighted spin-echo (SE) images of the entire thorax are initially acquired for the evaluation of suspected cardiac or paracardiac masses. In addition, such images are frequently acquired in the sagittal or coronal plane to delineate the regions that are displayed suboptimally in the transaxial plane, such as the diaphragmatic surface of the heart. Coronal images facilitate the evaluation of masses

FIG. 35.2. A: Axial contrast-enhanced CT image shows a right atrial mass (*arrowheads*) with a wide point of attachment to the wall. Note a second mass (*arrow*) within the right ventricle (*RV*). **B:** PET scan in the axial plane shows avid uptake of FDG in part of the atrial mass (*large arrow*) and in the ventricular mass (*small arrows*) patient with metastatic thyroid cancer. Note that part of the atrial mass (*arrowhead*) has no uptake due to tumor necrosis. *LV*, left ventricle.

FIG. 35.3. Angiosarcoma. ECG-gated spin-echo image in the coronal plane shows a large tumor in the right atrium extending through the atrial wall (*arrow*). The wide field of view of the coronal plane demonstrates the extent of this angiosarcoma.

FIG. 35.4. Angiosarcoma. ECG-gated spin-echo image in the coronal plane demonstrates a tumor (*T*) infiltrating through the right atrial cavity and extending around the superior vena cava (*arrows*).

involving the aortopulmonary window and pulmonary hili, and mediastinal masses that extend through the cervicothoracic junction. The wide field of view afforded by sagittal and coronal images can readily display the extent of tumors (Figs. 35-3 and 35-4). Contrast between intramural tumor and normal myocardium may be low on nonenhanced T1-weighted images. Transaxial T2-weighted SE images are acquired to enhance the contrast between myocardium and tumor tissue, which usually has a longer T2 relaxation time, and to delineate possible cystic or necrotic components of a mass. The comparison of signal intensities of a mass lesion

on T1-weighted and T2-weighted images may to a certain degree allow for tissue characterization. For example, lipomas have relatively high signal intensity on T1-weighted images and moderate signal intensity on T2-weighted images. Cystic lesions (filled with simple fluid) have low signal intensity on T1-weighted images and high signal intensity on T2-weighted images (Fig. 35-5). The administration of Gd-DTPA (gadolinium diethylenetriamine pentaacetic acid) usually improves the contrast between tumor tissue and myocardium on T1-weighted images and may facilitate tissue characterization. Hyperenhancement of tumor tissue with

A   B

FIG. 35.5. Pericardial cyst. ECG-gated spin-echo T1-weighted (**A**) and T2-weighted (**B**) images of a pericardial cyst (*C*). The simple fluid in the cyst has typical low signal on T1-weighted and homogeneous high signal on T2-weighted images.

FIG. 35.6. Angiosarcoma. ECG-gated spin-echo T1-weighted images before (**A**) and after (**B**) gadolinium chelate administration demonstrates hyperenhancement of the tumor (*T*) compared with the septal myocardium. The postcontrast image uses fat saturation.

MR contrast agents indicates either an enlarged extracellular space of tumor tissue in comparison with normal myocardium (Fig. 35-6) or a high degree of vascularization of the mass. Application of a fat-saturation sequence, which vitiates the bright signal of fat, is effective for the tissue characterization of lipomas (Fig. 35-7).

In patients with cardiac tumors, cine MRI provides valuable information regarding the movement of the cardiac mass relative to cardiovascular structures. Because cine MR images are acquired with gradient-echo or steady-state free precession (SSFP) sequences, a different contrast is obtained than with the SE technique. On SE images, flowing blood appears with low signal intensity, whereas gradient-echo or SSFP images display the blood pool with high signal intensity. Most studies using white blood imaging now use some form of SSFP sequence.

LOCATION OF CARDIAC AND PARACARDIAC MASSES

1. Intracavitary
2. Intramural
3. Intrapericardial—outer contour of pericardium with compression of adjacent cardiac chamber
4. Paracardiac or mediastirial (Fig. 35-8)

FIG. 35.7. Lipoma. ECG-gated spin-echo images in coronal plane, before (**A**) and after (**B**) fat saturation, of a mass situated above the left atrium (*LA*). Signal of the mass is suppressed with fat saturation.

Intracavitary

Intramural

Pericardial

Paracardiac

FIG. 35.8. Location of masses on tomographic imaging.

BENIGN PRIMARY CARDIAC TUMORS

About 80% of primary cardiac tumors are benign (Table 35-1). Although these tumors do not metastasize or invade locally, they may lead to significant morbidity and mortality by causing arrhythmias, valvular obstruction, or embolism. An intramyocardial location can interfere with normal conduction pathways and produce arrhythmias, obstruct coronary blood flow, or diminish compliance or contractility through replacement of myocardium. Both benign and malignant tumors have characteristic sites of origin (Table 35-2).

Myxoma

Myxoma is the most common benign cardiac tumor. It is located in the left atrium in 75% of cases and in the right atrium in 20% of cases. Multiple atrial myxomas may occur rarely, especially in Carney's syndrome. This tumor is usually spherical, but the shape may vary during the cardiac

cycle because of its gelatinous consistency. Left atrial myxomas are typically attached by a narrow pedicle to the area of the fossa ovalis (Fig. 35-9, A). Infrequently, myxomas have a wide base of attachment to the atrial septum (see Fig. 35-9, B). However, a wide mural attachment is more frequently encountered with malignant tumors. The extent of attachment may be difficult to assess for large tumors, which fill nearly the entire cavity so that they are compressed against the septum (Fig. 35-9, B). As a result, the tumor appears to have broad contact with the atrial septum on static MR images. Myxomas can grow through a patent foramen ovale and extend into both atria, a condition that has been described

TABLE 35.1 Primary Benign Cardiac Tumors

- Myxoma
  - usually attached to atrial septum
  - most frequently in LA
- Lipoma or lipomatous hypertrophy of atrial septum
- Papillary fibroelastoma
  - usually attach to valve (aortic valve most frequent)
- Rhabdomyoma
  - most common tumor in children
- Fibroma
- Pheochromocytoma
- Hemangioma

TABLE 35.2 Typical Sites of Origin of Cardiac Tumors

Tumor	Site(s)
• Myxoma	Left atrium 75%; right atrium 20%
• Lipoma	Right atrium; atrial septum
• Papillary fibroelastoma	Aortic valve 30%; mitral valve 2%; pulmonary valve 13%; tricuspid valve 17%
• Rhabdomyoma	Left and right ventricular myocardium
• Fibroma	Right ventricular wall and ventricular septum
• Pheochromocytoma	Peri-left atrium; retroaortic; aorticopulmonary window
• Hemangioma	Any cardiac chamber
• Angiosarcoma	Right atrium, pericardial cavity
• Rhabdomyosarcoma	Ventricular myocardium
• Lymphoma	Right atrium

FIG. 35.9. Myxomas. ECG-gated spin-echo images display two left atrial myxomas with a narrow point of attachment (pedicle; **A**) and a wide point of attachment (**B**) to the left side of the atrial septum.

as a "dumbbell" appearance. Cine MRI permits an evaluation of tumor motion and may help to identify the site and length of attachment of the tumor to the wall or walls of the cardiac chambers. With this technique, myxomas have been shown to prolapse through the funnel of the atrioventricular valve (Fig. 35-10) or into the corresponding ventricle during diastole. Rarely, myxoma can have a wide point of attachment to ventricular endocardium (Figs. 35-11 and 35-12).

Usually, myxomas display intermediate signal intensity (isointense to the myocardium) on T1-weighted SE images. On T2-weighted SE images, myxomas usually have higher signal intensity than myocardium. However, myxomas with very low signal intensity have also been observed. Fibrous stroma, calcification, and the deposition of paramagnetic iron following interstitial hemorrhage can reduce the signal intensity of the tumor on T2-weighted SE images. Rarely, myxomas have been reported to be invisible on SE images because of a lack of contrast with the dark blood pool. Such tumors can be delineated with cine MRI, on which they appear with high contrast against the surrounding bright blood. Most myxomas show increased signal intensity after the administration of Gd-DTPA on T1-weighted images (Fig. 35-13) and on delayed gadolinium-enhanced images, which is probably secondary to an increased interstitial space and, therefore, a larger distribution volume of the contrast agent within the tumor than in normal tissue.

FIG. 35.10. Myxoma. Cine MR images (balanced steady-state free precession) in the axial plane display a right atrial myxoma in diastole (**A**) and systole (**B**). The motion of the tumor is evident with movement into the tricuspid valve during diastole.

A   B

FIG. 35.11. Left ventricular myxoma. T1-weighted axial spin-echo images before (**A**) and after (**B**) the administration of gadolinium chelate show a tumor (*arrow*) with a wide point of attachment to the left ventricular (*LV*) endocardium. Tumor markedly enhances after contrast media. Fat saturation was used after gadolinium. *RV*, right ventricle.

Lipoma and Lipomatous Hypertrophy of the Atrial Septum

Lipomas are reported to be the second most common benign cardiac tumor in adults but may actually be the most common. If the mass projects into the right atrium, it is called

FIG. 35.12. Contrast-enhanced CT in the axial plane shows the left ventricular myxoma (*arrow*) with some enhancement of the central part of the tumor. *LV*, left ventricle; *RV*, right ventricle.

a lipoma, while lipomatous hypertrophy is confined to the atrial septum. They may occur at any age but are encountered most frequently in middle-aged and elderly adults. Lipomas consist of encapsulated mature adipose cells and fetal fat cells. The tumor consistency is soft, and lipomas may grow to a large size without causing symptoms. Lipomas are typically located in the right atrium (Fig. 35-14) or atrial septum. They arise from the endocardial surface and have a broad base of attachment. Lipomas have the same signal intensity as subcutaneous and epicardial fat on all MRI sequences. Because fat has a short T1 relaxation time, lipomas have high signal intensity on T1-weighted images, which can be suppressed with fat-saturating pulse sequences (see Fig. 35-14). Usually, they appear with homogeneous signal intensity but may have a few thin septations. They do not enhance after the administration of contrast. On T2-weighted images, lipomas have intermediate signal intensity.

Lipomatous hypertrophy of the atrial septum is considered to be an entity distinct from intracavitary lipoma. Lipomatous hypertrophy of the atrial septum is more common and is alleged to be a cause of supraventricular arrhythmias. Lipomatous hypertrophy is defined as a deposition of fat in the atrial septum around the fossa ovalis that exceeds 2 cm in transverse diameter. It spares the fossa ovalis, a characteristic feature that is clearly delineated with T1-weighted SE images (Fig. 35-15). Lipomatous hypertrophy has the same cellular composition as lipoma but is not encapsulated and infiltrates through the tissue of the atrial septum. It is not a true neoplasm. Fatty tissue may extend from the septum into both atria to a considerable degree. Signal intensity on MRI is similar to that of lipomas.

A   B

FIG. 35.13. Myxoma. ECG-gated spin-echo images of a myxoma before (**A**) and after (**B**) gado-linium chelate administration. Tumor (*arrows*) increases substantially in signal intensity.

Papillary Fibroelastoma

Papillary fibroelastomas constitute about 10% of benign primary cardiac tumors. These tumors consist of avascular fronds of connective tissue lined by endothelium. Papillary fibroelastomas are attached to the valves by a short pedicle in approximately 90% of cases. They usually do not exceed 1 cm in diameter. Papillary fibroelastomas have been found on the aortic (29%), mitral (2%), pulmonary (13%), and tricuspid (17%) valves. Right-sided tumors usually remain asymptomatic. Symptoms associated with fibroelastoma are related to embolization of thrombi, which may accumulate on the tumor. Because of their high content of fibrous tissue, they have low signal intensity on T2-weighted images. The diagnosis of these valvular tumors is challenging because of their small size, low contrast relative to the blood pool

A   B

FIG. 35.14. Lipoma. ECG-gated spin-echo images of a lipoma (*arrows*) of the right atrium without (**A**) and with (**B**) fat saturation prepulse sequence. With fat saturation, signal is depleted from the right atrial mass.

A   B

FIG. 35.15. Lipomatous hypertrophy (infiltration) of the atrial septum. ECG-gated T1-weighted spin-echo images before (**A**) and after (**B**) fat saturation show the atrial septum thickened by fatty infiltration. Signal of the fat is decreased on the fat-saturation image.

on SE images, and location on the rapidly moving valves. On cine MR sequences with improved homogeneity of the bright blood pool signal (SSFP sequence), visualization of valve motion during the cardiac cycle can be excellent. So, small masses attached to valves can be depicted with cine MRI. In most cases, signal intensity characteristics after the administration of Gd-DTPA are difficult to evaluate, so the differential diagnosis between thrombus and tumor may not be feasible. Cine MRI can be used to assess the effect of valvular tumors on valve function; it demonstrates jet flow caused by either obstruction or regurgitation.

Rhabdomyoma

Rhabdomyomas are the most common cardiac tumors in children, representing 40% of all cardiac tumors in this age group. Thirty to fifty percent of rhabdomyomas occur in patients with tuberous sclerosis. Rhabdomyomas may vary in size and are frequently multiple. They are characterized by an intramural location and involve equally the left and right ventricles (RV). Small, entirely intramural tumors may be difficult to identify. Larger tumors distort the shape of the myocardial wall or may bulge into the cavity. Larger tumors can also distort the epicardial contour of the heart. Rhabdomyomas may have a signal intensity similar to that of normal myocardium on SE images and may display hyperenhancement after the administration of gadolinium contrast.

Fibroma

Fibroma is the second most common benign cardiac tumor in children. It is a connective tissue tumor that is composed

of fibroblasts interspersed among collagen fibers. It arises within the myocardial walls. Unlike most other primary cardiac tumors, fibromas usually do not display cystic changes, hemorrhage, or focal necrosis, but dystrophic calcification is common. Fibromas may cause arrhythmias and have been reported to be associated with sudden death. Approximately, 30% of these tumors remain asymptomatic and may be discovered incidentally because of heart murmurs, ECG changes, or abnormalities on chest roentgenography. Fibromas occur most often within the septum or anterior wall of the RV and can reach a large diameter (Figs. 35-16 and 35-17). On T2-weighted MR images, they are characteristically hypointense to the surrounding myocardium, which is compatible with the short T2 relaxation time of fibrous tissue. On T1-weighted images, fibromas may appear isointense to the myocardium. Fibromas show hyperenhancement of the periphery of the tumor early after the administration of Gd-DTPA. Administration of Gd-DTPA has been effective for demarcating these intramural tumors more clearly from normal myocardium (see Figs. 35-16 and 35-17). Hyperenhancement of compressed myocardium at the margin of the tumor facilitates delineation of the borders of the tumor. Delayed (15 to 20 minutes after contrast administration) hyperenhancement of the entire mass has also been observed on the inversion recovery gradient echo (viability) sequence.

The differential diagnosis for intramural masses in children is rhabdomyoma versus fibroma. If the tumor is solitary and has low signal intensity on T2-weighted images, fibroma is more likely. If multiple tumors are present with high intensity on T2-weighted images, rhabdomyomas are the likely diagnosis.

A   **B**

FIG. 35.16. Fibroma. ECG-gated T1-weighted spin-echo images before (**A**) and after (**B**) gadolinium chelate administration show a fibroma (*T*) of the ventricular septum in a young child. There is hyperenhancement of the periphery (*P*) of the mass but no enhancement of the center (*C*).

Pheochromocytoma

Pheochromocytomas arise from neuroendocrine cells clustered in the visceral paraganglia in the wall of the left atrium, roof of the right and left atrium, atrial septum, behind the ascending aorta, and along the coronary arteries. Hypertension, the most common symptom, is related to catecholamine overproduction by the mass. The average age at diagnosis is 30 to 50 years.

Pheochromocytomas can be found at each of the above locations but are predominantly encountered in and around the left atrium (Figs. 34-18 and 34-19). Most are located outside of the cardiac chamber. They usually have a broad interface with the heart. Cardiac pheochromocytomas are usually benign. Pheochromocytomas are generally highly vascularized. The average size ranges from 3 to 8 cm at diagnosis. Pheochromocytomas are hyperintense to the myocardium on T2-weighted images and isointense or hyperintense on T1-weighted images (see Figs. 35-18 and 35-19). After Gd-DTPA administration, they show strong signal enhancement because of their high vascularity. Enhancement may be heterogeneous, with central nonenhancing areas, related to tumor necrosis. The combination of imaging findings, clinical symptoms, and biochemical evidence of catecholamine overproduction usually permits a confident diagnosis.

A   **B**

FIG. 35.17. Fibroma. ECG-gated T1-weighted spin-echo transaxial images before (**A**) and after (**B**) gadolinium chelate administration in an infant. The periphery of the huge mass shows hyperenhancement. The center of the mass shows low intensity on the cine MR image. The mass bulges off the free wall of the right ventricle.

FIG. 35.18. Pheochromocytoma. ECG-gated T1-weighted spin-echo images show a mass of high signal intensity (*M*) adjacent to the left atrium.

FIG. 35.19. Pheochromocytoma. ECG-gated T1-weighted image in coronal plane. The mass originates from the aortic body and is situated above the roof of the left atrium (*LA*). It has high signal intensity on T1-weighted images.

Hemangioma

Cardiac hemangiomas are composed of endothelial cells that line interconnecting vascular channels. These vascular cavities are separated by connective tissue. According to the size of the vascular channels, hemangiomas are divided into capillary, cavernous, or venous types. Calcification, which can easily be identified on CT, is often present in these tumors. Hemangiomas may involve the endocardium, myocardium, or epicardium. They have been found in all chambers and also the pericardium. On T2-weighted images, hemangiomas are hyperintense. On T1-weighted images, they are of intermediate signal intensity but can have higher intensity than myocardium (Fig. 35-20). Because of interspersed calcifications and possible flow voids at areas of blood flow in the channels of hemangiomas, they may have

FIG. 35.20. Hemangioma. T1-weighted (**top left**), T2-weighted fat saturation (**top right**), and T1-weighted after gadolinium chelate administration (**bottom left**) spin-echo images and a gradient-echo cine MR image (**bottom right**) demonstrate a large mass (*M*) originating in the septum and bulging into the right ventricular cavity. The mass has high signal on all sequences.

TABLE 35.3 Primary Malignant Cardiac Tumors

- Angiosarcoma (most frequent)
- Rhabdomyosarcoma
- Leiomyosarcoma
- Fibrosarcoma
- Liposarcoma
- Malignant histiosarcoma
- Osteochrondrosarcoma
- Lymphoma

TABLE 35.4 Imaging Features of Malignant Cardiac Tumors

1. Involvement of more than one cardiac chamber or chamber and attaching vessel.
2. Extension into pulmonary veins, vena cavae; pulmonary artery or aorta.
3. Wide point of attachment to wall of cardiac chamber(s).
4. Combined intramural and intracavitary components.
5. Necrosis within tumor.
6. Extension outside a cardiac chamber.
7. Hemorrhagic pericardial effusion.
8. Pulmonary metastasis(es).

inhomogeneous signal intensity. They usually show intense enhancement after the administration of gadolinium contrast because of their rich vascularity.

MALIGNANT PRIMARY CARDIAC TUMORS

One fourth of primary cardiac tumors are malignant; sarcomas represent the largest number, followed by primary cardiac lymphomas. The types of malignant cardiac tumor are indicated in Tables 35-3. The features of malignant cardiac tumors are the following: involvement of more than one cardiac chamber; extension into pulmonary veins, pulmonary arteries, or vena cavae; wide point of attachment to the wall of a chamber or chambers; necrosis within the tumor; extension outside the heart; and hemorrhagic pericardial effusion. A combined intramural and intracavitary location is another suggestive feature of malignant tumors (Fig. 35-21). MRI is effective for demonstrating invasion of the pericardium and extension into the pericardial fat (Figs. 35-3 and 35-22). Pericardial infiltration is displayed on MRI as a disruption, thickening, or nodularity of the

pericardium, often combined with pericardial effusion. Cardiac tamponade as a consequence of hemorrhagic pericardial effusion may be demonstrated as diastolic indentation of the right atrial free wall. Features of malignant tumors are summarized in Table 35-4.

Extension into the mediastinum and metastasis are also clear signs of malignancy. The organs most frequently involved are the lungs, pleurae, mediastinal lymph nodes, and liver. The rapid growth of malignant cardiac tumors may cause focal necrosis in the central part of the tumor. Necrotic areas are delineated as regions of lower signal intensity within a hyperenhancing mass after the administration of Gd-DTPA (Fig. 35-23).

Angiosarcoma

Angiosarcomas are the most common malignant cardiac tumors in adults and constitute one third of malignant

A

B

FIG. 35.21. Lymphoma. Coronal spin-echo (**A**) and gradient-echo (cine MR; **B**) images demonstrate a large mass (*M*), which involves the lateral wall of the left ventricle and extends into the left ventricular (*LV*) and atrial (*LA*) cavities.

A   B

FIG. 35.22. Rhabdomyosarcoma. Coronal (**A**) and transaxial after gadolinium chelate administration (**B**) spin-echo images. Coronal images show a loculated pericardial effusion (*E*) with high intensity on T1-weighted imaging (hemorrhagic effusion). The epicardial fat line (*arrows*) is disrupted by the tumor extending into the pericardial space. Transaxial image after contrast administration shows the tumor (*T*) demonstrated by the marked enhancement, whereas the pericardial fluid is not enhanced.

cardiac tumors (Figs. 35-3, 35-4, 35-24, and 35-25). They occur predominantly in men between 20 and 50 years of age. This entity has been divided into two clinicopathologic forms. Most frequently, angiosarcomas are found in the right atrium (see Figs. 35-3, 35-4, 35-24, and 35-25). In this form, no evidence of Kaposi sarcoma is found. Another form is characterized by involvement of the epicardium or pericardium in the presence of Kaposi sarcoma. This form is associated with the acquired immunodeficiency syndrome. Angiosarcomas consist of ill-defined anastomotic vascular spaces that are lined by endothelial cells and avascular clusters of moderately pleomorphic spindle cells

FIG. 35.23. Left ventricular myocardial sarcoma. Sagittal image after gadolinium chelate administration demonstrates enhancement of the mass (*arrows*) involving the diaphragmatic wall of the left ventricle (*LV*). The central necrotic region does not enhance. There is a large loculated pericardial effusion below the diaphragmatic wall.

FIG. 35.24. Angiosarcoma. ECG-gated spin-echo image demonstrates a mass filling most of the right atrium and extending through the atrial wall. The tumor has heterogeneous intensity on this T1-weighted image. High signal region (*arrow*) represents intratumoral hemorrhage.

FIG. 35.25. Angiosarcoma. T1-weighted spin-echo (**A**) and gradient-echo (**B**) images show components of the mass along the posterior right atrial wall and in the pericardial cavity. Note the sinuous regions in the pericardial mass, which represent vascular channels. These channels have high signal because of blood flow on the gradient-echo images (*arrows*). *RA*, right atrium; *RV*, right ventricle.

surrounded by collagen stroma. T1-weighted SE imaging usually demonstrates heterogeneous signal intensity of the tumor with focal areas of high signal intensity, which presumably represent hemorrhage (see Fig. 35-24). However, angiosarcomas can also have homogeneous signal intensity. After contrast administration, angiosarcomas show hyperenhancement. Some of the tumors show regions of low signal intensity on both T1- and T2-weighted images. These central regions have high signal intensity on cine gradient-echo images and represent vascular channels (see Fig. 35-25). This finding is often described as a "cauliflower" appearance. Cases with diffuse pericardial infil-

tration have been found to show linear hyperenhancement along vascular spaces.

Rhabdomyosarcoma

Rhabdomyosarcomas are the most common malignant cardiac tumors in children. They can arise anywhere in the myocardium and are often multiple. Their signal intensity on MRI is variable. Rhabdomyosarcomas may be isointense to the myocardium on T1- and T2-weighted images, but areas of necrosis can exhibit heterogeneous signal intensity and patchy hyperenhancement after Gd-DTPA administration

FIG. 35.26. Lymphoma. T1-weighted spin-echo image with fat saturation after gadolinium chelate administration at the level of the right atrium (**A**) and the right ventricle (**B**). A mass (*M*) invades the right atrial cavity and right ventricular wall. *RA*, right atrium; *RV*, right ventricle.

(see Fig. 35-22). Extracardiac extension into the pulmonary arteries and descending aorta has been clearly delineated with MRI.

Other Sarcomas (Fibrosarcoma, Osteosarcoma, Leiomyosarcoma, Liposarcoma)

Other possible primary sarcomas are fibrosarcomas, osteosarcomas, leiomyosarcomas, and liposarcomas. These all are rare tumors. The signal intensity characteristics of these entities are nonspecific. Most of these tumors show signal intensity isointense to normal myocardium on T1-weighted images and hyperintense on T2-weighted images. Most of these tumors show increased signal intensity on T1-weighted images after Gd-DTPA administration, so that the lesions are more conspicuous and the delineation of the tumor margins is increased.

Lymphoma

Primary cardiac lymphoma is less common than secondary lymphoma involving the heart, which usually represents the spread of non-Hodgkin's lymphoma. Primary lymphoma of the heart most often occurs in immunocompromised patients and is highly aggressive. Almost all primary cardiac lymphomas are B-cell lymphomas. Although primary cardiac lymphoma is rare, it is mandatory to consider this entity in the diagnosis of malignant cardiac tumors because early chemotherapy is usually effective. These tumors arise most often on the right side of the heart, especially in the right atrium, but have also been found in the other chambers (see Fig. 35-21). A large pericardial effusion is frequently present. Variable morphology of the masses has been described; both circumscribed polypoid and ill-defined infiltrative lesions have been reported. Lymphomas may appear hypointense to the myocardium on T1-weighted images and hyperintense on T2-weighted images. After Gd-DTPA administra-

FIG. 35.27. Mediastinal tumor (*T*) invading the pericardium and atrial walls. *LA*, left atrium; *RA*, right atrium.

tion, homogeneous or heterogeneous enhancement of the tumor, depending on the presence of necrosis, may be seen. Some lymphomas consist of a large extracardiac mediastinal mass as well as an invasive mass in the cardiac chambers (Fig. 35-26).

SECONDARY CARDIAC TUMORS

Secondary tumors of the heart and pericardium are about 40-fold more frequent than primary tumors. Three routes of spread to the heart can be discerned: (1) direct extension from intrathoracic tumors (mediastinum and lungs); (2) extension of abdominal malignancies through the inferior vena cava into the right atrium (renal, adrenal, and hepatic carcinomas); and (3) metastasis (Table 35-5).

TABLE 35.5 Secondary Cardiac Tumors
1. Direct extension from primary lung and mediastinal malignancy
• lung cancer
• malignant thymoma
• malignant mesothelioma
2. Inferior vena caval extension of abdominal malignancy
• hepatocellular carcinoma
• renal cell carcinoma
• adrenal carcinoma
3. Metastasis
• lung cancer
• breast cancer
• malignant melanoma
• lymphoma, leukemia
• sarcoma
• other

FIG. 35.28. Extension of lung cancer through left atrial wall.

FIG. 35.29. Metastasis to the left atrium. ECG-gated T1-weighted spin-echo transaxial images.

Direct Extension from Adjacent Tumors

Tumors of the lung and mediastinum can infiltrate the pericardium and heart directly (Figs. 35-27 and 35-28). It is important to recognize invasion of the heart because such a tumor is usually nonresectable. In mediastinal lymphoma, possible invasion of the pericardium can change the staging of the tumor. CT and MRI are effective for delineating paracardiac tumors and possible extension into the heart because of its wide field of view. CT and MRI clearly show extension of these tumors to the cardiac structures (Figs. 35-2, 35-27, and 35-28) and possible evidence of hemorrhagic or nonhemorrhagic pericardial effusion. These modalities are

FIG. 35.31. Renal cell carcinoma. Direct extension of mass (*M*) into the right atrium via inferior vena cava. *CS*, coronary sinus; *RA*, right atrium.

effective in demonstrating invasion of the pericardium and myocardium in advanced lung cancer.

Metastasis

Melanomas, leukemias, and lymphomas (see Fig. 35-26) are the tumors that most frequently metastasize to the heart, but cardiac metastases can arise from almost any malignant tumor in the body. Melanomas have the highest frequency of seeding into the heart and are frequently found in the heart at autopsy. The mechanism of metastatic spread of tumors to the heart is direct seeding to the endocardium, passage of tumor emboli through the coronary arteries, or retrograde lymphatic spread through bronchomediastinal lymphatic chan-

FIG. 35.30. Metastasis to right atrial appendage. ECG-gated T1-weighted spin-echo sagittal image shows a large mass (*M*) filling and expanding the right atrial appendage.

FIG. 35.32. Left ventricular thrombus after myocardial infarction. Transaxial gradient-echo (cine MR) image shows a low-intensity intracavitary mass (*arrow*).

A

B

FIG. 35.33. **A:** Cine MR image in the vertical long-axis plane shows apical wall thinning and mural thrombus (*arrow*). **B:** Delayed-enhancement image in the same plane shows transmural hyper-enhancement (*arrowheads*) consistent with prior myocardial infarction and a low-intensity mural thrombus (*arrow*). *LA*, left atrium; *LA*, left ventricle. Compliments of H. Sakuma, Mie, Japan.

nels. MRI is highly effective for delineating the location and extent of metastatic tumors in cardiac chambers (Figs. 35-29 and 35-30) and assessing potential respectability.

Transvenous Extension into the Heart

Another site for the entry of secondary tumors into the heart is tumor extension through the large veins connecting with cardiac chambers. Tumor thrombus arising from carcinoma of the kidney, liver, or adrenal gland can extend through the inferior vena cava into the right atrium (Fig. 35-31), and primary carcinoma of the lung and thymus can extend through the superior vena cava. Lung cancer can extend into the left atrium through a pulmonary vein. The evaluation of the possible attachment of such tumors to the atrial wall is mandatory for surgical planning. If the atrial walls are not infiltrated, complete resection of the tumor may still be possible.

INTRACARDIAC THROMBUS

Thrombus is the most common intracardiac mass, involving most frequently the LV or left atrium. Atrial thrombus is encountered in patients with mitral valve disease or atrial fibrillation. LV mural thrombus is associated with akinetic or dyskinetic regions of the ventricle. It is most often located in the LV at the site of myocardial infarction (Figs. 35-32, 35-33 and 35-34) or at the apex in dilated cardiomyopathy. However, any region of the ventricular cavity with static blood is prone to thrombus formation. CT and MRI are especially advantageous for detecting throm-

bus in the left atrial appendage, which may be difficult to assess using transthoracic echocardiography (Figs. 35-35 and 35-36).

On SE images, the signal intensity of thrombus can vary from low to high depending on age-related changes in the composition of the thrombus. The signal intensity

FIG. 35.34. Delayed-enhancement image in the axial plane shows a low signal intensity multilayered organized thrombus in the left ventricular apex (*arrow*). Note the transmural area of delayed enhancement in the apical and apical-septal regions (*arrowheads*).

A

B

FIG. 35.35. Left atrial appendage thrombus (**A**) and metastatic tumor of the right ventricle (**B**). Transaxial gradient echo (cine MR) image shows a mass (*M*) filling the left atrial appendage with low intensity. The mass (*M*) in the right ventricle has intermediate signal intensity.

of thrombus can vary with time since it is influenced by paramagnetic hemoglobin breakdown products, such as intracellular methemoglobin and hemosiderin, or superparamagnetic substances, such as ferritin. Fresh thrombus usually shows high signal intensity on T1- and T2-weighted SE images, whereas older thrombus has low signal intensity on T1- and T2-weighted images. Intracavitary high signal on SE images caused by slowly flowing blood may be difficult to distinguish from thrombus. However, this problem can be overcome by using cine MRI.

DIFFERENTIATION BETWEEN TUMOR AND BLOOD CLOT

The distinction between clot and tumor is usually made with gradient-echo sequences. The gradient-echo technique is more sensitive to susceptibility and T2* effects than is the SE technique (Table 35-6). As the various blood degeneration

FIG. 35.36. Axial image from a contrast-enhanced CT shows a filling defect within the left atrial appendage (*arrow*), with lobulated contour, consistent with a thrombus. Note the enlargement of the left atrium (*LA*) in this patient with atrial fibrillation.

TABLE 35.6 Distinguishing MR Imaging Features of Tumors Versus Clot

Tumor
- Medium signal on T1 and high signal on T2 SE
- Early enhancement after gadolinium chelate on T1 SE
- Shorter T1 nulling time than myocardium on delayed gadolinium-enhanced sequence (IRGRE)
- Higher signal than myocardium on cine GRE or cine SSFP

Clot
- Variable signal on SE depending on age
- No early enhancement after gadolinium chelate on T1 SE
- Longer T1 nulling time than myocardium on delayed gadolinium-enhanced sequence
- Lower signal than myocardium or cine GRE and cine SSFP

products pass through the different stages of magnetic susceptibility, they cause shortening of T2* relaxivity. The result is low signal intensity of the thrombus on cine MR images (see Figs. 35-32, 35-33, and 35-35). An exception to this generalization is fresh thrombus, which can have high signal intensity. Tumor tissue usually is hyperintense in comparison with myocardium and skeletal muscle on T2-weighted SE images and cine MR images. However, some myxomas containing substantial iron produce low signal and so mimic thrombus. Another method for differentiating between tumor and clot is to use Gd-DTPA-enhanced T1-weighted images. Thrombus does not enhance after the administration of Gd-DTPA, whereas tumors show enhancement (Fig. 35-13). Tumor can usually be differentiated from thrombus by using cine MR images and T1-weighted SE images after Gd-DTPA administration. Another approach is using the delayed gadolinium-enhanced sequence. At an inversion delay that nulls myocardial signal, the thrombus has even lower signal than myocardium (Figs. 35-33 and 35-34).

DIFERENTIATION OF CARDIAC MASSES FROM NORMAL ANATOMIC VARIANTS

A potential pitfall in the evaluation of intracardiac masses may arise from the misdiagnosis of normal anatomic variants, such as a prominent crista terminalis, eustachian valve, or Chiari network. The crista terminalis, a fibromuscular band extending between the ostia of the superior and inferior vena cavae on the posterior right atrial wall, represents a residuum of the septum spurium where the sinus venosus was incorporated into the right atrial wall. The Chiari network, a reticulum situated in the right atrium, is attached to the region of the crista terminalis and extends to the valves of the inferior vena cava and coronary sinus, or sometimes to the floor of the right atrium near the ostium of the coronary sinus. The Chiari network is derived from the valvulae venosi. These structures regress to variable degrees, and a nodule-like residue in the right atrium is visible on MRI in some patients. Awareness of these variants can prevent misinterpretation as mass lesions.

SELECTED READING

Araoz PA, Eklund HE, Welch TJ, et al. CT and MR imaging of primary cardiac malignancies. Radiographics 1999; 19:1421.

Araoz PA, Mulvagh SL, Tazlaar HD, et al. CT and MR imaging of benign primary cardiac neoplasms with echocardiographic correlation. Radiographics 2000; 20:1303.

Hoffmann U, Globits S, Schima W, et al. Usefulness of MRI of cardiac and paracardiac masses. Am J Cardiol 2003; 92:890.

Krombach GA, Saeed M, Higgins CB. Cardiac masses In: Higgins CB, de Roos A (eds). MRI and CT of Cardiovascular System. Philadelphia: Lippincott Williams & Wilkins, 2006:162.

Schvartzman PR, White RD. Imaging of cardiac and paracardiac masses. J Thorac Imaging 2000; 15:265.

Siripornpitak S, Higgins CB. MRI of primary malignant cardiovascular tumors. J Comput Assist Tomogr 1997; 21:462.

36

Magnetic Resonance Imaging of Congenital Heart Disease

CHARLES B. HIGGINS, KAREN ORDOVAS, AND GAUTHAM P. REDDY

The overall objectives of imaging in congenital heart disease (CHD) are the precise delineation of cardiovascular anatomy and the quantitative assessment of function. The evaluation of CHD was one of the first applications of cardiac magnetic resonance imaging (MRI) and continues to be one of its most important indications. MRI has significant advantages over other modalities, including echocardiography and angiography, for the definitive assessment of congenital cardiovascular anomalies. MRI does not require the use of a contrast agent or ionizing radiation. The absence of ionizing radiation is a major advantage of MRI in children, who in the past have been exposed to large does of radiation during cine angiography for initial diagnosis and postoperative monitoring.

The role of MRI has been greatly influenced by the perceived success of echocardiography as the primary noninvasive imaging technique in CHD. The major applications have been for lesions incompletely evaluated by echocardiography. However, substantial technological improvements, especially fast cine MRI using (steady-state free precessation [SSFP]) and noncontrast and contrast-enhanced magnetic resonance angiography (MRA), make MRI at least equal to echocardiography in the diagnosis of all types of CHD in children and adults. Echocardiography is still considered to be the more effective and easily applicable modality for infants. On the other hand, MRI is becoming recognized as more effective in adolescent and adult CHD and for follow-up of corrected complex anomalies.

MAJOR CLINICAL INDICATIONS

At present, the major indications for MRI in CHD are as follows:

1. Thoracic aortic anomalies, such as coarctation and arch anomalies
2. Pulmonary arterial anomalies and pulmonary atresia
3. Complex cyanotic disease, such as atresia of atrioventricular valves and double-inlet ventricles
4. Abnormalities of pulmonary venous connections
5. Postoperative evaluation of complex procedures
6. Coronary arterial anomalies
7. Adolescent and adult CHD
8. Monitoring regurgitation and ventricular function before and after surgery

TECHNIQUES

MRI studies are directed toward precise display of the cardiovascular anatomy and quantification of ventricular function and blood flow. An advantage of MRI in CHD is measurement of ventricular volumes and function using cine MRI and velocity-encoded (phase contrast) cine MRI.

For children younger than 8 to 10 years and children unwilling or unable to remain immobile and cooperative during imaging, light anesthesia without intubation is used. This is usually under the control of an anesthesiologist. The favored drug is intravenous propofol. Blood pressure, heart rate, and oxygen saturation are monitored during the procedure.

Anatomy

Assessment of anatomy is done with one or more of the following techniques: ECG-gated multislice spin-echo (black-blood images); breath-hold single-slice or multislice turbo spin-echo (black blood); balanced SSFP (white blood); and noncontrast and contrast-enhanced three-dimensional (3D) MRA. The latter technique is usually applied for the evaluation of anomalies of the great arteries, pulmonary veins, and surgical shunts.

Function

The techniques used in the evaluation of right and left ventricular function are generically called cine MRI. There are a multitude of cine MRI sequences; the most frequently applied one now is a balanced steady-state free precession (SSFP) sequence and real-time cine MRI. Because of optimized homogeneous contrast between cavitary blood and myocardium, balanced SSFP sequences (balanced fast field echo [FFE]; true fast imaging with steady precession [FISP]; and fast imaging employing steady-state acquisition [FIESTA]) are now preferred. The so-called real-time sequence may be advantageous in infants and young children who cannot hold their breath.

Cine MR images are used to quantify ventricular volumes and function. Right and left ventricular volumes are indexed to body surface areas (EDV/m² and ESV/m²).

FIG. 36.1. Postoperative tetralogy of Fallot. Sagittal cine MR images in systole (**left**) and diastole (**right**) demonstrate a signal void (*arrowhead*) projected into the pulmonary artery (pulmonary stenosis) and a signal void (*arrow*) into the right ventricle (pulmonary regurgitation).

A distinct advantage of MRI compared to echocardiography is its precision and reproducibility for quantifying right ventricular volume and function. For ventricular volumetrics, images are acquired in the cardiac short-axis plane.

Cine MR images are also used to evaluate valvular function. Planes approximately parallel to the valve leaflet or cusps can demonstrate valve motion, such as the horizontal long-axis plane for assessing mitral valve motion

and RV outlet plane for visualizing infundibular and pulmonary valvular stenosis. The high-velocity jet caused by valvular stenosis and regurgitation may be identified on cine MR images as a flow void (Fig. 36-1). However, flow voids may not be discernible if the echo time (TE) is less than 6 milliseconds on GRE cine and on balanced SSFP cine. On the latter cine, high flow velocity may cause increased signal.

Volume and Velocity of Blood Flow

Quantification of blood flow is done using velocity-encoded (VEC; phase contrast) MRI. In phase contrast imaging, the signal intensity signifies the velocity of blood at each pixel. ECG-gated phase contrast images can be produced in which each image shows the velocity at a different time in the cardiac cycle. Because these are cine-images, they can be referred to as VEC cine MRI. A region of interest drawn around a blood vessel will give the mean velocity within the vessel at that point in the cardiac cycle. The cross-sectional area of the vessel can be multiplied by the spatial mean velocity to obtain the flow in the blood vessel.

VEC cine MRI is used to measure valvular regurgitant volume (Fig. 36-2); differential flow in central pulmonary arteries; systemic to pulmonary shunt flow; flow through conduits (Rastelli and Fontan conduits); and collateral

FIG. 36.2. A: Postoperative tetralogy of Fallot. Sagittal spin-echo image (**top left**), axial magnitude image (**top right**), and phase images in systole (**bottom left**) and diastole (**bottom right**). Phase contrast images show forward flow in systole (dark voxels) and retrograde flow in diastole (bright voxels; *arrow*). Region of interest for flow measurements is shown on the pulmonary artery. **B:** Flow versus time curve displays the forward and retrograde flow in the pulmonary artery. Area under negative component of the curve yields a direct quantification of the volume of regurgitation.

flow in coarctation. By determining the voxel with the peak velocity just beyond a stenosis, this technique can estimate the peak gradient across a valvular or conduit stenosis.

ACYANOTIC LESIONS

Left-to-Right Shunts

Echocardiography provides essential diagnostic information in most left-to-right shunts. MRI is used for a few specific purposes. The major indications are for the following suspected lesions: sinus venosus atrial septal defect (ASD), partial anomalous pulmonary venous connection, and supracristal ventricular septal defect (VSD). A new indication in patients with ASD is to provide precise measurement of the defect and its location for planning of transcatheter ASD closure device placement. VEC cine MRI may also be employed to measure the systemic to pulmonary flow ratio.

Atrial Septal Defect

Spin-echo and cine MR images in the transaxial or four-chamber planes demonstrate the site of the ASD (Fig. 36-3). MR clearly depicts the defect in the portion of the septum separating the superior vena cava from the left atrium, which is diagnostic of a sinus venosus ASD (Fig. 36-4). It also shows the anomalous connection of the right upper lobe pulmonary vein to the superior vena cava adjacent to the septal defect. On spin-echo MR images, the thin fossa ovalis can be mistaken for an ASD. To avoid this error, the defect should

FIG. 36.4. Sinus venosus atrial septal defect. Cine MR images in three axial planes (**top row and bottom left**) and the coronal plane (**bottom right**) show the defect (*arrow*) in the portion of the atrial septum between the superior vena cava and the left atrium. The right upper lobe pulmonary vein (*arrowheads*) connecting at the junction of the superior vena cava (*SVC*) with the right atrium is associated with the sinus venosus defect. Coronal image shows the dilatation of the SVC at the site of connection of the anomalous pulmonary vein.

be evident at two adjacent anatomic levels or confirmed by a flow jet (void) across the defect on cine MRI.

Secundum ASD is situated in the middle of the atrial septum (Fig. 36-3). If very large, it may approach the aortic or mitral valve annulus (Fig. 36-5). Primum ASD is situated just adjacent to the atrioventricular valves (Fig. 36-6). A diagnostic characteristic of primum ASD is that the mitral and tricuspid valves are at the same level (distance) from the cardiac apex (Fig. 36-6). The demonstration of the location and size of an ASD is facilitated by cine MRI in the horizontal long-axis (four chamber) plane.

VEC (phase contrast) cine in a plane parallel to the ASD is used to determine the dimensions of the defect and if it is amenable for closing with an ASD closure device (Fig. 36-7). For this purpose, a low velocity encoding value (40 cm/s) is used in order to include flow at the margins of the defect. For placement of a closure device, the defect should be less than 3.5 to 4.0 cm in diameter. Cine MRI is also used to measure the distance of the margins of the defect from the mitral and aortic valves and pulmonary veins.

VEC cine MRI measurement in the main pulmonary artery and proximal ascending aorta can be used to calculate pulmonary to systemic flow ratio (Qp/Qs) (Fig. 36-8). The imaging planes are placed perpendicular to the direction of

FIG. 36.3. Secundum atrial septal defect. Cine MR image in the axial plane demonstrates the defect in the atrial septum (*arrowhead*). *RA*, right atrium; *LA*, left atrium.

FIG. 36.5. Large secundum atrial septal defect. Axial cine MR image shows a large secundum ASD (*arrow*) approaching the aortic valve annulus. *RA*, right atrium; *LA*, left atrium; *Ao*, aorta.

FIG. 36.6. Primum atrial septal defect. Axial cine MR image shows a defect in the primum atrial septum (*arrow*). The atrioventricular valve is attached to the fore-shortened ventricular septum (*arrowhead*).

blood flow in each artery using sagittal images to site their planes. Good correlations have been found for Qp/Qs, measured by VEC cine MR and oximetric samples acquired at cardiac catheterization.

Partial Anomalous Pulmonary Venous Connection

Partial anomalous pulmonary venous connection (PAPVC) produces volume overload of right-sided cardiac chambers. The hemodynamic are identical to ASD. The most common type is connection of right upper lobe pulmonary vein to superior vena cava. This type of connection can occur alone (Fig. 36-9) or accompany sinus venosus ASD (Fig. 36-4). Nearly equally frequent is left upper lobe vein drainage via a vertical vein to the left innominate vein (Fig. 36-10). There is an increased incidence of

secundum ASD as well as sinus venosus ASD in patients with PAPVC.

MRI and MRA are the procedures of choice for identifying the presence and connections of this anomaly. MRA is crucial in this regard (Figs. 36-9 and 36-10). The connection of the right-sided pulmonary veins to one or more veins that connect to the inferior vena cava (IVC) can be displayed in the scimitar syndrome (Fig. 36-11).

Cine MR is done in the horizontal long plane to exclude a concomitant ASD. Cine MRI is also performed in the short-axis plane in order to document the severity of right ventricular enlargement. VEC cine MR is performed perpendicular to the direction of flow in the proximal pulmonary artery and aorta, in order to calculate pulmonary to systemic flow ratio (Qp/Qs) (Fig. 36-8).

FIG. 36.7. ASD size. Magnitude (**left**) and phase (**right**) images from velocity-encoded cine MR sequence acquired parallel to the atrial septum (en face) delineates the flow through the defect (*arrows*) allowing precise measurement of the defect dimensions.

A   **B**

FIG. 36.8. A: Atrial septal defect. Magnitude (**left**) and phase (**right**) images from VEC cine MR in planes perpendicular to the long axis of the pulmonary artery (**top**) and the proximal ascending aorta (**below**). Regions of interest surround the aorta and pulmonary artery. **B:** Flow versus time curves for the aorta and pulmonary artery. Because of the left-to-right shunt, the area under the pulmonary artery curve is greater. The area under each curve provides a direct measurement of the pulmonary to systemic flow ratio (2.1:1).

Ventricular Septal Defect

MRI in the transaxial, horizontal long-axis, or four-chamber plane can precisely demonstrate the site of single or multiple VSDs (Fig. 36-12). Inlet VSD is situated just beneath the atrioventricular valves. The tricuspid and mitral valves are equidistant from the cardiac apex. This relationship and the defect are displayed optimally on cine MR in the horizontal long-axis plane. The supracristal VSD is characterized by a defect that lies between the right ventricular outlet and the base of the aorta (Fig. 36-13). On cine MR, a flow void apparently passes from the base of the aorta (it actually passes from just below the aortic valve) to the right ventricular outlet region and into the proximal pulmonary artery. VEC cine MRI can be used to calculate Qp/Qs and quantify the left-to-right shunt.

FIG. 36.9. Partial anomalous pulmonary venous connection. Contrast-enhanced 3D MRA shows anomalous connection of the right upper pulmonary vein (*arrow*) to the superior vena cava.

FIG. 36.10. Partial anomalous pulmonary venous connection. Contrast-enhanced 3D MRA shows anomalous connection of the left upper vein (*arrowhead*) to a vertical vein and the right upper vein (*arrow*) to the superior vena cava. *AO*, ascending aorta; *PA*, pulmonary artery; *SVC*, superior vena cava; *V*, vertical vein.

FIG. 36.11. Partial anomalous pulmonary vena connection in scimitar syndrome. Contrast-enhanced 3D MRA shows the scimitar vein (*arrow*) connecting with the inferior vena cava, hypoplastic right pulmonary artery, and dextroposition of the heart. *IVC*, inferior vena cava; *RA*, right atrium. (Courtesy of Gus Bis, Detroit, Michigan.)

Aorta to Right-sided Shunts

MRI is rarely used to demonstrate patent ductus arteriosus or aorticopulmonary window (Fig. 36-14). With recent improvements in coronary MRA, it is effective for demonstrating the presence and sites of emptying of coronary arteriovenous fistulas. MRI and MRA are very effective for demonstrating sinus of Valsalva aneurysms and fistulas.

Atrioventricular Septal Defect/Atrioventricular Canal (Endocardial Cushion Defect)

These terms denote a spectrum of abnormalities that have in common an abnormal septation between the atria and ventricles. They are also called endocardial cushion defects because the defects are considered to be abnormalities of the embryologic endocardial cushions, which grow together in the center of the heart and divide the atria from the ventricles.

In the normal heart, the atrioventricular septum separates the right atrium from the left ventricle. The atrioventricular septum lies between the more apically located normal

FIG. 36.12. Ventricular septal defect. Spin-echo (**left**) and gradient-echo (**right**) axial images show a defect in the perimembranous ventricular septum. A signal void at the defect is projected into the right ventricle.

tricuspid valve and mitral valve (Fig. 36-15). In all cases of atrioventricular septal defect, the tricuspid and mitral valves lie at the same level, and the atrioventricular septum is defective. This abnormal relationship can be shown on MRI in the transaxial or horizontal long-axis plane. In the mildest form of atrioventricular septal defect, the shunt is from the left ventricle to the right atrium, which can be evident on cine MR. In other cases, the atrial septum adjacent to the atrioventricular valve orifice may also be absent, resulting in an ostium primum ASD (Fig. 36-16). Some patients have an inlet VSD, usually located in the same axial image as the atrioventricular valve or valves. In the most severe cases, both the atrial and ventricular portions of the septum around the valve origins are absent, a condition referred to as complete atrioventricular canal. This creates a common atrioventricular valve orifice with continuous, common atrioventricular valve leaflets (Fig. 36-17).

Coarctation of the Aorta

MRI is the procedure of choice for definitive diagnosis and assessment of the severity of coarctation. MRI has been shown to be effective for preoperative assessment of coarctation and for postoperative evaluation of recurrent or persistent hypertension. To evaluate coarctation, spin-echo or cine MR sequences are obtained in the axial and oblique sagittal planes. The diameter of the narrowing can be precisely measured with MRI, especially with the use of thin (3-mm) sections through the center of the stenosis. Thin oblique sagittal images through the long-axis plane of the aorta show the diameter of the stenosis and provide an accurate measurement of its length (Fig. 36-18).

FIG. 36.13. Supracristal ventricular septal defect. Spin-echo (**left**) and cine MR (**right**) images in the axial plane demonstrate a defect (*white arrow*) in the outlet portion of the septum. A flow void (*black arrow*) projects into the upper region of the right ventricular outflow region.

FIG. 36.14. Aorticopulmonary window. Coronal (**left**) and axial (**center and right**) spin-echo images demonstrate a defect (*arrows*) between the proximal ascending aorta and the pulmonary artery. *Ao*, aorta; *RV*, right ventricular outlet region.

FIG. 36.15. Atrioventricular septum. Axial spin-echo image shows the small portion (*arrow*) of ventricular septum separating the left ventricle and the right atrium. Note the more ventral position of the tricuspid valve relative to the mitral valve.

FIG. 36.16. Primum atrial septal defect. Cine MR image in the horizontal long-axis plane shows a defect at the level of the septum primum (*arrow*). *RA*, right atrium; *LA*, left atrium.

FIG. 36.17. Atrioventricular canal (endocardial cushion) defect. Axial spin-echo image shows a large defect in the inlet portion of the ventricular septum. A single atrioventricular valve (*arrows*) spans the inlet of both ventricles.

FIG. 36.18. Coarctation of aorta. Axial (**left**) and oblique sagittal (**right**) spin-echo images. A line bisecting the ascending and descending aorta at the coarctation prescribes the oblique sagittal plane (long-axis plane of thoracic aorta). This latter image displays the coarctation site along with the arch.

FIG. 36.19. Coarctation of aorta. Contrast-enhanced 3D MRA in the sagittal plane shows a discrete juxtaductal coarctation (*arrow*) on the maximum intensity projection (**left**) and the volume-rendered 3D reconstruction (**right**).

The oblique sagittal images also display the dimension of aortic isthmus (region between the left subclavian artery and the ligamentum arteriosum) and the aortic arch. In some cases, a single 3-mm slice in this plane may not display the coarctation and arch because of tortuosity of the arch and proximal descending aorta, but the assessment can be done from adjacent images. Gadolinium-enhanced 3D MRA can display the entire thoracic aorta on a single image with the use of maximum intensity projection or volume-rendering reconstruction techniques (Fig. 36-19). Gadolinium-enhanced MRA is also effective for demonstrating collateral vessels (Fig. 36-20).

VEC cine MRI can be applied to demonstrate the presence of and estimate the volume of collateral circulation to

FIG. 36.20. Coarctation of aorta. Contrast-enhanced 3D MRA in the sagittal plane shows long-segment coarctation caused by Takayasu's arteritis. Note the abundant collateral arterial connections (*arrows*).

the descending aorta below the coarctation site (Fig. 36-21). This is accomplished by using two imaging planes perpendicular to the aorta; one is about 2 cm beyond the coarctation and the other at the level of the diaphragm. In the normal

A   B

FIG. 36.21. **A:** Coarctation of the aorta. Sites of planes for magnitude and phase images in the proximal (**top**) and distal aorta (**bottom**) used to estimate the volume of collateral flow. **B:** Flow versus time curves for the proximal and distal descending aorta show a larger flow volume in the distal compared with the proximal aorta caused by retrograde flow in aortic branches below the coarctation. The volume of collateral flow is estimated as the difference in flow volumes (areas under the curves) at the two sites.

aorta, volume flow is greater (about 5% to 7% higher) at the proximal site. On the other hand, in a hemodynamically significant coarctation, volume flow is greater at the diaphragm because of retrograde flow through the intercostal and mammary arteries and other collaterals into the distal aorta. The presence of greater volume flow at the diaphragmatic level is considered a functional indicator of hemodynamic significance of the coarctation. There is a rough linear relationship between the percentage of stenosis and the volume of collateral circulation. After stenting of the coarctation, VEC cine MRI has demonstrated reversal of the collateral flow since volume flow at the proximal site becomes greater than at the distal one.

Theoretically, VEC cine MRI can also be used to estimate the gradient across the coarctation. Using planes perpendicular and parallel to the coarctation, peak velocity of flow can be estimated. Applying the modified Bernoulli formula (peak pressure gradient = $4 \times [\text{peak velocity}]^2$), the peak gradient is estimated. The voxel (s) with highest velocity in systole can be identified on phase images in both planes. The highest in either plan is considered the peak velocity (Fig. 36-22).

Arch Anomalies

There are numerous types of arch anomalies resulting from abnormal resorption of the anterior or posterior segments of

FIG. 36.23. Double aortic arch. Spin-echo images in sagittal (**left**) and axial (**right**) planes display posterior compression of the trachea by a retroesophageal component (*arrow*) of a double arch. The axial plane shows that the right arch is the larger of the two and also shows a short atretic posterior segment (*arrowhead*) of the left arch.

the embryonic double-arch configuration. However, the only ones encountered with any frequency are complete (patent) double arch, double arch with atretic posterior component of the left arch (Fig. 36-23), right arch with aberrant (retroesophageal) left subclavian artery (Fig. 36-24), and left arch with aberrant right subclavian artery. The first three produce complete vascular rings that narrow the trachea and esophagus. Compression of the trachea is by the aortic component situated between the vertebral body and the esophagus. The vascular ring with right arch and aberrant left subclavian artery is completed by the posterior component that is tethered anteriorly by a left-sided ligamentum arteriosum. With mirror-image right aortic arch, the ligamentum courses between the left innominate artery and the proximal left pulmonary artery. On the other hand, with non–mirror-image right aortic arch, the ligamentum courses between the descending aorta and the proximal left pulmonary artery. At the site of attachment of the ligamentum, there is an enlargement or diverticulum of the descending aorta.

FIG. 36.22. Pressure gradient in aortic coarctation. Magnitude (**top left**) and phase (**top right**) images from VEC-MR acquisition perpendicular to the descending aorta in a level distal to the coarctation demonstrate an estimated pressure gradient of 21 mm Hg. Magnitude (**bottom left**) and phase (**bottom right**) images from an in-plane VEC-MR aligned to the descending aorta show an estimated pressure gradient of 33 mm Hg.

FIG. 36.24. Right aortic arch with aberrant left subclavian artery. Spin-echo axial images (**left**) show the right arch (*A*) and aberrant left subclavian artery (*arrowhead*). Another axial image shows the diverticulum (*arrow*) of the descending arch, which is the site of origin of the left subclavian artery.

FIG. 36.25. Branch pulmonary artery stenoses. Transaxial spin-echo images display stenosis (*arrow*) of the left pulmonary artery. Note the size of the right pulmonary artery (*arrowhead*) for comparison.

This localized dilatation tethered anteriorly by the posterior left-sided ligamentum is the structure that compresses the trachea and esophagus rather than the left subclavian artery itself. These anatomic arrangements can be readily discerned on MR images in the transaxial plane.

For the evaluation of arch anomalies, spin-echo images are acquired in sagittal (5-mm slice thickness) and transaxial (3-mm slice thickness) planes (see Fig. 36-23). These images display the aortic anomaly and verify that the anomalous component produces airway compression. Cine MR images may be used to display the pulsatile nature of the airway obstruction. In some cases, the site of maximal airway compression is at the carina or even involves a proximal bronchus.

Contrast-enhanced 3D MRA may be used to demonstrate the arch anomaly. The MRA acquisition is done in either the sagittal or coronal planes.

Pulmonary Arterial Anomalies

Pulmonary arterial anomalies are evaluated using spin-echo and cine MRI (Fig. 36-25) and contrast-enhanced 3D MRA (Fig. 36-26) for depicting morphology and VEC (phase

contrast) MRI for measuring blood flow. Spin-echo and cine MR images are acquired in the transaxial plane followed by images along the long axis of the right (oblique coronal plane) and left (oblique sagittal plane) pulmonary arteries. Contrast-enhanced 3D MRA is usually acquired in the coronal plane; a short acquisition period is optimal to depict the pulmonary arteries before enhancement of the left heart and aorta. VEC cine sequences are obtained perpendicular to the long axis of the right, left, and main pulmonary arterial segments.

Compared to echocardiography, MRI is more useful for examining the right and left pulmonary arteries, as well as the lobar and segmental arteries. MRI is especially useful for demonstrating central and peripheral pulmonary artery stenoses (see Fig. 36-27), absent pulmonary artery (Fig. 36-28), and pulmonary artery sling (Fig. 36-29). MRI and MRA are the preferred techniques for the evaluation of residual pulmonary arterial stenoses after repair of tetralogy of Fallot (Fig. 36-30).

The hemodynamic significance of pulmonary arterial stenoses is assessed by VEC cine MRI measurement of blood flow separately for each pulmonary artery (Fig. 36-30). Since flow is also measured for the main pulmonary artery, the

FIG. 36.26. Pulmonary valvular stenosis. 3D reconstructions from an MRA demonstrate enlargement of the main (*MPA*) and left (*LPA*) pulmonary arteries, with normal dimension of the right pulmonary artery (*RPA*).

FIG. 36.27. Branch pulmonary artery stenosis. Contrast-enhanced 3D MRA in the coronal plane shows stenosis (*arrow*) of the left pulmonary artery.

FIG. 36.35. Anomalous origin of the left coronary artery from the right coronary artery with a retroaortic course. Two adjacent sections from coronary MRA display the ectopic origin of the left coronary artery from the right coronary (*arrowhead*) and passage of the left artery behind the aorta (*arrow*).

coronary arteriography can demonstrate ectopic origin, it usually cannot confidently and precisely define the proximal course of the artery.

The current approach to coronary MRA employs a respiratory navigator-compensated 3D free-breathing technique. This technique displays clearly the origin of the coronary artery from the sinus of Valsalva and its proximal course. A single coronary artery may arise from either the right or left sinus of Valsalva, or both coronary arteries may arise individually from one sinus of Valsalva (Fig. 36-36). In a child with chest pain or syncope during exercise or aborted sudden death, coronary MRA must exclude a proximal interarterial course.

CYANOTIC LESIONS

Tetralogy of Fallot

Tetralogy of Fallot consists of obstruction to the right ventricular outlet region (usually multilevel), malalignment outlet VSD, enlarged aorta overriding the VSD, and a hypertrabeculated, hypertrophied right ventricle. These features are clearly defined on spin-echo and cine MR images (Fig. 36-37). Transaxial and oblique coronal images demonstrate the VSD and the position of the aorta overriding the defect. Cine MRI in the RVOT plane is usually optional for defining the narrowed infundibulum and in some cases stenotic annulus and or valve. Sagittal and transaxial images are used to assess the size of the main and central pulmonary arteries and to display focal stenoses. Imaging oriented in a plane parallel to the long axis of the right (oblique coronal plane) and left (oblique sagittal plane) pulmonary arteries is used to assess the severity of central pulmonary arterial stenoses, which are common in this anomaly.

FIG. 36.36. Ectopic origin of the right coronary artery with an interarterial course. Coronary MRA shows the origin of the right coronary artery (*arrow*) from the right end of the left sinus of Valsalva in a position where the proximal portion of the artery is compressed between the aorta and the right ventricular outlet region.

Contrast-enhanced 3D MRA is also employed to demonstrate pulmonary arterial stenoses and the systemic source of collateral flow to the lungs (Fig. 36-38). VEC cine MRI can be used to define differential blood flow to the two lungs.

Tetralogy of Fallot is usually repaired by relieving the pulmonic stenosis and closing the VSD. Stenosis of the main or branch arteries, the size of the right ventricle outflow tract, and

FIG. 36.37. Tetralogy of Fallot. Oblique coronal (**left**), sagittal (**center**), and axial (**right**) cine MR images show ventricular septal defect (*arrows*), aorta overriding the defect, and pulmonic stenosis (*arrowhead* on flow void).

FIG. 36.38. Pulmonary atresia with ventricular septal defect. Contrast-enhanced 3D MRA in the coronal plane displays several large systemic to pulmonary artery collaterals (*arrows*) arising from the descending aorta.

FIG. 36.39. Pulmonary atresia with ventricular septal defect. Spin-echo axial images arranged from caudal (**top left**) to cranial (**bottom right**) demonstrate a single large artery (aorta) at the base of the heart, which overlies the ventricular septal defect (*arrow*). Right ventricular wall is hypertrophied. Note the central confluence (*arrowhead*) of the right and left pulmonary arteries distal to the atretic segment.

the size of the right ventricle are important to assess in preoperative planning and are well delineated by MRI. Coronary anomalies may occur in patients with tetralogy of Fallot. The most important is the origin of the left anterior descending coronary artery from the right coronary artery with anomalous artery passing anterior to the right ventricle outflow tract. Adequate sizes of the central pulmonary arteries and the presence of a central confluence may signify that the patient with severe multilevel stenoses is a candidate for a Rastelli procedure connecting the right ventricle to the pulmonary artery.

Pulmonary Atresia

Pulmonary atresia with VSD is an extreme form of tetralogy of Fallot in which a direct connection from the right ventricle to the pulmonary arteries is lacking. On axial MRI, a solid layer of muscle in the region of the right ventricle outflow tract indicates an infundibulum with a blind end. No connection between the right ventricle and the pulmonary artery confluence (if present) is evident on sequential images (Fig. 36-39). The atresia can be focal, limited to the valve level, or more extensive. The length of the atresia can be determined by inspecting sequential axial tomograms. Focal membranous pulmonary atresia may be indistinguishable from severe stenosis on axial MR images because of partial volume averaging. The use of 3-mm-thick spin-echo images reduces partial volume effects. Cine MRI in the axial or sagittal planes can establish the presence or absence of flow across the valve. A markedly enlarged aorta is seen overriding a perimembranous VSD (see Fig. 37-39). Blood is usually delivered to the lungs via systemic to pulmonary

collateral channels, which can be seen as abnormal vessels originating from the descending aorta and traveling toward the lungs or connecting with the pulmonary arteries (see Fig. 36-38). These are shown best on contrast-enhanced 3D MRA (see Fig. 36-38).

The surgical correction of pulmonary atresia with VSD usually consists of placing a conduit from the right ventricle to the central pulmonary arteries (if present) or to a surgically created confluence of pulmonary arteries and larger systemic to pulmonary collateral vessels (unifocalization procedure). Therefore, it is important for the surgeon to know whether a native confluence of the pulmonary arteries is present, its size, and the number and size of collateral vessels. Axial plane MRI is excellent for defining the main pulmonary arteries. The collateral channels are especially well seen on contrast-enhanced MRA (see Fig. 36-38).

It is important to assess the sizes of the central pulmonary arteries in patients who have tetralogy of Fallot with severe stenosis or pulmonary atresia. Thin (3-mm) transaxial MR images can readily depict the sizes of the main, right, and left pulmonary arteries. The right pulmonary artery is observed on the image that contains the right main bronchus, coursing in front of the right bronchus, and the left pulmonary artery passes over the left main bronchus and is seen on the image containing the left bronchus or on the one just above. The identification of central pulmonary arteries and of a central confluence of the right and left pulmonary arteries is a unique capability of MRI since opacification of the vessels with contrast is not required. The pulmonary arteries are frequently hypoplastic, or the central or peripheral arteries may contain one or more stenoses.

Cine MRI and contrast-enhanced MRA can be used to identify the blood supply to the lungs. Pulmonary and bronchial arteries have bright signal on cine MRI. On transaxial images at the level of the carina, pulmonary arteries can be differentiated from bronchial arteries. Bronchial arteries or systemic to pulmonary artery collaterals arise from the aorta or its branches and are usually located dorsal to the bronchi, whereas pulmonary arteries are ventral to the bronchi. On occasion, a bronchial artery originating from a subclavian artery is seen ventral to the bronchi.

Pulmonary Atresia With Intact Ventricular Septum

A VSD is not identified in this form of pulmonary atresia with intact ventricular septum. In this variety of pulmonary atresia, MRI is effective for demonstrating the size of the RV, which varies from markedly hypoplastic to dilated (Figs. 36-40 and 36-41). The pulmonary arteries are usually normal or nearly normal in size and do not contain stenoses.

Cine MR images can be acquired in the short-axis plane to quantify the volumes of the right and left ventricles. The size of the right ventricle is critical for determination of the surgical approach. A right ventricle of adequate size is necessary to consider treatment with a conduit from the right ventricle to the pulmonary arteries.

Exit of blood from the right ventricle in this anomaly is by tricuspid regurgitation or retrograde flow through myocardial sinusoid and coronary arteries into the aorta. Cine MR can demonstrate and give some insight into the severity of tricuspid regurgitation.

FIG. 36.41. Pulmonary atresia with intact ventricular septum, status postvalvotomy. Axial cine MR images show a distorted right ventricle (*RV*) with lack of normal trabeculation (bald RV). *RA*, right atrium; *LV*, left ventricle.

Abnormalities of Ventriculoarterial Connections

These abnormalities consist of complete transposition of the great arteries (TGA), corrected transposition of the great arteries (CTGA), double-outlet right ventricle (DORV), and double-outlet left ventricle (Table 36-1). The last anomaly is

FIG. 36.40. Pulmonary atresia with intact ventricular septum after pulmonary valvotomy. Axial cine MR shows enlarged right-sided chambers as a consequence of the associated tricuspid regurgitation. *RA*, right atrium; *RV*, right ventricle.

TABLE 36.1 Summary of Anatomy of Ventriculoarterial Connection Abnormalities

Complete Transposition
Situs solitus (right atrium on right side of chest)
D-ventricular loop (right ventricle to the right of left ventricle)
d-TGA (aorta anterior and to right of pulmonary artery)

Corrected Transposition
Situs solitus
L-ventricular loop (right ventricle to the left of left ventricle)
l-TGA (aorta anterior and to the left of pulmonary artery)

Double-Outlet Right Ventricle
Aorta orifice >50% overlies the right ventricle
Pulmonary orifice >50% overlies the right ventricle
Subaortic, subpulmonary, doubly committed or noncommitted VSD

Double-Outlet Left Ventricle
Aorta orifice >50% overlies the left ventricle
Pulmonary orifice >50% overlies the left ventricle

Truncus Arteriosus
One enlarged great artery (truncus) overlies both ventricles
VSD immediately beneath orifice of truncus

FIG. 36.42. Right ventricular characteristics. Axial cine MR images from the level of the great vessels (**top left**) to the midventricular level (**bottom right**) show a hypertrophied systemic right ventricle (*RV*) in a patient with transposition of the great arteries. Note the muscular infundibulum (*I*), moderator band (*arrow*), and irregular surface of the ventricular septum (*arrowhead*) at the apical level. *Ao*, aorta; *PA*, pulmonary artery; *LV*, left ventricle.

FIG. 36.44. MRA status post atrial switch procedure. Gadolinium-enhanced MR angiography in the coronal plane is shown in a patient status post atrial switch procedure for correction of transposition of great arteries. The inferior vena cava (*IVC*) is dilated and connects to the inferior limb of the baffle (*B*), which is then attached to the mitral valve. The superior limb of the baffle is occluded (*arrow*). Note an enlarged azygos vein (*arrowhead*). *LV*, left ventricle; *PA*, pulmonary artery.

exceedingly rare. Truncus arteriosus will also be considered under this heading.

A critical step in evaluating these anomalies is determining the morphology of the ventricles. This is readily accomplished using transaxial images that show the characteristics of a right ventricle: infundibulum (tunnel of myocardium) separating the atrioventricular and semilunar valves; moderator band; and corrugated surface of the right ventricular aspect of the septum (Fig. 36-42). The left ventricle shows direct fibrous continuity between the two valves, the papillary muscles, and the smooth surface of the left ventricular aspect of the septum.

Ventriculoarterial connections can be concordant or discordant. Concordant connections are right ventricle to pulmonary artery and left ventricle to aorta. Discordant connections occur in a diverse group of anomalies in which the great arteries are inverted (transposition). Both great arteries arise predominantly from one of the ventricles

(double-outlet ventricle). The ventriculoarterial connections and the arterial relationships are depicted on coronal and transverse MR images.

A great artery is considered connected to a ventricle if more than half of its orifice arises from that ventricle. A series of transaxial images extending from the aortic arch to the diaphragm demonstrates these connections. The initial determination is to identify the aorta unequivocally by following one of the great arteries to the arch. If this great artery (aorta) connects to the right ventricle and the pulmonary artery to the left ventricle, then the diagnosis of complete TGA is established (Fig. 36-43 and 36-44). At the base of the heart, the aorta is anterior and to the right of the pulmonary artery in most cases and is called d-TGA. The transaxial images also demonstrate the position of the ventricles in relation to each other and their connections to the atria (atrioventricular connections). Typically, in the presence of situs solitus, the images show the right

FIG. 36.43. d-Transposition of great arteries. Spin-echo images arranged from cranial (**left**) to caudal (**right**) show the aorta (*Ao*) ventral and slightly to the right of the pulmonary artery (*PA*). The aorta is shown connecting to the right ventricle (*RV*) and the pulmonary artery to the left ventricle (*LV*). There is a baffle (Mustard procedure) in the atrium, separating the mitral valve from the pulmonary venous atrium (*PVA*). *RVOT*, right ventricular outflow track.

FIG. 36.45. l-Transposition of great arteries. Spin-echo axial images arranged from cranial (**left**) to caudal (**right**) demonstrate the aorta (*Ao*) ventral and to the left of the pulmonary artery. It is connected to the morphologic right ventricle (*RV*), which lies to the left of the left ventricle (*LV*). The right ventricle is connected to the left atrium. The pulmonary artery (*PA*) is connected to the left ventricle, which is connected to the right atrium. *RVOT*, right ventricular outflow track.

ventricle situated to the right of the left ventricle and connected to the right atrium (D-ventricular loop). If the ventricles are inverted, the right ventricle is to the left of the left ventricle and connected to the left atrium (L-ventricular loop). The most frequent types of TGA are complete TGA (situs solitus, D-ventricular loop, d-TGA; see Fig. 36-43 and 36-44) and corrected TGA (situs solitus, L-ventricular loop, l-TGA; Fig. 36-45). The latter anomaly is considered to be corrected (corrected transposition) in terms of

blood flow in the central circulation since systemic venous blood flows from the right atrium into the left ventricle and out to the pulmonary artery for normal oxygenation, precluding obligatory cyanosis. Transaxial MR images also demonstrate anomalies frequently associated with complete and corrected transposition, such as ASD, VSD, subvalvular and valvular pulmonic stenosis, tricuspid atresia, and Ebstein anomaly.

Transaxial MR images demonstrate connection of both great arteries to the right ventricle in DORV (Fig. 36-46). Rarely, both great arteries connect to the anatomic left ventricle, indicating double-outlet left ventricle. Transaxial images are very effective for demonstrating the relationship of the obligatory VSD to the great arteries in DORV. The defect may be just below the aortic orifice (subaortic VSD) or pulmonary artery orifice (subpulmonary VSD); beneath both orifices (doubly committed VSD); or removed some distance from both (noncommitted VSD).

FIG. 36.46. Double-outlet right ventricle. Spin-echo axial images arranged from cranial (**top left**) to caudal (**bottom right**). At the base of the heart, the aorta (*Ao*) and pulmonary artery (*PA*) lie side by side. Both great arteries are connected to the right ventricle (*RV*). There are coni beneath both great arteries, and trabeculation of the right ventricular side of the ventricular septum. *LV*, left ventricle.

FIG. 36.47. Truncus arteriosus, type I. Spin-echo images in the coronal (**left**) and axial (**right**) planes demonstrate a large single artery arising from the heart. The pulmonary artery (*arrow*) arises from the left side of the truncus, and the aortic arch is right-sided.

Truncus Arteriosus

Truncus arteriosus was classified by Collet and Edwards based on the origin of the pulmonary artery from the common arterial trunk. In type I, a septum divides the origin of the aorta and pulmonary trunk. In type II, the right and left pulmonary arteries are close to each other but arise separately from the pulmonary trunk. In type III, right and left pulmonary arteries arise further laterally. The lesion labeled type IV truncus is in fact pulmonary atresia with VSD rather than truncus arteriosus.

Axial, sagittal, and coronal MR images at the base of the heart can show the truncus arteriosus aligned over the VSD (Fig. 36-47). The origins of the main pulmonary artery from the truncus in type I can be delineated with MRI. Axial images can show the relative sizes of the ventricles. Because it can demonstrate a small infundibular chamber in pulmonary atresia, MRI can be used to distinguish truncus arteriosus from pulmonary atresia.

The relative sizes and confluence of the pulmonary arteries are useful pieces of information because surgical treatment involves excision of the pulmonary arteries from the common trunk and the creation of a conduit from the right ventricle to the pulmonary arteries (Rastelli procedure). Also important in the evaluation is the demonstration of a right aortic arch (35%) and other arch anomalies. Cine MRI and VEC cine MRI can be employed to identify and quantify the severity of truncal regurgitation. Cine MRI can also be used to quantify the volume and mass of the two ventricles.

ANALYSIS OF COMPLEX CONGENITAL HEART DISEASE USING MRI: SEGMENTAL APPROACH

The analysis of complex congenital heart disease requires a systematic approach. The approach most widely used today is the segmental one, in which the heart is partitioned into three main segments (atria, ventricles, and great vessels) and the connections between them (atrioventricular and ventric-

uloarterial connections). Transaxial images from the aortic arch to the upper abdomen clearly demonstrate the segmental cardiovascular anatomy and connections of one segment to the other (atrioventricular connections and ventriculoarterial connections) and the types of situs.

Visceroatrial Situs

The right atria and left atria are described by their morphologic structure and not necessarily their position (Table 36-2). An atrium with the morphologic features of a left atrium, which may rarely be located to the right of midline, is called a morphologic left atrium. Transaxial MR images can clearly depict the characteristic morphologic features of the atria.

The most definite features of the atria are the appendages. On an axial MR image, the right atrial appendage appears as a triangular structure with a broad-based opening into the right atrium. This is in distinction to the left atrial appendage, a long, narrow, finger-like projection with a narrow orifice. The atrial appendages are the most constant part of the atria, even in complex abnormalities. If the atrial appendages are difficult to identify, the next most reliable structure is the drainage of the IVC. The atrium connecting to the IVC is considered the morphologic right atrium. Superior vena caval and pulmonary venous drainage is variable and is not used to identify atrial morphology.

Ventricular Loop

Several morphologic features identify right versus left ventricle (Table 36-3).

The normal rightward bending of the primitive cardiac tube places the morphologic right ventricle on the right side of the heart. This rightward bending is called D-looping (D for dextro, right). If the primitive heart tube bends to the left, the result is called L-looping (L for levo, left), in which the morphologic right ventricle is placed on the left side of the heart. A heart with the morphologic right ventricle on the left side has an L-ventricular loop. In

TABLE 36.2 Identification and Position of Atria
Left atrium
"Finger-shaped" appendage
Narrow orifice of appendage
Right atrium
Triangular shaped appendage
Wide orifice of appendage
Connects to IVC
Right atrium on right side—situs solitus
Right atrium on left side—situs inversus
Bilateral morphologic right atria—right sidedness (frequently asplenia)
Bilateral morphologic left atria—left sidedness (frequently polysplenia)

TABLE 36.3 Morphologic Features of Ventricles
Right ventricle
Infundibulum
No fibrous continuity between atrioventricular and semilunar valves
Moderator band
Corrugated surface of ventricular septum near apex
Left ventricle
No infundibulum
Fibrous continuity between atrioventricular and semilunar valves
Papillary muscles
Smooth septal surface near apex

situs solitus, a D-loop is normal. In situs inversus, L-loop is normal.

Atrioventricular connections can be concordant or discordant. In normal, concordant atrioventricular connections, the right atrium is connected to the right ventricle and the left atrium to the left ventricle. The atrioventricular valves remain with their respective ventricles, regardless of the type of ventricular loop. The mitral valve resides with the left ventricle and the tricuspid valve is part of the right ventricle, except in patients with double-inlet ventricle. Identification of ventricular morphology indicates the type of atrioventricular valve within the ventricle.

Discordant atrioventricular connections are right atrium to left ventricle and left atrium to right ventricle. Congenitally corrected TGA is an example of an anomaly with atrioventricular discordance.

Great Artery Relationships

Transaxial images at the base of the heart clearly define the normal relationship of the pulmonary artery anterior and to the left of the aorta. Such images also identify concordant (aorta connected to left ventricle and pulmonary artery connected to right ventricle) and discordant (aorta connected to right ventricle and pulmonary artery connected to left ventricle) ventriculoarterial connections.

Complete TGA is an example of atrioventricular concordance and ventriculoarterial discordance. Corrected TGA is an example of atrioventricular and ventriculoarterial discordance. Double discordance results in blood flowing in a normal pattern serially through the pulmonary and systemic circulation.

ABNORMALITIES OF ATRIOVENTRICULAR CONNECTIONS

Discordant Atrioventricular Connections

The right atrium connects with the left ventricle and the left atrium connects with the right ventricle, constituting discordant connections, in corrected transposition (see Fig. 36-45). One of the most frequent anomalies in patients with situs inversus is corrected transposition. In this anomaly, the anatomic right atrium (situated left of midline) connects discordantly to the left ventricle and the anatomic left atrium (situated right of midline) connects to the right ventricle. Mirror-image dextrocardia occurs with situs inversus. In contrast, isolated dextrocardia consists of situs solitus with a right-sided cardiac apex (see Fig. 36-48).

Double-inlet Ventricle (Single Ventricle; Univentricular Heart)

This complex anomaly consists of one adequate-size ventricle and one rudimentary ventricle. The most frequent type

FIG. 36.48. Situs solitus with corrected transposition and isolated dextrocardia. Spin-echo axial images arranged from cranial (**top left**) to caudal (**bottom right**). The right atrium (*RA*) is right-sided and the left atrium (*LA*) is left-sided, indicating situs solitus. The right ventricle (*RV*) is positioned to the left of the left ventricle (*LV*). The aorta (*AO*) is anterior and leftward to the pulmonary artery (*PA*). Note the conus (*arrow*) and moderator band on the left-sided ventricle, indicating it is a morphologic right ventricle in an L-ventricular loop. Thus, this arrangement of connections is situs solitus, L-ventricular loop, l-transposition, which constitutes corrected TGA. The cardiac apex is right-sided, which indicates isolated dextrocardia.

is double-inlet left ventricle: both atrioventricular valves connect to the morphologic left ventricle. The enlarged left ventricle is attached to a rudimentary right ventricular outlet via a bulboventricular foramina. In many instances, l-TGA is an associated anomaly.

Cine MRI can provide a set of end-diastolic and end-systole images encompassing the entire heart; consequently, it is the optimal method for quantifying the volumes, mass, and function of the dominant and rudimentary ventricle. Volumetric data may be essential for surgical planning (Fontan procedure versus two-ventricle repair). After repair with Fontan procedure, cine MR is used to monitor the volumes and ejection fraction of the dominant ventricle.

Atresia of Atrioventricular Valve

Either the tricuspid or mitral valves can be atretic; tricuspid atresia is more frequent. Tricuspid atresia is associated with d-TGA in nearly 50% of patients. It is also frequently associated with valvular or subvalvular pulmonary stenosis or atresia. The right ventricle is invariably hypoplastic. Transaxial MR images demonstrate a bar of muscle and fat across the atrioventricular inlet of the right ventricle (Figs. 36-49 to 36-51). Both spin-echo and cine MR images display the degree of right ventricle hypoplasia, interatrial communication, VSD, and ventriculoarterial connections. In a few cases, a thick membrane separates the right atrium

FIG. 36.49. Classic Fontan procedure. Axial black-blood images from the level of the great vessels (**top left**) to the midventricular level (**bottom right**) in a patient with tricuspid atresia status post classic Fontan operation. The right pulmonary artery (*R*) connects to the right atrial appendage (*Ap*). A dominant left ventricle (*LV*) is seen. Note the fatty replacement of the right atrioventricular grove (*arrow*). *L*, left pulmonary artery; *Ao*, aorta; *RA*, right atrium.

and right ventricle (imperforate tricuspid valve). The atrial and ventricular septal openings permit systemic venous blood to flow into the ventricles.

MR is frequently used to evaluate tricuspid atresia after various stages of surgical correction. Spin-echo MR images

FIG. 36.51. Tricuspid atresia with Fontan. Axial images, from the ventricular level (**bottom right**) to the level of the great vessels (**top left**), show a Fontan conduit (*F*) connecting the inferior vena cava (*IVC*) to the right pulmonary artery (*RPA*). A Glenn shunt (*G*) connects the superior vena cava to the RPA. A dominant left ventricle (*LV*) is seen. *LPA*, left pulmonary artery; *RA*, right atrium; *LA*, left atrium.

and 3D contrast-enhanced MRA are effective for displaying the anatomy of the Glenn anastomosis (Fig. 36-51 and 36-52) and the Fontan procedure and the status of the central pulmonary arteries (Fig. 36-51 to 36-53). VEC cine MR may be employed to quantify blood flow in the Glenn shunt

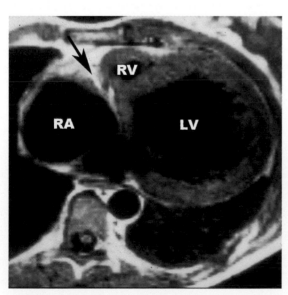

FIG. 36.50. Tricuspid atresia. Spin-echo axial image shows a bar of fat and muscle (*arrow*) separating the right atrium (*RA*) from the hypoplastic right ventricle (*RV*). The left ventricle (*LV*) is enlarged.

FIG. 36.52. Glenn shunt. Coronal (**upper left**) and axial spin-echo images from cranial (**top right**) to caudal (**bottom right**). The superior vena cava (*S*) is attached to the right pulmonary artery, with flow to both pulmonary arteries (bidirectional Glenn shunt). *PA*, pulmonary artery.

FIG. 36.53. Fontan procedure, extra-atrial type. Spin-echo coronal image shows the conduit (*arrows*) between the inferior vena cava and the right pulmonary artery (*RP*). The superior vena cava (*S*) is connected to the top of the right pulmonary artery (Glenn anastomosis). The conduit is located lateral to the right atrium (*R*), thus the connotation extra-atrial Fontan.

(superior vena cava), Fontan conduit (IVC to pulmonary artery conduit), and pulmonary arteries.

Ebstein Malformation

Ebstein malformation is a primary abnormality of the tricuspid valve in which the septal and anterior leaflets of the valve adhere to the right ventricle wall. The leaflets become free at a variable distance, at a location more apical than usual, so that the tricuspid valve orifice is displaced toward the apex. The right atrioventricular ring still defines the border of the anatomic right ventricle; however, because the valve orifice is more apical than usual, the functional part of the right ventricle is truncated. The portion of the right ventricle that is basal to the valve orifice becomes "atrialized," meaning that it functions as part of the atrium rather than as part of the right ventricle. The atrialized portion of the right ventricle is thin walled and nontrabeculated, and it may become dilated. Ebstein anomaly is frequently associated with an ASD.

MRI can demonstrate the position of tricuspid valve (Fig. 36-54), and cine MRI can be used to quantify chamber size and the ejection fraction of the functional right ventricle. Cine MR also demonstrates the systolic signal void projected into the right atrium, indicating tricuspid regurgitation, which is invariably present with this anomaly.

Hypoplastic Left Heart Syndrome

The term *hypoplastic left heart syndrome* refers to several different anomalies, all of which lead to underdevelopment of the left ventricle. It is usually caused by aortic stenosis or

FIG. 36.54. Ebstein anomaly. Gradient-echo axial image shows that the attachments of the septal leaflets (*black arrow*) of the tricuspid valve are displaced into the right ventricle. The level of the tricuspid annulus (*white arrow*) is the normal site of attachment. Right-sided chambers are enlarged due to tricuspid regurgitation. *RA*, right atrium; *aRV*, atrialized right ventricle; *fRV*, functional right ventricle.

atresia, mitral stenosis or atresia, or both. As in tricuspid atresia, the degree of ventricular hypoplasia varies, depending on the location and severity of the obstruction. For example, in mitral atresia without a large ASD and VSD, the left ventricle may be a small mass of muscle with no visible lumen (Fig. 36-55). On the other hand, if the mitral valve is patent and the problem is primarily one of aortic valvular hypoplasia, the left ventricle may be normal in size and hypertrophied. In all cases, the right atrium tends to be enlarged and the right ventricle to be dilated and hypertrophied. Axial MRI can readily depict the chamber enlargement and ventricular hypertrophy.

FIG. 36.55. Hypoplastic left heart syndrome. Spin-echo axial images demonstrate the severely hypoplastic ascending aorta (*arrow*) and lack of cavitation of the left ventricle (*L*) at the level displayed.

In most cases of hypoplastic left heart syndrome, little blood flows through the ascending aorta. Blood tends to flow from the pulmonary artery through the ductus arteriosus into the aorta, then in retrograde fashion to the aortic root to supply the coronary arteries. As a result, the ascending aorta is usually very small and the main pulmonary artery, which receives most of the cardiac output, is very large. The diameters of the great arteries are clearly defined on axial MR images.

Hypoplastic left heart syndrome is treated by the Norwood procedure, in which the large right ventricle is made to pump blood to the systemic circulation. This is accomplished by severing the main pulmonary artery and anastomosing the proximal pulmonary stump to the ascending aorta. The pulmonary circulation is reestablished by routing systemic blood into the pulmonary circulation, initially with a systemic to pulmonary shunt and later with a Fontan procedure. An important role for MRI in hypoplastic left heart syndrome has been the evaluation of the morphology and function of the various stages of the Norwood procedure.

Total Anomalous Pulmonary Venous Connection

In the embryo, the pulmonary veins grow from the lung buds and come together to form a confluence, which normally is incorporated into the posterior wall of the left atrium. However, if this confluence joins the circulatory system elsewhere, a situation is created in which the entire pulmonary venous return is anomalous: total anomalous pulmonary venous connection (TAPVC). TAPVC is usually classified according to the location of the venous insertion. It may be supracardiac (type I), in which the pulmonary venous confluence usually drains into the superior vena cava or an anomalous left-sided "vertical vein," which in turn drains into the left brachiocephalic vein. TAPVC at the cardiac level (type II) usually drains into the right atrium. In type III TAPVC, the pulmonary venous confluence drains below the diaphragm into the truncus venosus or the portal venous system. As the pulmonary veins pass below the diaphragm, obstruction to flow frequently results in pulmonary venous hypertension.

MRI has been shown to be highly accurate for the diagnosis of anomalous pulmonary venous connection. TAPVC can be diagnosed when MRI demonstrates that no pulmonary veins drain into the left atrium. Transaxial MRI and gadolinium-enhanced MRA can demonstrate the location of the anomalous connection along with enlargement of the superior vena cava or coronary sinus, or the presence of a common pulmonary vein posterior to or above the left atrium.

Situs Abnormalities

The right-sided abdominal and thoracic structures are usually on the same side as the morphologic right atrium; likewise, the left-sided organs are usually on the same side as the morphologic left atrium. In a developmental anomaly in which both atria have morphologic features of a right atrium (RA isomerism), the visceral and thoracic structures tend to be right sided.

Likewise, bilateral left atria (LA isomerism) are associated with bilateral left-sided visceral and thoracic structures.

The bronchi and pulmonary arteries have a characteristic relationship in isomerism syndromes. In RA isomerism, both lungs usually have three lobes and both bronchi have the pattern of a right bronchus—that is, the pulmonary artery runs in front of and beneath the main bronchus (a type of bronchus known as an eparterial bronchus) (Fig. 36-56). Right-sided isomerism is often associated with asplenia syndrome. The liver is large and crosses the midline, and the spleen is often absent.

In left-sided isomerism, both lungs have two lobes and both the right and left pulmonary arteries pass over their respective bronchi. This type of bronchial pattern is known as hyparterial because the bronchus passes below the pulmonary artery (Fig. 36-57). Left-sided isomerism is associated with polysplenia syndrome, characterized by multiple spleens. The IVC is frequently interrupted, with azygous continuation (Fig. 36-58).

Coronal and transaxial MR images are very effective for showing the anatomy of the pulmonary arteries in order to establish the diagnosis of isomerism. MRI also clearly defines the systemic, pulmonary venous anatomy and the morphology of the atrial appendages.

Postoperative Evaluation

MRI is excellent for the postoperative evaluation of CHD. The wide field of view permits effective depiction of complex repairs used to correct complex lesions.

Contrast-enhanced 3D MRA and tomographic images demonstrate surgical anastomoses, conduits, and shunts. Moreover, the 3D data set available from contiguous cine MR images at multiple phases in the cardiac cycle permits precise quantification of left and right ventricular volumes, mass, and

FIG. 36.56. Right-sided isomerism. Spin-echo axial image at the level of the main bronchi (*arrows*) shows that both pulmonary arteries are situated ventral to the bronchi.

FIG. 36.57. Left-sided isomerism. Spin-echo axial image at the level of the carina (*arrow*). Both pulmonary arteries course above the main bronchi.

function. Since cine MRI has high interstudy reproducibility, it is the best technique available for serial monitoring of ventricular volumes, mass, and function after surgery.

Spin-echo MRI and 3D contrast-enhanced MRA have demonstrated the anatomy of complex repairs such as the

FIG. 36.58. Polysplenia with interrupted inferior vena cava (IVC). Multiple axial cine MR images from the great vessels (**top left**) to the liver (**bottom left**) demonstrate a single ventricle (*SV*) and single atrium (*SA*). Note multiple hepatic veins (*arrows*) without an intrahepatic inferior vena cava (IVC). Azygous vein (*Az*) is dilated. Bilateral morphologic left pulmonary arteries (**top left**). Multiple spleens (*asterisks*) are seen in the axial black-blood image (**bottom right**). *Ao*, aorta.

FIG. 36.59. Norwood procedure. Spin-echo axial (**left**) and sagittal (**right**) images show the anastomosis of the proximal pulmonary artery (*P*) to the ascending aorta (*A*). Sagittal view shows the pulmonary artery (*P*) connected to a reconstructed distal ascending aorta (*A*) and arch. Blood flow to the distal pulmonary artery is reconstituted with a central shunt (not shown).

Norwood procedure for hypoplastic left heart (Fig. 36-59); the Jatene procedure (arterial switch) for TGA (Fig. 36-60); Senning and Mustard procedures (atrial baffle redirection of venous flow) for TGA (Fig. 36-44); the Fontan procedure for functional single ventricle (see Fig. 36-49 and 36-51); the Rastelli procedure for pulmonary atresia (Fig. 36-61); and various repairs of tetralogy of Fallot (see Figs. 36-1, 36-2, 36-61, and 36-62).

VEC cine MRI is employed for quantification of the volume and fraction of pulmonary regurgitation (see Fig. 36-2), volume flow through various components of the Fontan repair, and differential flow in the central pulmonary arteries (see Fig. 36-30). After various surgical procedures in cyanotic CHD, residual stenosis of the central pulmonary arteries is frequent. VEC cine MRI can be used to demonstrate disparity in flow between the right and left pulmonary arteries and changes after angioplasty.

FIG. 36.60. Jatene procedure. Spin-echo images in the sagittal (**left**) and axial (**right**) planes show the arterial correction. The aorta (*Ao*) above the anastomosis is situated between the right and left pulmonary arteries. This position can cause narrowing of the branch pulmonary arteries. *PA*, pulmonary artery.

FIG. 36.61. Rastelli procedure. Contrast-enhanced 3D MRA in oblique axial (**left**) and sagittal (**right**) planes shows a conduit (*C*) between the right ventricle (*R*) and the pulmonary artery (*P*). The oblique axial plane depicts a stenosis (*arrow*) of the right pulmonary artery.

Monitoring of Ventricular Function and Pulmonary Regurgitation in Postoperative tetralogy of Fallot (T of F)

Several surgical procedures are employed in total correction of T of F. Correction may be preceded by surgically creating a connection between the aorta and one of the central pulmonary arteries. This is usually done with a graft between the aorta or subclavian artery to the main or a central pulmonary artery. If the graft originates in the ascending aorta, it is called a central shunt. If the graft is between a subclavian artery and central pulmonary artery, it is called a modified Blalock-Tausing shunt. Alternatively, the subclavian artery contralateral to the aortic arch is directly anastomosed to the central pulmonary artery. At total correction, the shunt is closed and the VSD is closed. The RVOT obstruction is removed using one or more of several techniques: infundibulectomy, transannular patch, or conduit from right ventricular to the main or bifurcation of the pulmonary artery. (Fig. 36-1, 36-2, 36-61, and 36-62).

MRI is now used to identify, assess the severity, and monitor any residual abnormality (ies) and to quantify RV function. A typical study involves the following: axial spin-echo or cine MR images to evaluate anatomy; cine MR in the short-axis plane to quantify RV volumes and ejection fraction; cine MR in the RVOT plane to identify sites of RV infundibular, valvular, or supravalvular stenosis(es); contrast-enhanced MRA in coronal plane to evaluate stenosis of main, central or branch pulmonary arteries or in conduits; VEC (phase contrast) cine MR perpendicular to direction of flow in main, right, and left pulmonary arteries to quantify pulmonary regurgitation and differential pulmonary flow to the lungs. Delayed contrast-enhanced inversion recovery gradient echo sequence may be done to identify fibrosis (scar) at site of RV outlet resection (Fig. 36-63) or elsewhere in the ventricles.

The most frequent residual abnormality is moderate to severe pulmonary regurgitation. This nearly always presents after any repair but is particularly problematic after repair by transannular patch. Severity of regurgitation is stated as follows using regurgitation fraction: less than 20% is mild; 20% to 40% is moderate; greater than 40% is severe. Moderate and severe degrees always are associated with enlarged RV end-diastolic (>90 mL/m^2) and end-systolic volumes (>60 mL/m^2) (Fig. 36-64). End-diastolic volumes greater

FIG. 36.62. Tetralogy of Fallot with right ventricular outflow tract aneurysm. Short-axis cine MR image at end-diastole demonstrates aneurysm (*A*) of the right ventricular outflow tract and an overall enlarged right ventricle (*RV*).

FIG. 36.63. Tetralogy of Fallot after transannular patch. Cine MR (**left**) and delayed-enhancement (**right**) images in the short-axis plane show thinning of the right ventricular free wall (*arrowheads*) with associated delayed enhancement (*arrows*). These findings are consistent with myocardial scar related to the surgical procedure. *RV*, right ventricle; *LV*, left ventricle.

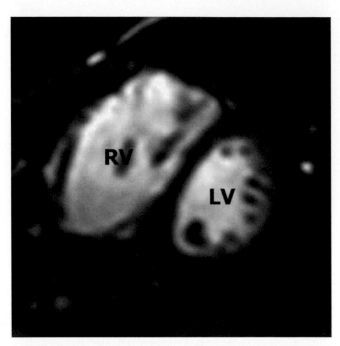

FIG. 36.64. Tetralogy of Fallot with pulmonary regurgitation. Short-axis cine MR image demonstrates an enlarged right ventricle (*RV*) due to the volume overload. The left ventricle (*LV*) is normal in size.

than 150 to 165 mL/m^2 and or end-systolic volume greater than 90 to 100 mL/m^2 are associated with reduced ejection fraction (<40%) and may prompt consideration of pulmonary valve replacement.

Residual or recurrent stenosis of the RV infundibulum, pulmonary valve, or valved conduit is also a frequent residual lesion. There may also be both residual stenosis and regurgitation. If stenosis is the dominant lesion, then the RV shows hypertrabeculation and hypertrophy. Moreover, the combination of stenosis and regurgitation produces less severe RV enlargement and better preservation of RV ejection fraction.

Regional contraction abnormalities of the RV are frequent after repair of tetralogy. Akinesis or dyskinesis of the RV outlet region can be displayed on cine MR images in the sagittal or RVOT planes. After placement of a generous outflow, track patch there may aneurysm of this region (Fig. 36-62). The inlet and body portions of the RV show no or less severe contractile dysfunction.

Adult Congenital Heart Disease

MRI is frequently used in the evaluation of CHD in grown-up children and adults. The major advantage for this purpose is precision and interstudy reproducibility of cine MRI for monitoring right and left ventricular volumes and ejection fraction. Additionally, VEC (phrase contrast) MRI is important for quantifying valvular regurgitation and flow in the pulmonary circulation.

Infrequently, MRI is used to initially identifying lesions, which have gone undetected in childhood. There are usually lesions, which have caused right-sided chamber enlargement in the adult. The most frequent is partial anomalous pulmonary venous connection, which is readily shown on contrast-enhanced MRA in the coronal plane. Occasionally, an ASD is not recognized until adulthood.

The most frequent use of MRI in adult CHD is to monitor the severity of a residual lesion after corrective surgery and to quantifying ventricular function. As discussed above, MRI is now universally employed to monitor pulmonary regurgitation and right ventricular function in postoperative tetralogy of Fallot.

There are several other complex operations for which monitoring of ventricular function is important. These are operations or lesions in which the right ventricular connects to the aorta and supports the systemic circulation. These include the following: atrial switch (Senning and Mustard procedures) for TGA; corrected transposition; single ventricle with RV configuration. The end stage of some operated CHD is right or biventricular failure. MRI is now used to monitor ventricular function in order to recognize the need for reoperation in order to avert such an outcome.

SELECTED READING

Araoz PA, Reddy GP, Higgins CB. Congenital heart disease: morphology and function. In: Higgins CB, de Roos A (eds). MRI and MRA of Cardiovascular System. Philadelphia: Lippincott Williams & Wilkins, 2002:302.

Kilner PJ. Adult congenital heart disease. In: Higgins CB, de Roos A (eds). MRI and MRA of Cardiovascular System. Philadelphia: Lippincott Williams & Wilkins, 2002:353.

Reddy GP, Higgins CB. Congenital heart disease: measuring physiology with MRI. Semin Roentgenol 1998; 33:228.

Roest AAW, Helbing WA, van der Wall EE, de Roos A. Postoperative functional evaluation of congenital heart disease. In: Higgins CB, de Roos A (eds). MRI and MRA of Cardiovascular System. Philadelphia: Lippincott Williams & Wilkins, 2002:339.

Magnetic Resonance Imaging of Ischemic Heart Disease

CHARLES B. HIGGINS, KAREN ORDOVAS, AND STEFANO MUZZARELLI

T he evaluation of ischemic heart disease (IHD) by noninvasive imaging techniques has usually involved nuclear imaging and echocardiography for initial diagnosis, monitoring, and assessment of severity. Coronary angiography has been employed for precise definition of coronary arterial stenoses and to guide therapeutic interventions. In the first two decades of cardiovascular magnetic resonance imaging (MRI), its application in IHD was meager. With the introduction of MR imagers adapted for cardiovascular imaging, however, the capability for the comprehensive evaluation of IHD has been demonstrated.

The comprehensive evaluation of IHD requires the following steps:

1. Detect and assess the severity of IHD
2. Define the coronary anatomy
3. Evaluate and monitor myocardial revascularization
4. Determine myocardial viability
5. Demonstrate complications of myocardial infarction

The role of MRI in accomplishing each of these tasks will be addressed. The evaluation of IHD by MRI remains technically complex because of the multitude of acquisition sequences used to accomplish a comprehensive evaluation. The various sequences will be described briefly in relation to the specific tasks.

DETECTION OF ISCHEMIC HEART DISEASE

The detection of IHD using noninvasive imaging employs two approaches: stress function and stress perfusion. Stress function is the major technique applied with echocardiography. Stress perfusion is the technique used with nuclear scintigraphy. It is generally felt that stress function has greater sensitivity and stress perfusion has better specificity. MRI uses both techniques for detecting and assessing the severity and extent of myocardial ischemia. The site of myocardial ischemia is assigned to a major coronary artery using the American Heart Association 17 segment model (Fig. 37-1). The 17 segments are evaluated by acquiring functional or perfusion images in multiple short-axis planes and the vertical long-axis planes. The apical segment (segment

17) of the left ventricle (LV) is assessed in the vertical long axis plane while the other 16 segments are inspected in three short-axis planes.

STRESS FUNCTION

Pharmacologic stress is employed to induce a regional contraction abnormality as a functional indicator of a hemodynamically significant coronary arterial stenosis. This is the method used to identify IHD by echocardiography. The pharmacologic stressor is usually an infusion of dobutamine. The dose is gradually increased to stimulate intermediate stress (20 µg/kg/min) and then peak stress (40 µg/kg/min). The maximum level of stress should achieve a heart rate equal to 85% of the maximum heart rate predicted for age. Atropine can be administered to achieve this heart rate.

Cine MRI is performed in the short-axis plane at multiple levels and vertical long-axis planes in the baseline state, at intermediate stress, and at peak stress using a balanced steady-state free precession sequence (variably named by the manufacturers as balanced fast field echo [balanced FFE], true fast imaging with steady precession [FISP], or fast imaging employing steady-state acquisition [FIESTA]). With these sequences, cine MR images consisting of 16 to 40 phases can be acquired at three anatomic locations in a breath-hold of 10 to 20 seconds (Fig. 37-2).

FIG 37.1. Seventeen-segment model suggested by the American Heart Association. The coronary artery territories are shown in the graph.

FIG 37.2. End-diastolic (**top**) and end-systolic (**bottom**) cine MR images in the short axis extending from apex (**left**) to base (**right**) of the ventricles.

Left ventricular dysfunction during stress is indicated by a segmental decrease in wall thickening, wall motion, or both (Fig. 37-3). The sensitivity and specificity for detecting a hemodynamically significant stenosis (greater than 50% reduction in luminal diameter) of the coronary artery subserving the dysfunctional segment are about 85%. This level of diagnostic accuracy is equivalent to stress echocardiography.

The rationale for stress function to identify a hemodynamically significant coronary arterial stenosis is that patients with such lesions have adequate blood flow in the resting (basal) state. However, when pharmacologic stress is applied flow may increase three- to fivefold in a normal artery. In the stenotic artery flow cannot increase to the appropriate level so regional myocardial contractile dysfunction is induced. Dobutamine is a secondary coronary vasodilator in that flow is stimulated by the beta sympathomimetic stimulation of myocardial contractility and heart rate; these effects increase myocardial oxygen consumption (demand) and consequently the need for increased coronary blood flow. Failure of coronary flow to rise to the appropriate demand is reflected in a regional contraction abnormality (decreased or no wall thickening or motion). Since myocardial ischemia is provoked by this test, careful patient monitoring is essential during this test (see Selected Reading for extensive discussion of the performance; safety precautions; and contraindications for this test).

Another approach for stress function is to administer a primary vasodilator such as dipyridmole or adenosine which increases coronary flow by directly dilating coronary arterioles (resistance vessels). In the presence of a hemodynamically significant stenosis, resistance vessels in the myocardium served by the coronary artery (conductance vessel) are already maximally dilated. Consequently, the primary vasodilator only increases flow to myocardium served by nonstenotic arteries and flow is stolen from the stenotic region inducing regional myocardial ischemia (coronary arterial steal). Dobutamine stress is superior to adenosine stress for inducing wall motion abnormalities.

Some studies have shown greater sensitivity, specificity, and diagnostic accuracy of dobutamine stress function MR compared to dobutamine stress echocardiography. Moreover, most patients with nondiagnostic dobutamine echocardiography had diagnostic stress MR studies. The provocation of regional myocardial dysfunction by dobutamine stress MR has been found to identify patients at risk of myocardial infarction and death.

STRESS PERFUSION

Pharmacologic stress is used to provoke a perfusion deficit in the myocardium supplied by a coronary artery with a hemodynamically significant stenosis. The pharmacologic agents used are dipyridamole and adenosine (primary vasodilators as described above). MR images are acquired

FIG 37.3. Patient with significant stenosis using steady state free precession (SSFP) two-chamber view at end-diastole (**left panel**) and end-systole (**right panel**). Note the wall-motion abnormality apical inferior at maximal stress. Normal wall motion at rest; 10 and 20 µg dobutamine. (From **Nagel E.** Left ventricular function in ischemic heart disease. In: Higgins CB, de Roos A (eds). MRI and CT of the Cardiovascular System, 2nd ed. Philadelphia: Lippincott Williams & Wilkins, 2006, with permission.)

FIG 37.4. Inversion recovery short-axis images before (**left**) and after the arrival of gadolinium chelate in the left ventricular cavity (**center**) and myocardium (**right**) demonstrate a large transmural perfusion deficit in the ventricular septum (*arrowhead*).

in the short-axis plane at three to five anatomic levels and at one vertical long-axis plane during the first passage of intravenously injected gadolinium chelate (0.03 to 0.05 mmol/kg). A saturation recovery or inversion recovery fast gradient-echo sequence is used to diminish the signal of myocardium before the arrival of the contrast. The images at each anatomic level are acquired at a rate of about 1 per second for about 30 seconds. A regional perfusion deficit is usually visible (Figs. 37-4 and 37-5). The defect may be subendocardial or nearly transmural. Quantitative analysis of the regional intensity-time curve during initial passage of the contrast can improve the diagnostic accuracy. The prime discriminatory parameter is the maximum upslope of the curve.

The sensitivity and specificity for identifying a hemodynamically significant stenosis are about 85%. The diagnostic accuracy of MR perfusion imaging has been found to be equal or better than single photon emission tomography and positron emission tomography. An expected advantage of MR perfusion imaging is greater sensitivity in detecting small subendocardial perfusion deficits (Fig. 37-5) and for demonstrating triple-vessel disease with diffuse myocardial ischemia (Fig. 37-6).

There are now both single center and multicenter studies comparing MR perfusion and radionuclide perfusion imaging. Receiver Operating Characteristic (ROC) curve analyses of sensitivity and specificity (Fig. 37-7) have shown better performance for MR perfusion in both single center and multicenter trials (see Selected Reading for details of these studies).

CORONARY FLOW RESERVE

Velocity-encoded (VEC; phase contrast) cine MR can be used to measure the flow velocity and flow volume of individual major coronary arteries. This is usually done using a breath-hold version of this sequence. This sequence provides a pair of images at approximately 12 to 16 phases of the cardiac cycle. The pair consists of magnitude and phase images acquired perpendicular to the direction of blood flow (Fig. 37-8). A set of images is acquired in the basal state and in the vasodilated state induced by dipyridamole or adenosine. From these images, peak velocity of flow can be calculated in each state (see Fig. 37-8). Coronary flow reserve is the ratio of maximal flow to basal flow. A normal value is designated as a ratio greater than 2.3 to 2.5. In the presence of a hemodynamically significant stenosis (more than 50% reduction in luminal diameter), it is lower than 2.3.

This technique can be used to demonstrate a hemodynamic stenosis before treatment. After stent placement, measurement of coronary flow reserve with MR can be used to monitor the coronary functional status in order to detect recurrence of stenosis.

Abnormal coronary flow and flow reserve may occur in myocardial and vascular diseases in the absence of a stenosis of the epicardial coronary arteries. VEC cine MR may be used to measure the average flow to the left ventricular myocardium by interrogating the flow in the coronary sinus. The coronary sinus conducts about 90% of the left ventricular myocardial flow. Since total coronary flow is proportional to left ventricular mass, total coronary flow is normalized to left ventricular mass to express the flow in mL/min/g myocardium. Left ventricular mass is measured from a stack of cine MR images encompassing the entire LV. The VEC images are acquired in the basal and vasodilated states to calculate coronary flow reserve. Abnormally low coronary flow reserve has been elicited by this method in patients with heart transplants, hypertrophic cardiomyopathy, and dilated cardiomyopathy.

FIG 37.5. Inversion recovery short-axis images at several time frames after administration of gadolinium chelate demonstrate a subendocardial perfusion deficit (*arrow*) in the posterior wall of the left ventricle. (Courtesy of Scott Flamm, M.D., Houston, Texas.)

FIG 37.6. Inversion recovery short-axis images before and at three time intervals after arrival of gadolinium chelate in the left ventricle show perfusion deficits around the entire circumference of the myocardium, indicating the likelihood of triple-vessel disease. (Courtesy of Hajime Sakuma, M.D., Mie, Japan.)

CORONARY ANATOMY

A number of MRI techniques have been explored for displaying coronary artery anatomy. These have included two- and three-dimensional (2D and 3D) acquisition techniques; breath-hold and free-breathing techniques; and white blood and black blood MR sequences. No technique has proved totally suitable, so experimentation continues with several imaging techniques. At present, 3D, free-breathing techniques with respiratory compensation seem to be most effective. The 3D data used to reconstruct the coronary arteries are restricted to a short period of the cardiac cycle (about 50 milliseconds) when there is little respiratory motion. Diaphragmatic motion is monitored (navigator echo) to minimize the effect of respiratory excursion of the heart. Data are used from only about the shallowest 10% of diaphragmatic motion. Conspicuity of the coronary arteries is augmented by applying various prepulses that reduce the signal of the surrounding fat and myocardial tissue.

Under optimized circumstances, impressive images of the coronary arteries can be produced using selected restricted volumes along the predicted course of the major coronary arteries or more recently using whole-heart coronary MRA (Fig. 37-9). However, the sensitivity and specificity for

demonstrating hemodynamically significant stenoses (more than 50% luminal narrowing) remain inadequate for routine clinical application. The sensitivities and specificities of MRA for this purpose are about 90% and 50%, respectively. However, coronary MRA has a good diagnostic accuracy for identifying left main stenosis and triple vessel disease. Importantly, a normal coronary MRA has nearly 100% negative predictive value for left main and triple-vessel disease.

Coronary CTA has become the procedure for assessment of coronary arterial stenoses; coronary MRA is used infrequently for this purpose. Its use is confined to identifying coronary arterial anomalies and for detecting and monitoring coronary arterial aneurysms in Kawasaki's disease.

Diagnostic accuracy of perfusion CMR vs. perfusion SPECT

(D)

1–3 vessel disease
CMR: 0.86 ± 0.06
P = 0.013 vs.all SPECT
P = 0.18 vs.gated SPECT
all SPECT: 0.67 ± 0.05
gated SPECT: 0.76 ± 0.08

J. Schwitter et al. European Heart Journal (2008) 29, 480–489

FIG 37.7. Comparison of the perfusion-CMRversus single-photon emission computed tomography performance. The area under the receiver operating characteristic curve for CMR is larger than for single-photon emission computed tomography (0.86 ± 0.06 vs. 0.67 ± 0.5, p = 0.013). Difference between perfusion-CMR and gated-single-photon emission computed tomography did not reach statistical significance. (From **Schwitter J, et al.** MR-IMPACT: comparison of perfusion-cardiac magnetic resonance with single-photon emission computed tomography for the detection of coronary artery disease in a multicentre, multivendor, randomized trial. Eur Heart J 2008; 29:480–489, with permission.)

Blood flow velocity curve

FIG 37.8. Top: Velocity-encoded cine MR in the short-axis plane consisting of magnitude (**left**) and phase (**right**) images. These images, acquired at 16 phases of the cardiac cycle, can be used to interrogate flow and flow velocity in the left anterior descending coronary artery (*arrow*). **Bottom:** Graph shows the velocity versus time curves for left anterior descending coronary artery flow velocity in the basal and vasodilated state provoked by dipyridamole.

EVALUATION OF MYOCARDIAL REVASCULARIZATION

MR techniques can be used to demonstrate the morphology and blood flow in revascularization conduits and internal mammary arterial and saphenous vein grafts. Contrast-enhanced 3D MRA during breath-holding can depict stenoses in the conduit. The hemodynamic significance of the

stenoses can be assessed using VEC (phase contrast) cine MR with the acquisition in a plane perpendicular to the long axis (flow direction) of the conduit. Revascularization conduits without stenoses, similar to normal coronary arteries, can be shown to have higher peak diastolic flow compared with systolic flow (diastole flow/systolic flow is greater than 1). Conduits with stenoses have higher systolic flow (diastolic flow/systolic flow less than 1), or essentially nonpulsatile flow patterns. Basal flow and coronary flow reserve have also been found to be lower in conduits with significant stenoses. However, basal flow is importantly influenced by the status of the myocardial vascular bed subserved by a bypass conduit and number of distal anastomoses. Frequently, coronary flow reserve is lower than 2.0 even in conduits without stnoses, since the distal native coronary arteries are not normal.

The status of the bypass conduits and native coronary arteries after stent placement is now usually evaluated using coronary CTA rather than contrast enhanced MR angiography or coronary MRA.

MYOCARDIAL VIABILITY

There are two approaches for determining regional myocardial viability after schemic injury using MR. One approach probes the contractile reserve of a dysfunctional segment of the LV using a low dose of a beta-adrenergic agonist, dobutamine (5 to 10 µg/kg/min). Cine MR performed in the basal state displays left ventricular segments with contractile dysfunction, usually severe hypokinesis or akinesis, which raises the question of residual viability in the segments. Under stimulation with a low dose of dobutamine, segments composed of mostly viable myocardium demonstrate improvement in wall motion and wall thickening (more than 2 mm) during systole. An additional sign of a segment with residual viability is end-diastolic wall thickness greater than 5.5 mm.

Another approach to viability assessment is delayed contrast enhancement. This approach employs an inversion recovery gradient-echo sequence with an inversion time set to attenuate the signal of normal myocardium at 10 to 15 minutes after contrast medium administration. At 10 to 15 minutes after intravenous administration of 0.15 to 0.2 mmol/kg gadolinium chelate, the MR sequence is done. At this time, the contrast is substantially cleared from viable myocardium, but nonviable myocardium (necrotic or fibrotic) shows delayed contrast enhancement (Fig. 37-10).

FIG 37.9. MRA of right and left coronary arteries using a balanced FFE sequence encompassing the whole heart. (Courtesy of Oliver Weber, PhD, San Francisco, California.)

FIG 37.10. Inversion recovery gradient-echo image in the short-axis plane using an inversion time, which attenuates the signal of normal myocardium. The image was acquired 15 minutes after intravenous administration of gadolinium chelate (0.2 mmol/kg). There is delayed (persistent) contrast enhancement of a septal myocardial infarction *(arrow)*. *LV*, left ventricle; *RV*, right ventricle.

FIG 37.11. Multilevel short-axis delayed gadolinium enhancement images showing an acute inferior myocardial infarction with microvascular obstruction. There is hyperenhancement of the periphery of the infarction. The endocardial center shows no enhancement due to microvascular obstruction. (Courtesy of H. Sakuma, Mie, Japan.)

Determination of regional myocardial viability has clinical importance, since segments determined to be nonviable do not benefit from revascularization. On the other hand, those determined to be viable demonstrate improved regional function after revascularization.

The delayed enhancement caused by acute or chronic myocardial infarction has two features which are characteristic: (1) always involves the subendocardial layer of myocardium; (2) corresponds to the distribution of one or more coronary arteries or branch arteries (Fig. 37-1). Delayed enhancement occurs with both acute (necrosis) and chronic (scar) myocardial infarctions. There may be homogeneous delayed enhancement in a LV myocardial segment or there may be enhancement along with subendocardial low signal (lack of delayed enhancement). The latter pattern is indicative of an acute infarct with microvascular obstruction (Fig. 37-11). Microvascular obstruction usually occurs with larger infarctions and infarctions in which coronary arterial reperfusion has been delayed (more than 2 hours). Microvascular obstruction is characterized by higher morbidity, mortality, occurrence of complications, and more severe LV remodeling. Indeed, a microvascular obstruction pattern of delayed enhancement is perhaps the strongest predictor for risk stratification after acute myocardial infarction.

Using cine MR to assess LV regional contraction and delayed enhancement MR imaging, it is possible to distinguish among various types of myocardial injury (Table 37-1). Stunned and hibernating myocardium show regional contractile dysfunction but no delayed enhancement. Acute and chronic infarction show regional dysfunction and delayed enhancement. Ischemic cardiomyopathy invariably shows some region(s) with subendocardial delayed enhancement. Idropathic dilated cardiomyopathy has delayed enhancement

TABLE 37.1 Types of Myocardial Injuries

Type	Regional Function	Delayed Hyperenhancement	Perfusion
Normal myocardium	Normal	No	Normal
Stunned myocardium	Dysfunction	No	Acute transient decrease
Hibernating myocardium (ischemic cardiomyopathy)	Dysfunction (regional or global)	No	Chronic decrease
Acute infarction (necrosis)	Dysfunction	Yes	Decreased till reperfusion
Chronic infarction	Dysfunction (wall thinning)	Yes	Decreased till reperfusion
Nonischemic cardiomyopathy	Global dysfunction	Infrequent—not subendocardial	Normal

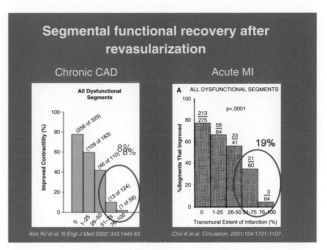

FIG 37.12. Short-axis and vertical long-axis delayed gadolinium enhancement images demonstrate a transmural infarction of the anterior region and a subendocardial infarction in the diaphragmatic-posterolateral region of the left ventricle. Time and extent of myocardial ischemia determines the transition from some degree of viability to transmural necrosis. (MR images are courtesy of S. Wolff, New York.)

FIG 37.13. Left: Graph showing the percent of dysfunctional segments with recovery in regional contractility versus transmural extent of delayed gadolinium enhancement after revascularization for chronic myocardial infarction. (From **Kim RJ, et al.** The use of contrast-enhanced magnetic resonance imaging to identify reversible myocardial dysfunction. New Engl J Med 2000; 343:1445–1453, with permission.) **Right:** Graph showing the percent of dysfunctional segments with recovery in regional contractility versus transmural extent of delayed gadolinium enhancement at late follow-up after acute myocardial infarction. (From **Choi K, et al.** Transmural extent of acute myocardial infarction predicts long-term improvement in contractile function. Circulation 2001; 104:1101–1107, with permission.) If there is greater than 50% transmurality, recovery occurred in 8% of chronic infarcts and 19% of acute infarcts.

in a minority of cases; the delayed enhancement is not subendocardial but rather usually mid wall in location.

The transmurality of delayed enhancement provides insight into the likelihood of recovery of regional contractile function after myocardial revascularization; subendocardial delayed enhancement indicates the likelihood of sufficient viability to result in recovery of contractile function while increasing transmurality indicates decreasing likelihood of recovery of function (Fig. 37-12). The critical value is less than 50% transmurality. In chronic infarcts, greater than 50% transmurality means about 10% of segment will recover function after revascularization (Fig. 37-13). For acute infarcts, greater than 50% transmurality means less than 20% chance of functional recovery in the subsequent 2 to 3 months.

Delayed enhancement in a distribution which does not include the subendocardium suggests an non-ischemic etiology. A midwall distribution might suggest idiopathic dilated cardiomyopathy while subepicardial distribution suggests myocarditis (see Chapter 33).

ACUTE MYOCARDIAL INFARCTION AND MYOCARDIAL SALVAGE

Myocardial edema occurs in the first week of acute myocardial infarction. The ischemic injury causes reversible or irreversible myocardial cellular increased permeability. This results in interstitial and intracellular edema. The regional myocardial edema produces increased signal on T2 weighted images. Triple inversion recovery spin echo sequences with inversion pulses for suppression of the signal intensity of fat

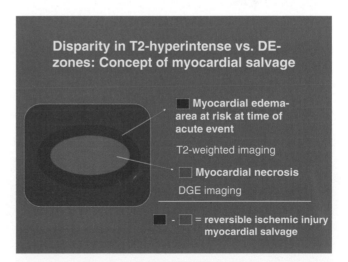

FIG 37.14. Diagram showing relationship between area of hyperintensity of ischemic region on T2 weighted image (myocardial edema) and area of delayed gadolinium hyperenhancement (myocardial necrosis) of the infarcted region. In the event of early reperfusion the difference between the areas represents salvage of ischemic myocardium (salvage area or salvage index).

FIG 37.15. Cine MR image in a transaxial plane shows a mural thrombus at the site of an anteroapical myocardial infarction.

and blood are used to provide improved contrast between normal and edematous myocardium without respiratory and blood flow signal artifacts.

The edematous myocardial region (increased T2 signal) has been shown to correspond to the region rendered ischemic (ischemic jeopardy zone) after coronary occlusion. Usually the area of delayed gadolinium enhancement (infarction) is smaller than the T2 hyperintense region (ischemic jeopardy zone). In patients who undergo early interventions (within 90 minutes) to open the occluded artery, there may be a much smaller infarct area compared to jeopardy zone. The difference between the two has been called the myocardial salvage index (Fig. 37-14).

COMPLICATIONS OF MYOCARDIAL INFARCTION

Cine MR or electrocardiogram-gated spin-echo images can demonstrate the complications that may be caused by myocardial infarction, such as true and false left ventricular aneurysms, mural thrombus (Fig. 37-15), and mitral regurgitation due to papillary muscle dysfunction or rupture. MR is particularly effective for demonstrating the narrow ostium between the left ventricular chamber and false aneurysm.

SELECTED READING

Baer FM, Schmidt M. Regional ventricular function in ischemic heart disease: determination of viability. In: Higgins CB, de Roos A (eds). MRI and CT of Cardiovascular System, 2nd ed. Philadelphia: Lippincott Williams & Wilkins, 2006:224.

Choi KM, Kim RJ, Gubernikoff G, et al. Transmural extent of myocardial infarction predicts long term improvement in contractile function. Circulation 2001; 104:1101.

Hundley WG, Hamilton CA, Thomas MS, et al. Utility of fast cine magnetic resonance imaging and display for the detection of myocardial ischemia in patients not well suited for second harmonic stress echocardiography. Circulation 1999; 100:1697.

Kim RJ, Elliott MD, Judd RM. Assessment of myocardial viability by contrast enhancement. In: Higgins CB, de Roos A (eds). MRI and CT of Cardiovascular System, 2nd ed. Philadelphia: Lippincott Williams & Wilkins, 2006:233.

Kim WY, Danias PG, Stuber M, et al. Coronary magnetic resonance angiography for the detection of coronary stenosis. N Engl J Med 2001; 345:1863.

Nagel E. Left ventricular function in ischemic heart disease. In: Higgins CB, de Roos A (eds). MRI and CT of Cardiovascular System, 2nd ed. Philadelphia: Lippincott Williams & Wilkins, 2006:215.

Nagel E, Klein C, Paetsch I, et al. Magnetic resonance perfusion measurements for the noninvasive detection of coronary artery disease. Circulation 2003; 108:432.

Sakuma H, Higgins CB. Coronary blood flow measurements. In: Higgins CB, de Roos A (eds). MRI and CT of the Cardiovascular System, 2nd ed. Philadelphia: Lippincott Williams & Wilkins, 2006:316.

Schwitter J. Myocardial perfusion in ischemic heart disease. In: Higgins CB, de Roos A (eds). MRI and CT of Cardiovascular System, 2nd ed. Philadelphia: Lippincott Williams & Wilkins, 2006:198.

Sechtem U, Baer FM, Voth E, et al. Stress functional MRI: detection of ischemic heart disease and myocardial viability. J Magn Res Imag 1999; 10:667.

Stuber M, Botnar RM, Kissinger KV, Manning WJ. Coronary MRA: technical approaches. In: Higgins CB, de Roos A (eds). MRI and MRA of the Cardiovascular System. Philadelphia: Lippincott Williams & Wilkins, 2003:252.

Watzinger N, Saeed M, Higgins CB. Tissue characterization in ischemic heart disease. In: Higgins CB, de Roos A (eds). MRI and CT of Cardiovascular System, 2nd ed. Philadelphia: Lippincott Williams & Wilkins, 2006:263.

38

Computed Tomography of Coronary Arteries and Ischemic Heart Disease

KAREN ORDOVAS, BRETT ELICKER, AND CHARLES B. HIGGINS

INTRODUCTION

More than 700,000 patients die each year from myocardial infarction (MI) in the United States. Approximately 50% of these patients have sudden death or MI as the first manifestation of coronary artery disease (CAD). Therefore, methods for early detection and risk stratification of CAD are extremely important. The most widely used risk stratification method is the Framingham score. This score provides an estimate of the risk of a major cardiac event occurring in the following 10 years based upon eight clinical and laboratory criteria including blood pressure, serum lipids, diabetes, and family history of CAD. As up to 50% of patients with MI have no Framingham risk factors, supplementary methods for detection and additional risk stratification for CAD are highly desirable.

The development of fast computed tomography (CT) scans with cardiac gating capabilities has made noninvasive visualization of the moving heart and coronary arteries possible. The first cross-sectional images of the coronary arteries were obtained for the purposes of calcium quantification using electron beam CT in the early 1980s. Subsequently, methods for coronary CT angiography have been developed, allowing not only visualization of the coronary lumen, but also assessment of the coronary wall and atherosclerotic plaque characteristics. Initial studies demonstrating the clinical utility of CT coronary imaging were performed using 16 slice multidetector CT (MDCT) scanners.

These showed a reasonable accuracy for the detection of significant coronary stenosis when compared to invasive coronary angiography. Most of the clinical studies, however, showing the highest accuracy of CTA for the detection of CAD have used 64 MDCT technology. More recently, new CT technology including 256 MDCT, 320 MDCT, dual energy, and dual source MDCT have shown significant improvement in coronary CTA image quality and are very promising tools for improved assessment of CAD including vessel wall imaging.

INDICATIONS

Multiple studies have been performed to assess the accuracy of coronary CT for the diagnosis of CAD using both 16 and 64 slice MDCT, and more recently dual source CT scanners.

The sensitivity, specificity, positive predictive value, and negative predictive value for the detection of significant coronary stenosis (greater than 50% luminal narrowing) have varied from 86% to 99%, 90% to 99%, 66% to 97%, and 92% to 100%, respectively (Table 38-1). The negative predictive value is the parameter that has been consistently high in these studies, with numbers approaching 100%. Applying this concept to clinical practice, the most important indication for coronary CTA is to exclude the presence of significant CAD.

Guidelines on appropriate criteria for the use of coronary CTA have been formulated by national and international radiology and cardiology societies (Table 38-2). In the outpatient setting, there is consensus that coronary CTA is indicated for patients who have a discrepancy between their pretest probability of having CAD based upon risk factors and clinical symptoms. For instance, coronary CTA is indicated for patients with a low risk of CAD who present with classic symptoms of angina. It may also be useful in patients who have moderate risk for CAD and present with equivocal symptomatology. Other accepted indications include coronary evaluation prior to major vascular surgery, aortic valvular replacement, and lung or liver transplant, among others.

In patients with acute chest pain, recent studies have shown that coronary CTA can accurately exclude acute coronary syndrome and can be used as a first line test leading to direct discharge from the emergency room. Coronary CTA has been used in patients with an intermediate risk for CAD presenting to the emergency room with chest pain and normal cardiac enzyme levels or normal/equivocal ECG findings. Recent studies in this particular clinical setting have shown that these patients can be safely discharged from the emergency room after a negative CTA or a CTA showing less than 25% stenosis of the coronary arteries. This approach has the potential to significantly reduce the cost of unnecessary hospital admissions for the diagnosis of possible acute coronary syndrome in patients with a low to intermediate risk for CAD. These patients account for the majority of those presenting with chest pain to emergency rooms. Guidelines on the use of CTA for acute chest pain have been recently published and recommend the use of this technique in patients with

TABLE 38.1 Accuracy of CT for Detection of Significant Coronary Artery Stenosis Compared to Conventional Coronary Angiography

Author	Scanner	n	Sensitivity (%)	Specificity (%)	PPV (%)	NPV (%)
Raff et al.	64 MDCT	70	86	95	66	98
Leschka et al.	64 MDCT	67	94	97	87	99
Mollet et al.	64 MDCT	51	99	95	76	99
Fine et al.	64 MDCT	66	95	96	97	92
Ropers et al.	64 MDCT	81	93	97	56	100
Ehara et al.	64 MDCT	69	90	94	89	95
Ong et al.	64 MDCT	134	82	96	79	96
Oncel et al.	64 MDCT	80	96	98	91	99
Meijboom et al.	64 MDCT	360	88	90	47	99
Weustink et al.	Dual-source CT	100	95	95	75	99
Kohnson et al.	Dual-source CT	35	88	98	78	99
Leber et al.	Dual-source CT	88	94	99	81	99
Ropers et al.	Dual-source CT	100	92	97	68	99
Brodoefel et al.	Dual-source CT	100	91	92	75	97

NPV, negative predictive value; PPV, positive predictive value.

intermediate pretest probability of CAD, negative enzymes, and negative or equivocal ECG. It should be mentioned that multiple trials using coronary CTA for the exclusion of acute coronary syndrome are ongoing and changes to the current guidelines should be expected in the near future.

ACQUISITION TECHNIQUES

Coronary CTA images are acquired using MDCT technology. The two major technical challenges of coronary CTA are obtaining optimal spatial and temporal resolution, and at the same time trying to minimize three-dimensional (3D) reconstruction artifacts. Spatial resolution is primarily a function of the physics of the scanner and currently is in the range of approximately 0.4 mm. The greater the number of detectors, the longer the z-axis length of coverage per unit time, allowing for acquisition of images covering the entire heart in only 1 to 2 beats. Reducing the number of heart beats used for full cardiac coverage significantly reduces or eliminates misregistration artifacts on reconstructed images.

TABLE 38.2 Clinical Indications for Coronary CTA

Detection of CAD
Acute chest pain
  Intermediate pretest probability of CAD, normal or equivocal ECG and negative serial enzymes
Chronic chest pain (angina)
  Intermediate pretest probability of CAD
  ECG uninterpretable
  Unable to exercise or equivocal test results
  Evaluation for coronary anomalies

Structure and function
Coronary artery mapping prior to repeat revascularization
Assessment of complex congenital heart disease

Fast acquisitions with high temporal resolution decrease motion artifacts and provide higher image quality. Temporal resolution is primarily a function of gantry rotation speed. Based upon half-rotation scanning time techniques, it takes a minimum of one half a gantry rotation to produce an entire 3D dataset. The newer generation of scanners has significantly faster gantry rotation speeds than previous generations and thus improved temporal resolution. With the introduction of dual source CT, two separate gantries have introduced the possibility of quarter-rotation scanning providing sufficient projection data to image the entire heart with a minimum temporal resolution of approximately 83 ms. That being said, reasonable image quality can still be obtained with 16-detector MDCT technology. Sixty-four MDCT technology is currently the most commonly used platform, since it provides a good balance of cost and image quality. Advantages of the most advanced CT scanners with state-of-the-art technology such as 256 MDCT, 320 MDCT, dual energy, and dual source scanners are of higher image quality with the possibility of image acquisition without pharmacologic heart rate control.

Cardiac Gating

CT with cardiac gating has allowed for imaging of the heart while minimizing the blurring artifacts caused by cardiac motion. Visualization of the beating cardiac structures can be obtained using either a prospective or retrospective gating technique (Fig. 38.1). With prospective cardiac gating, the images are only acquired during a predetermined phase of the cardiac cycle, usually end-diastole. Retrospective cardiac gating technique acquires data throughout the entire cardiac cycle and allows the diagnostician to select, after the acquisition, the phases of the cardiac cycle to be used for reconstruction of the images. Retrospective gating has two major advantages. First, the phase of the cardiac cycle in which

FIG. 38.1. Diagram demonstrates the principles of prospective and retrospective cardiac gating. The top image shows an ECG trace including three consecutive heart beats (R-R intervals). CT acquisition occurs only during a short predetermined diastolic period (gray square) with prospective cardiac gating. On the bottom image CT acquisition occurs throughout the entire cardiac cycle (gray strip) with retrospective gating.

the coronary arteries are best visualized can be used for the evaluation of stenoses and production of the 3D reconstructions. This is not always at a predetermined phase of the cardiac cycle. Also, with retrospective gating cine loops can be used for the assessment of ventricular and valvular function.

The other important difference between the two gating methods is the amount of radiation used. While prospective cardiac images can be obtained with very low radiation exposure, approaching 3 to 5 mSv, prospective images of the heart require a much higher radiation dose (approximately 12 to 15 mSv) that is similar to that used during invasive coronary angiography. Dual source CT with radiation reduction techniques has recently produced diagnostic CT coronary angiograms at less than 1 mSv.

Heart Rate Control

The optimal cardiac phase for imaging the coronary arteries is typically end-diastole. Patients with a low heart rate have a longer diastolic length than patients with fast heart rates. Therefore, heart rate management is essential for the acquisition of good quality coronary images. Beta-blockers are used to decrease the heart rate prior to a coronary CTA. In addition, these agents affect the heart rhythm and tend to stabilize the heart rate, which is essential for good image quality as imaging data is currently acquired over multiple cardiac cycles. It has been shown that patients with a heart rate lower than 60 bpm have significantly better image quality and less motion artifact compared to patients with higher heart rates. Various groups use oral β-blockers, intravenous β-blockers, or a combination of both. The most common protocol is to use oral β-blockers (Metoprolol 50 mg or Atenolol 100 mg) 1 hour prior to the imaging study, followed by intravenous fast acting β-blocker (usually Metoprolol) immediately before contrast administration if the heart rate is still above 60 bpm.

The Protocol

A complete cardiac CTA study starts with a noncontrast chest CT for the purposes of calcium scoring. These

are continuous axial images with 2.5 to 3 mm thickness encompassing the entire heart using prospective gating (R-R interval of 75%) and a small field of view (25 cm²).

The contrast enhanced CT images are then acquired with prospective or retrospective gating, with the minimum slice thickness available (0.625 mm for a 64 detector CT), encompassing the entire heart with a small field of view (25 cm²). Rotation speed and temporal resolution depend on patient's heart rate and scanner characteristics. Temporal resolution varies from 83 to 330 ms.

Contrast Injection

Optimal enhancement of the coronary arteries is the goal of contrast enhancement techniques for coronary CTA. In addition, avoiding streak artifact from dense contrast in the superior vena cava (SVC) and right atrium is essential for good visualization of the right coronary artery (RCA) in particular (Fig. 38.2). For this purpose, a saline flush is generally used after contrast administration in hopes of washing out the dense contrast in these chambers. A triple phase injection technique can also be used, consisting of standard concentration contrast followed by diluted contrast and finally a saline flush.

Good image quality can be obtained with either timing bolus or bolus tracking techniques. For bolus tracking, the region of interest is placed in the ascending aorta and the threshold is set for at least 100 HU. With the timing bolus technique, a test injection of 40 mL of contrast is administered followed by 40 mL of saline. This method allows for timing of not only the peak enhancement within the ascending aorta, but also for timing of peak enhancement of the SVC, which can be used to calculate the timing of the saline bolus. With both techniques, an injection rate of 5 mL/second is recommended.

IMAGE POSTPROCESSING

Calcium score. There are multiple commercially available softwares for postprocessing of the calcium score. Following the Agatston score protocol, any pixel within the coronary

A   **B**

FIG. 38.2. Timing of contrast enhancement. **A:** Poor timing of the contrast injection is seen in this case, resulting in dense contrast enhancement of the right atrium producing streak artifacts (*arrows*). Note the poor visualization of the right coronary artery (*arrowhead*) due to the artifact. **B:** Ideal contrast injection protocol for a coronary CTA shows well-opacified left-sided cardiac chambers and coronary arteries. Contrast has been washed out of the right-sided cardiac chambers from the saline flush.

arterial tree with a density higher than 130 HU is considered as containing calcium. A peak density factor is then multiplied to the area of calcification depending on the density of each of the identified pixels. The results are plotted against risk curves obtained from multiple cardiovascular disease population studies and the results are compared to an age and gender matched cohort. Results can be provided as an Agatston score (the most used parameter), calcium volume or volume score. Based on the calcium score and

the percentile compared to the population curves, the risk of an obstructive coronary lesion is estimated. The American Heart Association has proposed guidelines on reporting and clinical recommendations for calcium score studies.

Coronary CTA. The initial step for postprocessing of the coronary arteries is the selection of the cardiac phase with best image quality and least amount of motion artifact (Fig. 38.3). This is usually, but not always, approximately

A   **B**

FIG. 38.3. Cardiac phase selection. **A:** Axial coronary CTA image obtained at 50% of the R-R interval shows motion artifact precluding visualization of the right coronary artery (*arrow*). **B:** Image reconstruction at 70% of the R-R interval shows no motion artifact and clear visualization of the right coronary artery (*arrow*).

70% of the R-R interval. In some cases, different cardiac phases must be used in the reconstruction of the right and left coronary arteries. This is often necessary in patients with high heart rates. In these patients the best quality images are often found earlier in the cardiac cycle, around 45% of the R-R interval. When a prospective acquisition technique is used, reconstructions are limited to a small window of the cardiac cycle thus this technique is best reserved for patients with well controlled heart rates.

The most commonly used techniques for 3D reconstructions of the coronary arteries are 3D volume rendering, curved multiplanar reformated (MPR) image and cross-sectional images of the coronary arteries. Three-dimensional volume rendered reconstructions are useful for an overall depiction of the coronary artery anatomy and its relationship to the cardiac chambers (Fig. 38.4). It provides a good overview of the anatomy when bypass grafts are present. This technique is not particularly useful for visualization of specific coronary artery lesions. Curved MPR images are reconstructions performed in a plane aligned to the center of the coronary artery lumen. Multiple projections can be obtained encompassing 360 degrees of the vessel circumference, maintaining the plane aligned to the center of the coronary vessel (Fig. 38.5). This technique allows for accurate visualization of coronary lesions and depiction of the point of maximum stenosis. When a lesion is detected, cross-sectional images of the coronary artery can be obtained in a plane perpendicular to the curved maximum intensity projection (MIP) reconstruction plane, providing the best tool for determining the degree of stenosis (Fig. 38.6).

IMAGE INTERPRETATION

Most of the findings on a coronary CTA can be identified on the axial images. Three-dimensional reformations are excellent tools for focused problem solving and for precise measurement of the degree of coronary stenosis. An ideal reading session involves interactive use of 3D workstations. The most useful reformats are the curved multiplanar reconstructions and the cross-sectional coronary views.

A systematic and comprehensive approach to interpreting a coronary CTA study should include calcium scoring and evaluation of the coronary arteries, followed by an assessment of other cardiac and extracardiac findings.

Calcium Scoring

The use of calcium scoring for CAD risk stratification is based on multiple research studies which have shown a correlation between the amount of calcium present in the coronary arteries and likelihood of significant coronary stenosis/cardiac death. This association is independent of other traditional risk factors for CAD. The relative risk of cardiac death in patients with a calcium score greater than 160 compared to those with a calcium score less than 160 is approximately 4.2 (95% confidence interval 1.6–11.3). It is known that the extent of atherosclerotic disease correlates with the amount of calcium in the coronary arteries (Fig. 38.7). Although the absence of coronary calcification does not exclude the presence of soft atherosclerotic plaque, the likelihood of an obstructive lesion is very low in these patients. The negative

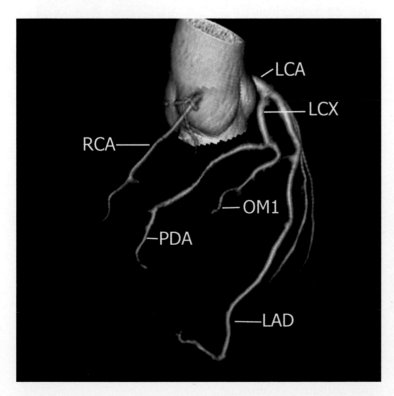

FIG. 38.4. Volume rendering. Three-dimensional volume rendered reconstruction of the coronary arteries. Note a very long left anterior descending (LAD) coronary artery with a transapical course. RCA, right coronary artery; LCA, left coronary artery; LCX, left circumflex coronary artery; OM1, first obtuse marginal branch of the left circumflex; PDA, posterior descending coronary artery.

FIG. 38.5. Curved multiplanar reformation (MPR) of the left anterior descending **(A)** and right coronary **(B)** arteries. Liner reformation of the curved MPR shows multiple images **(C–E)** obtained during rotation along the curved MPR plane.

FIG. 38.6. Curved multiplanar reformation of the left anterior descending coronary artery shows multiple calcified and non-calcified atherosclerotic plaques **(A)**. A plane (line) was prescribed for cross-sectional visualization of a calcified plaque. Cross-sectional reconstruction **(B)** shows an eccentric calcified plaque (*arrow*) with no significant luminal narrowing.

FIG. 38.7. Calcium score. Axial images from a two calcium score protocols in patients with no coronary calcium **(A and B)** and coarse coronary calcification (*arrows*) **(C and D)** with a calcium score of 500.

predictive value of coronary calcium screening is very high, with an estimated risk of 0.1% per year of developing a major cardiovascular event in 2 to 5 years.

Calcium score and Framingham risk assessment have similar accuracy in predicting major cardiovascular events in 10 years. The added value of calcium scoring to the Framingham risk is an approximate 15% increase in accuracy for predicting a major cardiovascular event. Patients with an intermediate risk of CAD based on the Framingham score are most likely to benefit from undergoing coronary calcium scoring. A recent study has shown that intermediate risk patients with a calcium score greater than 300, have the same

cardiovascular risk as patients in the high risk category and should be managed similarly. Additionally, this study showed that patients with an intermediate risk and a calcium score less than 300 have a low risk of cardiovascular events.

Coronary Artery Findings

Coronary assessment should begin by determining the coronary arterial dominance. A right dominant system is most common (80%) and characterized by a RCA which gives origin to both the posterior descending and posterolateral arteries (Fig. 38.8). A left dominant system, the second

A

B

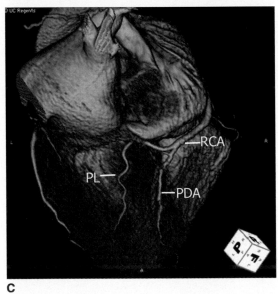

C

FIG. 38.8. Right dominant coronary circulation. Volume rendered reconstructions of the heart and coronary arteries displayed in anterior **(A)**, lateral **(B)**, and posterior **(C)** projections show the right coronary artery branching. In this right dominant coronary arterial circulation, the right coronary artery (RCA) bifurcates into a posterior descending coronary artery (PDA), which courses in the posterior interventricular grove, and a posterolateral coronary artery (PL) which supplies the inferior left ventricular region. M1, first acute marginal branch.

most common variant (15%), occurs when both the posterior descending and the posterolateral arteries originate from the left circumflex artery (Fig. 38.9). Finally a codominant circulation (5%) is seen when the posterior descending artery originates from the RCA and the posterolateral artery originates from the left circumflex artery (Fig. 38.10).

Coronary arterial anomalies. Assessment of the coronary artery ostia, course, and termination is essential for identification of coronary anomalies (Table 38-3). The most common coronary anomalies include anomalous origin of a coronary artery from the contralateral sinus of Valsalva or from the contralateral coronary artery. In this scenario, the proximal diameter and course of the anomalous vessel should be carefully evaluated. Possible anomalous courses include the pre-pulmonary, interarterial, septal, and retroaortic (Figs. 38.11 and 38.12). Among these anomalous courses, the most clinically significant is the interarterial course, also

called a "malignant" coronary anomaly. Patients with this abnormality, particularly when involving the left coronary system, are at risk for sudden death. Coronary arteries with an interarterial course are also typically intramural and demonstrate a long segment at their origin which runs within the wall of the aorta. In fact, it may be this long intramural course which predisposes patients with this anomaly to sudden death. CTA findings that are suggestive of an intramural course of an anomalous interarterial vessel include an acute angle at the vessel origin, proximal course parallel to the sinus of Valsalva, and narrowing of the ostium (Fig. 38.13). Treatment for an interarterial coronary artery includes bypass graft, unroofing of an intramural vessel, or reimplantation in the ascending aorta.

The most common course abnormality of the coronary arteries is a myocardial bridge. It consists of a segment of coronary artery which has an intramyocardial

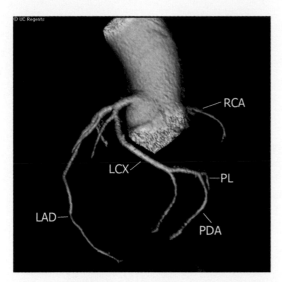

FIG. 38.9. Left dominant coronary circulation. Volume rendered reconstruction of the coronary arteries displayed in a posterior projection. Note that both the posterior descending (PDA) and posterolateral (PL) coronary arteries originate from the left circumflex artery (LCX). The right coronary artery (RCA) is a very short vessel, typical of left dominant coronary circulations. LAD, left anterior descending coronary artery.

course as opposed to the normal course in the epicardial fat (Fig. 38.14). It usually affects the mid segment of the left anterior descending artery. Myocardial bridges can be complete or incomplete, can have a deep course in the myocardium or be quite superficial and can involve a short or a long

FIG. 38.10. Co-dominant coronary circulation. Volume rendered reconstruction of the heart and coronary arteries displayed in a posterior projection. The posterior descending (PDA) coronary artery originates from the right coronary artery (RCA). The posterolateral coronary artery (PL) originates from the circumflex coronary artery.

TABLE 38.3 Coronary Anomalies

Anomalous origin
Single coronary ostium
Multiple coronary ostia
Ectopic origin coronary artery
    Contralateral sinus of Valsalva or non-coronary sinus
    Above the sinotubular junction
    Pulmonary artery

Anomalous course
Retroaortic
Prepulmonary
Interarterial
Septal
Myocardial bridging
Artery duplications

Anomalous termination
Coronary artery fistula
Coronary arcade
Extracardiac termination

coronary segment. Some patients may have ischemia due to arterial compression during systole. However, it is not clear what imaging findings correlate with the presence of myocardial ischemia.

Plaque and stenosis. The coronary arteries should then be assessed for the presence of wall abnormalities and luminal narrowing or dilatation. Abnormalities of the coronary artery wall include calcifications (calcified atherosclerotic plaque) and soft tissue attenuation thickening (soft atherosclerotic plaque) (Fig. 38.15). Soft atherosclerotic plaques have been associated with unstable disease and acute coronary syndrome, however it is not yet been documented that coronary CTA can accurately identify vulnerable plaques. Wall thickening with mixed components of calcified and non-calcified plaque is commonly seen. Lesions of the wall should be described based upon length and whether they are eccentric or circumferential. Finally, the precise location of the lesion in relationship to the coronary artery ostia and branches should be indicated. The most commonly used system for localization of a coronary artery lesion is the American Heart Association standard coronary segmentation (Fig. 38.16).

When coronary luminal narrowing is identified, grading of the percentage stenosis compared to the diameter of the normal coronary artery either proximal or distal to the lesion should be provided. The most useful images for establishing the severity of a coronary stenosis are the curved multiplanar reformations (MPRs) and the cross-sectional images of the coronary arteries. Although most available commercial workstations provide tools for quantification of a coronary stenosis, most readers provide a visual assessment of the degree of stenosis, which is usually classified as narrowing of 0 to 25%, 25 to 50%, 50 to 75%, 75 to 99% and coronary occlusion. A lesion causing more than 50% stenosis is considered hemodynamically significant.

Aneurysm and ectasia. Coronary artery dilatation can be classified as aneurysm or ectasia. The definition of a coronary

FIG. 38.11. Anomalous origin of the left coronary artery from the right coronary sinus (*R*) with four different anomalous courses: interarterial (between the aorta and the pulmonary artery [*PA*]) (*A*), retroaortic (*B*), pre-pulmonic (*C*), and septal (subpulmonic [beneath the right ventricular outflow tract]) (*D*). *L*, left coronary sinus, *N*, noncoronary sinus. Reproduced from **Kim SY, Seo JB, Do K-H, et al**. Coronary artery anomalies: classification and ECG-gated multi-detector row CT findings with angiographic correlation. Radiographics 2006; 26:317–333, with permission.

FIG. 38.12. Different courses of anomalous coronary arteries. **A:** Anomalous origin of the left main coronary artery (LCA) from the right sinus of Valsalva is noted in this maximum intensity projection reformation, with a retroartic course. **B:** Curved MPR shows an anomalous right coronary artery (RCA) from the left sinus of Valsalva, coursing between the ascending aorta (Ao) and the main pulmonary artery (MPA). **C:** Maximum intensity projection reformation shows an anomalous LCA from the right sinus of Valsalva coursing anterior (*arrow*) to the MPA in a pre-pulmonary course. **D:** Three-dimensional volume rendered reconstruction of the same patient as in **(C)** again shows the pre-pulmonary course of the LCA.

FIG. 38.13. Interarterial course of an anomalous coronary artery. **A:** Curved MPR shows an anomalous origin of the right coronary artery (RCA) from the left sinus of Valsalva, with an acute angle between the RCA and the aorta (Ao) and narrowing of the most proximal segment of the anomalous vessel (*arrow*). These findings are suggestive of an intramural coronary course. Cross-sectional reformations were obtained at the site of the right coronary artery narrowing **(B)** showing an elliptical shape of the vessel (*arrow*). Similar reconstruction obtained distal to the narrowing **(C)** depicts normal cross-sectional appearance of the right coronary artery (*arrow*). MPA, main pulmonary artery.

artery aneurysm is focal dilatation with a diameter 1.5 times greater than the adjacent normal of the coronary artery and involvement of less than 50% of the vessel length (Fig. 38.17). The term ectasia is used to described diffuse dilatation (>1.5 times the normal diameter) of the vessel that involves 50% or more of the length of the vessel. Aneurysms may be fusiform or saccular in shape and are usually due to atherosclerotic CAD or Kawasaki's disease (Table 38-4). The precise diameter and location of the coronary aneurysm is important in management decisions including stent placement and anticoagulation therapy. Positive remodeling is a type of ectasia seen with

CAD in which the vessel dilates in an effort to compensate for a decreased coronary flow due to atherosclerotic wall thickening (Fig. 38.18). An association between positive remodeling and unstable coronary lesions causing acute coronary syndromes has also been recently described in coronary CTA studies. A remodeling index can be calculated comparing the cross-sectional vessel area at the level of the dilatation to a normal reference area immediately proximal or distal to the area of remodeling.

Coronary bypass imaging. Coronary CTA may be used for visualization of graft anatomy before surgical intervention, assessment of graft stenosis or occlusion, and evaluation

FIG. 38.16. Diagram shows the standard American Heart Association coronary segmentation. Reproduced from **Scanlon PJ, Faxon DP, Audet A**. ACC/AHA guidelines for coronary angiography. A report of the American College of Cardiology/American Heart Association task force on practice guidelines (committee on coronary angiography) developed in collaboration with the Society for Cardiac Angiography and Interventions. JACC 1999; 33(6):1756–1824, with permission.

FIG. 38.14. Myocardial bridge. Curved multiplanar reformation of the left anterior descending coronary artery shows an intramyocardial course of the mid segment (*arrows*) consistent with a myocardial bridge.

A   B

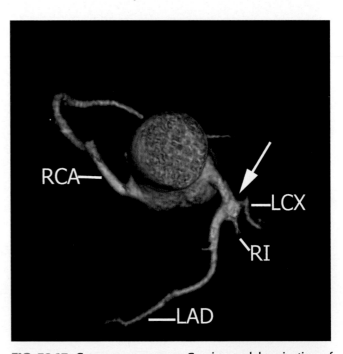

FIG. 38.15. Coronary atherosclerotic plaque. Curved multiplanar reformation **(A)** of the right coronary artery (RCA) shows multiple calcified plaques along the entire course of the artery. None of the plaques cause significant stenosis of the lumen. Curved MPR **(B)** of the left anterior descending artery (LAD) shows a concentric soft plaque (*arrows*) of the mid LAD segment, demonstrating approximately 50% stenosis of the lumen.

FIG. 38.17. Coronary aneurysm. Cranio-caudal projection of a volume rendered reconstruction shows a coronary aneurysm (*arrow*) at the site of the left main coronary artery trifurcation into left anterior descending (LAD), left circumflex (LCX), and ramus intermedius (RI). The aneurysm measures approximately 7 mm in diameter. RCA, right coronary artery.

TABLE 38.4 Causes of Coronary Aneurysm and Ectasia

Atherosclerosis
Kawasaki disease
Inflammatory disorders
   Takayasu's arteritis
   Systemic lupus erythematosus
   Wegener's granulomatosis
   Giant cell arteritis
   Others (Behçet's syndrome, sarcoidosis, rheumatoid arthritis, CREST syndrome, etc.)
Compensatory dilatation
   Post-stenotic dilatation
   Fistula
   Coronary anomalies (ALCAPA)
Miscellaneous connective tissue disorder
   Marfan's syndrome
   Ehlers-Danlos' syndrome
   Cystic medial necrosis
Mycotic
Trauma/Iatrogenic

FIG. 38.18. Positive remodeling. Curved multiplanar reformation of the right coronary artery (RCA) shows dilatation of the mid and distal RCA in addition to dilatation of the proximal posterior descending artery (PDA) in a patient with several risk factors for coronary artery disease. PL, posterolateral.

of disease in the native run-off vessels. The protocol differs from that used for the evaluation of native coronary arteries. A longer scan coverage is required, encompassing the aortic arch and the origin on the internal mammary arteries, which requires a different contrast injection protocol (Fig. 38.19). Evaluation of grafts is less susceptible to motion artifacts due to the relatively larger size of the vessels, particularly venous grafts, and greater distance from the cardiac surface (Fig. 38.20). One limitation specific to graft evaluation is streak artifact from

surgical clips which generate streak artifact and may limit the evaluation of certain graft segments (Fig. 38.21).

Graft occlusion is the most common acute complication after CABG (approximately 10% of cases). CTA will show lack of contrast enhancement in an enlarged or normal sized

FIG. 38.19. Field of view for different coronary CTA protocols. Scout images from coronary CTA studies demonstrate the typical field of view used to scan native coronary arteries **(A)** and patients with coronary artery bypass grafts **(B)**.

FIG. 38.20. Left internal mammary (LIMA) graft. Curved multiplanar reformation along the LIMA graft clearly depicts the entire course of the vessel. Note the proximity of the graft with the chondrosternal joints (*arrows*), which is useful information prior to re-sternotomy.

FIG. 38.22. Acute graft occlusion. Multiplanar reformation of a venous graft shows contrast enhancement of the proximal vessel up to the site of occlusion (*arrow*). Note the enlarged non-enhanced graft (*arrowheads*) distal to the occlusion. Ao, ascending aorta.

vessel (Fig. 38.22). In chronic graft occlusion, the vessel becomes atretic and a focal out-pouching at the level of the aortic anastomosis may be the only finding (Fig. 38.23). Graft stenosis is a common chronic complication, most frequently seen in venous grafts. One potential advantage of coronary

FIG. 38.21. Streak artifact. Multiplanar reformation is seen on the right internal mammary artery (RIMA) to right coronary artery graft. Note the streak artifact from the dense surgical clips (*arrows*) along the course of the graft, precluding the evaluation for graft stenosis at these levels.

FIG. 38.23. Chronic graft occlusion. Axial image from coronary CTA shows a chronic venous graft occlusion near the anastomosis with the ascending aorta. Note the focal out-pouching (*arrow*) at the level of the proximal anastomosis with no vessel seen distally.

CTA over invasive cardiac angiography is the detection of ostial stenosis. This may be obscured because of selective canulation of the grafts during cardiac catheterization, but typically can be clearly visualized with CTA (Fig. 38.24).

Cardiac Findings

Attention to the size and function of the cardiac chambers should be part of a comprehensive coronary CTA interpretation. In a prospectively gated study, when images are available only at end-diastole, it is possible to assess for cardiac chamber enlargement and myocardial hypertrophy (Fig. 38.25). A retrospectively gated cardiac study, on the other hand, can be reconstructed during multiple phases of the cardiac cycle, usually 10 phases, and visualized as cine loops. Cine loops are usually reconstructed in the most common cardiac planes named horizontal long axis, vertical long axis and short axis (Fig. 38.26). This provides an accurate depiction of biventricular size and function. There is good correlation of right and left ventricular ejection fractions when comparing coronary CTA with echocardiography. End-diastolic, end-systolic, and stroke volume indexes can also be calculated with cardiac CTA. The presence of wall thinning or aneurysm formation in the setting of prior MI can also be depicted (Fig. 38.27). Fatty replacement or calcification of the myocardium is usually seen in association with wall thinning. A myocardial perfusion defect can also be visualized with coronary CTA. The role of cardiac CT for myocardial imaging and specific protocols for this purpose will be further discussed later in this chapter. Finally, the cardiac chamber contents should be closely assessed for filling defects that could represent a thrombus or cardiac masses (Fig. 38.28).

In addition to the chambers, the cardiac valves can also be visualized on a cardiac CTA. Routine contrast injection tech-

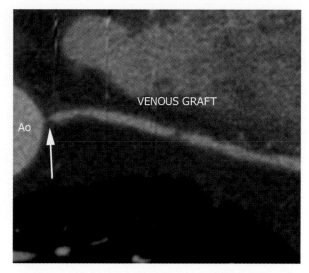

FIG. 38.24. Ostial graft stenosis. Curved multiplanar reformation of a venous graft shows diffuse thickening of the vessel wall with significant focal stenosis (*arrow*) at the site of anastomosis with the ascending aorta (Ao).

niques in coronary CTA are designed to minimize contrast enhancement of the right-sided chambers, thus there will be limited assessment of the tricuspid and pulmonic valves. If the primary indication of the cardiac CT is evaluation of valvular disease an alternative contrast injection protocol should be employed. In this case the injection rate should be slowed and should continue throughout the data acquisition in order to maximize opacification of both sides of the heart and allow assessment of all four cardiac valves. Cardiac CT images should be evaluated for the excursion of the valve leaflets, with particular interest in complete closure and wide

A   **B**

FIG. 38.25. **A:** Axial image at the end-diastolic cardiac phase shows a dilated left ventricle (LV) in a patient with dilated cardiomyopathy. Note the streak artifact (*arrow*) from the pacemaker leads within the right ventricle (RV). **B:** Horizontal long axis image at the end-diastolic phase shows concentric left ventricular hypertrophy (*asterisks*) in a patient with severe systemic hypertension. LV, left ventricle; RV, right ventricle.

A

B

C

FIG. 38.26. Cardiac planes. Thin maximum intensity projection reconstructions were obtained at the end-diastolic phase in the horizontal long axis **(A)**, vertical long axis **(B)**, and short axis **(C)** planes. LV, left ventricle; RV, right ventricle; LA, left atrium; RA, right atrium.

opening of the valve (Fig. 38.29). Valve leaflet thickening and calcification can be depicted with cardiac CTA (Fig. 38.30). In fact, the main role of cardiac CT for valve assessment is in patients with course leaflet calcification, when

echocardiography images are limited by calcium artifacts. Multiple studies have demonstrated the utility of cardiac CT for preoperative assessment of aortic valve leaflets, particularly prior to valve replacement surgery. Cardiac CT

FIG. 38.27. Left ventricular pseudoaneurysm. Coronal reformation from a cardiac CTA shows a focal pseudoaneurysm (A) in the inferior left ventricular wall in a patient with prior history of myocardial infarction. Note the narrow ostium of attachment (*arrow*) between the aneurysm and the left ventricle (LV), characteristic of a false aneurysm.

FIG. 38.28. Left ventricular thrombus. Axial image from a coronary CTA shows a low density intraluminal defect (*arrow*) within the left ventricle (LV) consistent with a thrombus. RV, right ventricle.

FIG. 38.29. Aortic valve. Thin maximum intensity projection reformations in a plane parallel to the aortic valve orifice (*arrow*) during end-diastole **(A)** and end-systole **(B)** show normal excursion of the aortic valve leaflets during the cardiac cycle.

can provide a 3D visualization of the valve components in relationship to the ascending aorta and origin of the coronary arteries.

FIG. 38.30. Aortic stenosis. Thin maximum intensity projection reformation in a plane parallel to the aortic valve orifice during end-systole shows course leaflet calcification (*arrow*) and limited opening of the aortic valve orifice, consistent with calcific aortic stenosis.

Extra-Cardiac Findings

Multiple studies have shown a high frequency of extra-cardiac findings on coronary CTA studies. A small percentage of these findings have been considered clinically significant and should prompt further imaging or may effect future management decisions. The small field of view used for cardiac studies partially encompasses the great mediastinal vessels, airways, lungs, chest wall, and superior abdomen. Although there has been extensive discussion in the literature regarding the advantages of routinely reconstructing the CT images with a large field of view for full visualization of the lungs and mediastinum, there are no guidelines established regarding this practice.

The most common extra-cardiac findings seen on a coronary CTA are mediastinal lymphadenopathy and lung nodules. Lung nodules, in particular, are important to detect on these studies given the association of smoking with CAD, placing selected patients at increased risk for lung cancer. Practice guidelines for lung nodule follow-up imaging should be followed when nodules are seen on a cardiac CT study.

RADIATION REDUCTION TECHNIQUES

Numerous recent reports have raised concern about radiation exposure with CT studies and the potential for radiation induced cancers. Particular interest has been given to the radiation involved in cardiac studies, including CTA of the heart. Despite the lack of definitive evidence linking low-level radiation exposure with cancer, multiple strategies have been recently developed to lower radiation exposure.

It is important to note that the risk/benefit ratio for each individual study should be judged on an individual basis. The best radiation reduction strategy is to avoid ordering a cardiac CT when there is no reasonable indication present or if it would not help guide patient management decisions.

Radiation exposure. The most useful parameter to assess radiation exposure resulting from a CT study is the effective radiation dose (e), which is expressed in millisieverts (mSv). It represents a whole-body radiation dose and is useful as a single measurement of the overall dose imparted by a CT scan. Effective dose is estimated by multiplying the individual dose to each organ by a tissue specific weighting factor and then summing these values. Effective dose in the chest may be estimated by multiplying the CT dose length product by 0.014.

Scan coverage. The radiation exposure is influenced by the scan coverage volume. Therefore, it is important to be very conservative in planning the coronary CTA acquisition and avoiding extra-coverage which will not provide any additional diagnostic information. Scout images are generally used for planning the coverage, which should start at the level of the carina and extend to the diaphragmatic level. However, if calcium screening images are available, those should be used for a more accurate determination of the scan length. For each 1 cm reduction in length, the radiation exposure will be reduced approximately 5%.

ECG-controlled tube current modulation. This technique maximizes the radiation during a specific cardiac phase, usually end-diastole, when image quality is expected to be the highest. It reduces radiation approximately 20% during the remaining phases of the cardiac cycle. With effective use of current modulation, the entire radiation exposure can be reduced by approximately 50%. It is important to mention that maximum benefit from current modulation is obtained when the heart rate is lowered to less than 60 bpm. Additionally, the stabilizing effects of β-blockage can avoid rhythm irregularities which could generate maximum radiation exposure in phases other than end-diastole.

Tube voltage. Recent studies have shown that decreasing tube voltage from 120 to 100 kV in non-obese patients is not accompanied by significant image degradation as previously believed. Since the radiation dose varies with the square of the tube voltage, a 50% reduction in radiation can be achieved using 100 kV instead of 120 kV. In very thin patients, reasonable image quality can be obtained with a tube voltage as low as 80 kV. New back-projection filters and reconstruction algorithms, like iterative reconstruction, have the potential of reducing noise and generating reasonable quality images with very low tube voltage.

Prospective gating. Robust prospective gating techniques have been recently introduced to coronary CTA technology, allowing for rapid acquisition of contrast enhanced images with temporal and spatial resolutions similar to retrospective gating. A specified phase of the R-R interval, usually mid-diastole, is determined prior to the acquisition and images are acquired in a step-and-shoot mode only during that predetermined cardiac phase. This technique has been shown to decrease radiation exposure from approximately 12 to 15 mSv with retrospective gating to approximately 1 to 5 mSv. The main disadvantage of this method is the inability to reconstruct images at multiple phases of the cardiac cycle in cases of suboptimal image quality in mid diastole. In addition, functional myocardial and valvular assessment cannot be obtained with prospective cardiac gating.

PITFALLS

Imagers should be aware of the possible pitfalls that can be generated by multiplanar reconstructions, simulating CAD in patients with normal coronary arteries. The most common pitfalls are motion artifact, streak artifact, blooming artifact, misregistration artifact, and reconstruction related artifacts.

Motion. Motion artifact is the most common pitfall in coronary imaging. When an object of interest is moving during data acquisition, images demonstrate ill-defined and blurred contours. As previously discussed, gating techniques with optimization of temporal resolution are necessary to obtain images without cardiac pulsation artifact. However, suboptimal heart rate control can generate images with a substantial amount of motion artifact, which can simulate coronary lesions (Fig. 38.31). The most important tool for correction of motion artifact is reconstruction of the images at multiple cardiac phases (multiple R-R intervals). Retrospectively gated cardiac studies can be reconstructed in any phase of the cardiac cycle, allowing for correction of motion artifacts in many cases. The coronary arteries should be evaluated on the phase that demonstrates the least amount of motion. However, when prospective gating technique is used, only limited phases at end-diastole are available for reconstruction and motion artifacts generally cannot be overcome.

Streak. Streak artifacts are low density radial lines originating from an area of very high density. This artifact can be caused by dense contrast enhancement, course calcifications, electrodes, cardiac lines, surgical clips, pacemakers or

FIG. 38.31. Motion artifact. Curved multiplanar reformation of the left anterior descending (LAD) coronary artery shows significant blurring of the coronary artery contours (*arrows*) due to motion artifact. Ao, ascending aorta.

FIG. 38.32. Blooming artifact. Curved multiplanar reformation of the left anterior descending (LAD) coronary artery shows extensive calcification (*arrows*) of the vessel simulating significant stenosis. The conventional angiogram (not shown) showed no lesions causing greater than 50% stenosis.

any other dense structure within or near the area of interest (Figs. 38.2 and 38.21). The low density lines can cause significant degradation of the images and sometimes generate uninterpretable studies. As described previously, contrast injection strategies to decrease contrast enhancement of the SVC and right atrium are used to minimize streak artifacts in the RCA territory.

Blooming. Blooming artifacts are caused by the volume averaging phenomenon. A very dense structure within a pixel will result in an overall increase in the density of the entire pixel. Consequently, a dense structure, smaller than the pixel size, will artifactually appear much larger than its true dimension. Applying this concept to the edges of a calcified plaque, we can assume that the visualized size of the calcification is greater than its true dimension (Fig. 38.32). Therefore, assessment of the severity of stenosis caused by

a calcified plaque should be interpreted with the knowledge that the stenosis is overestimated. This is one of the main limitations of coronary CTA. As the primary role of coronary CTA is to exclude significant CAD, patients with high calcium scores are not good candidates for this imaging method. The same concept applies to coronary stents. It has been shown that stents with thick struts and those that are located in a distal coronary branch are usually associated with greater blooming artifact and it may not be possible to accurately visualize the coronary lumen within the stent.

Multiple techniques have been used in an attempt to minimize blooming artifact from coronary stents and calcifications. Reduction of the field of view and consequently the pixel size can reduce blooming artifact (Fig. 38.33). Alternatively, sharp filters with edge enhancing properties can also minimize this artifact. The most promising technique for correction of blooming artifacts is the use of dual energy CT with calcium subtraction.

Misregistration. Another common pitfall is the misregistration artifact due to variations in heart rate between beats. Because of these variations, images acquired at different anatomic levels may be in slightly different phases of the cardiac cycle (Fig. 38.34). Although this artifact can simulate significant coronary stenosis, the classic appearance of a "stair-step" artifact is easily identifiable and the lesion can usually be recognized as a pitfall (Fig. 38.35). Similarly, misregistration artifacts can be seen when there is breathing variation during the CT acquisition. In these cases, the stair-step appearance extends throughout the entire field of view and can be best appreciated in the chest wall contour. Most postprocessing softwares allow for partial correction of a misregistration artifact by selecting different R-R intervals for different anatomical levels (Fig. 38.36).

Reconstruction-related artifact. The most common artifact due to the processing of the axial data to produce curved multi-planar reconstructions is seen when the plane of reconstruction is not aligned to the center of the coronary artery, but is eccentric to the coronary arterial lumen. This can simulate various degrees of stenosis or even coronary occlusion. Most workstations allow for manual correction of the curved MIP planes.

FIG. 38.33. Blooming artifact. Curved multiplanar reformations of the proximal left main coronary artery (LCA) processed using axial images with regular field of view (*left*) compared to axial images with a reduced field of view (*right*). Note that the blooming artifact seen on the left sided image (*arrowhead*) has been significantly reduced after the reduced field of view reconstruction, allowing for better visualization of the in-stent restenosis (*arrow*).

FIG. 38.34. Misregistration artifact. Cardiac image acquisition during three cardiac cycles (1, 2, and 3). Note that the cardiac cycles vary in length and therefore the phases of acquisition (black lines) occur in slightly different phases of ventricular contraction/relaxation. Consequently, the reconstructed image that corresponds to the second cardiac cycle shows the heart with a smaller volume than in cycles 1 and 3. The edge of the reconstruction shows the typical stair-step appearance (*arrows*) seen with the misregistration artifact.

Volume rendered 3D images can be misleading in the assessment of coronary stenosis. They usually overestimate the stenosis and should not be used alone for the identification of coronary lesions.

NEW APPLICATIONS

The use of cardiac CT for assessment of myocardial viability was initially described in the late 1970s. However, recent improvements in the temporal and spatial resolution of cardiac CT have motivated a growing interest in the applications of CT for myocardial imaging. The combined use of CTA in the detection of coronary anatomy and assessment of myocardial function/viability is likely to become a safe and attractive alternative to a combination of multiple traditional diagnostic tests.

FIG. 38.35. Misregistration artifact. Curved multiplanar reformation of the left anterior descending (LAD) coronary artery shows a misregistration artifact of the distal segment. Note the misleading appearance of a significant coronary stenosis (*arrow*) with a clear stair-step artifact (*arrowhead*) extending beyond the contour of the vessel.

Myocardial Perfusion

Coronary CTA has the potential to perform a combined evaluation of the coronary arteries and myocardial perfusion. Studies with combined coronary CTA and nuclear perfusion imaging have shown an incremental diagnostic value of the combined technique compared to each technique alone. Recent clinical studies have shown a good correlation between coronary CTA and SPECT nuclear myocardial perfusion for detection of myocardial ischemia.

Scanners with a wide range of detectors are able to acquire images of the entire heart during one heart beat, allowing for visualization of myocardial first pass perfusion in all myocardial segments. The capability of CT to identify and quantify reduced myocardial blood flow in areas of ischemic myocardium during stress has been shown in pre-clinical studies. Recent studies with dual energy CT have shown the feasibility of coronary CTA and perfusion imaging with one single acquisition, using different reconstruction methods (Fig. 38.37). Further clinical studies are required to support the widespread use of CTA for accurate assessment of myocardial perfusion.

FIG. 38.36. Curved multiplanar reformats of the left anterior descending (LAD) coronary artery before (*left*) and after (*right*) correction of the misregistration artifact. The image on the left shows a stair-step artifact (*white arrow*) simulating a coronary stenosis when reconstructed at 70% of the R-R interval. By selecting different phases of the cardiac cycle (70% and 80%) for different slabs of the reconstruction, the misregistration artifact can be corrected (*black arrow*).

A

B

C

D

E

FIG. 38.37. Images in 58-year-old woman with atypical chest pain and prior abnormal stress test. Contrast-enhanced retrospectively ECG-gated dual-source coronary CT angiogram obtained with dual-energy technique and displayed as **(A)** curved multiplanar reformation shows occlusion (*arrow*) of the mid left anterior descending (LAD), which is subsequently confirmed at **(B)** invasive coronary catheterization in left anterior oblique caudal projection. **C**: Prior rest perfusion SPECT in short-axis view shows corresponding fixed perfusion defect (*arrowheads*) in the anteroseptal myocardium. Dual-energy reconstruction of the same CT scan displayed in **(D)** short-axis view and as **(E)** 3D volume rendering from a caudal left anterior oblique perspective show corresponding lack of iodine-based contrast material in the anteroseptal left ventricular wall (*arrowheads* in **D**); **(E)** illustrates the anatomic relationship of LAD occlusion (*arrow*) to myocardial segments with decreased blood supply (*arrowheads*). Reproduced from **Bastarrika G, Lee YS, Huda W, et al**. CT of coronary artery disease. Radiology 2009; 253:317–338, with permission.

FIG. 38.38. Subacute infarction (*arrowheads*) on delayed enhancement multidetector CT (*left*) acquired 4 minutes after contrast injection and histologic slice at the same level died with TCC (2,3,5-Triphenylterazolium chloride) (*right*). Note the match between the extent of the infarction on CT and histology. Reproduced from **Furtado AD, Carlsson M, Wintermark M, et al**. Identification of residual ischemia, infarction and microvascular impairment in revascularized myocardial infarction using 64-slice MDCT. Contrast Media Mol Imaging 2008; 3:198–206, with permission.

Myocardial Viability

Similar to magnetic resonance viability imaging, cardiac CT can demonstrate increased delayed contrast enhancement of the myocardium in areas of non-viable tissue (Fig. 38.38). A few imaging studies have shown a good correlation between CTA and MRI in the detection of areas of delayed enhancement during different stages MI. However, it has been shown that CT systematically underestimates the infarct area in comparison to MRI. In the assessment of delayed enhancement on CT an additional acquisition is necessary after the coronary CT angiography has been performed, resulting in increased radiation exposure. The additional radiation exposure has been calculated as approximately 3.8 mSv for males and 2.8 mSv for females. Recently, low dose protocols for viability imaging with 64 MDCT have been reported with diagnostic image quality. The timing for optimal contrast between normal and abnormal myocardial enhancement varies in the literature from 5 to 15 minutes after the administration of the iodine-based contrast media. Encouraging animal studies with 320 MDCT have shown the feasibility of CT for the detection of delayed enhancement and definition of a peri-infarct zone.

SUGGESTED READING

Bastarrika G, Lee YS, Huda W, et al. CT of coronary artery disease. Radiology 2009; 253:317–338.

Bluemke DA, Achenbach S, Budoff M, et al. Noninvasive coronary artery imaging: magnetic resonance angiography and multidetector computed tomography angiography: a scientific statement from the American Heart Association Committee on cardiovascular imaging and intervention of the council on cardiovascular radiology and intervention, and the councils on clinical cardiology and cardiovascular disease in the young. Circulation 2008; 118:586–606.

Choi HS, Choi BW, Choe KO, et al. Pitfalls, artifacts, and remedies in multidetector row CT coronary angiography. Radiographics 2004; 24:787–800.

Furtado AD, Carlsson M, Wintermark M, et al. Identification of residual ischemia, infarction, and microvascular impairment in revascularized myocardial infarction using 64-slice MDCT. Contrast Media Mol Imaging 2008; 3:198–206.

Greenland P, LaBree L, Azen SP, et al. Coronary artery calcium score combined with Framingham score for risk prediction in asymptomatic individuals. JAMA 2004; 291:210–215.

Hendel RC, Patel MR, Kramer CM, et al. ACCF/ACR/SCCT/SCMR/ASNC/NASCI/SCAI/SIR 2006 appropriateness criteria for cardiac computed tomography and cardiac magnetic resonance imaging: a report of the American College of Cardiology Foundation Quality Strategic Directions Committee Appropriateness Criteria Working Group, American College of Radiology, Society of Cardiovascular Computed Tomography, Society for Cardiovascular Magnetic Resonance, American Society of Nuclear Cardiology, North American Society for Cardiac Imaging, Society for Cardiovascular Angiography and Interventions, and Society of Interventional Radiology. J Am Coll Cardiol 2006; 48:1475–1497.

Kim SY, Seo JB, Do KH, et al. Coronary artery anomalies: classification and ECG-gated multi-detector row CT findings with angiographic correlation. Radiographics 2006; 26:317–333; discussion 333–314.

Pletcher MJ, Tice JA, Pignone M, et al. What does my patient's coronary artery calcium score mean? Combining information from the coronary artery calcium score with information from conventional risk factors to estimate coronary heart disease risk. BMC Med 2004; 2:31.

Pugliese F, Cademartiri F, van Mieghem C, et al. Multidetector CT for visualization of coronary stents. Radiographics 2006; 26:887–904.

Stillman AE, Oudkerk M, Ackerman M, et al. Use of multidetector computed tomography for the assessment of acute chest pain: a consensus statement of the North American Society of Cardiac Imaging and the European Society of Cardiac Radiology. Eur Radiol 2007; 17: 2196–2207.

INDEX

Note: Page numbers followed by *f* indicate an illustration; page numbers followed by *t* indicate a table.